AF577108

Neurology – Laboratory and Clinical Research Developments Series

CEREBRAL ISCHEMIA IN YOUNG ADULTS: PATHOGENIC AND CLINICAL PERSPECTIVES

NEUROLOGY – LABORATORY AND CLINICAL RESEARCH DEVELOPMENTS SERIES

Intracranial Hypertension
Stefan Mircea Iencean and Alexandru Vladimir Ciurea
2009 ISBN: 978-1-60741-862-7

Cerebral Blood Flow Regulation
Nodar P. Mitagvaria and Haim (James) I. Bicher
2009 ISBN: 978-1-60692-163-0

Cerebral Ischemia in Young Adults: Pathogenic and Clinical Perspectives
Alessandro Pezzini and Alessandro Padovani (Editors)
2009 ISBN: 978-1-60741-627-2

Neurology – Laboratory and Clinical Research Developments Series

CEREBRAL ISCHEMIA IN YOUNG ADULTS: PATHOGENIC AND CLINICAL PERSPECTIVES

ALESSANDRO PEZZINI
AND
ALESSANDRO PADOVANI
EDITORS

Nova Biomedical Books
New York

For permission to use material from this book please contact us:
Telephone 631-231-7269; Fax 631-231-8175
Web Site: http://www.novapublishers.com

Library of Congress Cataloging-in-Publication Data

Cerebral ischemia in young adults : pathogenic and clinical perspectives / [edited by] Alessandro Padovani and Alessandro Pezzini.
p. ; cm.
Includes bibliographical references and index.
ISBN 978-1-60741-627-2 (hardcover)
1. Cerebral ischemia. 2. Young adults--Diseases. I. Padovani, Alessandro, 1959- II. Pezzini, Alessandro.
[DNLM: 1. Brain Ischemia. 2. Risk Factors. 3. Stroke. 4. Young Adult. WL 355 C41554 2009]
RC388.5.C39735 2009
616.8'1--dc22

2009012441

Published by Nova Science Publishers, Inc. ✢ New York

Contents

Preface

The literature concerning cerebral circulation, its control, its relation to the metabolism of the brain and its disorders, including cerebral ischemia, is very large and reflects an interest which goes back to Greek and Arabian medicine and which has greatly intensified, particularly over the past decades. Data of the literature remain, however, too sparse to propose a pragmatic approach to cerebral ischemia when affecting people at young age. As in many biological fields, there have been a limited number of imaginative and decisive studies; at the same time, very many studies merely served to perpetuate myths while in other areas it is clear that the proper questions have scarcely been formulated. A further difficulty for students attracted by "ischemic stroke at young age" depends on the fact that scientific contributions on this subject are scattered through a large number of journals, reflecting the background and interests of the Authors rather than the breadth of the subject.

The first purpose of this monograph has been therefore to bring together from such a literature a coherent account of how present concepts and approaches have developed. In this, we have been guided by what seems to us to be the important lines of investigation. Secondly, the evidence from studies which form the basis of our present understanding has been reviewed critically and, where possible, an attempt has been made to pose present controversies in terms which would be helpful in everyday clinical practice. This was made possible thanks to the efforts of well-established experts in stroke medicine in reviewing the latest advances in the field, with strong emphasis on pathogenesis, clinical presentation, and therapy.

This book is designed for use by physicians and other health professionals who deal with persons with ischemic stroke at young age at various stages of disease, including medical specialists in neurology, internal medicine, cardiology, and physical and rehabilitation medicine, and the basic scientists entering the field of research.

Chapter 1 provides an introduction to ischemic stroke in young adults with a particular focus on epidemiology, risk factors, and etiology. The influence of predisposing conditions on the occurrence of premature brain ischemia is covered in Chapters 2 - 8. Pregnancy and puerperium, as well as modern assisted reproductive technologies appear to be related to stroke occurrence, and many studies have investigated this; these are reviewed in Chapter 9. Non-atherosclerotic vasculopathies, including cervical artery dissection, the most frequent cause of ischemic stroke at young age, primary vasculitis of the central nervous system and other forms of cerebral vasculitis, and moyamoya disease are reviewed in Chapters 10 - 12. Chapters 13 and 14 deal with cardioembolic causes of ischemic stroke, while hematologic disorders predisposing to brain ischemia are discussed in Chapters 15 - 17. The genetics of ischemic stroke at young age, including single-gene disorders, polygenic stroke, and mithocondrial diseases are covered in Chapters 19 – 23. Long term prognosis after ischemic stroke and the contribution of rehabilitation at various stages of the recovery process in stroke survivors are reviewed in Chapters 24 and Chapter 25, respectively.

We are indebted to the contributing Authors who gave much of their time so freely in preparing material for this work, to the numerous Authors who contributed unpublished material or who gave permission for material to be reproduced, and to NOVA Science Publishers for taking on the publication of the book. Finally, and most importantly, we are grateful to you the reader for your interest in this work and trust that you will come to share our enthusiasm for this dynamic field.

January 2009

Alessandro Pezzini
Alessandro Padovani

List of Contributors

Gian Paolo Anzola, MD
Service of Neurology
Heart and Brain Department
S. Orsola Hospital FBF
Via Vittorio Emanuele II, 27
25100 Brescia, Italy

Marta Altieri, MD, PhD
Clinica Neurologica A
Department Neurological Sciences
University of Rome "La Sapienza"
Viale dell'Università, 30
00185 Rome, Italy

Brunilda Alushi, MD
Heart and Brain Department
S. Orsola Hospital FBF
Via Vittorio Emanuele II, 27
25100 Brescia, Italy

Anna Bersano, MD, PhD
Department of Neurological Sciences
University of Milan
Ospedale Maggiore Policlinico, Mangiagalli e Regina Elena, IRCCS
Via F. Sforza, 35
Milan, Italy

Marco Berti, MD
Heart and Brain Department
S. Orsola Hospital FBF
Via Vittorio Emanuele II, 27
25100 Brescia, Italy

Silvia Bianchi, PhD
Department of Neurological, Neurosurgical and Behavioural Sciences
Medical School
University of Siena
Viale Bracci, 2
53100 Siena, Italy

Maura Bragoni, MD, PhD
IRCCS Santa Lucia Foundation
Via Ardeatina, 306
00179 Rome, Italy

Tobias Brandt, MD
Kliniken Schmieder
Teaching Hospital of the University of Heidelberg
69115 Heidelberg, Germany

Cheryl D. Bushnell, MD, MHS
Department of Neurology
Wake Forest University Health Sciences
Medical Center Boulevard
Winston-Salem, NC 27157, USA

Patrícia Canhão, MD
Department of Neurosciences
Serviço de Neurologia
Hospital de Santa Maria
University of Lisboa
Lisboa, Portugal

Giorgio Caretta, MD
Department of Experimental and Applied Medicine
Section of Cardiovascular Diseases
Brescia University Medical School
P.le Spedali Civili, 1
25123 Brescia, Italy

Francesco Casilli, MD
Heart and Brain Department
S. Orsola Hospital FBF
Via Vittorio Emanuele II, 27
25100 Brescia, Italy

Valeria Caso, MD, PhD
Department of Neurological Rehabilitation
IRCCS San Raffaele Pisana
Via della Pisana 235
Rome, Italy

Maurizio Castellano, MD
Department of Medical and Surgical Sciences
Brescia University Medical School
2° Medicina
P.le Spedali Civili, 1
25123 Brescia, Italy

Paola Coiro, MD
IRCCS Santa Lucia Foundation
Via Ardeatina, 306
00179 Rome, Italy

Paolo Costa, MD
Department of Medical and Surgical Sciences
Neurology Clinic
Brescia University Medical School
P.le Spedali Civili, 1
25123 Brescia, Italy

Simona Costanzo, ScD
Laboratory of Genetic and Environmental Epidemiology, Research Laboratories
"John Paul II" Centre for High Technology Research, Care and Education in Biomedical Sciences
Catholic University, Largo Gemelli, 1
86100 Campobasso, Italy

Jeffrey M. Craig, MD
Department of Neurology
Wake Forest University Health Sciences
Medical Center Boulevard
Winston-Salem, NC 27157, USA

Domenico De Angelis, MD
IRCCS Santa Lucia Foundation
Via Ardeatina, 306
00179 Rome, Italy

Stéphanie Debette, MD, PhD
University Hospital
Department of Neurology, Stroke Department
F-59037 Lille, France

Giovanni de Gaetano, MD, PhD
Laboratory of Genetic and Environmental Epidemiology, Research Laboratories
"John Paul II" Centre for High Technology Research, Care and Education in Biomedical Sciences
Catholic University, Largo Gemelli, 1
86100 Campobasso, Italy

Elisabetta Del Zotto, MD
Department of Medical and Surgical Sciences
Neurology Clinic
Brescia University Medical School
P.le Spedali Civili, 1
25123 Brescia, Italy

Augusto Di Castelnuovo, ScD
Laboratory of Genetic and Environmental Epidemiology, Research Laboratories
"John Paul II" Centre for High Technology Research, Care and Education in Biomedical Sciences
Catholic University
Largo Gemelli, 1
86100 Campobasso, Italy

Vittorio Di Piero, MD, PhD
Clinica Neurologica A
Department Neurological Sciences
University of Rome “La Sapienza”
Viale dell’Università, 30
00185 Rome, Italy

Maria Benedetta Donati, MD, PhD
Laboratory of Genetic and Environmental Epidemiology, Research Laboratories
"John Paul II" Centre for High Technology Research, Care and Education in Biomedical Sciences
Catholic University
Largo Gemelli, 1
86100 Campobasso, Italy

Maria Teresa Dotti, MD
Department of Neurological, Neurosurgical and Behavioural Sciences
Medical School
University of Siena
Viale Bracci, 2
53100 Siena, Italy

Antonio Federico, MD
Department of Neurological,
Neurosurgical and Behavioural Sciences
Medical School
University of Siena
Viale Bracci, 2
53100 Siena, Italy

José M. Ferro, MD, PhD
Department of Neurosciences
Serviço de Neurologia
Hospital de Santa Maria
University of Lisboa
Lisboa, Portugal

Massimiliano Filosto, MD, PhD
Department of Medical and Surgical Sciences
Neurology Clinic
Brescia University Medical School
P.le Spedali Civili, 1
25123 Brescia, Italy

Francesca Romana Fusco, MD
IRCCS Santa Lucia Foundation
Via Ardeatina, 306
00179 Rome, Italy

Francesco Guercini, MD
Division of Internal and Cardiovascular Medicine
Stroke Unit
Santa Maria della Misericordia Hospital
University of Perugia
06126 Perugia, Italy

Giulio Giordano, MD
UOC di Onco-Hematology
"John Paul II" Centre for High Technology Research,
Care and Education in Biomedical Sciences
Catholic University
Largo Gemelli, 1
86100 Campobasso, Italy

Alessia Giossi, MD
Department of Medical and Surgical Sciences
Neurology Clinic
Brescia University Medical School
P.le Spedali Civili, 1
25123 Brescia, Italy

Caspar Grond-Ginsbach, PhD
Department of Neurology
University of Heidelberg
Im Neuenheimer Feld 400
D-69120 Heidelberg, Germany

Armin J Grau, MD, PhD
Department of Neurology
Klinikum der Stadt Ludwigshafen am Rhein
Ludwigshafen am Rhein, Germany

Kiyohiro Houkin, MD, PhD
Department of Neurosurgery
Sapporo Medical University
Sapporo, Japan

Licia Iacoviello, MD, PhD
Laboratory of Genetic and Environmental Epidemiology, Research Laboratories
"John Paul II" Centre for High Technology Research, Care and Education in Biomedical Sciences
Catholic University
Largo Gemelli, 1
86100 Campobasso, Italy

Satoshi Kuroda, MD, PhD
Department of Neurosurgery
Hokkaido University Graduate School of Medicine
North 15 West 7, Kita-ku
Sapporo 060-8638, Japan

Gian Luigi Lenzi, MD, FRSP
Clinica Neurologica A
Department Neurological Sciences
University of Rome "La Sapienza"
Viale dell'Università, 30
00185 Rome, Italy

Didier Leys, MD, PhD
University Hospital
Department of Neurology, Stroke Department
F-59037 Lille, France

Christoph Lichy, MD
Department of Neurology
University of Heidelberg
Im Neuenheimer Feld 400
D-69120 Heidelberg, Germany

Michelangelo Mancuso, MD, PhD
Department of Neuroscience
Neurological Clinic, University of Pisa
Via Roma 67
Pisa, Italy

Alessio Mercurio, MD
Clinica Neurologica A
Department Neurological Sciences
University of Rome "La Sapienza"
Viale dell'Università, 30
00185 Rome, Italy

Halvor Naess, MD, PhD
Department of Neurology
Haukeland University Hospital
University of Bergen
N-5021 Bergen, Norway

Pietro Offelli, MD
Department of Cardiothoracic and Vascular Sciences,
Clinical Cardiology, Thrombosis Centre
University of Padua
Ospedale 'Ex Busonera'
Via Gattamelata, 64
35128 Padova, Italy

Eustaquio Onorato, MD
Service of Neurology
Heart and Brain Department
S. Orsola Hospital FBF
Via Vittorio Emanuele II, 27
25100 Brescia, Italy

Gustavo Ortiz, MD
Jackson Memorial Hospital
University of Miami
Miller School of Medicine
Miami, FL 33136, USA

Maurizio Paciaroni, MD
Division of Internal and Cardiovascular Medicine
Stroke Unit
Santa Maria della Misericordia Hospital
University of Perugia
06126 Perugia, Italy

Alessandro Padovani, MD, PhD
Department of Medical and Surgical Sciences
Neurology Clinic
Brescia University Medical School
P.le Spedali Civili, 1
25123 Brescia, Italy

Frederik Palm, MD
Department of Neurology
Klinikum der Stadt Ludwigshafen am Rhein
Ludwigshafen am Rhein, Germany

Stefano Paolucci, MD
IRCCS Santa Lucia Foundation
Via Ardeatina, 306
00179 Rome, Italy

Vittorio Pengo, MD
Department of Cardiothoracic and Vascular Sciences,
Clinical Cardiology, Thrombosis Centre
University of Padua
Ospedale 'Ex Busonera'
Via Gattamelata, 64
35128 Padova, Italy

Pilar Peredo, MD
Department of Neurology
University of Heidelberg
Im Neuenheimer Feld 400
D-69120 Heidelberg, Germany

Alessandro Pezzini, MD
Department of Medical and Surgical Sciences
Neurology Clinic
Brescia University Medical School
P.le Spedali Civili, 1
25123 Brescia, Italy

Maria Paola Piras, MD
Heart and Brain Department
S. Orsola Hospital FBF
Via Vittorio Emanuele II, 27
25100 Brescia, Italy

Luca Pratesi, MD
IRCCS Santa Lucia Foundation
Via Ardeatina, 306
00179 Rome, Italy

Roberta Priori, MD
Rheumatology Unit
University of Rome "La Sapienza"
Viale dell'Università, 30
00185 Rome, Italy

Alejandro A. Rabinstein, MD
Department of Neurology
Mayo Clinic College of Medicine
200 First Street SW
Mayo W8,
Rochester, MN , 55905, USA

Riccardo Raddino, MD
Department of Experimental and Applied Medicine,
Section of Cardiovascular Diseases
Brescia University Medical School
P.le Spedali Civili, 1
25123 Brescia, Italy

Stefano Radicchia, MD
Division of Internal and Cardiovascular Medicine
Stroke Unit
Santa Maria della Misericordia Hospital
University of Perugia
06126 Perugia, Italy

Bianca Maria Ricerca, MD
Institute of Hematology
Università Cattolica del Sacro Cuore
Largo Agostino Gemelli, 8
00168 Rome, Italy

Sergio Storti, MD
Institute of Hematology
Università Cattolica del Sacro Cuore
Largo Agostino Gemelli, 8
00168 Rome, Italy

Bhomraj Thanvi, MD
Department of Integrated Medicine
University Hospitals of Leicester NHS Trust
Leicester Royal Infirmary
Leicester LE15WW, UK

Sean D. Treadwell, MD
Department of Integrated Medicine
University Hospitals of Leicester NHS Trust
Leicester Royal Infirmary
Leicester LE15WW, UK

Guido Valesini, MD
Rheumatology Unit
University of Rome “La Sapienza”
Viale dell’Università, 30
00185 Rome, Italy

Vincenzo Venturiero, MD, PhD
IRCCS Santa Lucia Foundation
Via Ardeatina, 306
00179 Rome, Italy

Enrico Vizzardi, MD
Department of Experimental and Applied Medicine,
Section of Cardiovascular Diseases
Brescia University Medical School
P.le Spedali Civili, 1
25123 Brescia, Italy

Irene Volonghi, MD
Department of Medical and Surgical Sciences
Neurology Clinic
Brescia University Medical School
P.le Spedali Civili, 1
25123 Brescia, Italy

In: Cerebral Ischemia in Young Adults
Editors: A. Pezzini and A. Padovani
ISBN 978-1-60741-627-2

Chapter 1

Epidemiology of Ischemic Stroke in Young Adults

Didier Leys [*] ***and Stéphanie Debette***
University Lille II (EA 2691), Department of Neurology,
Stroke Department, Lille, France

Abstract

The main differences between ischemic strokes occurring in young adults and those occurring later in life, are the breakdown of causes with a prominence of "unknown " and "other determined" causes, and an overall good outcome. Cervical-artery dissection is the leading cause of cerebral ischemia in young adults in western countries. The association of a patent foramen ovale and an interatrioseptal aneurysm is a marker of an increased risk of recurrence. Depending on how exhaustive the diagnostic work-up was, up to 50% of patients have no clearly identified cause. Mortality and recurrence rates are low, especially in patients with a negative diagnostic work-up, but epilepsy and behavioural changes are frequent sequelae.

Stroke is a major public health issue because of its frequency, the risk of death and residual physical cognitive or behavioural changes, and the risk of recurrent vascular events, either cardiac or cerebral [1-3]. Strokes occur at a mean age of 75 years in western countries, but they may also occur in young patients [4-7]. Most strokes occurring in young patients are ischaemic in origin: they account for 2 to 12% of all strokes [8,9]. Although young adults are at low risk for stroke, the public health impact is high because of the indirect costs due to the long period of lost productivity.

We will not cover in this chapter the issues of spinal strokes, perinatal strokes and strokes in children, cerebral venous thrombosis, silent strokes, and cerebrovascular disorders that are not associated with a stroke, such as cervical artery dissection revealed by cranial nerve palsies.

---

[*] Correspondence: Didier Leys, University Hospital, Department of Neurology, Stroke Department, F-59037 Lille, France. Tel. + 33 320 44 68 13, Fax: + 33 320 44 60 28. E-mail: dleys@chru-lille.fr.

Descriptive Epidemiology

Epidemiological data depend on the definition of "young". Three upper thresholds can be found in the literature, at 30, 45 and 55 years of age. The most frequently used upper age limit is 45 years. It is a good compromise between an age-category where common causes of cerebral ischemia are very rare, and a disorder that is quite frequent in specialised centres.

Incidence of Ischemic Stroke in the Young

The incidence of ischemic stroke in young people ranges between 60 and 200 new cases per year per million inhabitants [10], depending on the characteristics of the population and definition of young. The incidence of ischemic strokes increases exponentially with age even in young people [7,11]. This incidence of ischemic stroke remains stable over time and does not decline as does the incidence rate of ischemic stroke in older age-categories. The incidence is higher in non-industrialised countries and in black populations [4]. In young women, the incidence of ischemic strokes during pregnancy is around 43 per million deliveries, and is similar to that observed in non-pregnant women of similar age [12].

Prevalence of Ischaemic Stroke in the Young

The prevalence of stroke in western countries is about 2400 per million inhabitants but there are no data providing reliable prevalence rates before the age of 45 years.

Outcome after Ischemic Stroke in the Young

Studies that evaluated the long-term outcome after an ischemic stroke in stroke patients are heterogeneous and can hardly be compared. Their findings are influenced by the inclusion or not of all types of stroke including intracerebral ischemia [10,13-16], subarachnoid haemorrhages [10,13-15], and even sometimes transient ischemic attacks (TIA). Those studies used different thresholds of age to define "young", and often suffered recruitment bias when conducted in specialised centres [7,10,17,18]. Moreover, most studies were conducted in small samples, were retrospective, with patients lost to follow-up [13-15,18-21], excluded recurrent cases [10,13,15,22], or included only those who survived the acute stage, leading to a selection bias towards less severe cases, and therefore better outcomes.

Case Fatality

The case fatality rate is low at short- and intermediate- terms [7,8,10,13,14,17-20,23-27]. In the Lille cohort of 287 patients aged between 15 and 45 years, with a mean follow-up of 3 years and no lost to follow-up, the case fatality rate was 4.5% after 1 year, then 0.8% per year during the following two years [7]. Although there is no population-based study evaluating the incidence of malignant infarcts, it appears from hospital practice that malignant infarcts are much frequent in young adults. They are also more likely to benefit from hemicraniectomy than older subjects [28].

Recurrent Vascular Events

The risk of recurrent vascular events is low in young patients, but it depends mainly on the presumed cause of cerebral ischemia. In the Lille cohort the risk of recurrent stroke was 1.4% during the first year then 1.0% per year during the subsequent two years, and the risk of myocardial infarction was 0.2% per year [7]. In cervical artery dissections the risk of recurrent stroke is very low [2,29-32]. A negative diagnostic work-up and absence of risk factors, is also associated with a low risk of new events [7,33,34].

Epilepsy

Epilepsy is more frequent after an ischaemic stroke in a young patient than stroke recurrence: the risk at 3 years ranges between 5 and 7% [7,35]. Most patients with post stroke epilepsy have their first seizure during the first year after stroke [7,35].

Quality of Life

Even if most patients remain independent, many of them lost their job or divorced within 3 years after ischaemic stroke [7]. In the absence of a systematic evaluation it is difficult to identify the reason, but depression, fatigue, mild cognitive or behavioural changes, or alterations in social cognition are the most likely explanations. Ischaemic stroke in young people is frequently associated with a decline in quality of life that is not explained by handicap [5,7,24].

Pregnancy after an Ischemic Stroke

A multicenter French study [36] conducted in 373 consecutive women who have had an ischaemic stroke between 15 and 40 years of age and were followed-up for 5 years found an overall risk of recurrent stroke of 0.5% at year-5 (95% CI: 0.3-0.95) in periods without pregnancy and 1.8% (95% CI: 0.5-7.5) during pregnancy, without significant difference. Therefore young women who have had an ischemic stroke have an overall low risk of recurrence during a subsequent pregnancy and this risk does not significantly increase during pregnancy [36].

Risk Factors for Ischemic Stroke in the Young

Classical Risk Factors

Classical risk factors for stroke (arterial hypertension, smoking, diabetes mellitus, and hypercholesterolemia) are also risk factors for stroke in the young, but the attributable risk is lower than in older patients. They are frequent in patients with a negative diagnostic work-up [7].

More Specific Risk Factors in the Young

Oral Contraceptive Therapy

Oral contraceptive therapy increases the risk of ischemic stroke even in micro doses of oestrogens: the relative risk of cerebral ischemia is 2.3 (95% CI: 1.6-3.3) [37]. However the absolute risk is low,, with only an additional 4·1 ischemic strokes per 100 000 non-smoking, normotensive women using low dose oestrogen oral contraceptive [38]. The combination of oral contraceptive use with conventional vascular risk factors such as smoking, hypertension, hypercholesterolemia or obesity [37] and prothrombotic genetic variants [39,40] increases the risk of ischemic stroke.

Migraine

Migraine is associated with a relative risk of ischemic stroke of 3.5 with any type of migraine, 6 for migraine with aura [41], and even more in the presence of vascular risk factors. Case-control studies suggest that the association between migraine with aura and stroke is valid. In a recent population-based, case-control study of young African-American and white women, probable migraine with aura was significantly associated with increased odds of ischemic stroke, particularly stroke of undetermined origin, while no association was observed between probable migraine without visual aura and stroke [42]. This study also found that although smoking or OC use did not independently modify the effect of probable migraine with aura on stroke risk, these factors had a multiplicative effect on the risk of stroke [42].There is no convincing evidence on the mechanism that would be implied. The concept of migrainous infarct is still under debate: it requires exclusion of other causes and a typical temporal relationship [43]. The neurological deficit should be a prolongation of a typical aura.

HIV Infection

HIV infection is also associated with an increased risk of ischemic stroke. The mechanisms of stroke are multiple in HIV-infected patients, with an important role of vasculitis and hypercoagulability state [44].

Pregnancy

Pregnancy is classically associated with an increased risk of ischemic stroke [6,12,45,46]. However, data supporting this classical statement are scarce. A study conducted in high risk women, i.e. women who have already had an ischemic stroke, showed no significant increase in incidence of recurrent stroke during periods of subsequent pregnancy [36]. The main difference during pregnancy is the breakdown of aetiologies, with specific causes described above that do not exist or and other causes that are rare in non-pregnant women [46]. Stroke occurring during pregnancy is one of the leading cause of maternal death [47-49].

Genetic Factors

Genetic factors may predispose to ischemic stroke, in rare cases as part of a single gene disorder and more commonly as part of a multifactorial predisposition. The single gene disorders causing stroke are detailed in other parts of this chapter. In most cases of ischaemic stroke there is no evidence for an underlying monogenic disease, but both twin studies [50-52] and studies on the family history of stroke [53-61] suggest that genetic factors substantially contribute to stroke susceptibility, as part of a multifactorial predisposition. There is some evidence suggesting a stronger genetic component in stroke patients younger than 70 years [62-64]. Despite the very large number of genetic association studies published in the last decade [65-67], results remain inconclusive until now, as most associations could not be convincingly replicated. Several difficulties explain why genetic studies conducted up to now failed to identify genetic risk factors for ischemic stroke in the young or could not be replicated [68]: (i) most were conducted in small groups of patients and were therefore underpowered; (ii) the choice of controls was not always appropriate; (iii) heterogeneity of ischemic stroke was not always taken into account; (iv) the choice of genetic markers was not always appropriate. Besides, almost all studies were based on a candidate gene approach and were thus unable to identify novel genetic variants involved in unsuspected pathways, since they are based on what is already known or suspected about the pathophysiology of the disease [69]. Genome-wide association studies offer a solution to this problem by genotyping large numbers of SNPs distributed across the chromosomes without requiring any a priori hypothesis. This approach has recently been applied to a number of complex diseases with notable successes, e.g. identification of novel genes conferring increased risk of diabetes [70] and coronary heart disease [71,72] with replication in large independent populations. This new approach is currently being applied to ischemic stroke [73] and will hopefully substantially contribute to a better understanding of the genetic component of this disorder.

Aetiology of Ischemic Strokes in the Young

There are huge differences in the breakdown of aetiologies depending on the centres and countries where the data are collected [11,74]. Despite an extensive diagnostic work-up, the cause of cerebral ischemia remains undetermined in up to 45% of patients [75], often because it was not extensive enough or performed too late after the onset [76]. However, the proportion of patients with an undetermined cause decreases with increasing age [11]. The most frequent cause in western countries is CAD [11], and in non-industrialised countries valvulopathies and congenital cardiopathies. We will detail the aetiologies according to the TOAST classification [74] large-vessel atherosclerosis, atrial fibrillation and small-vessel occlusion are rare in young patients.

Large-vessel Atherosclerosis

Large-vessel atherosclerosis is found mainly in men and after the age of 35 years [11]. It has no specificity concerning the clinical presentation, diagnosis, and predisposing factors. Smoking is a major risk factor in this age-category, and a family history is frequent, suggesting a genetic predisposition [77].

Cardioembolism

High-risk Cardiopathies

- *Atrial fibrillation is associated* with a high risk of cerebral emboli when there are risk factors for stroke, especially high blood pressure, or an underlying cardiopathy, such as mitral stenosis. In the absence of evidence of atrial fibrillation on ECG, the search for atrial vulnerability provided results that are difficult to interpret in the absence of reliable controls. Most studies were conducted in too small cohorts, and lacked statistical power. The question of whether endovascular stimulation is useful remains unresolved, even in subgroups that may be at risk such as patients with interatrioseptal abnormalities [76]. *Intra-cardiac myxoma* is the most frequent intra-cardiac tumour. Its prevalence is 10 per million inhabitants and is usually located in the left atrium. In less than 50% of cases it leads to systemic emboli associated with fatigue, weight loss, fever, and sometimes cardiac signs such as dyspnoea, murmur or variations in blood pressure. Most myxomas remain asymptomatic and are revealed by an ischaemic stroke. The presence of facial lentiginosis (Carney syndrome, a rare autosomal dominant disorder) may be associated with a myxoma.
- *Papillary fibro-elastoma* is a benign tumour which is usually located on a cardiac valve difficult to distinguish from vegetations.
- *Congenital cardiopathies with cyanosis* are usually seen earlier in life and are rarely causes of ischaemic stroke in adults
- *The association patent foramen ovale (PFO) / inter-atrio septal aneurysm (ASIA)* in patients aged 55 years or less who have had an ischaemic stroke of unknown cause, is a marker of increased risk of recurrence under aspirin [78]. In the FOP-ASIA study [79], after 4 years of follow-up, the rate of recurrent strokes was 15.2 % (95% confidence interval [CI]: 1.8-28.6 %) in patients with PFO and ASIA, whereas it was only 2.3% (95% CI: 0.3-4.3 %) in those with isolated PFO, 4.2 % (95% CI: 1.8-6.6 %) in those without PFO and ASIA, and 0.0% in those with isolated ASIA. Therefore the coexistence of PFO and ASIA is associated with a 4.2-fold risk of recurrence (95% CI: 1.5-11.8). Ischemic stroke patients with coexistence of PFO and

ASIA have a higher risk of recurrence and are eligible for clinical randomised trials aiming at evaluating the safety and efficacy of PFO closure over anticoagulant or antiplatelet therapy.

- *Peripartum cardiomyopathies* are very rare in western countries but are reported quite frequently in sub-Saharan countries during the last month of pregnancy and during the post partum period [80,81]. The clinical presentation is that of a cardiac failure [80], often associated with cerebral emboli [80,81]. This disorder is multi-factorial and is associated with a high mortality rate.
- *Many other major cardiac causes* of cerebral ischaemia may be found in young adults, but they are not specific of this age-category: mitral stenosis mechanical prosthetic valves, infectious endocarditis, marastic endocarditis, intra-cardiac thrombus, acute myocardial infarction, ventricular akinesia, dilated cardiomyopathy, paradoxical emboli through a PFO or inter-atrial communication, complication of catheterism and cardiac surgery.

Low-risk Cardiopathies

- *Lone atrial fibrillation* is associated with a very low risk of cerebral emboli in young people when occurring in the absence of underlying cardiopathy (lone atrial fibrillation) and of vascular risk factors.
- *Mitral valve prolapse* is a protrusion of one or two mitral valves in the left atrium found in 2 to 6% of people in the community [79]. However, diagnostic criteria often lacked precision in studies and a causal relationship remains very controversial.
- *Isolated* ASIA is a protrusion of the atrial septum in either atrium. It is rare in the absence of PFO [33]. Diagnostic criteria are, on TEE, an excursion of 10 mm or more during cardiac contraction, and a basis of at least 15 mm [33]. Presence of ASIA is more frequent in young patients who had an ischemic stroke of unknown cause [33], but in the absence of associated PFO, the presence of an ASIA is not a marker of increased risk of recurrence [82].
- *Isolated patent foramen ovale* (PFO) is present in 10 to 20% of young patients with cerebral ischemia [33]. It may be familial, especially in women [33]. PFO consists of a communication between right and left atrium which becomes functional when the pressure in the right atrium becomes higher than in the left one (*e.g.* pulmonary embolism, Valsalva manoeuvre). PFO may be diagnosed by TTE or TEE with contrast, or transcranial Doppler with contrast. Evidence a right-to-left shunt by transcranial Doppler with contrast enhancement is, in most cases, a marker of the presence of a PFO. However, sometimes the cause of the right-to-left shunt is not a PFO but a pulmonary arteriovenous malformation, which is a rare disorder that occurs mainly in patients with Rendu-Osler-Weber disease. Evidence of a shunt without evidence of a PFO should therefore lead to a search for pulmonary arteriovenous malformation. When there is a causal relationship, possible mechanisms of cerebral ischemia are paradoxical emboli (requiring deep venous thrombosis, pulmonary embolism and cerebral ischemia without other potential cause), local thrombosis in the PFO (most likely hypothesis but almost never proven)

or paroxysmal atrial fibrillation [33]. However, the presence of a PFO is frequent in practice and the causal relationship is unlikely in many patients. The risk of recurrence after a first ischemic stroke in the presence of an isolated PFO does not differ from that of ischemic stroke patients of similar age who have no PFO [83]. A causal relationship will be proven only if on-going trials aiming at the closure of PFO show a clear reduction in the risk of recurrence after closure.

- *Many other minor or even disputable cardiac causes* of cerebral ischemia may be found in young adults, but they are not specific of this age-category or causes of ischemic stroke in children rather than in young adults: mitral calcification, bioprosthesis, aortic stenosis, bicuspid aortic valve, Lambl excrescence, etc.

Small-vessel Occlusion

Lacunar infarcts are small infarcts of less than 15 mm located in the deep white matter, basal ganglia and brainstem. They are the consequence of the occlusion of a single deep perforating intracerebral artery of less than 400 μm in diameter. These perforators have no collaterals and their occlusion always leads to an infarct. The short term outcome is usually good, but the risk is cognitive decline and dementia in case of recurrences.

Lipohyalinosis of the deep perforators. Arterial hypertension is the most important risk factor for lipohyalinosis of the deep perforators, but such hypertensive arteriolopathies are very rare before the age of 45 years.

CADASIL (Cerebral Autosomal Dominant Arteriopathy with Subcortical Infarcts and Leukoencephalopathy) is a genetic disorder of small deep perforating arteries identified on the basis of clinical, MRI and genetic criteria [81]. CADASIL is due to a mutation of the Notch3 gene on chromosome 19 [81], leading to an accumulation of granular osmiophilic material in the wall of small perforators leading to a progressive occlusion. CADASIL is associated with migraine with aura, depression, multiple subcortical infarcts and, at the end stage dementia with pseudobulbar palsy [7,30]. White matter changes are always already severe on MRI when the first symptoms occur usually during the 3rd decade of life [84,85], with characteristic features such as T2 hyperintensities in the anterior temporal white matter and the external capsule [86]. Death generally occurs within 20 years after the first symptoms [29,85].

Other Definite Causes of Cerebral Ischaemia

They are actually the most frequent causes of cerebral ischemia when a cause can be identified.

Diseases of Large Arteries

- *Cervical artery dissections* are the leading cause of cerebral ischemia in the young in western countries when a cause can be clearly identified [29,30]. The annual incidence of cervical artery dissections (CAD) in the general population is about 2.6 to 2.9 per 100,000 inhabitants [84,85] and CAD occurs at a mean age of 44 to 47 years [87,88]. In most cases no trauma can be identified, or the trauma is mild and a causal relationship between a trivial trauma and dissection is disputable [89]. It has been hypothesized that patients with CAD could have a constitutional, genetically determined, weakness of the vessel wall and that environmental factors such as acute infection or minor trauma could act as triggers [90,91]. Inherited connective tissue disorders, especially vascular Ehlers-Danlos syndrome, predispose to dissections but they are rare (although probably underdiagnosed). Familial cases are rare (<3%) [92,93], but in. 50% of CAD cases were shown to have connective tissue aberrations in their reticular dermis [90,94,95] the most common pattern being composite collagen fibrils and fragmentation of elastic fibres. These abnormalities seem to be transmitted according to an autosomal dominant pattern [96,97], without fulfilling the diagnostic criteria for known monogenic connective tissue disorders. The hypothesis that CAD is multifactorial and caused by genetic variants and environmental factors. Three genetic association studies [88,98,99] (of which 2 are overlapping [88,98]) have observed an association of the MTHFR 677TT genotype with CAD, [88,98,99]. Another study also found the 677TT genotype to be significantly more frequent in patients with multiple dissections, but the association with all CAD was not significant [100]. A positive association was also observed with a 2 base-pair deletion in the 3'UTR region of the COL3A1 gene, [101] and the E469K polymorphism in the ICAM-1 gene [102], but these have not yet been replicated. In a family-based study, tentative candidate loci were identified on chromosomes 15q24 and 10q26 in another family with inherited dermal connective tissue alterations [97], but the power of the analysis was insufficient to demonstrate linkage. Several other genetic studies on CAD yielded negative results, but they lacked statistical power. To overcome this difficulty, due to the low incidence of the disease, a large multicentre genetic association study is under way within the international CADISP-consortium (www.cadisp.org). Recurrences of stroke and of dissections are rare [103], and the overall outcome is good except when stroke was severe at the acute stage [104]. Nowadays the diagnosis is possible using exclusively non-invasive investigations, especially Doppler ultrasonography and MRI, both techniques being able to show the mural haematoma [104].

- *Post irradiation cervical arteriopathies* in young persons are often due to irradiation for haematological disorders, and less frequently to throat cancers. Patients always have radiodermitis in the area of irradiation. The arterial lesion is atheroma, irradiation being a local factor of atheroma. The outcome is usually more dependent on the underlying disorder that led to irradiation, than on irradiation arteriopathy per se [105].
- *Cervical fibromuscular dysplasia of cervical arteries* is associated with a low risk of ischaemic stroke except in case of dissection. It can be isolated or associated with other locations such as renal arteries. A monogenic mode of inheritance has been suggested in some cases [106] but the underlying genes are unknown.
- *Intra-cranial dissections* are very rare and difficult to diagnose. They are often revealed by cerebral ischemia, but may also lead to subarachnoid haemorrhage especially when located in the vertebro-basilar territory. Their prognosis is usually poor but benign cases, if they exist, may remain undiagnosed.

- *Moya-Moya disease* is a progressive intracranial vasculopathy that usually becomes symptomatic in children or young adults and may lead to ischemia, haemorrhage, or both. Angiography shows a tight stenosis or occlusion of the intracranial carotid arteries associated with intra-cerebral neo-vessels. Any disorder that can lead to progressive stenosis or occlusion of intracranial carotid arteries in children or in young adults may be a cause of Moya-Moya.
- *Secondary vasculitis occurring in a context of systemic disorder.* Such vasculitis may occur in a patient whose systemic disorder is already known, or be the first manifestation.
  - Systemic disorders where cerebral vasculitis is usually not the most prominent feature (panarteritis nodosa, Churg-Strauss syndrome, systemic lupus erythematosus, Sjögren syndrome, Behcet syndrome, sarcoidosis, Crohn disease, ulcerative rectocolitis) are usually diagnosed on the basis of other manifestations of the disease and, depending on the type of systemic disorder, either a neuropathological proof (*e.g.* sarcoidosis), or association of diagnostic criteria (*e.g.* systemic lupus erythematosus).
  - Takayasu disease is a chronic inflammatory arteriopathy that involves progressively the aorta and the brachiocephalic arteries. It occurs prominently in women before 45 years of age, and more frequently of Asian origin. Cerebral ischemia may be due to progressive stenosis or occlusion of the cervical artery when they arise from the aortic arch.
  - Buerger disease, so-called thromboangeiitis obliterans is a segmental inflammatory vasculitis involving arteries of intermediate and small calibres and also superficial veins. This is usually a disorder involving peripheral arteries, that may exceptionally involve cerebral arteries.
  - Eales disease is an inflammatory vasculitis that involves prominently retinal arteries and very rarely cerebral arteries. The causal relationship with cerebral ischemia is uncertain.
  - Acute multifocal placoid pigment epitheliopathy is a bilateral primary disorder that may rarely be associated with cerebral vasculitis and lead to permanent visual deficits [105]. The clinical picture is that of a decreased visual acuity and fever. The diagnosis is based on evidence of specific lesions at fundoscopy and inflammatory CSF. Intravenous corticosteroids and immunosuppressant therapy are requested [105].
  - Köhlmeier-Degos disease, or malignant atrophic papulosis is a systemic vasculitis that involves predominantly the skin. The severity of the disease is due to the consequences of the vasculitis involving the brain or the bowel.
- *Secondary vasculitis occurring in a context of infectious disorder.* Such vasculitis may occur in patients with bacterial infections (syphilis, tuberculosis, Lyme disease, etc.), viral infections (ophtalmic herpes zoster, HIV etc), parasites (malaria, cysticercosis, etc), or mycotic infections (aspergillosis, candidosis, cryptococcosis etc).
- *Primary vasculitis of the central nervous system* is a granulomatous inflammatory non-sarcoidosic non-infectious vasculitis with giant cells, restricted to the

leptomeningeal and cerebral arteries [105]. The incidence is approximately 2.4 new cases per year per million inhabitants [105]. They occur in both genders around 40 years of age. The first symptom is usually headache, followed by subacute focal neurological deficits, sometimes transient, and seizures [105]. Cerebral infarcts are usually multiple, cortical and sometimes associated with haemorrhages. Fever is possible. There is no systemic biological sign of inflammation. The CSF may be normal, but is usually characterised by an increased number of lymphocytes with or without oligoclonal bands. Brain imaging is suggestive when it shows (i) on CT or MRI scans multiple infarcts of small size in cortical areas, with or without associated haemorrhages, and (ii) on conventional angiography or MRA multiple beadings in intracranial arteries in various territories [107,108]. This finding is not specific and the diagnostic proof is provided by a biopsy of leptomeningeal arteries. In the absence of treatment (corticosteroids sometimes associated with cyclophosphamide for at least 1 year) or in case of failure of treatment, the outcome is poor with occurrence of cognitive decline, dementia and a high mortality rate [107,108]. It has been suggested that primary vasculitis of the central nervous system is a heterogeneous entity that consisting of several subsets of diseases [107,108].

- *Sneddon syndrome* is a potential cause of recurrent cerebral ischaemia. Each episode is usually of mild severity but their repetition may lead to dementia. This diagnosis should be discussed each time a young patient has recurrent episodes of cerebral ischaemia of mild severity associated with livedo racemosa, which is a purple livedo, involving the trunk and the most proximal part of the limbs, that does not disappear with cutaneous warming, as opposed to the more trivial livedo reticularis. Antiphospholipid antibodies are usually associated. Although there is not a high level of evidence, oral anticoagulation is recommended by experts.
- *Post partum cerebral angiopathy* is a rare entity that occurs usually in the first two weeks after delivery. Despite a severe clinical presentation, the outcome is usually excellent [107,108]. The clinical presentation consists of a combination of severe headache, vomiting, epileptic seizures, and focal neurological deficits [109]. The angiography (either conventional or magnetic resonance angiography) shows multiple beadings in large intracranial arteries that disappear spontaneously within a few weeks [109,110]. The pathophysiology may be a toxic angiopathy favoured by oestrogen withdrawal, the use of vasoconstrictive drugs and possibly bromocriptine [111].
- *Other acute reversible cerebral angiopathies* have been reported. They have the same clinical presentation and outcome as the post partum type. Possible aetiologies are toxic (vasoconstrictive drugs, illicit substances such cocaine or amphetamines), reversible hypertensive encephalopathies, pheochromocytoma, carcinoid tumours, or vasospasm after subarachnoid haemorrhage.
- *Eclampsia* is the main cause of maternal mortality and preterm birth in western countries [112,113]. The clinical presentation consists of headache, visual impairment, confusion or coma, epileptic seizures and focal neurological deficits [12]. The HELLP syndrome (Haemolysis; Elevated Liver enzymes, Low Platelets) is a subtype of eclampsia [114]. MRI shows in FLAIR sequences or in T2 sequences

multiple hyperintense signals, isolated or more frequently confluent, more prominent in posterior areas, bilateral, located at the junction between the cortex and the subcortical white matter [114]. These abnormalities completely disappear after a few days or weeks. Cerebral infarcts may lead to residual deficits, but in most patients who survive the acute stage the long term outcome is favourable [114].

– *Unruptured aneurysms of intracranial arteries* may be a cause of cerebral ischaemia secondary to a local intra-saccular thrombosis and subsequent distal emboli.

Haematological Diseases

– *Thrombotic thrombocytopenic purpura (Moschcowitz syndrome)* is a systemic disorder characterised by fever, renal failure, thrombocytopenia, and haemolytic anaemia with a negative Coombs test [115]. Cerebral infarcts are present in most cases [116]. The neurological manifestations may be the first manifestations of the disease [117]. The diagnosis is made easy by the determination of platelet count and search for schizocytes.
– *Haemoglobinopathies:*
  • Sickle cell disease is a cause of ischaemic stroke in children and young adults and during pregnancies [117].
  • Beta thalassemia is also a possible cause of cerebral ischemia
– Nocturnal paroxysmal haemoglobinuria (Marchiafava-Micheli disease)
– Congenital thrombophilia: deficits in proteins C and S, or antithrombin III, resistance to activated protein C, mutation of factor V Leiden, and mutation of the thrombin gene are clearly proven causes of cerebral venous thrombosis, but their role in arterial ischemia remains disputable [117].
– Acquired thrombophilia: antiphospholipid syndrome. This is a cause of arterial and venous occlusions, recurrent spontaneous miscarriages, and biological changes such as thrombocytopenia, false positivity of syphilis serology, and activated cephalin time increase. It may be associated with a clearly defined systemic disorder such as systemic lupus erythematosus, or be primary. Cerebral ischemia may be due to various mechanisms: prothrombotic state, Libman-sachs endocarditis, or early atheroma.
– Other haematological causes of cerebral ischemia in young people are polycythemia, iron-deficiency anaemia, leukaemia, thrombocytemia, hypereosinophilic syndrome, endovascular lymphoma, disseminated intravascular coagulation, and hyperviscosity syndromes.

Metabolic Disorders

– *Fabry disease* is an X-linked recessive lysosomal storage disease resulting from deficient alpha-galactosidase, caused by a mutation in the GLA gene. It causes an endothelial vasculopathy followed by cerebral ischemia [117]. The incidence of the disease is estimated at 1/40,000 (www.orpha.net). A few female cases have been reported [117]. Various types of mutations have been identified. The clinical picture associates episodes of unexplained fever, cutaneous angiokeratomas located in the trunk and proximal part of limbs, crisis of painful acroparesthaesia of feet and hands, corneal opacities, hypohydrosis, and later in the time-course of the disease cardiac and renal failure. Ischemic strokes occur during the 4th decade and are often associated with headache. Strokes are more prominent in the vertebrobasilar territory. The possible mechanisms of ischaemic stroke are dolichomega intracranial arteries, occlusions of the deep perforating arteries due to the accumulation of sphingolipids, cardiopathies, and prothrombotic state. The frequency of the disorder has been found to be of 1.2% in young ischemic stroke patients with a negative diagnostic work-up in a large German study [118], but this rate has never been confirmed thereafter. It is however important to recognise such cases because of possible therapeutic consequences with infusion of alpha-galactosidase [118], although the effect on stoke prevention is not clearly demonstrated. The diagnosis is performed on the basis of a low plasma alpha-galactosidase activity or mutation in the alpha-GAL gene in men, and only by identification of the mutation in women [118].

- *Homocystinuria* has a prevalence of 1/344,000 based on data from newborn screening (www.orpha.net), but this is probably an underestimation, as prevalence rates of up to 1 out of 20,500 have been described in some European countries [119]. One third of patients has a venous or arterial event during his / her life. Homocystinuria includes a group of heritable, mostly autosomal recessive, diseases causing high plasma concentrations of homocysteine and homocystinuria. The most frequent cause is a mutation in the CBS gene on chromosome 21. A toxicity of homocysteine on the endothelium leading to thrombosis has been suggested, but the mechanism of stroke occurrence is not fully understood yet. Homocystinuria ought to be distinguished from the much more frequent mild increase in plasma homocysteine (>15 μmol/l) which is more a risk factor than a cause of ischemic stroke. Folic acid supplementation reduces the serum level of homocysteine, but whether it also reduces the rate of vascular events remain to be proven.
- *MELAS syndrome (Mitochondrial Encephalopathy with Lactic Acidosis and Stroke-like episodes)* is a mitochondriopathy due to several types of mutation in the mitochondrial DNA. The major clinical features are, in a patient before 30 years of age, progressive deafness, stroke-like episodes (usually transient, located in posterior regions, and not confined to vascular territories) seizures, cognitive impairment and recurrent episodes of headache and vomiting. Progressive external ophtalmoplegia with ptosis, muscular pain at exercise, lactic acidosis after exercise, presence of ragged red fibres on the muscular biopsy, cataract, hypogonadism, diabetes mellitus, hypothyroidism, and cardiomyopathy are the other manifestations of the disease. The diagnosis needs evidence of the mitochondrial DNA mutation.

Non-cruoric Emboli

- *Gas emboli* occur during caesarean sections, traumatic deliveries, subclavian catheter accidents, gynaecologic and cardiac surgery or diving accidents [12,120]. The clinical picture consists of acute respiratory failure and acute diffuse encephalopathy, preceded by severe anxiety and dyspnoea [121]. In a few minutes the patient develops tachycardia, seizures and coma, leading to death [122]. As soon as the diagnosis is suspected the patient should be turned to the left side.
- *Amniotic emboli* occur after difficult deliveries in presence of a vaginal lesion. The patient develops acute pulmonary oedema and seizures [123].
- *Fat emboli* occur in long bones fractures or liposuction surgery [123].

Choriocarcinoma is a malignant trophoblastic tumour occurring in 1 pregnancy out of 40000. Lesions of the arterial wall may lead to cerebral ischemia without metastasis [123].

Rare Causes of Cerebral Ischemia in Young People of Undetermined Mechanism

- *Sweet syndrome (acute febrile neutrophilic dermatosis)* is a dermatologic disorder characterised by multiple pustulae and painful purple skin lesions where a neutrophilic infiltration can be found [124]. This dermatologic disorder has accompanying features of systemic inflammation such as fever, conjunctivitis or other types of ocular inflammation, and arthritis [125], They occur mainly around the age of 40 years and may be associated with cancer [126]. Cerebral ischemia may occur but a causal relationship is not proven.
- *Kawasaki syndrome* is a panarteritis of arteries of intermediate and small calibre occurring mainly in children, that leads to coronary or cerebral artery occlusions,.
- *Susac's syndrome* (or Sicret syndrome) is a rare disease occurring in young women of unknown pathogenesis consisting of a triad with retinal arterial occlusion, hearing loss by cochlear ischemia and diffuse vascular encephalopathy.
- *HERNS syndrome (Hereditary Endotheliopathy with Retinopathy and Stroke)* is an autosomal dominant hereditary syndrome consisting of retinopathy, nephropathy, and ischemic stroke, leading to blindness. Fundoscopic examination reveals a typical vasculopathy.

Cerebral Ischemia of Undetermined and Unknown Causes

Before classifying a patient in this category it is important to be sure that the diagnostic work-up has been extensive enough and repeated over time. Sometimes the aetiology is found during the follow-up.

Conclusion

Aetiologies of ischemic stroke in the young are multiple and the outcome is usually good. New causes should now be identified.

References

[1] Bamford J, Sandercock P, Dennis M, Burn J, Warlow C. Classification and natural history of clinically identifiable subtypes of cerebral infarction. *Lancet.* 1991;337:1521-1526

[2] Hankey GJ, Warlow CP. Treatment and secondary prevention of stroke: Evidence, costs, and effects on individuals and populations. *Lancet.* 1999;354:1457-1463

[3] Murray CJ, Lopez AD. Global mortality, disability, and the contribution of risk factors: Global burden of disease study. *Lancet.* 1997;349:1436-1442

[4] Bonita R. Epidemiology of stroke. *Lancet.* 1992;339:342-344

[5] Carolei A, Marini C, Di Napoli M, Di Gianfilippo G, Santalucia P, Baldassarre M, De Matteis G, di Orio F. High stroke incidence in the prospective community-based l'aquila registry (1994-1998). First year's results. *Stroke.* 1997;28:2500-2506

[6] Giroud M, Milan C, Beuriat P, Gras P, Essayagh E, Arveux P, Dumas R. Incidence and survival rates during a two-year period of intracerebral and subarachnoid haemorrhages, cortical infarcts, lacunes and transient ischaemic attacks. The stroke registry of dijon: 1985-1989. *Int. J. Epidemiol.* 1991;20:892-899

[7] Leys D, Bandu L, Henon H, Lucas C, Mounier-Vehier F, Rondepierre P, Godefroy O. Clinical outcome in 287 consecutive young adults (15 to 45 years) with ischemic stroke. *Neurology.* 2002;59:26-33

[8] Bogousslavsky J, Pierre P. Ischemic stroke in patients under age 45. *Neurol. Clin.* 1992;10:113-124

[9] Naess H, Nyland HI, Thomassen L, Aarseth J, Nyland G, Myhr KM. Incidence and short-term outcome of cerebral infarction in young adults in western norway. *Stroke.* 2002;33:2105-2108

[10] Marini C, Totaro R, Carolei A. Long-term prognosis of cerebral ischemia in young adults. National research council study group on stroke in the young. *Stroke.* 1999;30:2320-2325

[11] Putaala J, Metso AJ, Metso TM, Konkola N, Kraemer Y, Haapaniemi E, Kaste M, Tatlisumak T. Analysis of 1008 consecutive patients aged 15 to 49 with first-ever ischemic stroke: The helsinki young stroke registry. *Stroke.* 2009;40:1195-2203

[12] Sharshar T, Lamy C, Mas JL. Incidence and causes of strokes associated with pregnancy and puerperium. A study in public hospitals of ile de france. Stroke in pregnancy study group. *Stroke.* 1995;26:930-936

[13] Leno C, Berciano J, Combarros O, Polo JM, Pascual J, Quintana F, Merino J, Sedano C, Martin-Duran R, Alvarez C, et al. A prospective study of stroke in young adults in cantabria, spain. *Stroke.* 1993;24:792-795

[14] Nencini P, Inzitari D, Baruffi MC, Fratiglioni L, Gagliardi R, Benvenuti L, Buccheri AM, Cecchi L, Passigli A, Rosselli A, et al. Incidence of stroke in young adults in florence, italy. *Stroke*. 1988;19:977-981

[15] Marini C, Totaro R, De Santis F, Ciancarelli I, Baldassarre M, Carolei A. Stroke in young adults in the community-based l'aquila registry: Incidence and prognosis. *Stroke*. 2001;32:52-56

[16] Qureshi AI, Safdar K, Patel M, Janssen RS, Frankel MR. Stroke in young black patients. Risk factors, subtypes, and prognosis. *Stroke*. 1995;26:1995-1998

[17] Ferro JM, Crespo M. Prognosis after transient ischemic attack and ischemic stroke in young adults. *Stroke*. 1994;25:1611-1616

[18] Chancellor AM, Glasgow GL, Ockelford PA, Johns A, Smith J. Etiology, prognosis, and hemostatic function after cerebral infarction in young adults. *Stroke*. 1989;20:477-482

[19] Bogousslavsky J, Regli F. Ischemic stroke in adults younger than 30 years of age. Cause and prognosis. *Arch Neurol*. 1987;44:479-482

[20] Neau JP, Ingrand P, Mouille-Brachet C, Rosier MP, Couderq C, Alvarez A, Gil R. Functional recovery and social outcome after cerebral infarction in young adults. *Cerebrovasc. Dis*. 1998;8:296-302

[21] Johnson DM, Kramer DC, Cohen E, Rochon M, Rosner M, Weinberger J. Thrombolytic therapy for acute stroke in late pregnancy with intra-arterial recombinant tissue plasminogen activator. *Stroke*. 2005;36:e53-55

[22] Camerlingo M, Casto L, Censori B, Ferraro B, Caverni L, Manara O, Finazzi G, Radice E, Drago G, De Tommasi SM, Gotti E, Barbui T, Mamoli A. Recurrence after first cerebral infarction in young adults. *Acta Neurol. Scand*. 2000;102:87-93

[23] Hoffmann M. Stroke in the young in south africa--an analysis of 320 patients. *S. Afr. Med. J*. 2000;90:1226-1237

[24] Kappelle LJ, Adams HP, Jr., Heffner ML, Torner JC, Gomez F, Biller J. Prognosis of young adults with ischemic stroke. A long-term follow-up study assessing recurrent vascular events and functional outcome in the iowa registry of stroke in young adults. *Stroke*. 1994;25:1360-1365

[25] Kwon SU, Kim JS, Lee JH, Lee MC. Ischemic stroke in korean young adults. *Acta Neurol. Scand*. 2000;101:19-24

[26] Lisovoski F, Rousseaux P. Cerebral infarction in young people. A study of 148 patients with early cerebral angiography. *J. Neurol. Neurosurg. Psychiatry* 1991;54:576-579

[27] Nayak SD, Nair M, Radhakrishnan K, Sarma PS. Ischaemic stroke in the young adult: Clinical features, risk factors and outcome. *Natl. Med. J. India* 1997;10:107-112

[28] Vahedi K, Hofmeijer J, Jüttler E, Vicaut E, George B, Algra A, Amelink GJ, Schmiedeck P, Schwab S, Rothwell PM, Bousser MG, van der Worp HB, Hacke W. Early decompressive surgery in malignant infarction of the middle cerebral artery: A pooled analysis of three randomised controlled trials. *Lancet Neurol*. 2007;6:215-222

[29] Touzé E, Gauvrit JY, Moulin T, Meder JF, Bracard S, Mas JL. Risk of stroke and recurrent dissection after a cervical artery dissection: A multicenter study. *Neurology* 2003;61:1347-1351

[30] Leys D, Moulin T, Stojkovic T, Begey S, Chavot D. Follow-up of patients with history of cervical-artery dissection. *Cerebrovasc. Dis*. 1995;5:337-340

[31] Pozzati E, Giuliani G, Acciarri N, Nuzzo G. Long-term follow-up of occlusive cervical carotid dissection. *Stroke* 1990;21:528-531

[32] Schievink WI, Mokri B, O'Fallon WM. Recurrent spontaneous cervical-artery dissection. *N. Engl. J. Med*. 1994;330:393-397

[33] Mas J, Arquizan C, Lamy C, Zuber M, Cabanes L, Derumeaux G, Coste J, Group. FTPFOAASAS. Recurrent cerebrovascular events in young adults with patent foramen ovale, atrial septal aneuvrysm or both. *N. Engl. J. Med.*. 2001;345:1740-1746

[34] Waje-Andreassen U, Naess H, Thomassen L, Eide GE, Vedeler CA. Arterial events after ischemic stroke at a young age: A cross-sectional long-term follow-up of patients and controls in western norway. *Cerebrovasc. Dis*. 2007;24:277-282

[35] Lamy C, Domigo V, Semah F, Arquizan C, Trystram D, Coste J, Mas JL. Early and late seizures after cryptogenic ischemic stroke in young adults. *Neurology*. 2003;60:400-404

[36] Lamy C, Hamon JB, Coste J, Mas JL. Ischemic stroke in young women: Risk of recurrence during subsequent pregnancies. French study group on stroke in pregnancy. *Neurology* 2000;55:269-274

[37] Kemmeren JM, Tanis BC, van den Bosch MA, Bollen EL, Helmerhorst FM, van der Graaf Y, Rosendaal FR, Algra A. Risk of arterial thrombosis in relation to oral contraceptives (ratio) study: Oral contraceptives and the risk of ischemic stroke. *Stroke* 2002;33:1202-1208

[38] Gillum LA, Mamidipudi SK, Johnston SC. Ischemic stroke risk with oral contraceptives: A meta-analysis. *Jama*. 2000;284:72-78

[39] Slooter AJ, Rosendaal FR, Tanis BC, Kemmeren JM, van der Graaf Y, Algra A. Prothrombotic conditions, oral contraceptives, and the risk of ischemic stroke. *J. Thromb. Haemost*. 2005;3:1213-1217

[40] Pezzini A, Grassi M, Iacoviello L, Del Zotto E, Archetti S, Giossi A, Padovani A. Inherited thrombophilia and stratification of ischaemic stroke risk among users of oral contraceptives. *J. Neurol. Neurosurg. Psychiatry*. 2007;78:271-276

[41] Tzourio C, Kittner SJ, Bousser MG, Alperovitch A. Migraine and stroke in young women. *Cephalalgia* 2000;20:190-199

[42] MacClellan LR, Giles W, Cole J, Wozniak M, Stern B, Mitchell BD, Kittner SJ. Probable migraine with visual aura and risk of ischemic stroke: The stroke prevention in young women study. *Stroke* 2007;38:2438-2445

[43] Silberstein SD, Olesen J, Bousser MG, Diener HC, Dodick D, First M, Goadsby PJ, Gobel H, Lainez MJ, Lance JW, Lipton RB, Nappi G, Sakai F, Schoenen J, Steiner TJ. The international classification of headache disorders, 2nd edition (ichd-ii)--revision of criteria for 8.2 medication-overuse headache. *Cephalalgia*. 2005;25:460-465

[44] Ortiz G, Koch S, Romano JG, Forteza AM, Rabinstein AA. Mechanisms of ischemic stroke in hiv-infected patients. *Neurology* 2007;68:1257-1261

[45] Stirling Y, Woolf L, North WR, Seghatchian MJ, Meade TW. Haemostasis in normal pregnancy. *Thromb. Haemost*. 1984;52:176-182

[46] Davie CA, O'Brien P. Stroke and pregnancy. *J. Neurol. Neurosurg. Psychiatry* 2008;79:240-245
[47] Bouvier-Colle MH, Varnoux N, Costes P, Hatton F, et le groupe d'experts sur la mortalité maternelle. Mortalité maternelle en france. Fréquence et raisons de sa sous-estimation dans la statistique des causes médicales de décès. *J. Gynecol. Obstet. Biol. Reprod. (Paris)*. 1991;20:885-891
[48] Gibbs CE. Maternal death due to stroke. *Am. J. Obstet Gynecol*. 1974;119:69-75
[49] Kaunitz AM, Hughes JM, Grimes DA, Smith JC, Rochat RW, Kafrissen ME. Causes of maternal mortality in the united states. *Obstet Gynecol*. 1985;65:605-612
[50] de Faire U, Friberg L, Lundman T. Concordance for mortality with special reference to ischaemic heart disease and cerebrovascular disease. A study on the swedish twin registry. *Prev. Med*. 1975;4:509-517
[51] Brass LM, Isaacsohn JL, Merikangas KR, Robinette CD. A study of twins and stroke. *Stroke* 1992;23:221-223
[52] Bak S, Gaist D, Sindrup SH, Skytthe A, Christensen K. Genetic liability in stroke: A long-term follow-up study of danish twins. *Stroke* 2002;33:769-774
[53] Vitullo F, Marchioli R, Di Mascio R, Cavasinni L, Pasquale AD, Tognoni G. Family history and socioeconomic factors as predictors of myocardial infarction, unstable angina and stroke in an italian population. Progetto 3a investigators. *Eur. J. Epidemiol*. 1996;12:177-185
[54] Liao D, Myers R, Hunt S, Shahar E, Paton C, Burke G, Province M, Heiss G. Familial history of stroke and stroke risk. The family heart study. *Stroke* 1997;28:1908-1912
[55] Welin L, Svardsudd K, Wilhelmsen L, Larsson B, Tibblin G. Analysis of risk factors for stroke in a cohort of men born in 1913. *N. Engl. J. Med*. 1987;317:521-526
[56] Touzé E, Rothwell PM. Heritability of ischaemic stroke in women compared with men: A genetic epidemiological study. *Lancet Neurol*. 2007;6:125-133
[57] Kiely DK, Wolf PA, Cupples LA, Beiser AS, Myers RH. Familial aggregation of stroke. The framingham study. *Stroke* 1993;24:1366-1371
[58] Hassan A, Sham PC, Markus HS. Planning genetic studies in human stroke: Sample size estimates based on family history data. *Neurology* 2002;58:1483-1488
[59] Caicoya M, Corrales C, Rodriguez T. Family history and stroke: A community case-control study in asturias, spain. *J. Epidemiol. Biostat*. 1999;4:313-320
[60] MacClellan LR, Mitchell BD, Cole JW, Wozniak MA, Stern BJ, Giles WH, Brown DW, Sparks MJ, Kittner SJ. Familial aggregation of ischemic stroke in young women: The stroke prevention in young women study. *Genet. Epidemiol*. 2006;30:602-608
[61] Jood K, Ladenvall C, Rosengren A, Blomstrand C, Jern C. Family history in ischemic stroke before 70 years of age: The sahlgrenska academy study on ischemic stroke. *Stroke* 2005;36:1383-1387
[62] Flossmann E, Schulz UG, Rothwell PM. Systematic review of methods and results of studies of the genetic epidemiology of ischemic stroke. *Stroke* 2004;35:212-227
[63] Schulz UG, Flossmann E, Rothwell PM. Heritability of ischemic stroke in relation to age, vascular risk factors, and subtypes of incident stroke in population-based studies. *Stroke* 2004;35:819-824

[64] Jerrard-Dunne P, Cloud G, Hassan A, Markus HS. Evaluating the genetic component of ischemic stroke subtypes: A family history study. *Stroke* 2003;34:1364-1369

[65] Bersano A, Ballabio E, Bresolin N, Candelise L. Genetic polymorphisms for the study of multifactorial stroke. *Hum. Mutat.* 2008;29:776-795

[66] Dichgans M. Genetics of ischaemic stroke. *Lancet Neurol.* 2007;6:149-161

[67] Hassan A, Markus HS. Genetics and ischaemic stroke. *Brain* 2000;123 (Pt 9):1784-1812

[68] Dichgans M, Markus HS. Genetic association studies in stroke: Methodological issues and proposed standard criteria. *Stroke* 2005;36:2027-2031

[69] Zondervan KT, Cardon LR. Designing candidate gene and genome-wide case-control association studies. *Nat Protoc.* 2007;2:2492-2501

[70] Zeggini E, Scott LJ, Saxena R, Voight BF, Marchini JL, Hu T, de Bakker PI, Abecasis GR, Almgren P, Andersen G, Ardlie K, Bostrom KB, Bergman RN, Bonnycastle LL, Borch-Johnsen K, Burtt NP, Chen H, Chines PS, Daly MJ, Deodhar P, Ding CJ, Doney AS, Duren WL, Elliott KS, Erdos MR, Frayling TM, Freathy RM, Gianniny L, Grallert H, Grarup N, Groves CJ, Guiducci C, Hansen T, Herder C, Hitman GA, Hughes TE, Isomaa B, Jackson AU, Jorgensen T, Kong A, Kubalanza K, Kuruvilla FG, Kuusisto J, Langenberg C, Lango H, Lauritzen T, Li Y, Lindgren CM, Lyssenko V, Marvelle AF, Meisinger C, Midthjell K, Mohlke KL, Morken MA, Morris AD, Narisu N, Nilsson P, Owen KR, Palmer CN, Payne F, Perry JR, Pettersen E, Platou C, Prokopenko I, Qi L, Qin L, Rayner NW, Rees M, Roix JJ, Sandbaek A, Shields B, Sjogren M, Steinthorsdottir V, Stringham HM, Swift AJ, Thorleifsson G, Thorsteinsdottir U, Timpson NJ, Tuomi T, Tuomilehto J, Walker M, Watanabe RM, Weedon MN, Willer CJ, Illig T, Hveem K, Hu FB, Laakso M, Stefansson K, Pedersen O, Wareham NJ, Barroso I, Hattersley AT, Collins FS, Groop L, McCarthy MI, Boehnke M, Altshuler D. Meta-analysis of genome-wide association data and large-scale replication identifies additional susceptibility loci for type 2 diabetes. *Nat. Genet.* 2008;40:638-645

[71] Samani NJ, Erdmann J, Hall AS, Hengstenberg C, Mangino M, Mayer B, Dixon RJ, Meitinger T, Braund P, Wichmann HE, Barrett JH, Konig IR, Stevens SE, Szymczak S, Tregouet DA, Iles MM, Pahlke F, Pollard H, Lieb W, Cambien F, Fischer M, Ouwehand W, Blankenberg S, Balmforth AJ, Baessler A, Ball SG, Strom TM, Braenne I, Gieger C, Deloukas P, Tobin MD, Ziegler A, Thompson JR, Schunkert H. Genomewide association analysis of coronary artery disease. *N. Engl. J. Med.* 2007;357:443-453

[72] McPherson R, Pertsemlidis A, Kavaslar N, Stewart A, Roberts R, Cox DR, Hinds DA, Pennacchio LA, Tybjaerg-Hansen A, Folsom AR, Boerwinkle E, Hobbs HH, Cohen JC. A common allele on chromosome 9 associated with coronary heart disease. *Science* 2007;316:1488-1491

[73] Matarin M, Brown WM, Scholz S, Simon-Sanchez J, Fung HC, Hernandez D, Gibbs JR, De Vrieze FW, Crews C, Britton A, Langefeld CD, Brott TG, Brown RD, Jr., Worrall BB, Frankel M, Silliman S, Case LD, Singleton A, Hardy JA, Rich SS, Meschia JF. A genome-wide genotyping study in patients with ischaemic stroke: Initial analysis and data release. *Lancet Neurol.* 2007;6:414-420

[74] Adams HP, Jr., Bendixen BH, Kappelle LJ, Biller J, Love BB, Gordon DL, Marsh EE, 3rd. Classification of subtype of acute ischemic stroke. Definitions for use in a multicenter clinical trial. Toast. Trial of org 10172 in acute stroke treatment. *Stroke* 1993;24:35-41

[75] Oliviero U, Orefice G, Coppola G, Scherillo G, Ascione S, Casaburi C, Barbieri F, Sacca L. Carotid atherosclerosis and ischemic stroke in young patients. *Int. Angiol.* 2002;21:117-122

[76] Berthet K, Lavergne T, Cohen A, Guize L, Bousser MG, Le Heuzey JY, Amarenco P. Significant association of atrial vulnerability with atrial septal abnormalities in young patients with ischemic stroke of unknown cause. *Stroke* 2000;31:398-403

[77] Arquizan C, Coste J, Touboul PJ, Mas JL. Is patent foramen ovale a family trait? A transcranial doppler sonographic study. *Stroke* 2001;32:1563-1566

[78] Demakis JG, Rahimtoola SH, Sutton GC, Meadows WR, Szanto PB, Tobin JR, Gunnar RM. Natural course of peripartum cardiomyopathy. *Circulation* 1971;44:1053-1061

[79] Homans DC. Peripartum cardiomyopathy. *N Engl J Med.* 1985;312:1432-1437

[80] Chabriat H, Vahedi K, Iba-Zizen MT, Joutel A, Nibbio A, Nagy TG, Krebs MO, Julien J, Dubois B, Ducrocq X, et al. Clinical spectrum of cadasil: A study of 7 families. Cerebral autosomal dominant arteriopathy with subcortical infarcts and leukoencephalopathy. *Lancet* 1995;346:934-939

[81] Joutel A, Corpechot C, Ducros A, Vahedi K, Chabriat H, Mouton P, Alamowitch S, Domenga V, Cecillion M, Marechal E, Maciazek J, Vayssiere C, Cruaud C, Cabanis EA, Ruchoux MM, Weissenbach J, Bach JF, Bousser MG, Tournier-Lasserve E. Notch3 mutations in cadasil, a hereditary adult-onset condition causing stroke and dementia. *Nature* 1996;383:707-710

[82] Procacci PM, Savran SV, Schreiter SL, Bryson AL. Prevalence of clinical mitral-valve prolapse in 1169 young women. *N. Engl. J. Med.* 1976;294:1086-1088

[83] Lucas C, Goullard L, Marchau M, Jr., Godefroy O, Rondepierre P, Chamas E, Mounier-Vehier F, Leys D. Higher prevalence of atrial septal aneurysms in patients with ischemic stroke of unknown cause. *Acta Neurol. Scand.* 1994;89:210-213

[84] Giroud M, Fayolle H, Andre N, Dumas R, Becker F, Martin D, Baudoin N, Krause D. Incidence of internal carotid artery dissection in the community of dijon. *J. Neurol. Neurosurg. Psychiatry* 1994;57:1443

[85] Lee VH, Brown RD, Jr., Mandrekar JN, Mokri B. Incidence and outcome of cervical artery dissection: A population-based study. *Neurology* 2006;67:1809-1812

[86] O'Sullivan M, Jarosz JM, Martin RJ, Deasy N, Powell JF, Markus HS. Mri hyperintensities of the temporal lobe and external capsule in patients with cadasil. *Neurology* 2001;56:628-634

[87] Gallai V, Caso V, Paciaroni M, Cardaioli G, Arning E, Bottiglieri T, Parnetti L. Mild hyperhomocyst(e)inemia: A possible risk factor for cervical artery dissection. *Stroke* 2001;32:714-718

[88] Pezzini A, Del Zotto E, Archetti S, Negrini R, Bani P, Albertini A, Grassi M, Assanelli D, Gasparotti R, Vignolo LA, Magoni M, Padovani A. Plasma homocysteine concentration, C677T MTHFR genotype, and 844ins68bp CBS genotype in young

adults with spontaneous cervical artery dissection and atherothrombotic stroke. *Stroke* 2002;33:664-669

[89] Guillon B, Berthet K, Benslamia L, Bertrand M, Bousser MG, Tzourio C. Infection and the risk of spontaneous cervical artery dissection: A case-control study. *Stroke* 2003; 34:e79-81

[90] Brandt T, Orberk E, Weber R, Werner I, Busse O, Muller BT, Wigger F, Grau A, Grond-Ginsbach C, Hausser I. Pathogenesis of cervical artery dissections: Association with connective tissue abnormalities. *Neurology* 2001;57:24-30

[91] Schievink WI. Spontaneous dissection of the carotid and vertebral arteries. *N. Engl. J. Med.* 2001;344:898-906

[92] Schievink WI, Mokri B, Piepgras DG, Kuiper JD. Recurrent spontaneous arterial dissections: Risk in familial versus nonfamilial disease. *Stroke* 1996;27:622-624

[93] Baumgartner RW, Arnold M, Baumgartner I, Mosso M, Gonner F, Studer A, Schroth G, Schuknecht B, Sturzenegger M. Carotid dissection with and without ischemic events: Local symptoms and cerebral artery findings. *Neurology* 2001;57:827-832

[94] Brandt T, Hausser I, Orberk E, Grau A, Hartschuh W, Anton-Lamprecht I, Hacke W. Ultrastructural connective tissue abnormalities in patients with spontaneous cervicocerebral artery dissections. *Ann. Neurol.* 1998;44:281-285

[95] Ulbricht D, Diederich NJ, Hermanns-Le T, Metz RJ, Macian F, Pierard GE. Cervical artery dissection: An atypical presentation with ehlers-danlos-like collagen pathology? *Neurology* 2004;63:1708-1710

[96] Grond-Ginsbach C, Klima B, Weber R, Striegel J, Fischer C, Hacke W, Brandt T, Hausser I. Exclusion mapping of the genetic predisposition for cervical artery dissections by linkage analysis. *Ann Neurol.* 2002;52:359-364

[97] Wiest T, Hyrenbach S, Bambul P, Erker B, Pezzini A, Hausser I, Arnold ML, Martin JJ, Engelter S, Lyrer P, Busse O, Brandt T, Grond-Ginsbach C. Genetic analysis of familial connective tissue alterations associated with cervical artery dissections suggests locus heterogeneity. *Stroke* 2006;37:1697-1702

[98] Pezzini A, Grassi M, Del Zotto E, Giossi A, Monastero R, Dalla Volta G, Archetti S, Zavarise P, Camarda C, Gasparotti R, Magoni M, Camarda R, Padovani A. Migraine mediates the influence of C677T MTHFR genotypes on ischemic stroke risk with a stroke-subtype effect. *Stroke* 2007;38:3145-3151

[99] Arauz A, Hoyos L, Cantu C, Jara A, Martinez L, Garcia I, Fernandez Mde L, Alonso E. Mild hyperhomocysteinemia and low folate concentrations as risk factors for cervical arterial dissection. *Cerebrovasc. Dis.* 2007;24:210-214

[100] Kloss M, Wiest T, Hyrenbach S, Werner I, Arnold ML, Lichy C, Grond-Ginsbach C. MTHFR 677tt genotype increases the risk for cervical artery dissections. *J. Neurol. Neurosurg. Psychiatry.* 2006;77:951-952

[101] von Pein F, Valkkila M, Schwarz R, Morcher M, Klima B, Grau A, Ala-Kokko L, Hausser I, Brandt T, Grond-Ginsbach C. Analysis of the col3a1 gene in patients with spontaneous cervical artery dissections. *J. Neurol.* 2002;249:862-866

[102] Longoni M, Grond-Ginsbach C, Grau AJ, Genius J, Debette S, Schwaninger M, Ferrarese C, Lichy C. The icam-1 e469k gene polymorphism is a risk factor for spontaneous cervical artery dissection. *Neurology* 2006;66:1273-1275

[103] Marcel M, Leys D, Mounier-Vehier F, Bertheloot D, Lartigau E, Pruvo JP, Al-Koussa M, Chevalier D, Henon H. Clinical outcome in patients with high-grade internal carotid artery stenosis after irradiation. *Neurology* 2005;65:959-961

[104] O'Halloran HS, Berger JR, Lee WB, Robertson DM, Giovannini JA, Krohel GB, Meckler RJ, Selhorst JB, Lee AG, Nicolle DA, O'Day J. Acute multifocal placoid pigment epitheliopathy and central nervous system involvement: Nine new cases and a review of the literature. *Ophthalmology* 2001;108:861-868

[105] Salvarani C, Brown RD, Jr., Calamia KT, Christianson TJ, Weigand SD, Miller DV, Giannini C, Meschia JF, Huston J, 3rd, Hunder GG. Primary central nervous system vasculitis: Analysis of 101 patients. *Ann. Neurol.* 2007;62:442-451

[106] Perdu J, Boutouyrie P, Bourgain C, Stern N, Laloux B, Bozec E, Azizi M, Bonaiti-Pellie C, Plouin PF, Laurent S, Gimenez-Roqueplo AP, Jeunemaitre X. Inheritance of arterial lesions in renal fibromuscular dysplasia. *J. Hum. Hypertens.* 2007;21:393-400

[107] Janssens E, Hommel M, Mounier-Vehier F, Leclerc X, Guerin du Masgenet B, Leys D. Postpartum cerebral angiopathy possibly due to bromocriptine therapy. *Stroke* 1995;26:128-130

[108] Rascol A, Guiraud B, Manelfe C, Clanet M. *Accidents vasculaires cérébraux de la grossesse et du post-partum.* Paris, France; 1979.

[109] Goldenberg RL, Culhane JF, Iams JD, Romero R. Epidemiology and causes of preterm birth. *Lancet.* 2008;371:75-84

[110] Sibai B, Dekker G, Kupferminc M. Pre-eclampsia. *Lancet.* 2005;365:785-799

[111] Barton JR, Sibai BM. Care of the pregnancy complicated by hellp syndrome. *Obstet Gynecol. Clin. North Am.* 1991;18:165-179

[112] Fredriksson K, Lindvall O, Ingemarsson I, Astedt B, Cronqvist S, Holtas S. Repeated cranial computed tomographic and magnetic resonance imaging scans in two cases of eclampsia. *Stroke* 1989;20:547-553

[113] Digre KB, Varner MW, Osborn AG, Crawford S. Cranial magnetic resonance imaging in severe preeclampsia vs eclampsia. *Arch Neurol.* 1993;50:399-406

[114] Garg AX, Suri RS, Barrowman N, Rehman F, Matsell D, Rosas-Arellano MP, Salvadori M, Haynes RB, Clark WF. Long-term renal prognosis of diarrhea-associated hemolytic uremic syndrome: A systematic review, meta-analysis, and meta-regression. *Jama* 2003;290:1360-1370

[115] Amlie-Lefond C, Sebire G, Fullerton HJ. Recent developments in childhood arterial ischaemic stroke. *Lancet Neurol.* 2008;7:425-435

[116] Douay X, Lucas C, Caron C, Goudemand J, Leys D. Antithrombin, protein c and protein s levels in 127 consecutive young adults with ischemic stroke. *Acta Neurol. Scand.* 1998;98:124-127

[117] Rolfs A, Bottcher T, Zschiesche M, Morris P, Winchester B, Bauer P, Walter U, Mix E, Lohr M, Harzer K, Strauss U, Pahnke J, Grossmann A, Benecke R. Prevalence of fabry disease in patients with cryptogenic stroke: A prospective study. *Lancet.* 2005; 366:1794-1796

[118] Corson SL. Venous air and gas emboli in operative hysteroscopy. *J. Am. Assoc. Gynecol. Laparosc.* 2002;9:106; author reply 106

[119]Gaustadnes M, Ingerslev J, Rutiger N. Prevalence of congenital homocystinuria in denmark. *N. Engl. J. Med.* 1999;340:1513

[120]Levy R, Furman B, Hagay ZJ. Fetal bradycardia and disseminated coagulopathy: Atypical presentation of amniotic fluid emboli. *Acta Anaesthesiol. Scand.* 2004; 48:1214-1215

[121]Mentz HA. Fat emboli syndromes following liposuction. *Aesthetic. Plast. Surg.* 2008

[122]Weir B, MacDonald N, Mielke B. Intracranial vascular complications of choriocarcinoma. *Neurosurgery* 1978;2:138-142

[123]Cohen PR. Sweet's syndrome--a comprehensive review of an acute febrile neutrophilic dermatosis. *Orphanet. J. Rare Dis.* 2007;2:34

[124]De Rosa G, Pardeo M, Rigante D. Current recommendations for the pharmacologic therapy in kawasaki syndrome and management of its cardiovascular complications. *Eur. Rev. Med. Pharmacol. Sci.* 2007;11:301-308

[125]Reiniger IW, Thurau S, Haritoglou C, Hilgert E, Dichgans M, Klopstock T, Kampik A. Susac-syndrom: Fallberichte und literaturubersicht. *Klin. Monatsbl. Augenheilkd.* 2006;223:161-167

[126]Jen J, Cohen AH, Yue Q, Stout JT, Vinters HV, Nelson S, Baloh RW. Hereditary endotheliopathy with retinopathy, nephropathy, and stroke (herns). *Neurology* 1997;49:1322-1330

In: Cerebral Ischemia in Young Adults
Editors: A. Pezzini and A. Padovani

ISBN 978-1-60741-627-2

Chapter 2

Conventional Risk Factors

Maurizio Castellano*
Dipartimento di Scienze Mediche e Chirurgiche, Medicina Interna,
Università degli Studi di Brescia, Italia

Abstract

Cerebral ischemia accounts for approximately 80% of strokes and is determined by atherosclerotic processes in most patients. Accordingly, ischemic stroke shares to a large extent the same pathogenic mechanism and the same risk factors underlying other cardiovascular diseases, such as coronary heart disease.

Extensive epidemiological investigation has clearly established that hypertension, dyslipidemia, diabetes mellitus and cigarette smoking are independent risk factors for cardiovascular disease; on the basis of such time-honored associations these four conditions have been labeled as "conventional" risk factors, as opposed to other predisposing conditions more recently assessed or showing weaker association. With specific regard to ischemic stroke, other conditions (such as atrial fibrillation) are traditionally associated to the occurrence (or recurrence) of the disease, but they are usually not regarded as "conventional" risk factors *sensu stricto* and will be considered elsewhere in this book. This chapter will deal with the role of conventional risk factors, as defined above, in the development of ischemic strokes, with particular attention to those occurring in young adults.

---

* Correspondence: Maurizio Castellano, Professor of Internal Medicine, Department of Medical and Surgical Sciences, Brescia University Medical School, 2^ Medicina, Spedali Civili, I-25100 Brescia, Italy. Phone +39-030-3995276, Fax +39-030-3384348, E-mail: castella@med.unibs.it.

Hypertension

High blood pressure represents the single most important risk factor for stroke. Hypertension can promote earlier development and more severe extent of atherosclerotic lesions, but it can also act through different mechanisms, such as direct endothelial damage with local thrombi formation. Degenerative changes of arterial wall can predispose to the development of hemorrhagic strokes as well.

The strict association between raised blood pressure values and the risk of stroke is well documented. Epidemiological data from the Framingham study clearly show that the incidence of ischemic stroke is increased by 50% in subjects with stage 1 hypertension (140 to 159 mm Hg of systolic blood pressure, SBP) and up to 300% in persons with stage 2 (160-179 mm Hg SBP) or 3 hypertension (SBP ≥180 mm Hg) [1]. Furthermore, a collaborative meta-analysis of prospective observational studies of the associations of usual blood pressure with common causes of death [2] involved 120 000 deaths at ages 40–89 years among one million participants in 61 cohorts and showed that the relationship of stroke mortality to usual blood pressure is strong and direct at all ages, with no evidence of a threshold at any age (Figure 1).

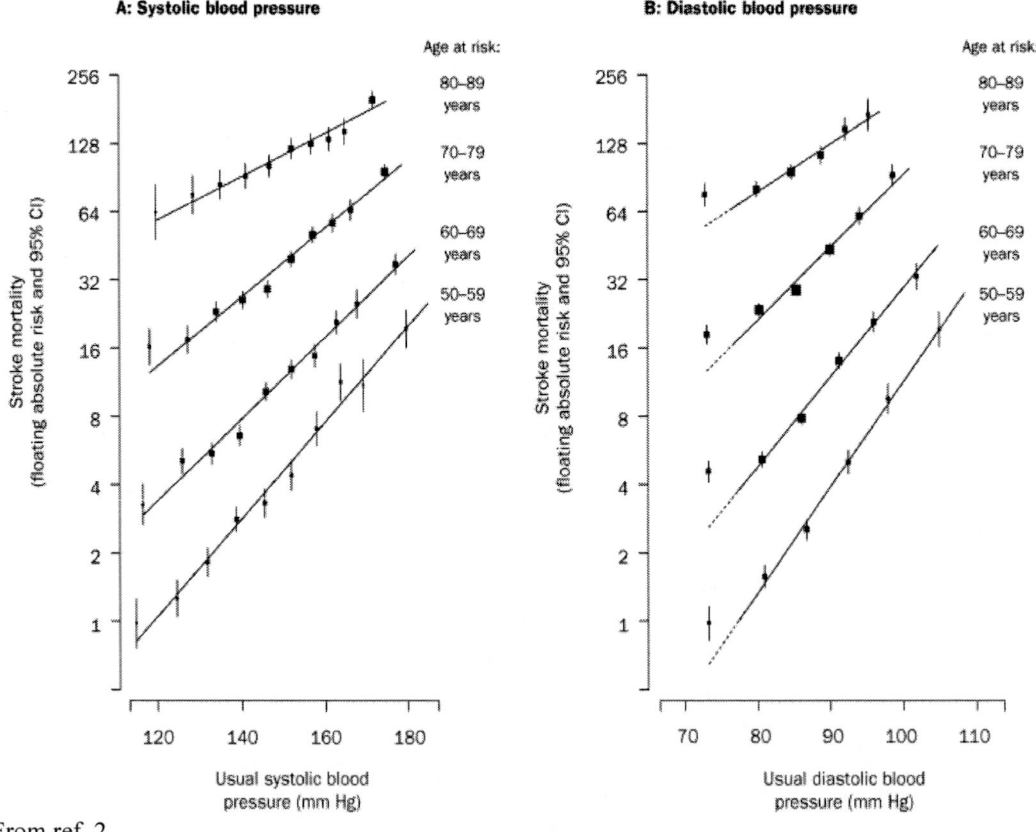

From ref. 2.

Figure 1. Stroke mortality rate in each decade of age according to usual blood pressure at the start of that decade.

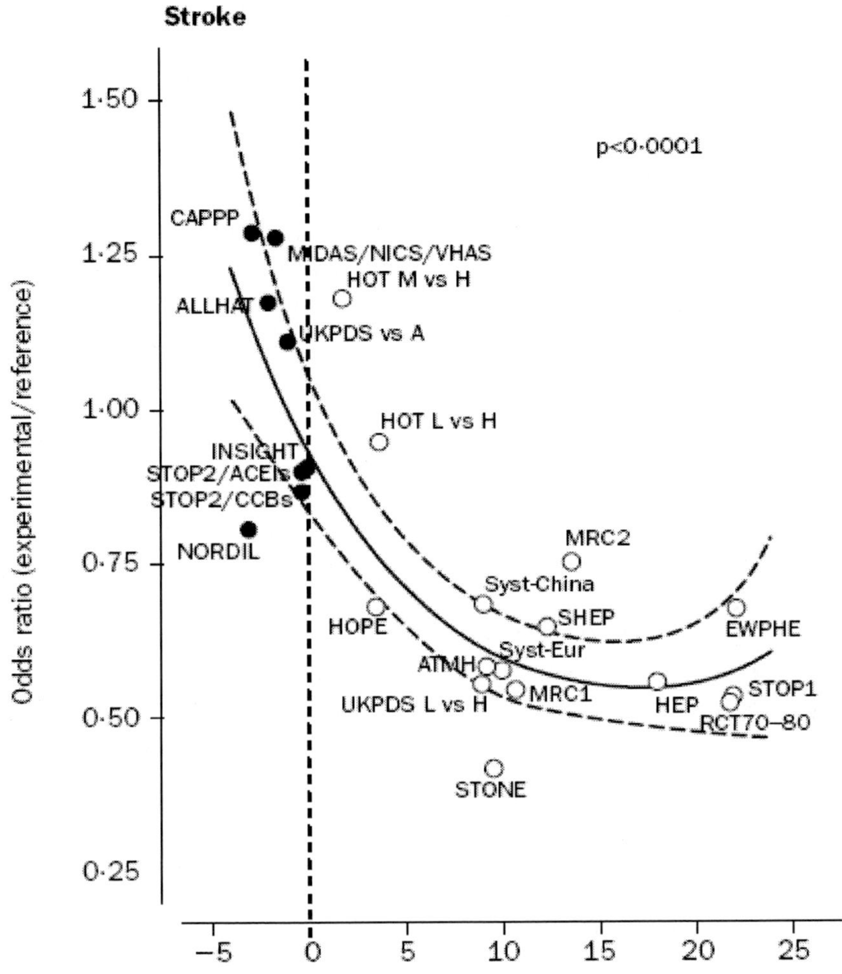

From ref. 9.

Figure 2. Relation between odds ratios for fatal and non-fatal stroke and corresponding differences in systolic blood pressure. Odds ratios were calculated for experimental versus reference treatment. Blood pressure differences were calculated by subtracting achieved levels in experimental groups from those in reference groups. Negative differences indicate tighter blood pressure control on reference treatment. Regression lines were plotted with 95% CI and were weighted for the inverse of the variance of individual odds ratios. Closed symbols denote trials that compared new with old drugs.

Stroke is much more common in old age than in middle age and the absolute annual difference in stroke death associated with a given difference in blood pressure increases with increasing age; however, the strength of the association between the proportional risk of stroke death and usual blood pressure is even more evident at younger ages: for each 20 mm Hg lower usual systolic blood pressure, the risk of stroke was 33% lower in those aged 80-89 but 62% lower in those aged 50-59. The central role of hypertension as a risk factor for ischemic stroke at young age is specifically supported also by a few studies [3-6] conducted in populations of different ethnic background, reporting odds ratio values for hypertension ranging from about 2 up to 7.

To confirm that the epidemiological association of arterial hypertension with ischemic stroke is expression of a true causal relationship, multiple clinical trials have shown that antihypertensive treatment is able to consistently reduce the incidence of ischemic stroke in hypertensive patients; this was first demonstrated in stage 2-3 hypertension, but then confirmed also in subjects with stage 1 hypertension. Different overviews and metanalyses [7-9] have clearly shown that antihypertensive treatment is associated to a risk reduction for stroke of about 30%, that such benefit is related to the degree of blood pressure level reduction (Figure 2), and that no major differences between different classes of drugs can be observed. In addition, no strong evidence that protection against major vascular events afforded by different drug classes varies substantially with age have been reported [9].

Diabetes

The pathophysiological link between diabetes and increased risk of ischemic stroke is not completely understood, but the underlying mechanisms most likely involve changes in both large and small cerebral blood vessels and may include excess glycation, endothelial damage and dysfunction, increased platelet aggregation, impaired fibrinolysis, and insulin resistance [10-12]. In addition, diabetic patients very often present associated dyslipidemia and hypertension, that contribute to the development of atherosclerotic lesions.

Most epidemiological studies, with few exceptions, have indicated that type 2 diabetes mellitus is an important risk factor for ischemic stroke, although relative risks associated to this condition have varied widely in different reports, from about 1.5 to 5 [13-23]. Despite such a large variability, it is probably correct to state that patients with type 2 diabetes have approximately twice the risk of ischemic stroke as compared to non diabetic subjects. On the other hand, the association with hemorrhagic stroke is more controversial, since available studies [13,18,24-28] report conflicting results of positive and negative association, while some investigations even seems to indicate a protective role of diabetes for non ischemic strokes.

Much less studies have examined the risk of stroke in patients with type 1 diabetes [27-29]. A cohort study of more than 23,000 type 1 diabetic patients (Diabetes UK Cohort), followed-up for an average of 17 years reported cerebrovascular mortality rates higher than the corresponding rates in the general population [27]. When stratified by age, the standard mortality rates were highest in the 20- to 39-year age group, while both sexes were almost equally affected, with slightly higher risk in females. A subsequent study examined the Nurses' Health Study prospective cohort, consisting of about 116,000 female registered nurses aged 30–55 years, with a 24-year follow-up [30]. The risk of total stroke was sixfold higher in women with type 1 and twofold higher among women with type 2 diabetes than for nondiabetic women in age-adjusted models. The age-adjusted RR of thrombotic stroke was eightfold higher in type 1 and threefold higher in type 2 diabetes. The risk of stroke was already present in women with duration of type 2 diabetes of 5 years or less, but there was a progressive increase of the risk paralleling the duration of the disease (Figure 3). Type 1 diabetes was also significantly associated with the age-adjusted risk of hemorrhagic stroke (RR, 4.5), but type 2 diabetes was not (RR, 1.1).

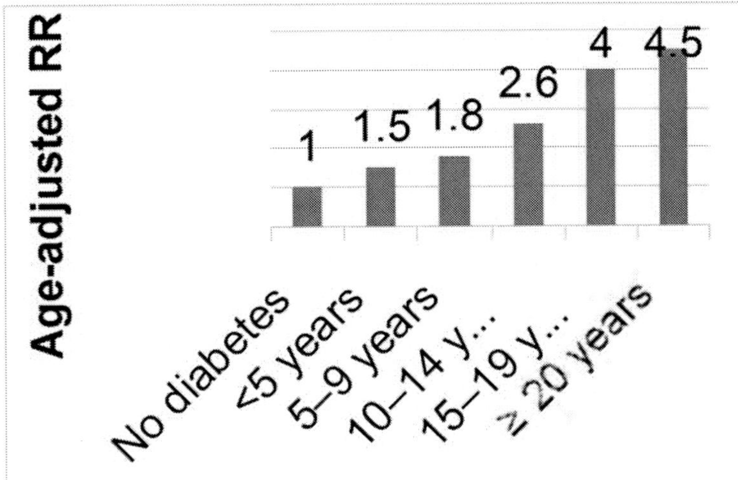

From ref. 30.

Figure 3. Age adjusted relative risk of ischemic stroke (24-years follow-up) according to duration of type 2 diabetes mellitus in Nurses' Health Study.

Despite some evidence that, in addition to the risk associated with overt diabetes, a graded rise in cardiovascular risk may also occur with dysglycemic conditions below the definition of overt diabetes, such as impaired fasting glucose (IFG), impaired glucose tolerance (IGT) or increasing levels of hemoglobin A1c [31,32], very little data confirm that these conditions may actually increase the risk of ischemic stroke, particularly in the young. Beside some indirect studies reporting an association between glycosylated hemoglobin level and carotid atherosclerosis in non diabetic subjects [33,34], it has been observed that nondiabetic patients with previous TIA or minor ischemic stroke have a nearly doubled risk of incident stroke in presence of IGT as compared with those with normal glucose levels (hazard ratio 1.8) [35]. On the other hand, a report from the HERS trial of 2763 postmenopausal women with known CHD followed for 6.8 years showed that IFG was not predictive of the risk of stroke or transient ischemic attack [36].

Once again, the identification of diabetes as a risk factor, even after statistical adjustement for potential confounders, cannot completely exclude that its effects on cardiovascular disease, and ischemic stroke in particular, may be mediated by the clustering of hypertension, dyslipidemia, and hyperglycemia rather than by hyperglycemia per se. As a matter of fact, rigorous control of blood pressure and lipids has proven to be critically important to reduce the risk of stroke in patients with diabetes [37], whereas information on the effect of glycemic control is rather limited. Strict glycemic control does reduce the risk of microvascular complications (retinopathy, nephropathy, and neuropathy) in diabetic patients, but its link with macrovascular complications and related hard cardiovascular events, at least for type 2 diabetes, is less clear. Several clinical trials, such as DCCT [38], VACSDM [39], UKPDS [40], ACCORD [41] and ADVANCE [42] failed to show any benefit of intensive glycemic control on macrovascular outcomes; results from ACCORD even suggests an adverse outcome in older patients with longstanding type 2 diabetes at high risk for cardiovascular disease [41]. From these findings it cannot be extrapolated whether a benefit in terms of reducing ischemic stroke will eventually be demonstrated in a subset of younger patients with diabetes under intensive glycemic control.

Smoking

Cigarette smoking in general and some specific components of cigarette smoke affect a number of basic pathophysiologic processes at the critical interface between circulating blood components and the inner arterial wall that may favor the development of ischemic stroke [43]. Smoking causes endothelial injury and cell dysfunction and produces a substantial shift in the hemostatic balance at the endothelium, leading to atherosclerosis and its thrombotic complications. Furthermore, components of cigarette smoke diminish the ability of the blood to carry oxygen. On the other hand, the mechanisms by which smoking contributes to hemorrhagic stroke are less clear.

The overall result of this constellation of toxic effects may account for the well-documented relationship between smoking and subclinical and clinical manifestations of atherosclerosis. In particular, smoking is a well established risk factor for both ischemic stroke and hemorrhagic stroke. The epidemiologic association was clearly assessed in early 60', with the first Report of the Advisory Committee on Smoking and Health to the Surgeon General of the USA Public Health Service [44]; this comprehensive review was followed and updated by 27 other reports, the latter being published in 2004 [43], that provide a substantial body of epidemiological and clinical evidence supporting several firm conclusions.

First, smoking is clearly associated with an increase in both the incidence of and mortality from both ischemic stroke and subarachnoid hemorrhage; A meta-analysis reviewed 32 case-control and cohort studies and documented that cigarette smoking increased the risk of stroke by an estimated 50 percent, although the effect differs according to stroke subtype: the RR for ischemic stroke was 1.9, and 2.9 for subarachnoid hemorrhage, but no elevation in risk was found for cerebral hemorrhage [45].

Second, there is a clear dose-response relationship between the increased risk and the average number of cigarettes smoked per day. For example, the U.S. Physicians Study showed that compared with lifetime non-smokers, current smokers of 1 to 19 cigarettes/day presented an age-adjusted relative risk for stroke incidence of 2.02, whereas smokers of 20 or more cigarettes/day had an adjusted risk of 2.52 [46]. Similar findings were obtained in the Nurses' Health Study [30], where he risk of stroke increased with the number of cigarettes smoked daily, and most recently in a cohort study involving almost 170,000 Chinese men and women aged 40 years and over, followed for an average of 8.3 years [47].

Third, the smoking-associated risk of stroke is particularly elevated in younger persons [48,49]. The relative risk of ischemic stroke, as well as of other cardiovascular events, is much greater in younger versus older smokers, primarily because cardiovascular events are rare in young nonsmokers (Figure 4). Although the relative risk declines considerably with age, the absolute excess mortality caused by smoking rises progressively with age, which makes important for clinicians to promote smoking cessation even in elderly smokers.

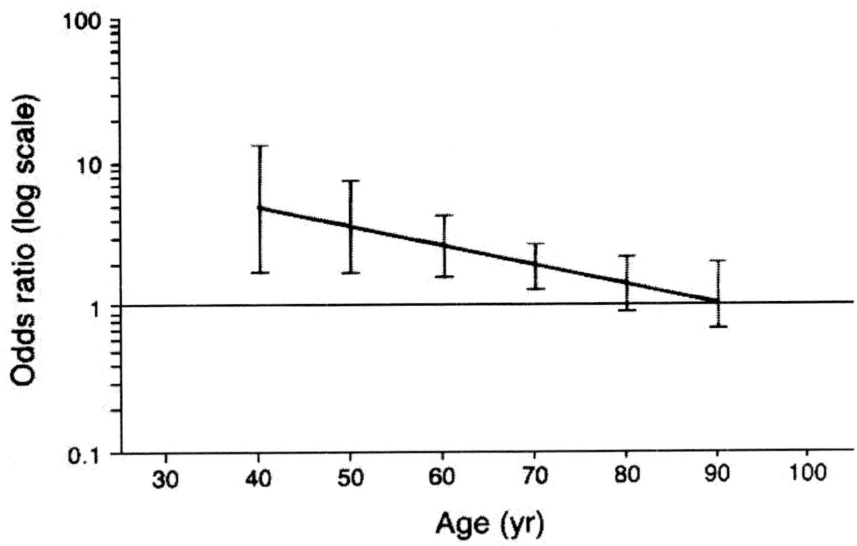

From ref. 49.

Figure 4. Odds ratios of current cigarette smoking for ischemic stroke by age with 95% confidence intervals.

Fourth, more recent studies (e.g., The Cancer Prevention Study II, CPS-II 1982–1986) tend to show a higher relative risk of stroke in relation to smoking than did earlier studies (CPS-I 1959–1965) [50].

Fifth, and more relevant to support the causal role of smoking in the epidemiological association, the elevated risk of stroke declines after smoking cessation. There are no randomized controlled trials of smoking cessation for stroke prevention, but several observational studies confirm the beneficial effect of quitting [51-53]. A recent analysis of the Nurses' Health Study found that women who quit smoking experienced a rapid decline in the risk of death from stroke, reaching 42% within 5 years after stopping smoking [54]. Similarly, in the Physicians' Health Study [46], male ex-smokers had a lower relative risk of total nonfatal stroke (RR, 1.2) than physicians currently smoking less than 20 and more than 20 cigarettes daily, (RR, 2.0 and 2.5, respectively). Lightwood and Glantz demonstrated that the decline in relative risk for stroke after smoking cessation follows an exponential decay curve: the curve flattens out within 4 years after quitting but the risk remains elevated as compared to lifetime non-smokers [55]. The observation that the benefits of cessation begin almost immediately when a smoker quits is consistent with the pathophysiologic mechanisms supposedly at play: improvement in coagulation parameters, lipid profile and hemodynamic variables [56-61]. In the recent study conducted by Kelly and colleagues in the Chinese population, the relative risk of stroke incidence and mortality in current smokers as compared with ever smokers were 1.28 and 1.13 in men and 1.25 and 1.19 in women, respectively, and there appeared to be a dose–response relationship with the number of cigarettes smoked per day and with duration of smoking [47].

Smoking also potentiates the effects of other stroke risk factors, such as oral contraceptive use (see chapter 6).

Dyslipidemia

The rationale for a potential role of dyslipidemia in the pathogenesis of ischemic stroke is quite straightforward: in fact, increased total cholesterol and/or low density lipoprotein (LDL) cholesterol, as well as reduced levels of high density lipoprotein (HDL) cholesterol, are well established pro-atherogenic risk factors. In addition, both low HDL cholesterol and high total to HDL cholesterol ratio favor the development of carotid atherosclerosis [62-64].

However, the relationship between serum cholesterol concentration and incidence of ischemic stroke is still unclear and inconsistent. The first available information, derived from the Framingham Study showed no clear association between total cholesterol levels and vascular disease of the brain [65]. The subsequent Honolulu Heart Study did not show a significant association with cerebral infarction but an inverse relationship with intracerebral hemorrhage [66]. At the end of the 90's, the large Multiple Risk Factor Intervention Trial, conducted in more than 350,000 men, reported that death from nonhemorrhagic strokes were correlated with elevated cholesterol, whereas serum cholesterol levels under 160 mg/dL increased the risk of fatal intracranial hemorrhage, particularly in hypertensive subjects [67].

In 1995, after a series of conflicting findings, a review of 45 prospective observational cohort studies involving 450,000 subjects, with more than 13,000 subjects experiencing a stroke over an average follow-up of 16 years [68], concluded that there was no association between serum cholesterol and stroke except in those under 45 years of age (Figure 5). Most of the observed stroke were fatal but details about stroke subtypes were not available for analysis, so that it cannot be excluded that a negative association for hemorrhagic stroke may have masked a positive association for ischemic stroke.

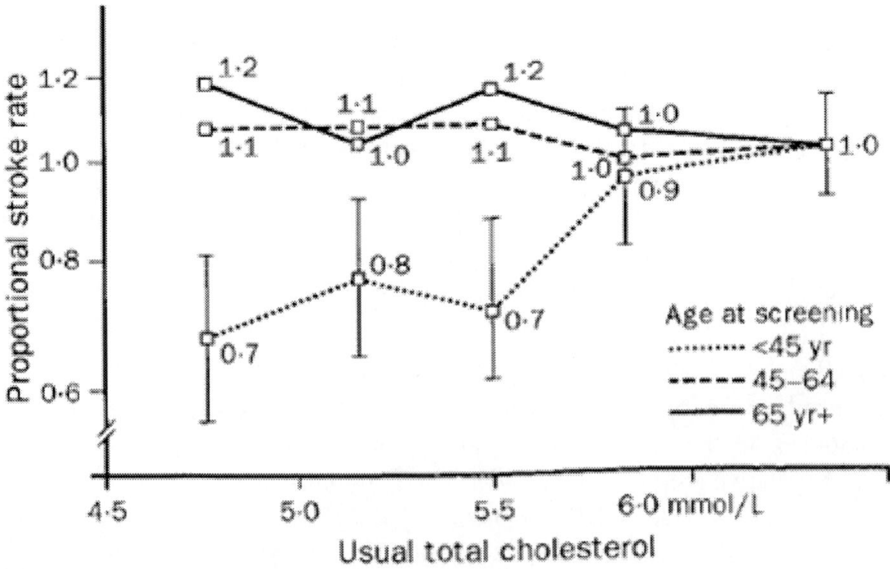

From ref. 68.

Figure 5. Relationship between proportional risk of stroke, total cholesterol levels and age in the Prospective Studies Collaboration metanalysis.

Subsequent studies confirmed a general heterogeneity of results. The Eastern Stroke and Coronary Heart Disease Collaborative Research Group study examined approximately 70,000 subjects of Asian descent and found that decreasing cholesterol levels showed only a nonsignificant trend toward a decreased risk of ischemic stroke and an increased risk of hemorrhagic stroke [69]. On the other hand, the Asia Pacific Cohort Studies Collaboration, which included over 350,000 individuals, found a 25% increase in ischemic stroke rates for every 1 mmol/L (38.7-mg/dL) increase in total cholesterol [70]. Other conflicting results were obtained in Caucasians, with the Eurostroke project (22,183 subjects, 34% female) reporting only a trend toward increased risk with 6% more cases of cerebral infarction for every 1-mmol/L increase in total cholesterol [71], while the US Women's Pooling Project (24,343 women at risk) found a 25% increased risk of fatal ischemic stroke for each 1-mmol/L increase in total cholesterol in women 30 to 54 years of age [72].

Another prospective study that compared cases of ischemic stroke (n = 1,242) and hemorrhagic stroke (n = 313) with controls (n = 6,455), showed that elevated total cholesterol and lower HDL levels were associated with an increased risk of ischemic stroke, especially for large artery atherosclerotic and lacunar stroke subtypes [73].

In summary, epidemiologic studies have not conclusively found dyslipidemia to play a major role in ischemic stroke, although there is some evidence suggesting it may be a risk factor particularly for large artery atherosclerotic and lacunar stroke subtypes, and in young subjects.

Clinical trials with lipid-lowering drugs have also obtained controversial results: dietary or drug intervention (fibrates and resins) other than statins seem not able to reduce the risk of stroke in subjects with elevated cholesterol levels [74], whereas treatment with HMG CoA reductase inhibitors consistently decreases the risk of stroke. This conclusion is supported by a meta-analysis and systematic review of randomized trials that compared statin drug treatment with placebo or standard care for all-stroke prevention: in 11 trials (n = 58,604) evaluating nonhemorrhagic stroke, the pooled relative risk for statin treatment was 0.81 [75]. Only one trial (SPARCL) examined the impact of statins on secondary stroke prevention, showing that atorvastatin was associated with a reduction in fatal or nonfatal stroke, the primary endpoint, of about 15% [76]. However, a post hoc analysis of this trial found that statin treatment was associated with an increased risk of hemorrhagic stroke (hazard ratio, 1.66). While these data do not establish that statin therapy increases the risk of hemorrhagic stroke in all patients with prior stroke or prior hemorrhagic stroke, they are congruent with some epidemiological studies suggesting an inverse association between cholesterol and hemorrhagic stroke.

The different results accomplished by non-statin versus statin treatment in terms of stroke prevention, as well as the efficacy of statin irrespective of serum cholesterol concentrations strongly suggest that the protective effects of this class of drugs are not mediated by cholesterol lowering per se, but by other properties of statins, possibly involving plaque stabilization, reducing inflammation, slowing carotid arterial disease progression, improving endothelial function, decreased thrombogenicity and also potential direct neuroprotective effects [78-79].

Conclusion

Despite the proliferation of "new" risk factors for the development of ischemic stroke, a vast amount of epidemiological, experimental and clinical data indicate that the so-called "conventional" risk factors remain on the whole the most important predictors of the disease. The correction of the hemodynamic, biochemical or behavioral abnormalities underlying such risk factors is associated to a significant reduction of the risk itself, and the benefit of therapeutic interventions in the prevention of ischemic stroke appears even more relevant when multiple risk factors are treated. This seems to be particularly the case in the young population, at least in terms of relative risk, because at this stage the influence of the crucial, unmodifiable risk factor, i.e. aging, is not overwhelming.

Acknowledgments

This work was supported by the Ministero dell'Università e della Ricerca: Programmi di Ricerca Scientifica di Rilevante Interesse Nazionale (n. 2004060749 e n. 2005069333_003); Fondazione della Comunità Bresciana Onlus and the European Community Network of Excellence: Integrating Genomics, Clinical Research and Care in Hypertension "InGenious HyperCare" 2006-2010.

References

[1] Kannel WB. Hypertension as a risk factor: The Framingham contribution, In: Birkenhager WH, Robertson JIS, Zanchetti A, editors. Handbook of Hypertension, vol. 22. Elsevier B.V.; 2004. p. 129-42.

[2] The Prospective Studies Collaboration. Age-specific relevance of usual blood pressure to vascular mortality: a meta-analysis of individual data for one million adults in 61 prospective studies. *Lancet*, 360: 1903–1913, 2002.

[3] You RX, McNeil JJ, O'Malley HM, Davis SM, Thrift AG, Donnan GA. Risk factors for stroke due to cerebral infarction in young adults. *Stroke* 1997; 28:1913-8.

[4] Kittner SJ, Stern BJ, Wozniak M, Buchholz DW, Earley CJ, Feeser BR, Johnson CJ, Macko RF, McCarter RJ, Price TR, Sherwin R, Sloan MA, Wityk RJ. Cerebral infarction in young adults: the Baltimore-Washington Cooperative Young Stroke Study. *Neurology* 1998; 50: 890–894.

[5] Nightingale AL, Farmer RD. Ischemic stroke in young women: a nested case-control study using the UK General Practice Research Database. *Stroke* 2004; 35: 1574–1578.

[6] Lipska K, Sylaja PN, Sarma PS, Thankappan KR, Kutty VR, Vasan RS, Radhakrishnan K. Risk factors for acute ischaemic stroke in young adults in South India. *J. Neurol. Neurosurg. Psychiatry* 2007; 78: 959-63.

[7] Collins R, Peto R, MacMahon S, Hebert P, Fiebach NH, Eberlein KA, Godwin J, Qizilbash N, Taylor JO, Hennekens CH. Blood pressure, stroke, and coronary heart

disease. Part 2, Short-term reductions in blood pressure: Overview of randomised drug trials in their epidemiological context. *Lancet* 1990; 335:827.

[8] Staessen JA, Wang JG, Thijs L. Cardiovascular protection and blood pressure reduction: a meta-analysis. *Lancet* 2001; 358: 1305–15

[9] Blood Pressure Lowering Treatment Trialists' Collaboration. Effects of different regimens to lower blood pressure on major cardiovascular events in older and younger adults: meta-analysis of randomised trials. *BMJ* 2008;336;1121-1123.

[10] Beckman JA, Creager MA, Libby P: Diabetes and atherosclerosis: epidemiology, pathophysiology, and management. *JAMA* 287:2570–2581, 2002.

[11] Monkovsky BN, Ziegler D: Stroke in patients with diabetes mellitus. *Diabetes Metab. Res. Rev.* 20:268–287, 2004.

[12] Idris I, Thomson GA, Sharma JC: Diabetes mellitus and stroke. *Int. J. Clin. Pract.* 60:48–56, 2006.

[13] Jorgensen H, Nakayama H, Raaschou HO, Olsen TS: Stroke in patients with diabetes: the Copenhagen Stroke Study. *Stroke* 25:1977–1984, 1994.

[14] Lehto S, Ronnemaa T, Pyorala K, Laakso M: Predictors of stroke in middle-aged patients with non-insulin-dependent diabetes. *Stroke* 27:63–68, 1996

[15] Davis TM, Millns H, Stratton IM, Holman RR, Turner RC: Risk factors for stroke in type 2 diabetes mellitus: United Kingdom Prospective Diabetes Study (UKPDS). *Arch Intern. Med.* 159:1097–1103, 1999.

[16] Folsom AR, Rasmussen ML, Chambless LE Howard G, Cooper LS, Schmidt MI, Heiss G: Prospective associations of fasting insulin, body fat distribution, and diabetes with risk of ischemic stroke: the Atherosclerosis Risk in Communities (ARIC) Study investigators. *Diabetes Care* 22:1077–1083, 1999.

[17] Rodriguez BL, D'Agostino R, Abbott RD, Kagan A, Burchfiel CM, Yano K, Ross GW, Silbershatz H, Higgins MW, Popper J, Wolf PA, Curb JD: Risk of hospitalized stroke in men enrolled in the Honolulu Heart Program and the Framingham Study: a comparison of incidence and risk factor effects. *Stroke* 33:230–236, 2002

[18] Kissela BM, Khoury J, Kleindorfer D, Woo D, Schneider A, Alwell K, Miller R, Ewing I, Moomaw CJ, Szarflaski JP, Ebel J, Shukla R, Broderick JP: Epidemiology of ischemic stroke in patients with diabetes: the greater Cincinnati/Northern Kentucky Stroke Study. *Diabetes Care* 28:355–359, 2005.

[19] Iso H, Imano H, Kitamura A, Sato S, Naito Y, Tanigawa T, Ohira T, Yamagishi K, Iida M, Shimamoto T: Type 2 diabetes and risk of non-embolic ischemic stroke in Japanese men and women. *Diabetologia* 47:2137–2144, 2004

[20] Lawes CM, Parag V, Bennett DA, Suh I, Lam TH, Whitlock G, Barzi F, Woodward M; Asia Pacific Cohort Studies Collaboration: Blood glucose and risk of cardiovascular disease in the Asia Pacific region. *Diabetes Care* 27:2836–2842, 2004.

[21] Almdal T, Scharling H, Jensen JS, Vestergaard H: The independent effect of type 2 diabetes mellitus on ischemic heart disease, stroke, and death: a population-based study of 13,000 men and women with 20 years of follow-up. *Arch Intern. Med.* 164:1422–1426, 2004.

[22] Davis PH, Dambrosia JM, Schoenberg BS, Schoenberg DG, Pritchard DA, Lilienfeld AM, Whisnant JP: Risk factors for ischemic stroke: a prospective study in Rochester, Minnesota. *Ann. Neurol.* 22:319–327, 1987

[23] Haheim LL, Holme I, Hjermann I, Leren P: Risk factors of stroke incidence and mortality: a 12-year follow-up of the Oslo Study. *Stroke* 24:1484–1489, 1993

[24] D'Agostino RB, Wolf PA, Belanger AJ, Kannel WB: Stroke risk profile: adjustment for antihypertensive medication: the Framingham Study. *Stroke* 25:40–43, 1994.

[25] Knekt P, Reunanen A, Aho K, Heliovaara M, Rissanen A, Aromaa A, Impivaara O: Risk factors for subarachnoid hemorrhage in a longitudinal population study. *J. Clin. Epidemiol.* 44:933–939, 1991.

[26] Megherbi SE, Milan C, Minier D, Couvreur G, Osseby GV, Tilling K, Di Carlo A, Inzitari D, Wolfe CD, Moreau T, Giroud M; European BIOMED Study of Stroke Care Group: Association between diabetes and stroke subtype on survival and functional outcome 3 months after stroke: data from the European BIOMED Stroke Project. *Stroke* 344:688–694, 2003.

[27] Laing SP, Swerdlow AJ, Carpenter LM, Slater SD, Burden AC, Botha JL, Morris AD, Waygh NR, Gatling W, Gale EA, Patterson CC, Qiao Z, Keen H: Mortality from cerebrovascular disease in a cohort of 23 000 patients with insulin-treated diabetes. *Stroke* 34:418–421, 2003.

[28] Fuller JH, Stevens LK, Wang SL: Risk factors for cardiovascular mortality and morbidity: the WHO Multinational Study of Vascular Disease in Diabetes. *Diabetologia* 44 (Suppl. 2):S54–S64, 2001.

[29] Deckert T, Poulsen JE, Larsen M: Prognosis of diabetics with diabetes onset before the age of thirty-one. *Diabetologia* 14:363–370, 1978.

[30] Janghorbani, M, Hu, FB, Willett, WC, et al. Prospective study of type 1 and type 2 diabetes and risk of stroke subtypes: the Nurses' Health Study. *Diabetes Care* 2007; 30:1730.

[31] Singer DE; Nathan DM; Anderson KM; Wilson PW; Evans JC Association of HbA1c with prevalent cardiovascular disease in the original cohort of the Framingham Heart Study. *Diabetes* 1992 Feb;41(2):202-8.

[32] Blake GJ; Pradhan AD; Manson JE; Williams GR; Buring J; Ridker PM; Glynn R. Hemoglobin A1c level and future cardiovascular events among women. *Arch Intern. Med.* 2004 Apr 12;164(7):757-61.

[33] Vitelli LL; Shahar E; Heiss G; McGovern PG; Brancati FL; Eckfeldt JH; Folsom AR. Glycosylated hemoglobin level and carotid intimal-medial thickening in nondiabetic individuals. The Atherosclerosis Risk in Communities Study. *Diabetes Care* 1997 Sep;20(9):1454-8.

[34] Jorgensen L; Jenssen T; Joakimsen O; Heuch I; Ingebretsen OC; Jacobsen BK. Glycated hemoglobin level is strongly related to the prevalence of carotid artery plaques with high echogenicity in nondiabetic individuals: the Tromso study. *Circulation* 2004 Jul 27; 110(4): 466-70. Epub 2004 Jul 12.

[35] Vermeer SE; Sandee W; Algra A; Koudstaal PJ; Kappelle LJ; Dippel DW. Impaired glucose tolerance increases stroke risk in nondiabetic patients with transient ischemic attack or minor ischemic stroke. *Stroke* 2006; 37: 1413-7.

[36] Hulley S, Grady D, Bush T, Furberg C, Herrington D, Riggs B, Vittinghoff E. Randomized trial of estrogen plus progestin for secondary prevention of coronary heart disease in postmenopausal women. Heart and Estrogen/progestin Replacement Study (HERS) Research Group. *JAMA* 1998;280:605-13.

[37] Goldstein LB, Adams R, Alberts MJ, Appel LJ, Brass LM, Bushnell CD, Culebras A, DeGraba TJ, Gorelick PB, Guyton JR, Hart RG, Howard G, Kelly-Hayes M, Nixon JV, Sacco RL; American Heart Association; American Stroke Association Stroke Council. Primary prevention of ischemic stroke: a guideline from the American Heart Association/American Stroke Association Stroke Council: cosponsored by the Atherosclerotic Peripheral Vascular Disease Interdisciplinary Working Group; Cardiovascular Nursing Council; Clinical Cardiology Council; Nutrition, Physical Activity, and Metabolism Council; and the Quality of Care and Outcomes Research Interdisciplinary Working Group. *Circulation* 2006; 113: e873-923.

[38] The Diabetes Control and Complications Trial Research Group. Effect of intensive diabetes management on macrovascular events and risk factors in the Diabetes Control and Complications Trial. *Am. J. Cardiol.* 1995; 75:894.

[39] Abraira C; Colwell J; Nuttall F; Sawin CT; Henderson W; Comstock JP; Emanuele NV; Levin SR; Pacold I; Lee HS. Cardiovascular events and correlates in the Veterans Affairs Diabetes Feasibility Trial. Veterans Affairs Cooperative Study on Glycemic Control and Complications in Type II Diabetes. *Arch Intern. Med.* 1997 Jan 27; 157(2): 181-8

[40] UK Prospective Diabetes Study (UKPDS) Group. Intensive blood-glucose control with sulphonylureas or insulin compared with conventional treatment and risk of complications in patients with type 2 diabetes (UKPDS 33). *Lancet* 1998; 352: 837-53.

[41] The Action to Control Cardiovascular Risk in Diabetes Study Group. Effects of Intensive Glucose Lowering in Type 2 Diabetes. *N. Engl. J. Med.* 2008; 358: 2545-59.

[42] http://www.advance-trial.com/static/html/healthcare/home.asp (accessed September 8, 2008)

[43] Report of the Advisory Committee to the Surgeon General of the Public Health Service, 2004. http://www.cdc.gov/tobacco/data_statistics/sgr/sgr_2004/index.htm#full (accessed September 8, 2008).

[44] U.S. Department of Health, Education, and Welfare. Smoking and Health: Report of the Advisory Committee to the Surgeon General of the Public Health Service. Washington: U.S. Department of Health, Education, and Welfare, Public Health Service, 1964. PHS Publication No. 1103.

[45] Shinton R, Beevers G. Meta-analysis of relation between cigarette smoking and stroke. *British Medical Journal* 1989;298: 789–94.

[46] Robbins AS, Manson JE, Lee IM, Satterfield S, Hennekens CH. Cigarette smoking and stroke in a cohort of U.S. male physicians. *Annals of InternalMedicine* 1994;120(6): 458–62.

[47] Kelly TN, Gu D, Chen J, Huang JF, Chen JC, Duan X, Wu X, Chen CS, He J. Cigarette smoking and risk of stroke in the Chinese adult population. *Stroke* 39, 1688–1693 (2008).

[48] J.P. Whisnant, MD; D.O. Wiebers, MD; W.M. O'Fallon, PhD; J.D. Sicks, MS; and R.L. Frye, MD A population-based model of risk factors for ischemic stroke: Rochester, Minnesota. *Neurology*, Volume 47(6), December 1996, pp 1420-1428.

[49] Bhat VM, Cole JW, Sorkin JD, Wozniak MA, Malarcher AM, Giles WH, Stern BJ, Kittner SJ. Dose-response relationship between cigarette smoking and risk of ischemic stroke in young women. *Stroke* 2008 Sep;39(9):2439-43.

[50] Garfinkel L. Selection, follow-up, and analysis in the American Cancer Society prospective studies. *Natl. Cancer Inst. Monogr.* 1985;67:49-52.

[51] Kawachi I, Colditz GA, Stampfer MJ, Willett WC, Manson JE, Rosner B, Speizer FE, Hennekens CH. Smoking cessation and decreased risk of stroke in women. *JAMA* 1993; 269:232-236.

[52] Wolf PA, D'Agostino RB, Kannel WB, Bonita R, Belanger AJ. Cigarette smoking as a risk factor for stroke. The Framingham Study. *JAMA* 1988; 259:1025-1029.

[53] Wannamethee, SG, Shaper, AG, Whincup, PH, Walker, M. Smoking cessation and the risk of stroke in middle-aged men. *JAMA* 1995; 274:155-160.

[54] Kenfield S, Stampfer M, Rosner B, Colditz G. Smoking and smoking cessation in relation to mortality in women. *JAMA* 2008; 299:2037–2047.

[55] Lightwood JM, Glantz SA. Short-term economic and health benefits of smoking cessation: myocardial infarction and stroke. *Circulation* 96(4), 1089–1096,1997.

[56] Hunter KA, Garlick PJ, Broom I, Anderson SE, McNurlan MA. Effects of smoking and abstention from smoking on fibrinogen synthesis in humans. *Clin. Sci.*; 100: 459–465, 2001.

[57] Terres W, Becker P, Rosenberg A. Changes in cardiovascular risk profile during the cessation of smoking. *Am. J. Med.* 97(3), 242–249 (1994).

[58] Morita H, Ikeda H, Haramaki N, Eguchi H, Imaizumi T. Only two-week smoking cessation improves platelet aggregability and intraplatelet redox imbalance of long-term smokers. *J. Am. Coll. Cardiol.* 45(4), 589–594 (2005).

[59] Eliasson B, Hjalmarson A, Kruse E, Landfeldt B, Westin A. Effect of smoking reduction and cessation on cardiovascular risk factors. *Nicotine Tob. Res.* 3(3), 249–255 (2001).

[60] Stubbe I, Eskilsson J, Nilsson-Ehle P. High-density lipoprotein concentrations increase after stopping smoking. *Br. Med. J.* (Clin. Res. Ed.) 284(6328), 1511–1513 (1982).

[61] Oren S, Isakov I, Golzman B et al. The influence of smoking cessation on hemodynamics and arterial compliance. *Angiology* 57(5): 564–568, 2006.

[62] Ford CS, Crouse JR 3rd, Howard G, Toole JF, Ball MR, Frye J. The role of plasma lipids in carotid bifurcation atherosclerosis. *Ann. Neurol.* 1985; 17:301-303.

[63] van Merode, T, Hick, P, Hoeks, APG, Reneman, RS. Serum HDL/total cholesterol ratio and blood pressure in asymptomatic atherosclerotic lesions of the cervical carotid arteries in men. *Stroke* 1985; 16:34-38.

[64] MacMahon S, Sharpe N, Gamble G, Hart H, Scott J, Simes J, White H, on behalf of the LIPID Trial Research Group. Effects of lowering average or below-average cholesterol levels on the progression of carotid atherosclerosis: Results of the LIPID atherosclerosis substudy. *Circulation* 1998; 97:1784-1790.

[65] Kannel WB, Dawber TR, Cohen ME, McNamara PM. Vascular disease of the brain—epidemiologic aspects: the Framingham Study. Am J Public Health. 1965;55:1355-1366.

[66] Kagan A, Popper JS, Rhoads GG. Factors related to stroke incidence in Hawaiian Japanese men, the Honolulu Heart Study. *Stroke* 1980;11:14-21.

[67] Iso H, Jacobs DR Jr, Wentworth D, Neaton JD, Cohen JD. Serum cholesterol levels and six-year mortality from stroke in 350,977 men screened for the multiple risk factor intervention trial. *N. Engl. J. Med.* 1989; 320:904-910.

[68] Prospective Studies Collaboration. Cholesterol, diastolic blood pressure, and stroke: 13 000 strokes in 450 000 people in 45 prospective cohorts. *Lancet;* 346: 1647-1653, 1995.

[69] Blood pressure, cholesterol, and stroke in eastern Asia. Eastern Stroke and Coronary Heart Disease Collaborative Research Group. *Lancet* 1998; 352:1801-1807.

[70] Zhang X, Patel A, Horibe H, Wu Z, Barzi F, Rodgers A, MacMahon S, Woodward M; Asia Pacific Cohort Studies Collaboration. Cholesterol, coronary heart disease, and stroke in the Asia Pacific region. *Int. J. Epidemiol.* 2003; 32: 563–572.

[71] Bots ML, Elwood PC, Nikitin Y, Salonen JT, Freire de Concalves A, Inzitari D, Sivenius J, Benetou V, Tuomilehto J, Koudstaal PJ, Grobbee DE. Total and HDL cholesterol and risk of stroke. EUROSTROKE: a collaborative study among research centres in Europe. *J. Epidemiol. Community Health* 2002; 56 (suppl 1): i19–i24.

[72] Horenstein RB, Smith DE, Mosca L. Cholesterol predicts stroke mortality in the Women's Pooling Project. *Stroke* 2002; 33: 1863–1868.

[73] Tirschwell DL, Smith NL, Heckbert SR, Lemaitre RN, Longstreth WT Jr, Psaty BM. Association of cholesterol with stroke risk varies in stroke subtypes and patient subgroups. *Neurology* 2004; 63:1868-1875.

[74] Corvol JC, Bouzamondo A, Sirol M, Hulot JS, Sanchez P, Lechat P. Differential effects of lipid-lowering therapies on stroke prevention: a meta-analysis of randomized trials. *Arch Intern. Med.* 2003; 163:669-676.

[75] O'Regan C, Wu P, Arora P, Perri D, Mills EJ. Statin therapy in stroke prevention: a meta-analysis involving 121,000 patients. *Am. J. Med.* 2008; 121:24-33.

[76] Amarenco P, Bogousslavsky J, Callahan A 3rd, Goldstein LB, Hennerici M, Rudolph AE, Sillesen H, Simunovic L, Szarek M, Welch KM, Zivin JA; Stroke Prevention by Aggressive Reduction in Cholesterol Levels (SPARCL) Investigators. High-dose atorvastatin after stroke or transient ischemic attack. *N. Engl. J. Med.* 2006; 355(6):549-59.

[77] Vaughan, CJ, Gotto, AM Jr, Basson, CT. The evolving role of statins in the management of atherosclerosis. *J. Am. Coll. Cardiol.* 2000; 35:1-10.

[78] Maron, DJ, Fazio, S, Linton, MF. Current perspectives on statins. *Circulation* 2000; 101:207-213.

[79] Martí-Fàbregas J, Gomis M, Arboix A, Aleu A, Pagonabarraga J, Belvís R, Cocho D, Roquer J, Rodríguez A, García MD, Molina-Porcel L, Díaz-Manera J, Martí-Vilalta JL. Favorable outcome of ischemic stroke in patients pretreated with statins. *Stroke* 2004; 35:1117-1121.

In: Cerebral Ischemia in Young Adults
Editors: A. Pezzini and A. Padovani

ISBN 978-1-60741-627-2

Chapter 3

Migraine and Ischemic Stroke

Alessandro Pezzini,*[*1] *Elisabetta Del Zotto,*[1,2] *Alessia Giossi,*[1] *Irene Volonghi,*[1] *Paolo Costa,*[1] *and Alessandro Padovani*[1]

1. Dipartimento di Scienze Mediche e Chirurgiche,
Clinica Neurologica, Università degli Studi di Brescia, Brescia, Italia
2. Dipartimento di Scienze Biomediche e Biotecnologie,
Università degli Studi di Brescia, Brescia, Italia

Abstract

Numerous epidemiological observations reporting high prevalence of migraine among young individuals with stroke as well as dysfunction of cerebral arteries during migraine attacks, prompt speculation on the existence of a co-morbidity between the two disorders. The recent finding of silent infarct-like brain lesions in migraineurs reinforced this hypothesis and raised questions on whether migraine may be a *progressive* disorder, rather then simply an episodic disorder.

Stroke can occur during the course of migraine attacks with aura, supporting the assumption of a causal relation between the two diseases. Migraine may accentuate other existing risk factors for stroke, and both jointly increase the risk of cerebral ischemia outside of migraine attacks. In this regard, the role of migraine might be that of predisposing condition for cerebral ischemia. Migraine and ischemic stroke may be the end phenotype of common pathogenic mechanisms. Evidence of a migraine-stroke relation in cases of specific disorders such as CADASIL and MELAS strongly supports this concept. Finally, acute focal cerebral ischemia can trigger migraine attacks, and, thus, migraine may be the consequence of stroke. In the present chapter we will review contemporary epidemiological studies, discuss potential mechanisms of migraine-induced stroke and co-morbid ischemic stroke, and pose new research questions.

[*] Correspondence: Alessandro Pezzini, Clinica Neurologica, Università degli Studi di Brescia, P.le Spedali Civili, 1, 25100 Brescia, Italia. Tel: +39.030.399 5631 – 5632, Fax: +39.030.399 5027. e-mail: ale_pezzini@ hotmail. com.

Introduction

Migraine is a common, chronic, multifactorial neurovascular disease characterized by severe attacks of headache and autonomic nervous system dysfunction (migraine without aura; MO). Neurological aura symptoms (migraine with aura; MA) are present in a percentage of patients which varies, according to the ascertainment criteria and the study design, from up to one-third in population-based studies to lower frequency in clinic-based studies [1-3].

Although migraine attacks may be acutely disabling, the traditional view is that they do not result in long-term consequences to the brain. Against this assumption, new data have emerged which emphasize the high prevalence of migraine among young individuals with stroke as well as a dysfunction of cerebral arteries during migraine attacks and the finding of silent infarct-like brain lesions in migraineurs, thus leading to the hypothesis that a co-morbidity between migraine and cerebral ischemia exists [4]. A careful evaluation of the existing data on the relation between migraine and stroke raises more questions than providing a clear picture.

In the present chapter we will review contemporary epidemiological studies, discuss potential mechanisms of migraine-induced stroke and co-morbid ischemic stroke and pose new research questions.

Migraine as a Risk Factor for Ischemic Stroke

The first epidemiological suggestion that migraine may be an independent risk factor for stroke came from the Collaborative Group for the Study of Stroke in Young Women, published in 1975, which showed a doubling of the relative risk of stroke with migraine compared with neighbour controls [5]. Since then, the association of migraine with the risk of stroke has been investigated in several observational studies (Table 1), most of which have been summarized in a recent meta-analysis [6]. According to this meta-analysis, the pooled relative risk of ischemic stroke among patients with any type of migraine is 2.16 (95% CI, 1.89 to 2.48). The relative risk for people with MA and MO are 2.27 (95% CI, 1.61 to 3.19) and 1.83 (95% CI, 1.06 to 3.15), respectively. However, as opposed to the MA-ischemic stroke association which was consistently confirmed by subsequent observational studies, two prospective and one case-control studies recently published and not included in the meta-analysis did not show any increased risk of cerebral ischemia in patients with MO [7-9]. A stronger predisposing effect of MA was also observed in a recent analysis of the UK-based General Practice Research Database [10]. Therefore, it seems at least unlikely that MA and MO are equally associated with ischemic stroke. At present, as the association is not as robust, whether MO should be considered a stroke risk factor remains unclear.

No difference in the pooled risk was found stratifying analysis by age. Otherwise, all the analysed studies found an increased risk in young women (RR 2.76; 95% CI, 2.17 to 3.52 for women younger than 45 years). Moreover, users of oral contraceptives had an approximately eight-fold increase in the risk of stroke compared with those not using these agents (RR 8.72; 95% CI, 5.05 to 15.05).

Table 1. Risk of ischemic stroke according to type of migraine in epidemiological studies

Authors, year	Methodology	Population	Subjects' characteristics	Patients with migraine	Migraine Status			Adjustment for covariates and confounders	Notes
				ischaemic stroke cases (%): controls (%)	Any RR (95% CI)	MA RR (95% CI)	MO RR (95% CI)		
Collaborative Group for the Study of Stroke in Young Woman, 1975 [5]	Case-control study	Women aged 14-44yrs	430 stroke cases, 429 hospital control subjects and 451 neighbor controls	48 (34.2) : 234 (26.5)	2.0 (1.2 to 3.3)*	NS	NS	Age, contraceptives, smoking	* RR calculated for ischemic stroke using neighbor controls for comparison
Henrich and Horwitz, 1989 [114]	Case-control study	Men and Women aged 15-65 yrs	89 ischemic stroke cases, 178 hospital controls	17 (19.1): 20 (11.2)	1.8 (0.9 to 3.6)	2.6 (1.1 to 6.6)	1.3 (0.5 to 3.6)	NS	
Marini et al, 1993 [115]	Case-control study	Men and Women aged 15-44 yrs	308 ischemic stroke or TIA cases, 308 hospital controls and 308 population controls	46 (14.9): 57 (9.2)*	1.91 (1.05 to 3.5)	14.85 (1.8 to 124)	1.6 (0.9 to 3.0)	Diet, obesity, alcohol, smoking, contraceptives, hypertension, diabetes, paroxysmal disorders, hematocrit, cholesterol, triglycerides, HDL, cardiac and carotid abnormalities	* from ischemic stroke and TIA cases
Tzourio et al, 1993 [59]	Case-control study	Men and Women aged18-80yrs	212 ischemic stroke cases, 212 hospital controls	41 (19.3): 34 (16)	1.3 (0.8 to 2.3)	1.3 (0.5 to 3.8)	0.8 (0.4 to 1.5)	NS	
Lidegaard, 1995 [116]	Case-control study	Women aged 15-44yrs	497 stroke cases, 1370 population controls	64 (12.9): 66 (4.8)	2.8 *	NS	NS	Hypertension, other predisponsing diseases	* 95% CI not reported; p< 0.01;
Tzourio et al, 1995 [60]	Case-control study	Women aged <45yrs	72 ischemic stroke cases, 173 hospital controls	43 (59.7): 52 (30)	3.5 (1.8 to 6.4)	6.2 (2.1 to 18)	3.0 (1.5 to 5.8)	Age, smoking, hypertension, contraceptives	
Carolei et al, 1996 [117]	Case-control study	Men and Women aged 15-44 yrs	308 ischemic stroke or TIA cases, 591 hospital controls and population controls	24 (13.9): 34 (10.3)	1.3 (0.7 to 2.4)	1.0 (0.5 to 2.0)	8.6 (1.0 to 75)	Obesity, alcohol, smoking, hypercholesterolaemia, hypertrigliceridaemia, low HDL-cholesterol, age, contraceptives, hypertension, diabetes	
Haapaniemi et al, 1997 [118]	Case-control study	Men and Women aged 16-60 yrs	506 ischemic stroke cases, 345 hospital controls	86 (17): 42 (12.2)	2.1 (1.05 to 2.9)*	NS	NS	Hypertension, cardiac disease, current smoking, diabetes, alcohol, age, body mass index	* RR reported for male subgroup
Chang et al, 1999 [119]	Case-control study	Women aged 20-44 yrs	291 ischemic, hemorragic or unclassified arterial stroke cases, 736 hospital controls	26 (30.2): 26 (11.8)	3.5 (1.3 to 9.6)	3.81 (1.3 to 11.5)	2.9 (0.7 to 13.5)	Hypertension, smoking, education, family history of migraine, alcohol, social class	
Donaghy et al, 2002 [120]	Case-control study	Women aged 20-44 yrs	86 ischemic stroke cases, 214 hospital controls	26 (30.2): 26 (12.1)	NS	8.4 (2.3 to 30.1)	2.2 (0.5 to 10.1)	NS	
Schwaag et al, 2003 [121]	Case-control study	Men and Women aged <46 yrs	160 ischemic stroke and TIA cases, 160 hospital controls	37 (23.1): 20 (12.5)*	2.1 (1.2 to 3.8)*	NS	NS	NS	* from ischemic stroke and TIA cases
Nightingale et al, 2004 [122]	Nested case-control study	Women aged 15-49 yrs	190 ischemic stroke cases, 1129 population controls	16 (8.4): 44 (3.9)	2.3 (1.04 to 5.2)	NS	NS	NS	
Kurth et al, 2005 [7]	Cohort study	Women aged 45 yrs or older partecipants of the Women's Health Study (WHS)	39754 subjects (385 ischemic, hemorragic or unclassified stroke cases)	41 (13.2): 5126 (13)	1.4 (0.97 to 1.9)*	1.7 (1.1 to 2.7)*	1.1 (0.7 to 1.8)*	Age, hypertension, menopausal status, contraceptives, alcohol, randomized aspirin assignment, exercise, body mass index, smoking, postmenopausal hormone therapy, diabetes, cholesterol	* calculated as Hazard Ratio (95% CI) for ischemic stroke
MacClellan et al, 2007 [9]	Case-control study	Women aged 15-49 yrs	386 ischemic stroke cases, 614 population controls	180 (47%):254 (42%)	NS	1.5 (1.1 to 2.0)	1.0 (0.6 to 1.5)	Age, race, geographic region, study period	
				Patients with ischemic stroke migraine cases (%): controls (%)					
Buring et al, 1995 [123]	Cohort study	Male physicians aged 40-84 yrs participants to the Physicians' Health Study	22071 subjects (1479 migraine sufferers)	17 (1.1): 154 (0.7)	2.0 (1.1-3.6)	NS	NS	Age, smoking, cholesterol, diabetes, hystory of angina, body mass index, parental hystory of premature MI, alcohol, excercise, randomized treatment assignment, hypertension,	
Merikangas et al, 1997 [16]	Cross sectional study	Population-based national probability sample	12220 subjects (1109 migraine sufferers)	NS	2.1 (1.5 to 2.9)*	NS	NS	Age, sex, smoking, hypertension, diabetres, cholesterol, heart condition, alcohol	* from all stroke cases
Velentgas et al, 2004 [96]	Cohort study	Population from United Health Care	260822 (130411 migraine sufferers)	216 (0.16): 98 (0.07)*	1.6 (1.3 to 2.1)*	NS	NS	Age, sex, year of cohort entry, comorbidities in years prior to study entry, contraceptives, estrogen replacement therapy	* from all stroke cases
Hall et al, 2004 [97]	Cohort study	Population from General Practice Research Database	140814 subjects (63575 migraine sufferers)	71 (0.11): 31 (0.04)	2.5 (1.6 to 3.8)	NS	NS	Hypertension, diabetes, cardiac disease, obesity, hypercholesterolemia, oral contraceptive, smoking	
Stang et al, 2005 [8]	Cohort study	Men and women aged 45-64 yrs participants to the Atherosclerosis Risk in the Communities (ARIC) Study	12750 subjects (1015 migraine sufferers)	NS	NS	2.8 (1.6 to 4.9)	0.8 (0.4 to 1.7)	Age, sex, race/center, hypertension medication use, aspirin use, NSAID use, systolic blood pressure, diabetes, parental hystory of migraines, smoking, pack-years of smoking, cholesterol	
Kurth et al, 2007 [15]	Cohort study	Men aged 40-84 yrs participants to the Physicians' Health Study	20084 subjects (1449 migraine sufferers)	51 (3.5): 699 (3.7)	1.1 (0.8 to 1.5)*	NS	NS	Age, hypertension, diabetes, smoking, exercise, body mass index, alcohol, cholesterol, parental hystory of MI before age 60 yrs, randomized treatment assignments	* calculated as Hazard Ratio (95% CI) for ischemic stroke
Becker et al, 2007 [10]	Cohort study	Population from General Practice Research Database	103376 subjects (51688 migraine suffers)	137 (0.2): 63 (0.12)*	2.7 (1.9-3.9)*	14.5 (4.4 to 47.9)*	2.6 (1.8 to 3.7)*	Age, gender, general practice, calendar time, BMI, smoking, diabetes, hypertension, dyslipidemia	* from all stroke cases

NS, not specified; MI, myocardial infarction; RR, relative risk.

In line with this observation, recent data from the Stroke Prevention in Young Women Study (SPYW) showed a higher risk of stroke in women with probable migraine with visual aura who were cigarette smokers and oral contraceptive users and further reinforced the hypothesis that specific subgroups of patients in which the migraine-stroke pathogenic link is more expressed might be identified [9].

Is this enough to conclude that migraine is a risk factor for stroke? As pointed out by many Authors, most of these studies are subjects to several limitations. First, in most of the considered studies, a consistent definitions for migraine is lacking. Accurate diagnosis of migraine is important to avoid non-differential misclassification of exposure, which will bias the risk estimate towards showing no association. If this is the case, however, we cannot but assume that the increased risk of stroke emerging from the pooled analysis of data from observational studies is rather an underestimation of the effect. As such, it should be retained as an argument in favour of the reported association between migraine and stroke. Furthermore, in case-control studies an *interviewer bias* and a *recall bias* can arise as possible consequences of the retrospective design. Second, potential bias in the selection of patients should be taken into account. At least theoretically, a *referral bias* may exist if stroke patients with migraine would be referred to the recruiting centres more frequently than stroke cases without migraine, or if the investigators were more prone to include stroke cases with migraine than without migraine. A further selection bias could be the consequence of a stroke-migraine misdiagnosis. As TIA are sometimes difficult to distinguish from an attack of MA, especially when the aura occurs without headache, and migraine with prolonged neurological aura (lasting longer than 24 hours) may mimic stroke, the end results of such misclassifications would be an over-estimation of the prevalence of migraine in cases and, therefore, an overestimation of the risk. Third, in some of the studies the influence of several confounders on the final results was not considered, while others were not controlled for. These include, for example, the use of medications with a potential effect on stroke risk (i.e anti-hypertensive agents), or risk factors for both migraine and stroke, such as anti-phospholipids antibodies. Finally, most studies are limited to younger individuals (aged 45 years or younger) leaving the association between migraine and stroke among the elderly unclear and ignoring the fact that migraine may start later in life.

With regard to this last observation, two prospective studies recently examined this relation. Data from 39,876 US female health professionals aged 45 or older included in the Women's Health Study after a mean of 9 years of follow-up showed that MA increased 1.5-fold the risk of total stroke after adjusting for potential confounders of age, hypertension, menopausal status, contraceptive use, and alcohol consumption (HR 1.53; 95% CI 1.02 to 2.31) and a 1.7-fold the risk of ischemic stroke (HR 1.71; 95% CI 1.11 to 2.66) when compared to participants without migraine [7]. In contrast, there was no association between MO and total stroke or ischemic stroke. This association between MA and cerebrovascular disease as well as with ischemic stroke was confirmed in a large cohort of individuals $\geq$ 55 years of age at the time of migraine assessment, who participated to the Atherosclerosis Risk in Communities (ARIC) Study [8].

Taken together, these findings provide arguments to the assumption that migraine may have some influence on stroke risk even in older subgroups. However, effect modification by age is evident from prospective data, the risk of stroke being higher in younger age groups and decreasing over time, with no increased risk among the elderly (age 60 or older) according to case-control analyses [11]. Whether this is the consequence of the greater effect of other major risk factors for ischemic stroke with increasing age or of their interaction with the mechanism by which migraine may lead to stroke remains to be determined.

The association between migraine and increased prevalence of cardiovascular risk factors and the observation that the vascular dysfunction of migraine may also extend to coronary arteries [12], has recently led to speculation that migraine, especially MA, may not only be associated with increased risk of stroke but also with other vascular events. To address this specific issue, data from two large-scale prospective cohorts of apparently healthy subjects, one including women aged 45 or older participating in the Women's Health Study (WHS), and the other including men aged 40 to 84 years participating in the Physicians' Health Study (PHS), were recently analyzed [13]. Data from the 27 840 women included in the WHS indicated an association between overall migraine and major ischemic cardiovascular disease after a mean of 10 years of follow-up. Such an increased risk for any ischemic vascular events was only apparent for women with MA, and turned out to be approximately two-fold higher compared to that observed in women who did not report any history of migraine after adjustment for traditional cardiovascular risk factors. In contrast, no increased risk for any ischemic vascular events was observed in women who reported MO [14].

With regard to men, data from the 20 084 male physicians included in the PHS indicated an association between overall migraine and major cardiovascular disease. Compared to non-migraineurs, men who reported migraine had an increased risk for major cardiovascular disease, ischemic stroke, myocardial infarction, coronary revascularization, angina, and ischemic cardiovascular death. As to stroke, men who were younger than 55 years of age had increased risk of stroke which was not apparent in the older age group [15], thus suggesting an age-dependent effect of migraine on disease risk.

At least theoretically, it cannot be excluded that the relation between migraine and stroke might be just one aspect of a more generalized effect of chronic non-specific headache. Actually, the evaluation of cross-sectional data from the first US National Health and Nutrition Examination Survey (NHANES I) showed a 1.5-fold increased risk of stroke in both patients with migraine and patients with severe non-specific headache compared to the subjects without these conditions [16]. More recently, in a prospective cohort study derived from the FINRISK study, Jousilahti et al. found a significant association between chronic non-specific headache and stroke among men [17]. However, because of the diagnostic criteria adopted in the NHANES I study, it is likely that most cases of severe non-specific headache were actually migraine sufferers. Similarly, the lack of a precise definition of migraine represents a major limitation for a correct interpretation of the data proposed by Jousilahti and co-workers. These drawbacks, in association with recent data from large, prospective cohorts, showing no association between non-migraine headache and stroke, make the hypothesis of a major effect of any non-specific headache on the risk of cerebral ischemia very unlikely.

Table 2. Differential diagnosis of multi-focal white matter lesions

Hypoxic/ischemic

- Acquired
  - Small vessel ischemic disease (hypertension, diabetes)
  - Embolic: cardiac, atheromatous
  - Unknown mechanism: Alzheimer disease, migraine
- Hereditary
  - Cerebral autosomal dominant arteriopathy with subcortical infarcts (CADASIL)
  - Mitochondrial encephalopathy with lactic acidosis and stroke (MELAS)
  - Fabry's disease
  - Cerebrotendineous xanthomatosis
  - Familial hyperlipidemia
  - Phenylketonuria
  - Adrenoleukodystrophy

Inflammatory

- Multiple sclerosis and variants
- Primary CNS vasculitis
- Secondary CNS vasculitis (lupus, antiphospholipid antibody syndrome, Sjogren syndrome, Bechet syndrome)
- Sarcoidosis
- Susac's syndrome

Infectious/post-infectious

- Viral: HIV, progrssive multifocal leucoencephalomyelopathy (PML)
- Spirochetal: Lyme disease, syphilis
- Acute demyelinating encephalmyelopathy (ADEM), subacute sclerosing postinfectious encephalitis (SSPE)
- Granulomatous (tubercolosis)
- Fungal (coccidiomycosis)

Toxic/metabolic

- Central pontine myelinolysis
- Carbon monoxide intoxication
- Radiation-induced
- Inhaled solvents, heroin
- Vitamin B12 deficiency

Neoplastic

- Primary central nervous system malignancy
- Metastatic disease
- Lymphoma

Other

- Prominent Virchow-Robin spaces

Classification of Migraine-related Stroke

One of the most relevant drawback in unrevealing the complex relation between migraine and cerebral ischemia is the lack of consistency in the definition of migraine-related stroke. In the attempt to categorize this entity, 4 major issues might be considered [18]. First, cerebral ischemia can occur in the course of an attack of MA, causing true migraine-induced infarction. Second, migraine and stroke share a common underlying disorder, that increases the risk of both diseases. Third, migraine might cause stroke only because other risk factors for stroke are present to interact with the migraine-induced pathogenesis. Fourth, stroke may mimic migraine.

Migraine-induced Stroke: The Migrainous Infarction

It has long been recognized that, although a rare event, stroke may occur during the course of a migraine attack with aura. This phenomenon suggests a causal relationship between migraine and stroke.

According to the International Headache Society (IHS) migraine classification, "migrainous infarction" is defined as a stroke occurring during a typical attack of MA [3]. Patients have a history of MA and the neurological deficits occur in the same vascular distribution as the aura and are associated with an ischemic brain lesion in a suitable territory demonstrated by neuroimaging. A major criterion of this cause of infarction is that other possible causes are excluded by appropriate investigations. However, which investigations should be done and when is not clear. The absence of causes other than migraine does not necessarily imply that migraine is the cause, given that about half of the ischemic strokes in young adults have no detectable cause.

Furthermore, stroke has been reported in persons experiencing MO, and in two large series this was more common than infarcts during attacks of MA [19,20]. Criteria for true migraine-induced stroke should include potentially modifying risk factors that might be present and that are critical to understanding the mechanisms. Finally, the definition of migrainous stroke, with the stipulation that the present MA attack is typical of previous attacks is also biased towards posterior cerebral artery (PCA) territory infarcts, since most aura are visual in nature.

According to large series, the incidence of migrainous infarction [16, 20-23] varies between 0.5 to 1.5% of all ischemic strokes and 10 to 14% of ischemic strokes in young patients. The incidence of migraine-related infarction (per 100000 persons per year) was estimated at 1.44 (95% CI, 0 to 3.07) from the Oxfordshire Community Stroke Project prospective registry, and at 1.7 from a retrospective review of Mayo Clinic records from nearly 5000 migraineurs aged <50 years [24, 25]. In series published since the introduction of the IHS criteria, the percentage of stroke in persons aged <45 years attributed to migrainous infarction ranges from 1.2% to 14% [21, 22, 26, 27]. The clinical features typifying migrainous stroke included female sex, mean age in the low-to-mid-30s, a history of cigarette smoking and ischemic involvement of the PCA territory [21].

In summary, IHS criteria might be too strict for a correct diagnosis of migrainous infarction. In spite of the limitations inherent in the diagnostic criteria and the consequent weakness of the epidemiologic studies, it seems reasonable to assume that migrainous infarction does not account for all strokes occurring during migraine attacks, and, overall, it is responsible for only a minority of migraine-related infarcts.

Symptomatic Migraine

Migraine and Stroke Share a Common Cause

Ischemic stroke and migraine are major clinical features of some specific syndromes: cerebral autosomal dominant arteriopathy with subcortical infarcts and leucoencephalopathy (CADASIL), mitochondrial myopathy, encephalopathy, lactic acidosis, and stroke-like episodes (MELAS), cerebroretinal vasculopathy (CRV) and hereditary endotheliopathy with retinopathy, nephropathy, and stroke (HERNS). The coexistence of ischemic stroke and migraine in the context of a syndrome characterized by peculiar phenotype, proven inherited background and chronic alterations of the wall of cerebral small vessel arteries suggests a common pathogenic mechanism shared by these two conditions.

CADASIL is an autosomal dominant disease of vascular and smooth muscle cells due to Notch-3 mutations [28], characterized by leucoencephalopathy, small deep infarcts, and subcortical dementia. MA is usually the first manifestation, presenting about 15 years before stroke and before the appearance of MRI signal abnormalities. MA is present in one third of symptomatic subjects and its frequency can vary greatly among the affected pedigrees. In 40% of families, more than 60% of symptomatic subjects had a history of MA [29, 30] and within some families, MA is the most important clinical aspect of the phenotype. The frequency of attacks of basilar migraine, or hemiplegic migraine, or migraine with prolonged aura, or isolated aura, according to the IHS diagnostic criteria, is noticeably high [30, 31]. The mechanism underlying MA in CADASIL is not clear. Presenting 10-20 years before ischemic manifestations, MA is not the consequence of subcortical infarcts. In CADASIL absence of difference in the frequency and distribution of white-matter abnormalities between patients with and without MA suggests that chronic subcortical hypoperfusion is also unlikely. Another hypothesis is that MA directly relates to dysfunction of smooth muscle cells of meningeal and cortical vessels, triggering cortical spreading depression (CSD) [32]. Furthermore, if the cells signalling abnormalities (resulting from the mutation) extend and reach neurons, the resulting hyperexcitable membrane instability could predispose to CSD.

Cerebroretinal vasculopathy (CRV) and hereditary endotheliopathy with retinopathy, nephropathy, and stroke (HERNS) are two rare inherited conditions characterized by a primary microangiopathy of the brain in combination with vascular retinopathy. A distinctive feature of CRV and HERNS is the presence of progressive subcortical contrast-enhancing lesions with surrounding oedema (psudotumours) typically located within the fronto-parietal white matter. Migraine is a clinical finding in some cases, also including progressive visual loss, seizures, focal neurologic deficits of sudden onset (stroke-like), cognitive worsening, renal insufficiency and proteinuria.

Mitochondrial myopathy, encephalopathy, lactic acidosis, and stroke-like episodes (MELAS) is associated to several mutations in mitochondrial DNA (mtDNA). The phenotypic expression is highly variable ranging from asymptomatic state to severe childhood multisystem disease with lactic acidosis. Recurrent episodes of headache (mostly migraine) are part of the clinical spectrum.

Migraine is also a clinical finding of other mitochondrial disorders such as Leber's hereditary optic neuropathy, myoclonic epilepsy with ragged-red fibers, and a syndrome characterized by neuropathy, ataxia, and retinitis pigmentosa [33, 34].

Migraine is also part of the clinical spectrum of hereditary haemorragic teleangiectasia (HHT; Osler-Weber-Rendu disease), an autosomal dominant vascular dysplasia characterized by a high prevalence of vascular malformations in various organs, including lung, liver, kidney, and brain, as well as by mucocutaneous teleangiectasias [35].

MA is classically related to cerebral arteriovenous malformations (AVMs). In most of these cases, MA ceasing after removal of AVM has been documented, consistent with the definition of symptomatic migraine, but there are also sparse reports of cases unchanged after surgery [36]. The possibility of a causal relation is indirectly supported by the side of aura, being contralateral to the AVMs and the side of headache, being ipsilateral to the AVMs, as well as by the coexistence of MA and arteriovenous shunts in leptomeningeal angiomatosis (Sturge-Weber syndrome) [37].

Migraine Mimic: Migraine as a Consequence of Ischemic Stroke

Stroke due to acute structural disease is accompanied by headache and neurological signs and symptoms indistinguishable from those of migraine. This entity might be termed a "migraine mimic". Spontaneous cervical artery dissection (sCAD) is a good example of a migraine mimic, expecially because patients with migraine are at increased risk of dissection. These symptomatic migraine attacks might be more common than migraine-induced ischemic insults [38]. Cerebral infarction can thus present with migraine attacks at onset, which should not be confused with migrainous infarction. The reported frequency of stroke-related headache ranges from 7% to 65% [39, 40]. A stronger association was observed among younger female individuals whose ischemic event was located in the vertebrobasilar territory, and with a personal history of migraine. Unfortunately, no precise data are available on the specific frequency of migraine cases caused by cerebral infarction.

Coexisting Ischemic Stroke and Migraine

Because of the high frequency of migraine in young adults, the possibility that this condition can coexist with ischemic stroke without contributing to stroke occurrence cannot be ruled out, in spite of the apparent increased risk of stroke in migraineurs. As the etiology of these strokes is probably multifactorial, identification and management of other established risk factors should be pursued with particular vigilance in all migraine sufferers.

Diffuse white Matter Lesions in Migraineurs

Abnormalities of uncertain clinical significance are frequent findings on brain MRI scans of patients with migraine. The most common abnormality is white matter lesions (WMLs), typically multiple, small, punctate hyperintensities occurring in the deep or periventricular white matter and often seen on T2-weighted or Fluid-Attenuated Inversion Recovery (FLAIR) images. Not infrequently, these WMLs may cause uncertainty for physicians and anxiety for patients and can lead to a variety of diagnostic tests and treatments [41]. In a small minority of cases, the number, distribution, and location of WMLs may lead to the diagnosis of an underlying disease of which migraine may be but one symptomatic manifestation.

The clinical history, presence or absence of cardiovascular risk factors, family history, physical examination, and specific neuroimaging features assist clinicians in narrowing the differential diagnosis in these cases, whereas, in selected circumstances, specific biochemical and genetic testing, and further neuroimaging are necessary.

WMLs are common in the general population, occurring in approximately 10% of individuals in the fourth decade of life and up to 80% of individuals in the eight decade [42]. Several reports suggest that the prevalence and the number of WMLs on brain MRI scan increase with advancing age, vascular risk factors (diabetes, smoking, hypercholesterolemia, hypertension), cardiovascular disease, stroke, and dementia [43, 44]. The prevalence of WMLs in migraine ranges from 6% to 40% [45, 46]. Suggested variables that might influence this association are the quality of MR imaging equipment and sequences used, patient age, migraine type and frequency, and the presence or absence of vascular risk factors.

Results of a recent meta-analysis showed a 4-fold increased prevalence of WMLs on MRI scan in patients with migraine in contrast to non-migraineurs age- and sex-matched controls (OR, 3.9; 95% CI, 2.26 to 6.72). The risk of WMLs in migraineurs appears to be independent on both age and vascular risk factors [47]. The recently published Cerebral Abnormalities in Migraine, an Epidemiological Risk Analysis (CAMERA) study supports the observation that some migraineurs are at increased risk for subclinical infarct-like brain lesions [48]. This cross-sectional prevalence study evaluated a population-based sample of Dutch adults aged 30 to 60 years. Randomly selected patients with MA (n = 161), MO (n = 134) and age- and sex-matched controls (n = 140) underwent brain MRI. Overall, there was no significant difference between patients with migraine and controls in prevalence of infarct-like lesions (8.1% versus 5.0%). However, patients with migraine had a higher prevalence of such lesions than controls in the cerebellum (5.4% versus 0.7%, $P = 0.02$; adjusted OR 7.1; 95% CI, 0.9 to 55.0). The adjusted OR was higher for individuals with MA and migraine attack frequency of one or more per month (OR 15.8; 95% CI, 1.8 to 140). The study found no association between severity of periventricular WMLs and migraine, irrespective of sex, migraine frequency, or migraine subtype. An increased risk for deep WMLs load was observed in women (OR 2.1; 95% CI, 1.0 to 4.1) and in subjects with attack frequency of ≥ 1 per month. Conversely, the prevalence of deep WMLs in male migraineurs did not differ from controls [48].

Overall, the study showed that patients with MA have a 12-fold increased risk of cerebellar infarct-like lesions, and that female migraineurs had more supratentorial deep

WMLs than non-migraineurs. The risk of lesions increased with attack frequency, independent on cardiovascular risk factors.

Further analyses of the infarct-like lesions observed in the CAMERA study were subsequently performed, in which topographic details of these parenchimal defects were systematically characterized to better define their pathophysiology [49, 50]. The combination of vascular distribution, deep border zone location, shape, size and imaging characteristics on MRI makes it likely that these lesions have an infarct origin. If these lesions are true vascular infarcts, it might be that a combination of (possibly migraine-related) hypoperfusion and embolism is the likeliest mechanism, and not atherosclerosis or small-vessel disease. However, as there are no post-mortem studies identifying the pathology of these MRI findings, their etiology is unknown. Interestingly, a case patient with migraine who developed what appeared to be cerebellar infarcts on MRI, but whose lesions vanished on repeat imaging, which questions an ischemic pathology, has been reported [51].

Is Migraine a Progressive Disorder?

The evidence of WMLs in migraineurs opens the issue of whether migraine may be a *progressive* disorder in some way, rather then simply an episodic disorder. The natural history of migraine is to decrease in severity and to abate and disappear in later life, suggesting a non-progressive course. However, in a population sample, Scher et al [52] showed that over the course of one year, 3% of individuals with episodic headache (headache frequency 2-104 days per year) progressed to chronic daily headache (attacks frequency >180 days per year). This population-based result is compatible with findings from a case-control study and numerous clinic-based observation studies [53].

Imaging results suggesting progressive brain changes in migraine are particularly interesting in light of these epidemiological results. However, these data should be interpreted cautiously because numerous factors, other than the presumed progressive course of the disease, may contribute to "chronification" of episodic migraine. Among them, one of the most common modifiable factors for transformation, occurring in approximately one third of patients developing chronic daily headache, is analgesic overuse. The evidence that chronic daily headache may spontaneously revert to episodic in some cases is a further argument against the hypothesis of migraine as a progressive disorder [53]. Finally, as the migraine-stroke relation seems to be subtype specific, the influence being prominent for MA and negligible for MO, one might speculate that migraine is a progressive disorder only in a specific sub-group of subjects. Therefore, whether migraine causes permanent, progressive brain lesions is not definitively established and there is no data over whether lesions in the brain produce chronic migraine. Only a longitudinal study would give information on accumulation of lesion load that would provide evidence for a progressive course.

How Can Migraine Lead to Ischemic Stroke?

So far, no fully convincing evidence has been produced to explain the exact mechanism of the increased risk of ischemic stroke in migraine. Numerous hypotheses have been raised including vasospasm, endothelial dysfunction, congenital thrombophilia, platelet hyperaggregability, association with cardiac abnormalities, among others.

A first hypothesis is that stroke can occur during the course of migraine attacks with aura (migraineus stroke). Migraine is considered to be a neurovascular disorder, in which arterial constriction and decreased blood flow to the posterior circulation are consequences of a spreading wave of neuronal depression in the cerebral cortex. In this regard, CSD may induce short-lived increases in cerebral blood flow (CBF) and tissue hyperoxia [54] followed by a more profound oligemia and consequent increased intraparenchymal vascular resistance [55]. Thus, low flow in major intracerebral vessels may be due to increased downstream resistance, not major intracranial arterial vasospasm. Essentially, a low CBF and neuronally mediated vasodilatation could cause sluggish flow in large intracerebral vessels during the aura of migraine. When combined with factors predisposing to coagulopathy, such as dehydration hyperviscosity, or intravascular thrombosis, migraine-induced cerebral infarction could occur, although rarely. Neurogenically mediated inflammatory responses accompanying vasodilation of extra-parenchymal vessels caused by release of vasoactive peptides, nitric oxide (NO), activation of cytokines, and up-regulation of adhesion molecules also predispose to intravascular thrombosis [56]. This could explain why migraine-induced stroke usually respects intracranial arterial territories while aura involves more widespread brain regions. In addition, frequent aura, if due to CSD, could induce cytotoxic cell damage and gliosis based on glutamate release or excess intracellular calcium accumulation [57]. Thus, a persistent neurological deficit could be due to selective neuronal necrosis. Finally, vasospasm, the result of the release of vasoconstrictive molecules, including endothelin and serotonin, once thought to be the mechanism of migraine aura, has been implicated in migrainous infarction, although documented cases are rare.

Experimental data also point towards activation of the thrombotic cascade during the course of a migraine attack. In fact, platelets and mast cells have been shown to release platelet-activating factor (PAF), a potent inducer of platelet activation and aggregation, also involved in the release of von Willebrand Factor (vWF), and indirectly in the activation of the platelet IIb/IIIa receptor, crucial for binding fibrinogen, thus leading to primary haemostasis [58]. Increased plasma levels of these molecules have been observed during the course of migraine attacks compared with those in the interictal phases.

However, these mechanisms hold only for the so-called migraineus strokes, which, as defined by IHS criteria, is a rare event. Therefore, its low incidence can not explain the increased risk of stroke in migraine. Further, ischemic strokes mostly occur between migraine attacks [59, 60].

A second hypothesis is that the migraine-ischemic stroke pathway is modulated by the intervention of common risk factors. In this regard, different case control studies have observed that patent foramen ovale (PFO) is significantly more common in patients who suffered MA than in patients without migraine [61, 62]. Similarly, in patients with ischemic stroke, MA is twice as prevalent in patients with PFO than in those without [63, 64]. Several observational studies, from both single and multi-centre experiences, suggest PFO closure to reduce the frequency of migraine attacks. In particular, among migraineurs this might be proposed for those patients in the MA subgroup and might indirectly reduce the risk of stroke, in spite of the small stroke predisposing effect of PFO and some recent findings indicating no stronger association between MA and ischemic stroke among women with PFO compared with women without [9]. However, these reports present some limitations including retrospective design which implicates recall bias, absence of control group, placebo effect that can result in a up to 70% reduction of attacks frequencies [65, 66], administration of aspirin after PFO closure and its potential prophylactic effect [67]. Paradoxical embolism is suggested to be the causal link between migraine and PFO, but insufficient data are available to substantiate the hypothesis that migraine frequency (and, indirectly, ischemic stroke risk) is reduced by PFO closure. The only way to address this issue is by randomization. At present, only one prospective, randomised, double-blind trial on the therapeutic effect of PFO device closure on MA patients compared to sham has been conducted (Migraine Intervention with STARFlex® Technology, MIST). In the MIST trial, 73 patients underwent a sham operation and 74 patients had their PFO closed. The primary endpoint of the study, complete elimination of headache, was not achieved, as 3 patients in the treatment group *vs* 3 patients in the sham group had complete resolution of migraine. In contrast, one of the pre-planned secondary endpoints of the MIST trial showed that patients who underwent PFO closure had a 37% reduction in median total migraine headache days compared with 26% in the sham group ($p = 0.027$), apparently suggesting some benefits of treatment [68]. However, correction for multiple comparison was not applied, making such findings unsubstantiated [69]. A more comprehensive analysis of current data is desirable to provide information about how to identify patients who may have an improvement of their migraine, and a large number of patients with longer follow-up seems necessary. A second MIST trial is expected soon [70]. Based on all these findings, the possibility of a PFO-migraine-ischemic stroke triangular association remains matter of speculation.

Though unproven, these observations prompt to speculation that migraine might be a predisposing condition for specific pathogenic subtypes of ischemic stroke, particularly in young patients. In the last years, some observations have suggested migraine as a predisposing conditions for sCAD, one of the most common causes of stroke in young patients. In two French case-control studies migraine resulted twice as common in patients with sCAD than in patients whose ischemic stroke was not related to a CAD [71, 72], and this association was stronger and more significant in patients with dissections involving multiple vessels. A large Italian case-control study confirmed these findings [73]. The mechanism by which migraine may affect the risk of sCAD is unknown. A common generalized vascular disorder is hypothesized to be a predisposing condition for both diseases. Recent observations of increased activity of serum elastase, a metallopeptidase which degrades specific elastin-type aminoacid sequences, in migraineurs suggest a possible extracellular matrix degradation [74] which might facilitate sCAD occurrence. Furthermore, in line with previous observations of altered common carotid artery distensibility in patients with sCAD [75], Lucas and co-workers recently reported that the endothelium-dependent vasodilatation assessed in the brachial artery is significantly impaired in these subjects [76]. Similar vascular changes have been observed in migraine patients during interictal periods

[77] and replicated in a recent cross-sectional study in migraineurs of recent onset, thus excluding possibility of bias due to longstanding history of migraine and repeated exposure to vasoconstrictor drugs [78]. Finally, the analysis of small families has shown that the structural abnormalities related to sCAD might be familial and follow an autosomal dominant pattern of inheritance [79, 80]. This implicates that genetically determined alterations of the extracellular matrix may play a crucial pathogenic role and that candidate genes involved in the regulation of the endothelial and the vessel wall functions, might increase susceptibility to both conditions [81-83].

A third hypothesis is that a number of predisposing conditions may be operant in increasing the risk of ischemic stroke in migraine, particularly in young women. Hormonal status seems to play a pathogenic role in the development of MO, but not of MA that, as a matter of fact, represents the situation where the incidence of ischemic stroke is higher [84]. Inconsistent results have been also found for the various biological or clinical markers of thrombotic risk studied so far [85, 86], such as platelet activation, factor V Leiden mutation [86], von Willebrand factor [87], prothrombin factor 1.2 [88], platelet leucocyte aggregation [89], antiphospholipid antibodies [90, 91], and livedo reticularis [92].

In contrast, there is mounting evidence that migraine may be a risk factor for endothelial dysfunction, which may represent a link to ischemic stroke and heart disease. Endothelial dysfunction is characterized by reduction in bioavailability of vasodilator (such as NO), increase in endothelial-derived contracting factors, and consequent impairment of the reactivity of the microvasculature. It also comprises endothelial activation, characterized by a procoagulant, proinflammatory and proliferative state, which, in turns, predisposes to ischemia. Endothelial dysfunction is mediated by increased oxidative stress, an important promotor of the inflammatory process [93],proposed in the pathogenesis of migraine. In fact, compared to migraine-free controls, oxidative stress markers have been found to be higher in migraineurs, even during the interictal period, thus yielding support to the association.

A fourth hypothesis is that the migraine-stroke link is caused by the effects of specific medications. Actually, drugs used in migraine, such as triptans and ergot alkaloids, have been investigated as a possible risk factor for ischemic events. Cardiovascular safety of migraine treatments has been brought forward by their vasoconstrictive action and by reported cases of stroke, myocardical infarction and ischemic heart disease after triptan and ergotamine use [94, 95]. Moreover, an increased number of white matter abnormalities [48] and mortality [96] have been found in patients taking ergotamine. In the last years large-scaled studies have investigated the risk of ischemic events and death in patients with triptan and ergotamine-treated migraine. Data from General Practice Research Database in the United Kingdom showed that in general practice triptan treatment did not increase the risk of ischemic events [97]. Similarly, this finding was confirmed by a wide retrospective cohort study from a health care provider in USA [96]. This study also investigated the rates of vascular events in relation to ergotamine use finding no association. Recently, a retrospective nested case-control study using data from the PHARMO Record Linkage System conducted in Netherlands investigated whether overuse of triptans and ergotamina is associated with an increased risk of ischemic events [98]. Results showed that overuse of triptan, neither in the general populations nor in those using cardiovascular drugs increases the risk of cerebral, cardiovascular or peripheral ischemic events. In contrast, ergotamine overuse increases significantly the risk of ischemic complications (OR 2.55; 95% CI, 1.22 - 5.36) especially in patients concomitantly using cardiovascular drugs (OR 8.52; 95% CI, 2.57 - 28.2). However, therapeutic doses of either triptans or ergotamines were not associated with an increased risk of ischemic vascular events. Overall, these findings suggest that triptan use and even triptan overuse are safe in general, although heighten the risk of ischemic complications due to ergotamine overuse, likely in relation to its greater vasoconstrictive properties.

Finally, migraine and cerebral ischemia might be linked *via* genetic pathways.

Genetic Influence on Migraine-stroke Relation

Over the last years, evidence from twin and family history studies, though not entirely consistent, have supported the notion that genetic predisposition plays a major role in the occurrence of both migraine and ischemic stroke [99].

Monogenic Forms of Migraine

Although many chromosomal regions have been reported to be possibly involved in migraine occurrence, the mutations in three genes for familial hemiplegic migraine (FHM) represent the only established monogenic cause of migraine so far. FHM is a subtype of MA characterized by an autosomal dominant pattern of inheritance and at least some degree of weakness (hemiparesis) during the aura. In spite of these clinical markers, a broad variability is the rule: age at onset, frequency, duration and features of attacks may be different from one patient to another, even among affected members from a given family who carry the same mutation in the same gene [100, 101], and less frequent features such as cerebellar ataxia, which occurs in some families, minor head trauma as triggering factor and severe attacks with impairment of consciousness have been also reported. Furthermore, the majority of FHM patients also experience attacks of typical MA and MO. Thus, it seems reasonable to assume that FHM represents one side of the spectrum that at the other end is formed by the common forms of migraine and, as a consequence, a valid model to study genetic factors of migraine in general as well as the relation between migraine and ischemic stroke.

To date, three different genes responsible for different subtypes of FHM have been identified. FHM1 is caused by mutations in the *CACNA1A* gene, located on chromosome 19p13, encoding the pore-forming α_{1A} subunit of $Ca_v2.1$ (P/Q type) voltage-gated neuronal calcium channels [102]. FHM2 is caused by mutations in the *ATP1A2* gene, located on chromosome 1q23 [103], encoding the α_2 subunit of sodium-potassium pump ATPases. FHM3 is caused by mutations in the *SCN1A* gene, located on chromosome 2q24 [104], encoding the $\alpha 1$ subunit of the neuronal voltage-gated sodium channel $Na_v1.1$ that is crucial in the generation and propagation of action potentials.

Overall, the common consequence of FHM1, FHM2, and FHM3 mutations seems to lead to increased levels of glutamate and potassium in the synaptic cleft causing an increased propensity to CSD. Whether this might also increase the propensity to cerebral ischemia is unknown.

Similarly, the contribution of FHM genes in common forms of migraine (MO and MA) remains unclear [105]. A recent study showed no linkage to the *CACNA1A* and *ATP1A2* genes in families with apparently autosomal dominant mode of inheritance of MA [106], while a case-control study investigating the role of the *ATP1A2* gene in MA did not find evidence for an association [107].

Polygenic Forms of Migraine

The recent diffusion of powerful new technologies of gene analysis along with the possibility to use informatics resources that provide genome-wide sequence and variant data, has fostered an effective and challenging approach to complex diseases. Among these, genetic association studies are retained as a powerful instrument to identify small relative risks. Based on the results of such analyses, several specific genetic variants have been implicated in migraine susceptibility, which can be gathered into 3 main streams [105]. The first group includes genes involved in neurotransmitter-related pathway, such as genes encoding for dopamine D2 receptor (DRD2), human serotonin transporter (HSERT), catechol-O-methyltransferase (COMT), and dopamine β-hydroxylase (DBH). The second group includes genes involved in vascular function, such as 5,10-methylene-tetrahydrofolate reductase (MTHFR), angiotensin I-converting enzyme (ACE) and endothelin type A (ETA) receptor. The third group includes genes involved in hormonal function, such as estrogen receptor 1 (ESR1), progesterone receptor (PGR) and androgen receptor (AR).

Several candidate genes for migraine are also good candidate for cerebral ischemia (Table 3). Among them, in spite of the inconsistent results of some studies exploring the hypothesis of a link between this marker and migraine [108], the C677T polymorphism of the MTHFR gene seems particularly promising, because of its probable independent effect on ischemic stroke risk [109].

In this regard, we recently reported the results of a genotype-migraine-stroke interaction study in which the TT-genotype of the C677T MTHFR polymorphism was found to be associated to both diseases and influence their relation [110]. Applying a mediation modelling strategy on a group of patients with sCAD, a group of young patients whose ischemic stroke was unrelated to a sCAD (non-CAD), and a group of control subjects, we found that both migraine and the TT-genotype were significantly associated to the group of patients with ischemic stroke as compared to controls, with a stronger stroke subtype specific effect for sCAD. These findings suggest that migraine may act as mediator in the MTHFR-ischemic stroke pathway with a more prominent effect in the subgroup of patients with sCAD, and prompt speculating that the C677T MTHFR polymorphism may be one of the hitherto unknown factors linking migraine to cerebral ischemia. These findings have been replicated in a separate analysis of the Women's Health Study data [111].

Although genes involved in the migraine-stroke relation remain to be fully elucidated, we believe this methodological approach may shed light into the pathophysiological pathways linking the two disorders, and eventually result in new and individualized therapeutic strategies.

Table 3. Association studies of candidate genes for migraine also analysed as candidate genes for ischemic stroke

Gene	Polymorphism	Authors, year	Methodology	Results	Comments	Migraine status			
						Any headache RR (95% CI)	MA+MO RR (95% CI)	MA RR (95% CI)	MO RR (95% CI)
MTHFR	C677T	Kowa et al, 2000 [124]	Case-control study: 74 M cases (22 MA, 52 MO), 47 TH cases, 261 controls	positive	No association with TH		2.4 (1.2 to 4.8)	6.5 (2.5 to 16.8)	1.2 (0.5-3.2)
		Kara et al, 2003 [][125]	Case-control study: 102 M cases (23 MA, 70 MO, 9 TH cases), 136 controls	positive	Joint effect with A1298C MTHFR	5.7 (1.2 to 27.4)		3.0 (0.2 to 35.0)	7.4 (1.5 to 36.8)
		Lea et al, 2004 [126]	Unrelated case-control analysis: 270 M cases (170 MA), 270 controls	positive	MA association was confirmed in an indipendent family-based analysis of 92 migraine pedigrees.		1.9 (1.1 to 3.0)	2.5 (1.4 to 4.7)	NS
		Oterino et al, 2004 [127]	Case-control study: 230 M cases (152 MO, 78 MA), 204 controls	negative	Significant difference comparing MA vs MO (OR:2.3 (95% CI 1.0 to 5.2); tendency for higher frequency of T allele in MA vs MO and CO		0.8 (0.4 to 1.5)	1.4 (0.6 to 2.9)	0.6 (0.3 to 1.2)
		Oterino et al, 2005 [128]	Case-control study: 329 M cases (138 MA, 191 MO), 237 controls	negative	Significant difference comparing MA vs MO (OR:3.2 (95% CI 1.6 to 6.6); significant interaction effect with TS and MTHFD1, no interaction with MS		NS	NS	NS
		Scher et al, 2006 [83]	Cohort study:1625 subjects (1212 non migraineurs, 226 MO cases, 187 MA cases)	positive				2.0 (1.2 to 3.4)	0.8 (0.4 to 1.4)
		Bottini et al, 2006 [129]	Case-control study: 45 M cases (33 MA, 12 MO), 66 controls	negative	Young patients <18 yrs		2.3 (0.8 to 6.73)	2.4 (0.7 to 7.6)	
		Todt et al, 2006 [130]	Case-control study: 656 MA cases, 625 controls	negative	Confirmed in an indipendent family-based association study in 155 MA trios.			0.8 (0.6 to 1.2)	
		Kaunisto et al, 2006 [132]	Case-control study: 898 MA cases, 900 controls	negative				0.9 (0.8 to 1.1)	
		de Tommaso et al, 2007 [131]	Case-control study: 105 M cases (90 MO, 15 MA), 97 controls	positive					
		Pezzini et al, 2007 [110]	Case-control study: 206 M cases (106 MO, 100 MA), 105 controls	positive	Significant difference comparing MA vs MO (OR:2.2 (95% CI 1.0 to 4.8))			2.5 (1.1 to 5.6)	1.1 (0.5 to 2.6)
	A1298C	Kara et al, 2003 [125]	Case control study: 102 M cases (23 MA, 70 MO, 9 TH cases), 136 controls	positive	Joint effect with C677T MTHFR	8.9 (1.9 to 40.8)		14.1(2.4 to 82.3)	7.44 (1.5-36.9)
		Bottini et al, 2006 [129]	Case-control study: 45 M cases (33 MA, 12 MO), 66 controls	negative	Young patients <18 yrs		4.9 (0.8 to 37.3)	5.6 (0.9 to 45)	NS
		Kaunisto et al, 2006 [132]	Case-control study: 898 MA cases, 900 controls	negative				0.9 (0.8 to 1.1)	
MS	D919G	Oterino et al, 2005 [128]	Case-control study: 329 M cases (138 MA, 191 MO), 237 controls	negative	No interaction with C677T MTHFR		NS	NS	NS
FVL	A1698T	Bottini et al, 2006 [129]	Case-control study: 45 M cases (33 MA, 12 MO), 66 controls	negative	Young patients <18 yrs		1.5 (0.2 to 10.9)	2.1 (0.3 to 15)	
PRT	G20210A	Bottini et al, 2006 [129]	Case-control study: 45 M cases (33 MA, 12 MO), 66 controls	negative	Young patients <18 yrs		2.4 (0.3 to 14.2)	1 (0.1 to 11.4)	
ACE	I/D	Paterna et al, 1997 [133]	Case-control study: 191 MO cases, 201 controls	positive	DD genotype				
		Paterna et al, 2000 [134]	Case-control study: 320 MO cases, 201 controls	positive	DD genotype				
		Kowa et al, 2005 [135]	Case-control study: 54 MA cases, 122 MO, 78 TH, 248 controls	positive	No association with TH			1.8 (1.2 to 2.7)	1.2 (0.9 to 1.6)
		Lea et al, 2005 [136]	Case-control study: 270 M cases (100 MO, 170 MA), 270 controls	positive	ID/DD genotypes. Interaction with TT677 MTHFR in M group and MA subgroup, none in MO group		1.6 (1 to 2.7)	NS	NS
		Kara et al, 2007 [137]	Case-control study: 180 M cases (109 MO, 59 MA, 2 CM, 10 BM), 210 controls	positive	D allele in M group. Higher frequency in M group of combined genotypes DD/5A5A and ID/5A5A				

Table 3. Association studies of candidate genes for migraine also analysed as candidate genes for ischemic stroke (Continued)

Gene	Polymorphism	Authors, year	Methodology	Results	Comments	Migraine status			
						Any headache RR (95% CI)	MA+MO RR (95% CI)	MA RR (95% CI)	MO RR (95% CI)
APOE	apoε2/ε3/ε4	Rainero et al, 2002 [138]	Case-control study: 241 M cases (135 MO, 18 MA, 88 MO+TH), 587 controls	positive	No allelic association. ε2/ε4 genotype associated with M and in subtype analysis with mix group (MO+TH)				
ESR1	G594A	Colson et al, 2004 [139]	Population-based case-control study with two indipendent groups: 274 M cases, 274 controls and 300 M cases, 300 controls	positive	Results confirmed in both groups. OR calculated combining the datasets		1.9 (1.4 to 2.7)	1.9 (1.4 to 2.8)	1.8 (1.1 to 2.9)
		Kaunisto et al, 2006 [132]	Case-control study: 898 MA cases, 900 controls	negative				1.1 (0.9 to 1.2)	
		Oterino et al, 2006 [140]	Case-control study: 367 M cases, 232 controls	negative	Interaction effect with C325G				
	C325G	Colson et al, 2006 [150]	Case-control study: 240 M cases, 240 controls	negative					
		Oterino et al, 2006 [140]	Case-control study: 367 M cases, 232 controls	positive	C352C genotype in women (OR 3.2 (95% CI 1.3 to 8.1); interaction effect with G594A				
	Pvu II C/T	Colson et al, 2006 [150]	Case-control study: 240 M cases, 240 controls	negative					
eNOS	Glu298Asp	Griffiths et al, 1997 [142]	Case-control study: 91 M cases, 85 controls	negative					
		Borroni et al, 2006 [141]	Case-control study: 156 M cases (103 MO, 53 MA), 125 controls	positive	Significant difference comparing MA vs MO (OR:3.0 (95%CI 1.2 to 7.5);		NS	2.2 (1.0 to 5.0)	1.1 (0.8 to 1.8)
MMP3	11715A/6A	Kara et al, 2007 [137]	Case-control study: 180 M cases (109 MO, 59 MA, 2 CM, 10 BM), 210 controls	positive	5A5A genotype in M group. Higher frequency in M group of combined genotypes DD/5A5A and ID/5A5A				
HFE	C282Y	Rainero et al, 2006 [143]	Case-control study: 256 M cases (225 MO, 31 MA), 237 controls	negative					
	H63D	Rainero et al, 2006 [143]	Case-control study: 256 M cases (225 MO, 31 MA), 237 controls	negative	D63D genotype associated with late onset and high frequency of migraine attacks				
TNF alfa	G308A	Trabace et al, 2002 [144]	Case-control study: 47 MO cases, 32 MA cases, 101 controls	negative					
		Rainero et al, 2004 [146]	Case-control study: 299 M cases (261 MO, 38 MA), 306 controls	positive	Significant difference comparing MA vs MO (OR: 2.4 (95%CI 1.0 to 5.9);		2.8 (1.9 to 4.3)	1.3 (0.6 to 3.1)	3.3 (2.1 to 5.2)
		Mazaheri et al, 2006 [145]	Case-control study: 221 MO cases, 183 controls	positive					3,5 (2.3 to 5.4)
TNF beta		Trabace et al, 2002 [144]	Case-control study: 47 MO cases, 32 MA cases, 101 controls	positive	TNFB*2 allele associated with MO				
LDLR	TA(n)	Curtain et al, 2004 [147]	Case-control study: 244 M cases (151 MA, 96 MO), 242 controls	negative					
		Mochi et al, 2003 [148]	Case-control study: 360 M cases (140 MA, 220 MO), 200 controls	positive	Association with MO cases.				
	G142A	Mochi et al, 2003 [148]	Case-control study: 360 M cases (140 MA, 220 MO), 200 controls	negative					
IL6	G174C	Rainero et al, 2003 [149]	Case-control study: 268 M cases (141 MO, 29 MA, 98 MO+TH), 305 controls	negative					

M = migraine; MO = migraine without aura; MA = migraine with aura; TH = tension-type headache; NS = not specified; MTHFR = 5,10-methylenetetrahydrofolate reductase; MS = methionine synthase; TS = thymidylate synthase; MTHFD1 = methylenetetrahydrofolate dehydrogenase; FVL = factor V Leiden; PRT = protrombin; ACE = angiotensin converting enzyme; APOE = apolipoprotein E; eNOS = endothelial nitric oxide synthase; LDLR = low-density lipoprotein receptor; TNF = tumor necrosis factor; IL6 = interleukin 6; ESR1 = estrogen receptor 1; MMP-3 = matrix metalloproteinase 3; HFE = haemochromatosis.

Practical implications

The identification of susceptibility factors linking migraine to ischemic stroke is still in its early stages and, thus, in the short term, it will be impossible to stratify migraine sufferers and identify those at highest risk of stroke occurrence. At present, available data support the following recommendations:

1) emphasis on identification and treatment of modifiable vascular risk factors, such as smoking, hypertension, diabetes, and hypercholesterolemia, is warranted in migraineurs, expecially those with MA.
2) Because of the potential synergistic effect of several migraine-specific drugs with vasoconstrictive action, including triptans, and traditional predisposing conditions in increasing the risk of ischemic stroke, subjects with major cardiovascular risk factors should be encouraged to adopt migraine prophylactic strategies. This approach should be also recommended to those subjects with a personal history of prior ischemic (cerebral and/or myocardial) disease. Drugs that can decrease the risk of stroke (i.e, anti-hypertensives) are valid pharmacological options in these cases, whereas NSAIDs or combination analgesics should be considered an alternative acute treatment approach. Triptans are also contraindicated in patients with hemiplegic and basilar migraine.
3) Estrogen-containing oral contraceptives should not be prescribed to women with MA, particularly when they have major vascular risk factors or are aged $\geq$ 35 years.
4) There is no direct evidence that PFO closure is effective for MA prophylaxis and, indirectly, for primary prevention of stroke and, as a consequence, this procedure cannot be recommended for MA prophylaxis. Positive results from small observational studies need to be confirmed in the setting of a randomized, unbiased, placebo-controlled study with adequate power. Whether anti-platelet agents might be an effective preventive measure in these subjects remains to be determined.
5) Patients with migrainous stroke should undergo the same diagnostic work-up and receive the same pharmacological treatment of any ischemic stroke in the young, both in the acute phase and at follow-up.
6) The possibility that migraine may be conceptualized not just as an episodic disorder but as a chronic-episodic and sometimes chronic-progressive disorder remains an attracting hypothesis, at present. When proven, this shift in conceptualization would implicate that the goals of treatment may also shift. Preventing disease progression in migraine has already been added to the traditional goals of relieving pain and restoring patients' ability to function [112, 113]. If the brain lesions of migraineurs have a significant clinical correlate, preventing the accumulation of brain lesions may become an additional goal of treatment. The association of stroke with frequency of migraine attacks suggests that migraine, especially MA, prophylaxis may actually reduce migraine-related stroke risk, and opens the issue of whether prophylactic drugs that decrease such a risk (i.e, antihypertensives) might be the best option in these cases. At present, data are too limited to recommend the use of antiplatelet drugs to reduce the risk of stroke in migraineurs. Emerging treatment

strategies to prevent disease progression, including risk factor modification, preventive therapies, and the early use of acute treatments, will be an important focus for future investigations [53, 112].

Conclusion

Strong arguments support the hypothesis that the relationship between stroke and migraine is more than coincidental. The link between MA and cerebral ischemia, indicated by epidemiological observations, appears to be stronger among young but may persist in the elderly. In contrast, the evidence is very weak for MO. Although recent findings suggest the hypothesis of migraine as a progressive brain disorder, data are still too scarce to draw any conclusion. Identifying the population with migraine at highest risk of stroke should be the first step toward risk reduction and the goal of future research. At present, from the available data, the overall absolute risk of stroke among young migraine patients seems to be fairly low.

References

[1] Lipton RB, Stewart WF, Diamond S, Diamond ML, Reed M. Prevalence and burden of migraine in the United States: data from the American Migraine Study II. *Headache* 2001;41:646-657

[2] Launer LJ, Terwindt GM, Ferrari MD. The prevalence and characteristics of migraine in a population-based cohort: the GEM study. *Neurology* 1999;53:537-542

[3] Headache Classification Committee of the International Headache Society. The international Classification of Headache Disorders, 2nd edition. *Cephalalgia* 2004;24:1-160

[4] Lipton RB, Silberstein SD. Why study the comorbidity of migraine? *Neurology* 1994;44(suppl 7):S4-5

[5] Collaborative Group of the Study of Stroke in Young Women. Oral contraceptives and stroke in young women. *JAMA* 1975;231:718-722

[6] Etminan M, Takkouche B, Isorna FC, Samii A. Risk of ischemic stroke in people with migraine: systematic review and meta-analysis of observational studies. *BMJ* 2005;330:63-65

[7] Kurth T, Slomke MA, Kase CS, Cook NR, Lee IM, Gaziano JM, Diener HC, Buring JE. Migraine, headache, and the risk of stroke in women. A prospective study. *Neurology* 2005;64:1020-1026

[8] Stang PE, Carson AP, Rose KM, Mo J, Ephross SA, Shahar E, Szklo M. Headache, cerebrovascular symptoms, and stroke. The Atherosclerosis Risk in Communities Study. *Neurology* 2005;64:1573-1577

[9] MacClellan LR, Giles W, Cole J, Wozniak M, Stern B, Mitchell BD, Kittner SJ. Probable migraine with visual aura and risk of ischemic stroke: the Stroke Prevention in Young Women Study. *Stroke* 2007;38:2438-2445

[10] Becker C, Brobert GP, Almqvist PM, Johansson S, Jick SS, Meier CR. Migraine and the risk of stroke, TIA, or death in the UK. *Headache* 2007;47:1374-1384

[11] Mosek A, Marom R, Korczyn AD, Bornstein N. A history of migraine is not a risk factor to develop an ischemic stroke in the elderly. *Headache* 2001;41:399-401

[12] Uyarel H, Erden I, Cam N. Acute migraine attack, angina-like chest pain with documented ST-segment elevation and slow coronary flow. *Acta Cardiol.* 2005;60:221-223

[13] Kurth T. Migraine and ischaemic vascular events. *Cephalalgia* 2007;27:967-975

[14] Kurth T, Gaziano JM, Cook NR, Logroscino G, Diener HC, Buring JE. Migraine and risk of cardiovascular disease in women. *JAMA* 2006;296:283-291

[15] Kurth T, Gaziano JM, Cook NR, Bubes V, Logroscino G, Diener HC, Buring JE. Migraine and risk of cardiovascular disease in men. *Arch Intern. Med.* 2007;167:795-801

[16] Merikangas KR, Fenton BT, Cheng SH, Stolar MJ, Rish N. Association between migraine and stroke in a large-scale epidemiological study of the United States. *Arch Neurol.* 1997;54:362-368

[17] Jousilahti P, Tuomilehto J, Rastenyte D, Vartiainen E. Headache and the risk of stroke: a prospective observational cohort study among 35,056 Finnish men and women. *Arch Intern. Med.* 2003;163:1058-1062

[18] Welch KMA. Stroke and migraine. The spectrum of cause and effect. *Funct Neurol.* 2003;183:121-126

[19] General discussion. Migraine and stroke: a review of the cerebral blood flow. *Cephalalgia* 1998;18:22-25

[20] Linetsky E, Leker RR, Ben-Hur T. Headache characteristics in patients after migrainous stroke. *Neurology* 2001;57:130-132

[21] Arboix A, Massons J, Garcia-Eroles L, Oliveres M, Balcells M, Targa C. Migrainous cerebral infarction in the Sagrat Cor Hospital of Barcelona stroke registry. *Cephalalgia* 2003;23:389-394

[22] Kittner SJ, Stern BJ, Wozniak M, Buchholz DW, Earley CJ, Feeser BR, Johnson CJ, Macko RF, McCarter RJ, Price TR, Sherwin R, Sloan MA, Wityk RJ. Cerebral infarction in young adults: the Baltimore-Washington Cooperative Young Stroke Study. *Neurology* 1998;50:890-894

[23] Sochurkova D, Moreau T, Lemesle M, Menassa M, Giroud M, Dumas R. Migraine history and migraine-induced stroke in the Dijon stroke registry. *Neuroepidemiology* 1999;18:85-91

[24] Henrich JB, Sandercock PAG, Warlow CP, Jones LN. Stroke and migraine in the Oxfordshire Community Stroke Project. *J. Neurol.* 1986;23:257-262

[25] Broderick JP, Swanson JW. Migraine-related stroke: clinical profile and prognosis in 20 patients. *Arch Neurol.* 1987; 44:868-871

[26] Sacquegna T, Andreoli A, Baldrati A, Lamieri C, Guttmann S, de Carolis P, Di Pasquale G, Pinelli G, Testa C, Lugaresi E. Ischemic stroke in young adults: the relevance of migrainous infarction. *Cephalalgia* 1989;9:255-258

[27] Kristensen B, Malm J, Carlberg B, Stegmayr B, Backman C, Fagerlund M, Olsson T. Epidemiology and etiology of ischemic stroke in young adults aged 18 to 44 years in Northern Sweden. *Stroke* 1997;28:1702-1709

[28] Joutel A, Corpechot C, Ducros A, Vahedi K, Chabriat H, Mouton P, Alamowitch S, Domenga V, Cecillion M, Marechal E, Maciazek J, Vayssiere C, Cruaud C, Cabanis EA, Ruchoux MM, Weissenbach J, Bach JF, Bousser MG, Tournier-Lasserve E. Notch 3 mutations in CADASIL, a hereditary adult-onset condition causing stroke and dementia. *Nature* 1996;383:707-710

[29] Chabriat H, Vahedi K, Iba-Zizen MT, Joutel A, Nibbio A, Nagy TG, Krebs MO, Julien J, Dubois B, Ducrocq X, et al. Clinical spectrum of CADASIL: a study of 7 families. *Lancet* 1995;346:934-939

[30] Verin M, Rolland Y, Landgraf F, Chabriat H, Bompias B, Michel A, Vahedi K, Martinet JP, Tourier-Lasserve E, Lemaitre MH. New phenotype of the cerebral autosomal dominant arteriopathy mapped to chromosome 19: migraine as the prominent clinical feature. *J. Neurol. Neurosurg. Psychiatry* 1995;59:579-585

[31] Chabriat H, Tournier-Lasserve E, Vahedi K, Leys D, Joutel A, Nibbio, Escaillas JP, Iba-Ziben MT, Bracard S, Tehindrazanarivelo A, et al. Autosomal dominant migraine with MRI white-matter abnormalities mapping to the CADASIL locus. *Neurology* 1995; 45:1086-1091

[32] Vahedi K, Chabriat H, Levy C, Joutel A, Tournier-Lasserve E, Bousser MG. Migraine with aura and brain magnetic resonance imaging in patients with CADASIL. *Arch Neurol.* 2004; 61:1237-1240

[33] Ferrari MD, Haan J. The genetics of headache. In: Silberstein SD, Lipton RB, Dalessio DJ, eds. *Wolff's headache and other head pain*, 7th ed. New York: Oxford University Press, 2001

[34] Haan J, Terwindt GM, Ferrari MD. Genetics of migraine. *Neurol Clin.* 1997;15:43-60

[35] Guttmacher AE, Marchuk DA, White RI. Hereditary hemorrhagic teleangiectasia. *N. Engl. J. Med.* 1995;333:918-924

[36] Has DC. Arteriovenous malformations and migraine: case reports and analysis of the relationship. *Headache* 1991;31:509-513

[37] Chabriat H, Pappata S, Traykov L, Kurtz A, Bousser MG. Angiomatose de Sturge-Weber responsible d'une hémiplégie sans infarctus cérébral en fin de grossesse. *Rev. Neurol.* 1996;152:536-541

[38] Olesen J, Friberg I, Olsen TS, Andersen AR, Lassen NA, Hansen PE, Karle A. Ischemia-induced (symptomatic) migraine attacks may be more frequent than migraine-induced ischemic insults. *Brain* 1993;116:187-202

[39] Grau AJ, Weimer C, Buggle F, Heinrich A, Goertler M, Neumaier S, Glahn J, Brandt T, Hacke W, Diener HC. Risk factors, outcome, and treatment in subtypes of ischemic stroke: the German stroke data bank. *Stroke* 2001;32:2559-2566

[40] Kolominsky-Rabas PL, Weber M, Gefeller O, Neundoerfer B, Heuschmann PU. Epidemiology of ischemic strroke subtypes according to TOAST criteria: incidence, recurrence, and long-term survival in ischemic stroke subtypes: a population-based study. *Stroke* 2001;32:2735-2740

[41] McDonald IG, Daly J, Jelinek VM, Panetta F, Gutman JM. Opening Pandora's box: the unpredictability of reassurance by a normal test result. *BMJ* 1996;313:329-332

[42] Fazekas F. Magnetic resonance signal abnormalities in asymptomatic individuals: their incidence and functional correlates. *Eur. Neurol* 1989;29:164-168

[43] de Groot JC, de Leeuw FE, Oudkerk M, van Gijn J, Hofman A, Jolles J, Breteler MM. Cerebral white matter lesions and cognitive function: the Rotterdam Scan Study. *Ann. Neurol.* 2000;47:145-151

[44] Vermeer SE, Prins ND, den Heijer T, Hofman A, Koudstaal PJ, Breteler MM, Rotterdam Scan Study. Silent brain infarcts and the risk of dementia and cognitive decline. *N. Engl. J. Med.* 2003;348:1215-1222

[45] Fazekas F, Koch M, Schmidt R, Offenbacher H, Payer F, Freidi W, Lechner H. The prevalence of cerebral damage varies with migraine type: a MRI study. *Headache* 1992;32:287-291

[46] Gozke E, Ore O, Dortcan N, Unal Z, Cetinkaya M. Cranial magnetic resonance imaging findings in patients with migraine. *Headache* 2004;44:166-169

[47] Swartz RH, Kern RZ. Migraine is associated with MRI white matter abnormalities: a meta-analysis. *Arch Neurol.* 2004;61:1366-1368

[48] Kruit MC, van Buchem MA, Hofman PAM, Bakkers JT, Terwindt GM, Ferrari MD, Launer LJ. Migraine as a risk factor for subclinical brain lesions. *JAMA* 2004;291:427-434

[49] Kruit MC, Launer LJ, Ferrari MD, van Buchem MA. Infarcts in the posterior circulation territory in migraine. The population-based MRI CAMERA study. *Brain* 2005; 128: 2068-2077

[50] Kruit MC, Launer LJ, Ferrari MD, van Buchem MA. Brain stem and cerebellar hyperintense lesions in migraine. *Stroke* 2006;37:1109-1112

[51] Rozen TD. Vanishing cerebellar infarcts in a migraine patient. *Cephalalgia* 2007;27:557-560

[52] Scher AI, Steward WF, Ricci JA, Lipton RB. Factors associated with the onset and remission of chronic daily headache in a population-based study. *Pain* 2003;106:81-89

[53] Scher AI, Lipton RB, Steward W. Risk factors for chronic daily headache. *Curr. Pain Headache Rep.* 2002;6:486-491

[54] Cao Y, Welch KM, Aurora S, Vikingstad EM. Functional MRI-BOLD of visually triggered headache in patients with migraine. *Arch Neurol.* 1999;56:548-554

[55] Cutrer FM, Sorensen AG, Weisskoff RM, Ostergaard L, Sanchez del Rio M, Lee EJ, Rosen BR, Moskowitz MA. Perfusion-weighted imaging defects during spontaneous migrainous aura. *Ann Neurol.* 1998;43:25-31

[56] Bolay H, Reuter U, Dunn AK, Huang Z, Boas DA, Moskowitz MA. Intrinsic brain activity triggers trigeminal meningeal afferents in migraine model. *Nat. Med.* 2002; 8: 136-142

[57] Welch KMA, Ramadan NM. Mitochondria, magnesium and migraine. *J. Neurol. Sci.* 1995; 134:9-14

[58] McCrary JK, Nolasco LH, Hellums JD, Kroll MH, Turner NA, Moake JL. Direct demonstration of radiolabeled von Willebrand factor binding to platelet glycoprotein Ib and IIb-IIIa in the presence of shear stress. *Ann. Biomed. Eng.* 1995;23:787-793

[59] Tzourio C, Iglesias S, Hubert JB, Visy JM, Alperovitch A, Tehindrazanarivelo A, Biousse V, Woimant F, Bousser F. Migraine and risk of ischemic stroke: a case-control study. *BMJ* 1993;307:289-292

[60] Tzourio C, Tehindrazanarivelo A, Iglesias S, Alperovitch A, Chedru F, d'Anglejan-Chatillon J, Bousser MG. Case-control study of migraine and risk of ischemic stroke in young women. *BMJ* 1995;310:380-383

[61] Anzola GP, Magoni M, Guindani M, Rozzini L, Dalla Volta G. Potential source of cerebral embolism in migraine with aura: A transcranial Doppler study. *Neurology* 1999; 52:1622-1625

[62] Del Sette M, Angeli S, Leandri M, Ferriero GL, Finocchi C, Gandolfo C. Migraine with aura and right-to-left shunt on transcranial Doppler: a case-control study. *Cerebrovasc. Dis*. 1998;8:327-330

[63] Lamy C, Giannesini C, Zuber M, Arquizan C, Meder JF, Trystram D, Coste J, Mas JL. Clinical and imaging findings in cryptogenic stroke patients with and without patent foramen ovale: the PFO-ASA study. *Stroke* 2002;33:706-711

[64] Sztajzel R, Genoud D, Roth S, Mermillod B, Floch-Rohr J. Patent foramen ovale, a possible cause of symptomatic migraine: a study of 74 patients with acute ischemic stroke. *Cerebrovasc. Dis* 2002;13:102-106

[65] Migraine-Nimodipine European Study Group M. European multicenter trial of nimodipine in the prophylaxis of common migraine (migraine without aura). *Headache* 1989; 29:633-638

[66] Migraine-Nimodipine European Study Group M. European multicenter trial of nimodipine in the prophylaxis of classic migraine (migraine with aura). *Headache* 1989; 29:639-642

[67] Diener HC, Hartung E, Chrubasik J, Evens S, Schoenen J, Eikermann A, Latta G, Hauke W, Study Group. A comparative study of acetylsalycilic acid and metoprolol for the prophylactic treatment of migraine. A randomized, controlled, double-blind, parallel group phase III study. *Cephalalgia* 2001;21:120-128

[68] Dowson A, Mullen MJ, Peatfield R, Muir K, Khan AA, Wells C, Lipscombe SL, Rees T, De Giovanni JV, Morrison WL, HIldick-Smith D, Elrington G, Hillis WS, Malik IS, Rickards A. Migraine Intervention with STARFlex Technology (MIST) Trial. A prospective, multicenter, double-blind, sham-controlled trial to evaluate the effectiveness of patent foramen ovale closure with STARFlex septal repair implant to resolve refractory migraine headache. *Circulation* 2008;117:1397-1404

[69] Tepper SJ, Sheftell FD, Bigal ME. The patent foramen ovale-migraine question. *Neurol. Sci*. 2007; 28:S118-S123

[70] Knopf D. Innovation in intervention summit. *JACC*. 2006;47:9-12

[71] D'Anglejan-Chatillon J, Ribeiro V, Mas JL, Youl BD, Bousser MG. Migraine: a risk factor for dissection of cervical arteries. *Headache* 1989;29:560-561

[72] Tzourio C, Benslamia L, Guillon B, Aidi S, Bertrand M, Berthet K, Bousser MG. Migraine and the risk of cervical artery dissection: a case-control study. *Neurology* 2002;59:435-437

[73] Pezzini A, Granella F, Grassi M, Bertolino C, Del Zotto E, Immovilli P, Bazzoli E, Padovani A, Zanferrari C. History of migraine and the risk of spontaneous cervical artery dissection. *Cephalalgia* 2005;25:575-580

[74] Tzourio C, El Amrani M, Robert L, Alperovitch A. Serum elastase activity is elevated in migraine. *Ann. Neurol.* 2000;47:648-651

[75] Guillon B, Tzourio C, Biousse V, Adrai V, Bousser MG, Touboul PJ. Arterial wall properties in carotid artery dissection. An ultrasound study. *Neurology* 2000;55:663-666

[76] Lucas C, Lecroart JL, Gautier C, Leclerc X, Dauzat M, Leys D, Deklunder G. Impairment of endothelial function in patients with spontaneous cervical artery dissection: evidence for a general arterial wall disease. *Cerebrovasc. Dis.* 2004;17:170-174

[77] de Hoon JN, Willigers JM, Troost J, Struijker-Boudier HA, Van Bortel LM. Cranial and peripheral interictal vascular changes in migraine patients. *Cephalalgia.* 2003;23:96-104

[78] Vanmolkot FH, Van Bortel LM, de Hoon JN. Altered arterial function in migraine of recent onset. *Neurology* 2007;68:1563-1570

[79] Grond-Ginsbach C, Klima B, Weber R, Striegel J, Fischer C, Hacke W, Brandt T, Hausser I. Exclusion mapping of the genetic predisposition for cervical artery dissection by linkage analysis. *Ann. Neurol.* 2002;52:359-364

[80] Hausser I, Muller U, Engelter S, Lyrer P, Pezzini A, Padovani A, Moormann B, Busse O, Weber R, Brandt T, Grond-Ginsbach C. Different types of connective tissue alterations associated with cervical artery dissection. *Acta Neuropathol.* 2004;107:509-514

[81] Kloss M, Wiest T, Hyrenbach S, Werner I, Arnold ML, Lichy C, Grond-Ginsbach C. MTHFR 677TT genotype increases the risk for cervical artery dissections. *J. Neurol. Neurosurg. Psychiatry* 2006;77:951-952

[82] Pezzini A, Del Zotto E, Archetti S, Negrini R, Bani P, Albertini A, Grassi M, Assanelli D, Gasparotti R, Vignolo LA, Magoni M, Padovani A. Plasma homocysteine concentration, C677T MTHFR genotype and 844ins68bp CBS genotype in young adults with spontaneous cervical artery dissection and atherothrombotic stroke. *Stroke* 2002;33:664-669

[83] Scher AI, Terwindt GM, Verschuren WMM, Kruit MC, Blom HJ, Kowa H, Frants RR, van den Maagdenberg AMJM, Van Buchem M, Ferrari MD, Launer LJ. Migraine and MTHFR C677T genotype in a population-based sample. *Ann. Neurol.* 2006;59:372-375

[84] Bousser MG. Estrogens, migraine and stroke. *Stroke* 2004;35:2652-2656

[85] Crassard, I, Conard J, Bousser MG. Migraine and haemostasis. *Cephalalgia* 2001;21:630-636

[86] Kern RZ. Migraine-stroke: a causal relationship, but which direction? *Can. J. Neurol. Sci.* 2004;31:451-459

[87] Soriani S, Borgna-Pignatti C, Trabetti E, Casartelli A, Montagna P, Pignatti PF. Frequency of factor V Leiden in juvenile migraine with aura. *Headache* 1998;38:779-781

[88] Hering-Hanit R, Friedman Z, Schlesinger I, Ellis M. Evidence for activation of the coagulation system in migraine with aura. *Cephalalgia* 2001;21:137-139

[89] Zeller JA, Frahm K, Baron R, Stingele R, Deuschl G. Platelet-leukocyte interaction and platelet activation in migraine: a link to ischemic stroke? *J. Neurol. Neurosurg. Psychiatry* 2004;75:984-987

[90] Cervera R, Piette JC, Font J, et al, Euro-Phospholipid Project Group. Antiphospholipid syndrome: clinical and immunologic manifestations and pattern of disease expression in a cohort of 1000 patients. *Arthritis Rheum.* 2002;46:1019-1027

[91] Tietjen GE, Day M, Norris L, Aurora S, Halvorsen A, Schultz LR, Levine SR. Role of anticardiolipin antibodies in young persons with migraine and transient focal neurologic events: a prospective study. *Neurology* 1998;50:1433-1440

[92] Tietjen GE, Al Qasmi MM, Shukairy MS. Livedo reticularis and migraine: a marker for stroke risk? *Headache* 2002;42:352-355

[93] Bonetti PO, Lerman LO, Lerman A. Endothelial dysfunction: a marker of atherosclerotic risk. *Arterioscl Thromb. Vasc. Biol.* 2003;23:168-175

[94] Tfelt-Hansen P, Saxena PR, Dahlőf C, Pascual J, Lainez M, Henry P, Diener H, Schoenen J, Ferrari MD, Goadsby PJ. Ergotamine in the acute treatment migraine. A review and European consensus. *Brain* 2000;123:9-18

[95] Mueller L, Gallagher RM, Ciervo CA. Vasospasm-induced myocardial infarction with sumatriptan. *Headache* 1996;97:162-164

[96] Velentgas P, Cole JA, Mo J, Sikers CR, Walker AM. Severe vascular events in migraine patients. *Headache* 2004;44:642-651

[97] Hall GC, Brown MM, Mo J, MacRae KD. Triptans in migraine: the risk of stroke, cardiovascular disease, and death in practice. *Neurology* 2004;62:563-568

[98] Wammes-van der Heijden EA, Rahimtoola H, Leufkens HGM, Tijssen CC, Egberts AC. Risk of ischemic complications related to the intensity of triptan and ergotamine use. *Neurology* 2006;67:1128-1134

[99] Ferrari MD. Heritability of migraine. Genetic findings. *Neurology* 2003;60:S15-S20

[100] Ducros A, Denier C, Joutel A, Cecillon M, Lescoat C, Vahedi K, Darcel F, Vicaut E, Bousser MG, Tournier-Lasserve E. The clinical spectrum of familial hemiplegic migraine associated with mutations in a neuronal calcium channel. *N. Engl. J. Med.* 2001;345: 17-24

[101] Terwindt GM, Ophoff RA, Haan J, Vergouwe MN, Van Eijk R, Frants RR, Ferrari MD. Variable clinical expression of mutations in the P/Q-type calcium channel gene in familial hemiplegic migraine. *Neurology* 1998;50:1105-1110

[102] Ophoff RA, Terwindt GM, Vergouwe MN, Van Eijk R, Oefner PJ, Hoffmann SM, Lamerdin JE, Mohrenweisser HW, Bulman DE, Ferrari M, Haan J, Lindhout D, Van Ommen, Hofker MH, Ferrari MD, Frants RR. Familial hemiplegic migraine and episodic ataxia type-2 are caused by mutations in the Ca^{2+} channel gene CACNL1A4. *Cell* 1996;87:543-552

[103]De Fusco M, Marconi R, Silvestrini L, Atorino L, Rampoldi L, Morgante L, Ballabio A, Aridon P, Casari G. Haploinsuficiency of ATP1A2 encoding Na^{+}/K^{+} pump alpha2 subunit associated with familial hemiplegic migraine type 2. *Nat. Genet.* 2003;33:192-196

[104]Dichgans M, Freilinger T, Eckstein G. Mutation in the neuronal voltage-gated sodium channel SCN1A in familial hemiplegic migraine. *Lancet* 2005;336:371-377

[105]Colson NJ, Fernandez F, Lea RA, Griffiths LR. The search for migraine genes: an overview of current knoweledge. *Cell Mol. Life Sci.* 2007;64:331-344

[106]Kirchmann M, Thomsen LL, Olesen J. The CACNA1A and ATP1A2 genes are not involved in dominantly inherited migraine with aura. *Am. J. Med. Genet. B Neuropsychiatr. Genet.* 2006; 141;250-256

[107]Netzer C, Todt U, Heinze A, Freudenberg J, Zumbroich V, Becker T, Goebel I, Olraun H, Kubish C. Haplotype-based systematic association studies of ATPA1A2 in migraine with aura. *Am. J. Med. Genet B Neuropsychiatr. Genet.* 2006;141;257-260

[108]Rubino E, Ferrero M, Rainero I, Binello E, Vaula G, Pinessi L. Association of the C677T polymorphism in the MTHFR gene with migraine: a meta-analysis. *Cephalalgia* 2007 (in press)

[109]Casas PJ, Bautista LE, Smeeth L, Sharma P, Hingorani AD. Homocysteine and stroke: evidence on a causal link from Mendelian randomization. *Lancet* 2005;365:224-232

[110]Pezzini A, Grassi M, Del Zotto E, Giossi A, Archetti S, Dalla Volta G, Monastero R, Iacoviello L, Camarda C, Gasparotti R, Camarda R, Padovani A. Migraine mediates the influence of the C677T MTHFR genotypes on ischemic stroke risk with a stroke-subtype effect. *Stroke* 2007;38:3145-3151

[111]Schürks M, Zee RYL, Buring JE, Kurth T. Interrelationship among the MTHFR 677 C>T polymorphism, migraine, and cardiovascular disease. *Neurology* 2008;71:505-513

[112]Loder E, Biondi D. Disease modification in migraine: a concept that has come of age? *Headache* 2003;43:135-143

[113]Silberstein SD. Practice parameter: evidence-based guidelines for migraine headache (an evidence-based review): report of the Quality Standard Subcommittee of the American Academy of Neurology. *Neurology* 2000;55:754-763

[114]Henrich JB, Horwitz RI. A controlled study of ischemic stroke risk in migraine patients. *J. Clin. Epidemiol.* 1989;42:773-780

[115]Marini C, Carolei A, Roberts RS, Prencipe M, Gandolfo C, Inzitari D, Landi G, De Zanche L, Sconditti U, Fieschi C. Focal cerebral ischemia in young adults: a collaborative case-control study. *Neuroepidemiology* 1993;12:70-81

[116]Lidegaard O. Oral contraceptives, pregnancy and the risk of cerebral thromboembolism: the influence of diabetes, hypertension, migraine and previous thrombotic disease. *Br. J. Obstet Gynaecol.* 1995;102:153-159

[117]Carolei A, Marini C, De Matteis G. History of migraine and the risk of cerebral ischemia in young adults. *Lancet* 1996;347:1503-1506

[118]Haapaniemi H, Hillbom M, Juvela S. Life-style associated risk factors for acute brain infarction among persons of working age. *Stroke* 1997;28:26-30

[119]Chang CL, Donaghy M, Poulter N. Migraine and stroke in young women: case-control study. *BMJ* 1999;318:13-18

[120]Donaghy M, Chang CL, Poulter N. Duration, frequency, recency, and type of migraine and the risk of ischemic stroke in women of childbearing age. *J. Neurol. Neurosurg. Psychiatry* 2002;73:747-750

[121]Schwaag S, Nabavi DG, Frese A, Husstedt IW, Evers S. The association between migraine and juvenile stroke: a case-control study. *Headache* 2003;43:90-95

[122]Nightingale AL, Farmer RD. Ischemic stroke in young women: a nested case-control study using the UK general practice research database. *Stroke* 2004;35:1574-1578

[123]Buring JE, Hebert P, Romero J, Kittross A, Cook N, Manson J, Peto R, Hennekens C. Migraine and subsequent risk of stroke in the Physicians' Health Study. *Arch Neurol.* 1995;52:129-134

[124]Kowa H, Yasui K, Takeshima T, Urakami K, Sakai F, Nakashima K. The homozygous C677T mutation in the methylenetetrahydrofolate reductase gene is a genetic risk factor for migraine. *Am. J. Med. Genet.* 2000;96:762-764

[125]Kara I, Sazci A, Ergul E, Kaya G, Kilic G. Association of the C677T and A1298C polymorphisms in the 5,10 methylenetetrahydrofolate reductase gene in patients with migraine risk. *Brain Res. Mol. Brain Res.* 2003;111:84-90

[126]Lea RA, Ovcaric M, Sundholm J, MacMillan J, Griffiths LR. The methylenetetrahydrofolate reductase gene variant C677T influences susceptibility to migraine with aura. *BMC Med.* 2004;2:3

[127]Oterino A, Valle N, Bravo Y, Munoz P, Sáncez-Velasco P, Ruiz-Alegia C, Castello J, Leyva-Cobián F, Vadillo A, Pascual J. MTHFR T677 homozygosis influences the presence of aura in migraineurs. *Cephalalgia* 2004;24:491-494

[128]Oterino A, Valle N, Pascual J, Bravo Y, Munoz P, Castillo J, Ruiz-Alegria C, Sanchez-Velasco P, Leyva-Cobian F, Cid C. Thymidilate synthase promoter tandem repeat and MTHFD1 R653Q polymorphisms modulate the risk for migraine conferred by the MTHFR T677 allele. *Mol. Brain Res.* 2005;139:163-168

[129]Bottini F, Celle ME, Calevo MG, Amato S, Minniti G, Montaldi L, Di Pasquale D, Cerone R, Veneselli E, Molinari AC. Metabolic and genetic risk factorsfor migraine in children. *Cephalalgia* 2006;26:731-737

[130]Todt U, Freudenberg J, Goebel I, Netzer C, Heinze A, Heinze-Kuhn K, Gobel H, Kubish C. MTHFR C677T polymorphism and migraine with aura. *Ann. Neurol.* 2006; 60:621-622

[131]De Tommaso M, Difruscolo O, Sardaro M, Losito L, Serpino C, Pietrapertosa A, Santeramo MT. Influence of MTHFR genotype on contingent negative variation and MRI abnormalities in migraine. *Headache* 2007;47:253-265

[132]Kaunisto MA, Kallela M, Hamalainen E, Kilpikari R, Havanka H, Harno H, Nissila M, Sako E, Ilmavirta M, Liukkonen J, Teirmaa H, Tornwall O, Jussila M, Terwilliger J, Farkkila M, Kaprio J, Palotie A, Wessman M. Testing of variants of the MTHFR and ESR1 genes in 1798 Finnish individuals fails to confirm the association with migraine with aura. *Cephalalgia* 2006;26:1462-1472

[133]Paterna S, Di Pasquale, D'Angelo A, Cottone C, Seidita G, Cardinale A, Parrinello G, Ferrari G, Licata G. Migraine without aura and ACE-gene deletion polymorphism: is there a correlation? *Cardiovasc. Drugs and Therapy* 1997;11:603-604

[134]Paterna S, Di Pasquale, D'Angelo A, Seidita G, Tuttolomondo A, Cardinale A, Maniscalchi T, Follone G, Giubilato A, Tarantello M, Licata G. Angiotensin-converting enzyme gene deletion polymorphism determines an increase in frequency of migraine attacks in patients suffering from migraine without aura. *Eur. Neurol.* 2000;43:133-136

[135]Kowa H, Fusayasu E, Ijiri T, Ishizaki K, Yasui K, Nakaso K, Kusumi M, Takeshima T, Nakashima K. Association of the insertion/deletion polymorphism of angiotensin-I converting enzyme of migraine with aura. *Neurosci. Lett.* 2005;374:129-131

[136]Lea RA, Ovcaric M, Sundholm J, Solyom L, MacMillan J, Griffiths LR. Genetic variants of angiotensin converting enzyme and methylenetetrahydrofolate reductase may act in combination to increase migraine susceptibility. *Mol. Brain Res.* 2005;136:112-117

[137]Kara I, Ozkok E, Aydin M, Orhan N, Cetinkaya Y, Gencer M, Kilic G, Tireli H. Combined effects of ACE and MMP-3 polymorphisms on migraine development. *Cephalalgia* 2007;27:235-243

[138]Rainero I, Grimaldi LM, Salani G, Valfrè W, Savi L, Rivoiro C, Gentile S, Pinessi L. Apolipoprotein E gene polymorphisms in patients with migraine. *Neurosci. Lett.* 2002; 317:111-113

[139]Colson NJ, Lea RA, Quinlan S, Macmillan J, Griffiths LR. The estrogen receptor 1 G594A polymorphism is associated with migraine susceptibility in two indipendent case/control group. *Neurogenetics* 2004;5:129-133

[140]Oterino A, Pascual J, Ruiz de Alegria C, Valle N, Castillo J, Bravo Y, Gonzales F, Sanchez-Velasco P, Cayon A, Leyva-Cobian F, Alonso-Arranz A, Munoz P. Association of migraine and ESR1 G325C polymorphism. *Neuroreport* 2006;17:61-64

[141]Borroni B, Rao R, Liberini P, Venturelli E, Cossandi M, Archetti S, Caimi L, Padovani A. Endothelial nitric oxide synthase (Glu298Asp) polymorphism is an independent risk factor for migraine with aura. *Headache* 2006;46:1575-1579

[142]Griffiths LR, Nyholt DR, Curtain RP, Goadsby PJ, Brimage PJ. Migraine association and linkage studies of an endothelial nitric oxide synthase (NOS3) gene polymorphism. *Neurology* 1997;49:614-617

[143]Rainero I, Rubino E, Rivoiro C, Valfrè W, Binello E, Zampella E, De Martino P, Gentile S, Fenoglio P, Savi L, Gallone S, Pinessi L. Haemochromatosis gene (HFE) polymorphisms and migraine: an association study. *Cephalalgia* 2006;27:9-13

[144]Trabace S, Brioli G, Lulli P, Morellino M, Giacovazzo M, Cicciarelli G, Martelletti P. Tumor necrosis factor gene polymorphism in migraine. *Headache* 2002;42:341-345

[145]Mazaheri S, Hajilooi M, Rafiei A. The G-308A promoter variant of the tumor necrosis factor-alpha gene is associated with migraine without aura. *J. Neurol.* 2006;253:1589-1593

[146]Rainero I, Grimaldi LME, Salani G, Valfrè W, Rivoiro C, Savi L, Pinessi L. Association between the tumour necrosis factor-alpha –308 G/A gene polymorphism and migraine. *Neurology* 2004;62:141-143

[147]Curtain R, Lea RA, Quinlan S, Bellis C, Tajouri L, Hughes, MacMillan J, Griffiths LR. Investigation of the low-density lipoprotein receptor gene and cholesterol as a risk factor for migraine. *J. Neurol. Sci.* 2004;227:95-100

[148]Mochi M, Cevoli S, Cortelli P, Pierangeli G, Scapoli C, Soriani S, Montagna P. Investigation of an LDLR gene polymorphism (19p13.2) in susceptibility to migraine without aura. *J. Neurol. Sci.* 2003;213:7-10

[149]Rainero I, Salani G, Valfrè W, Savi L, Rivoiro C, Ferrero M, Pinessi L, Grimaldi LME. Absence of linkage between the interleukin-6 (-174 G/C) polymorphism and migraine. *Neurosci. Lett.* 2003;343:155-158

[150]Colson NJ, Lea RA, Quinlan S, Griffiths LR. No role for estrogen receptor I gene intron I Pvu II and exon 4 C325G polymorphisms in migraine susceptibility. *BMC Medical Genetics* 2006;7:12

In: Cerebral Ischemia in Young Adults
Editors: A. Pezzini and A. Padovani

ISBN 978-1-60741-627-2

Chapter 4

Oral Contraceptives and the Risk of Stroke: Epidemiology, Pathophysiologic Mechanisms and Risk Reduction

Jeffrey M. Craig and Cheryl D. Bushnell*
Department of Neurology, Wake Forest University Health Sciences, Winston-Salem, NC

Abstract

Oral contraceptives (OCPs) were first introduced to the market in 1960. Today, more than 100 million women worldwide rely upon OCPs for contraception. The initial preparations contained high estrogen doses and were associated with an increase in incidence of venous thromboembolism, coronary artery disease, and stroke. Even with newer generation OCPs that contain lower-dose estrogen and different progestins, an increased risk of stroke exists--approximately a two to five times greater risk than nonusers. Because the overall incidence of stroke among young women is relatively small (6 to 21 cases per 100,000 women-years), the absolute risk with OCP use is small and may be lower than that due to pregnancy, an important consideration when prescribing. There are many potential mechanisms by which OCPs promote stroke. There is evidence that OCPs alter coagulation, fibrinolytic, and prothrombotic factors. They also alter the endothelium, increase blood pressure, and alter metabolism of lipids and carbohydrates. There is also some evidence that OCPs activate the immune system. The significance of these effects with regard to stroke risk is poorly understood. However, there is evidence that certain populations--those with hypertension, who smoke, are over age 35, are obese, have migraine headache (particularly with aura), or have thrombophilic disorders--may be at higher risk of stroke while taking OCPs. It is also important to remember that these drugs have numerous noncontraceptive health benefits,

* Correspondence: Cheryl D. Bushnell, Medical Center Boulevard, Winston-Salem, NC 27157, Phone: (336) 716-2357, Fax: (336) 716-9489, Email: cbushnel@wfubmc.edu.

such as a reduced risk of endometrial and ovarian cancer, endometriosis, ovarian cysts, and a lower risk of osteoporosis as a result of improved bone mineral density. Given the many potential health benefits of OCPs, the overall small incidence of stroke in users, and a similar or higher risk of stroke in pregnancy, physicians and patients must decide whether the small absolute stroke risk is acceptable when discussing treatment. If, after discussing the risks and benefits, OCPs are prescribed, then it is important to recognize and optimally manage stroke risk factors. This practice will further reduce the risk of stroke in young women.

Introduction

Oral contraception has been available in the United States since 1960 [1]. Australia and many European nations approved oral contraception a few years later [1]. The advent of the oral contraceptive pill (OCP) was - and continues to be - laden with controversy from social, religious, legal, and medical perspectives. Despite these controversies, use of OCPs increased markedly in the early years. In 1961, an estimated 408,000 women in the United States were taking OCPs, a number which grew to 3.8 million by 1965 [1]. By 1967, the worldwide estimate of OCP use was more than 12.5 million [1]. Today it is estimated that 100 million women worldwide use oral contraception [2]; and one in four women have relied upon OCPs at some point for contraception [3]. Eight percent of married women worldwide use OCPs, making it the third most commonly used family planning method among married women. When China and India, the two most heavily populated nations, are excluded, the worldwide use of OCPs among married women increases to twelve percent [3]. Aside from China and India, OCP use is the top contraceptive method among married women in both developed and developing nations. Use of OCPs is even higher among unmarried women worldwide.

The use of supra-physiologic levels of sex steroid hormones has raised concerns regarding the safety of OCPs, including the potential for problems with future pregnancies and the potential risk of cancer with long-term exogenous hormone use [1]. Furthermore, shortly after OCPs became available to the public, cases of venous thromboembolism, myocardial infarctions, and stroke were tied to the use of these drugs[1].

Over the next four decades, numerous studies were undertaken in an attempt to elucidate the true risk of stroke and cardiovascular disease with OCP use [4,5]. The results of these studies are controversial, with most studies showing an increased risk of cerebrovascular events associated with OCPs, while other studies demonstrate little or no increased risk. The controversy is further amplified by the dramatic evolution of oral contraceptives--in terms of components and doses--since they first became available.

The purpose of this chapter is to explore the epidemiology of cerebrovascular disease associated with OCP use, as well as to understand the pathophysiologic mechanisms by which OCPs contribute to stroke. We will additionally discuss the different types of hormonal contraception currently available and the evidence that exists regarding their association with stroke. Finally, we will consider comorbidities that increase the likelihood of stroke in young women taking OCPs and evaluate current screening recommendations.

Types of Oral Contraceptives

Because OCPs are so commonly used, it is important to understand the mechanisms of action and potential benefits and risks. The estrogen component of OCPs inhibits release of follicle stimulating hormone (FSH), thereby preventing development of the ovum [6]. The progestin component acts to increase the viscosity of cervical mucous, prevent ovulation, and reduce tubal mobility [7]. It also induces changes in the endometrium that may prevent implantation or survival of the fertilized egg [6].

The chief purpose of OCPs is to prevent undesired pregnancy; and there is very high efficacy of most preparations. With perfect compliance to the prescribed regimen, less than two percent of OCP users become pregnant per year [8]. Because ideal compliance does not always occur, the actual failure rate ranges from three to eight percent [6,9]. The potential benefits of OCPs extend beyond prevention of pregnancy. Users of combined OCPs are significantly less likely than never-users to develop ovarian or endometrial cancers [10]. OCP use also helps control menorrhagia, dysmenorrhea, Mittelschmerz, and premenstrual syndrome [11,12]. OCPs are associated with reduced incidence of benign breast diseases such as fibrocystic disease and fibroadenomatous disease, endometriosis, recurrent ovarian cysts, and uterine fibroids [12-14,69]. Prolonged use of OCPs containing estrogen may improve bone mineral density and prevent osteoporosis [15]. OCPs reduce the incidence and severity of acne [7]. Some have suggested that the overall health benefits of OCPs may prevent up to 50,000 hospitalizations per year [6].

OCPs have undergone changes in the estrogen and progestin doses and types over time to reduce severe side effects. The earliest (first-generation) preparations contained either ethinylestradiol or mestranol as the estrogen component and either norethisterone or norethynodrel as the progestin component, both in high doses. The first commercially available OCP, Anovlar®, consisted of 150 mcg of mestranol. The ethinylestradiol dose in first-generation OCPs was typically ≥50 mcg. Second-generation OCPs typically contain lower estrogen doses (30 to 40 mcg), and the progestin components include levonorgestrel, norgestrel, norgestimate (whose active metabolite is levonorgestrel), norethindrone acetate, or ethynodiol diacetate. The third-generation OCPs have further reduced estrogen doses (20 to 40 mcg) combined with desogestrel or gestodene as the progestin components. Virtually all combined OCPs today contain ethinylestradiol as the estrogen component.

The progestins vary in their degree of androgenicity. Progestin-induced metabolic abnormalities related to increased androgenicity have been associated with an increased risk of atherosclerosis and therefore may play a role in increased stroke risk. Also, androgenicity may play a role in altering carbohydrate metabolism. In descending order, the androgenicity of selected progestins is gestodene, levonorgestrel, norgestrel, desogestrel norethindrone acetate, ethynodiol diacetate, norgestimate, and norethynodrel [11,16].

One of the most common adverse effects that occurs with OCP use is venous thromboembolism. Three studies published in late 1995 cited a significantly increased risk of venous thromboembolism in patients taking third-generation OCPs compared to those of the second-generation [17-19]. Several subsequent studies supported these findings [20,21], yet others reported conflicting results. Farmer et al. noted no difference in incidence of venous thromboembolism before and after the 1995 "pill scare" that resulted in a dramatic decrease in prescribing of third-generation OCPs in the United Kingdom. They concluded that there was no evidence to suggest that third-generation OCPs confer greater risk of venous thromboembolism than earlier preparations. Furthermore, studies evaluating hemostatic effects of second- and third-generation OCPs have demonstrated no clinically significant differences [22,23].

Heinemann notes three biases associated with earlier studies that suggested an increased risk of venous thromboembolism associated with third-generation OCPs [24]. First, women prescribed third-generation OCPs were more likely to have cardiovascular risk factors, suggesting that women with known increased risk were switched from second- to third-generation OCPs in an attempt to reduce OCP-associated cardiovascular risks. This leads to the second bias, the "healthy user" effect. Switching at-risk patients from second- to third-generation OCPs would effectively lower the overall incidence of thromboembolism in second-generation users and increase it in third-generation users. Finally, he notes referral bias in that at-risk women (who may be more common in the third-generation OCP group compared to the second-generation group for the reasons stated above) are more likely to be evaluated for cardiovascular symptoms. The relative risk of venous thromboembolism with second- and third-generation OCPs continues to be debated.

Epidemiology – Studies

The incidence of stroke specifically among young women is estimated to be between 6 and 21 cases per 100,000 person-years [25-28]. Shortly after the introduction of OCPs, concerns were raised regarding the role they seemed to play in several cases of venous thromboembolism, myocardial infarction, and stroke in young women using these drugs. One of the earliest studies demonstrated a 10-fold increased incidence (47 per 100,000 versus 5 per 100,000) in venous thromboembolism in OCP users compared to nonusers [29]. In the same study, women diagnosed with cerebral thrombosis were significantly more likely to have used OCPs than those without cerebral thrombosis (controls). A follow-up study echoed these results [30]. A case series in the United Kingdom demonstrated that between 1954 and 1963, 25 women (2 to 3 per year) under age 45 presented with "cerebral artery insufficiency" [31]. Between 1963 and 1974, a total of 83 cases occurred; and 62 of them had been taking OCPs.

Since then, numerous studies have been undertaken to assess the risk of stroke in women using OCPs (see Table 1). Data from such studies and others have led to several adjustments in the estrogen dose in OCPs, as well as the pursuit of newer and safer progestin components. Despite the newer formulations, there is still controversy over whether these drugs pose a significant risk of stroke.

A study done in seven Italian cities between 1984 and 1988 found 160 women less than 45 years of age who had strokes or transient ischemic attacks (TIA) [32]. Eighty women were less than age 35 and eighty were age 35 or older. The use of OCP was 17.5% among those less than 35 years and only 7.5% among those over age 35. The study noted that below age 35, women (61% of cases) were more likely than men to suffer stroke or TIA.

Table 1. Oral contraceptives and stroke risk

Study	Study Type	Location	Cases (n)	Controls (n)	Ages	OCP type	OR (95% CI)
Hannaford et al.	Nested case-control	United Kingdom	253	759	21-70 (median 45.4)	All generations	Ever- vs. never-users: 1.5 (1.1-2.0) Current vs. never-users: 2.5 (1.5-4.0)
Heinemann et al.	Case-control	United Kingdom, Germany, France, Switzerland, Austria	220	775	16-44	All generations	Any OCP type: 2.34 (1.72-3.17) Generation: First: 2.89 (1.48-5.63) Second: 2.09 (1.44-3.05) Third: 1.21 (0.76-1.94)
Kemmeren et al.	Population-based case-control	9 centers in the Netherlands	203	925	18-49	All generations	Any OCP type: 2.3 (1.6-3.3) Generation: First: 1.7 (0.7-4.4) Second: 2.0 (1.2-3.5) Third: 2.0 (1.2-3.5) Estrogen dose: 50 mcg: 2.7 (1.0-7.6) 30 mcg: 2.4 (1.4-4.1)
Lidegaard et al.	Case-control	Denmark	626 (212 current OCP users)	4054 (1208 current OCP users)	15-44	All generations, Low- and high- dose estrogen or progestin-only	Generation: First: 4.5 (2.6-7.7) Second: 2.2 (1.6-3.0) Third: 1.4 (1.0-1.9) Estrogen dose: 50 mcg: 4.5 (2.6-7.7) 30-40 mcg: 1.6 (1.3-2.0) 20 mcg: 1.7 (1.0-3.1) Progestin-only: 1.0 (0.3-3.0)
Nightingale et al.	Nested case-control	United Kingdom	190	1129	15-49	Any	Current (vs. noncurrent): 2.3 (1.15-4.59)

Table 1. Oral contraceptives and stroke risk (Continued)

Study	Study Type	Location	Cases (n)	Controls (n)	Ages	OCP type	OR (95% CI)
Petitti et al.	Population-based case-control	California, USA	295	885	18-44	Low-estrogen	Current use (vs. no use): Ischemic: 0.65 (0.25-1.70) Hemorrhagic: 1.02 (0.37-2.82)
Schwartz et al.	Population-based case-control	King, Pierce, and Snohomish counties, Washington, USA	162	485	18-44		Current use (vs. no use): Ischemic: 0.89 (0.27-2.94) Hemorrhagic: 0.93 (0.37-2.31)
Siritho et al.	Case-control	Melbourne, Australia	234	234	15-55	Any	Ever-user: 1.00 (00.52-1.86) Current user: 1.62 (0.69-3.83)
WHO Collaborative Study	Hospital-based case-control	21 centers in Europe, Africa, Asia, and Latin America	697	1962	20-44	All generations, low- and high-dose estrogen	Europe: 2.99 (1.65-5.40) Non-Europe 2.93 (2.15-4.00)

In 1994, a group in the United Kingdom published a case-control study examining the association between OCP use and stroke [5]. This report was based upon data from the Royal College of General Practitioners' Oral Contraception Study and included all women in the study who had a first-ever stroke (253 cases) and 759 stroke-free controls. Their data demonstrated a 2.5-fold increased odds of stroke in current users compared to those who never used OCPs (OR 2.5; 95% CI, 1.5 to 4.0). They additionally demonstrated the role that the estrogen component of OCPs plays in stroke risk. OCPs containing greater than 50 micrograms were associated with a nearly 6-fold increased risk (OR 5.8; 95% CI, 1.5 to 22.8); and those containing 50 μg posed a 3-fold increased risk of stroke (OR 2.9; 95% CI, 1.7 to 5.0). No statistically significant risk increase was observed in preparations containing less than 50 μg of estrogen (OR 0.6; 95% CI, 0.1 to 2.9). They concluded that the risk of stroke was incrementally increased with the dose of estrogen in OCPs.

The growing concern over the risk of stroke associated with OCP use led to the initiation of the World Health Organization Collaborative Study of Cardiovascular Disease and Steroid Hormone Contraception [33]. This study, performed in 21 centers in Europe, Latin America, Asia, and Africa between 1989 and 1993, included 697 stroke cases (most women 20 to 44 years of age; ages 15 to 49 in 3 centers) and 1,962 controls. They found a 3-fold increased odds of ischemic stroke in Europe (OR 2.99; 95% CI, 1.65 to 5.40) and a similar risk in developing nations (OR 2.93; 95% CI, 2.15 to 4.00). In Europe, low-dose estrogen was not associated with a significantly increased risk of ischemic stroke (OR 1.53; 95% CI, 0.71 to 3.31) but, similar to the UK study, high-dose estrogen was associated with a 5-fold increased risk (OR 5.3; 95% CI, 2.56 to 11.0).

There was no significant difference in stroke risk between various estrogen doses in developing nations, but the risk was roughly two times higher than low-dose estrogen OCPs in Europe. This may have been due in part to less frequent screening practices before prescribing in developing nations. Another study also reported a dose-response between increasing estrogen doses and stroke risk [34]. The odds ratios of stroke with 50 micrograms, 30-40 micrograms, 20 micrograms, and progestin-only preparations were 4.5 (95% CI, 2.6 to 7.7), 1.6 (95% CI, 1.3 to 2.0), 1.7 (95% CI, 1.0 to 3.1), and 1.0 (95% CI, 0.3 to 3.0), respectively. In a multi-national European case-control study, Heinemann et al. examined the impact on stroke risk of the duration of OCP use, as well as of first, second, and third-generation progestin preparations. They found a nearly 4-fold increased risk of stroke among current OCP users versus nonusers (adjusted OR 3.6; 95% CI, 2.4 to 5.4) [35,36]. They also found no association with stroke risk based on duration of use and no difference between third- versus second-generation OCPs. However, first-generation OCPs (considered in the study to include all preparations with 50 μg of ethinylestradiol, regardless of progestin component) were reportedly associated with a higher risk of stroke than second- and third-generation OCPs (it should be noted that no direct comparisons between first- and second-generation or first- and third-generation OCPs were reported in the study). The risk of stroke related to second- *vs* third-generation OCPs has also been examined. The Transnational Study Group found no significant difference in the risk of stroke between second- and third-generation OCP users [36]. Further, they found that the presence of cardiovascular risk factors were the most important determinants of stroke risk, regardless of the type of OCP used. The WHO Collaborative Study found no difference between stroke risks among different generations of OCPs with similar estrogen doses in Europe; however, there was an increased stroke risk among second-generation OCP users in developing nations, whereas third-generation users had no difference in risk compared with nonusers [33]. Of note, they attributed the increased risk among second-generation users to increased cardiovascular risk factors compared to other groups. The RATIO Study reported no difference between second- and third-generation OCPs on stroke risk [37]. A Danish case-control study noted a 61 percent higher risk of stroke in second-generation OCP users than third-generation users [34]. At a minimum, third-generation OCPs appear to be as safe as--if not safer than--second-generation OCPs in terms of stroke risk.

The majority of studies have demonstrated a significant association between OCP use and stroke risk [37-43], but not all of them. The Melbourne Risk Factor Study Group found no association between use of low-dose combined OCPs and stroke in young women [44]. Furthermore, Kemmeren et al. found that although OCP use was associated with increased stroke risk, the estrogen dose did not affect this risk [37]. They also observed a lower risk with first-generation OCPs compared to second- and third-generation OCPs, in contrast to the findings of Heinemann et al. [35]. Of note, there are multiple limitations of the studies examining the risk of ischemic stroke with OCP use. Most of these studies [4,33,45] were case-control or case series by design, which are limited because of their retrospective case ascertainment and the subsequent bias. Cohort studies, which are commonly prospective, may be less biased [46-48]. Many have been limited by their small size. Also, some studies included formulations of OCPs that do not reflect current prescribing patterns. Some studies included transient ischemic attacks (TIAs) [26,32] while others excluded them [33]. The majority of studies selected ischemic strokes only and excluded hemorrhagic strokes. There has only been one prospective cohort study published, and this study demonstrated an increased risk of hemorrhagic--but not ischemic--stroke in Chinese women taking OCPs long-term [40].

In attempts to combine smaller cohorts to determine the summary OR of stroke with OCPs, a pooled analysis and three meta-analyses have been performed. The pooled analysis combined two studies from the United States, and found no statistically significant difference in stroke risk among low-dose OCP users and those who never used OCPs (OR 0.66; 95% CI, 0.29 to 1.47) [50]. Contrary to the pooled analysis, the first meta-analysis included 16 studies done between 1960 and 1999, and estimated a 2.75-fold increased risk of stroke with current OCP use (OR 2.75; 95% CI, 2.24 to 3.38) [51]. The risk was lower for lower-dose estrogen preparations, as well as for newer-generation progestins. The second meta-analysis, which included 20 studies from 1970 to 2000 found no increased risk of stroke when assessing cohort studies but an increased risk (OR 2.13, 95% CI, 1.59 to 2.86, $p < .001$) in case-control studies [4]. It is important to note that, of the cohort studies included in the meta-analysis, only two reported results by stroke type, with two grouping all stroke types together. Therefore, the risk was only significant for thrombotic, but not hemorrhagic, stroke based on the cohort study that specified stroke type. They concluded that there is no clear evidence for increased risk of stroke associated with OCP use. They cited methodological limitations such as the lack of documentation for how stroke was defined, diagnosed, and verified, and the lack of blinding of investigators as to OCP use. Furthermore, they noted differences in definitions of "current use" of OCPs, as well as the fact that some studies compared current users to former users while others compared them to never-users. The last meta-analysis of studies from 1980 to 2002 found a statistically significant increased stroke risk in current OCP users (OR 2.12; 95% CI, 1.56 to 2.86) [52]. Of note, they evaluated only studies of low-dose combined OCPs (second- and third-generation). They found that both second- and third-generation OCPs were associated with significantly increased stroke risk (OR 2.54, 95% CI 1.96 to 3.28; and 2.03, 95% CI 1.15 to 3.57, respectively). No randomized-controlled trials have been done to evaluate the risk of stroke associated with OCP use. We are left to rely upon case series, case-control studies, and a small number of cohort studies. The results of these studies are at times conflicting, though most support a small increased risk of stroke associated with OCP use. The meta-analyses that have been done have not clarified the confusion. The incidence of stroke in the young is relatively low, as is the proportion of young women taking OCPs. These factors make it difficult to perform large studies during a short follow-up period. Furthermore, the components of combined OCPs have changed over the past 40 years and may continue to change in the future, possibly reducing the clinical relevance of older data as prescribing patterns continue to evolve.

Available data from the developed and developing nations of the world demonstrate some difference in stroke risk associated with OCP use--whether by overall stroke risk or by type of stroke [37]. These differences may be attributable to screening and prescribing practices, education, genetic factors, or prevalence of comorbidities that vary by region. A few specific additional factors have been delineated from various studies that are felt to increase the risk of stroke among young women taking OCPs (discussed below). There are data demonstrating that screening for some of these comorbidities (for example, hypertension) decreases the risk of stroke in young women.

Epidemiology - Stroke Mechanisms

Oral contraceptives have been associated with strokes that occur by multiple mechanisms. These include thromboembolic, intracerebral hemorrhage, subarachnoid hemorrhage, cerebral venous thrombosis, and arterial dissection.

Thromboembolic Stroke

Thromboembolic stroke is the most common cause of stroke in young women, comprising 50 to 70 percent of cases [36]. Below the age of 35 women are more likely than men to suffer ischemic stroke. This is felt by many to be due to the use of OCPs and the increased prevalence of migraine headaches among women, though other factors likely also play a role [32]. The risk of thromboembolic stroke seems to be lower in patients taking combined OCPs containing lower-dose estrogen and newer-generation progestins than those taking earlier preparations. Furthermore, there is ample evidence that OCP users with other cardiovascular risk factors (hypertension, smoking, and thrombophilic disorders) or migraine headaches with aura have substantially increased risk of stroke.

Hemorrhagic Stroke

Hemorrhagic stroke includes both intracerebral hemorrhage (ICH) and subarachnoid hemorrhage (SAH). There are fewer studies directly evaluating the risk of ICH among OCP users compared to ischemic stroke and SAH. Most studies [50,53,54,87] demonstrate no statistically significant risk of ICH in OCP users compared to nonusers. The WHO Collaborative Study found an overall slightly increased risk of hemorrhagic stroke (both intracerebral and subarachnoid) with OCP use [45]. However, this risk was not statistically significant in Europe but was for developing countries. Women under age 35 were not at increased risk in either group. Over age 35, women in Europe were at increased risk of SAH, whereas women in developing nations were at increased risk of both ICH and SAH. They further noted an increased risk of hemorrhagic stroke in current OCP users with history of hypertension (above the risk with hypertension in non-users) that was statistically significant in both Europe and developing nations. Concomitant smoking and OCP use significantly increased hemorrhagic stroke risk in both Europe and developing nations. The noted increased risk in developing nations was echoed by Li et al. [40]. In their large prospective cohort study in China, they noted an incidence of hemorrhagic stroke higher than that for ischemic stroke (34.74 versus 11.25 cases per 100,000 person-years, respectively). The relative risk of hemorrhagic stroke in OCP users (past or present) versus intrauterine device (IUD) users was 2.72 (95% CI, not reported); and this risk increased to 4.20 (95% CI, 2.11 to 8.36) among current OCP users. They noted that many women with hypertension in this region of China were undiagnosed, and that when women who reported hypertension during follow-up visits were excluded, the risk was still double that of IUD users.

Numerous studies have specifically addressed the concern that OCPs increase the risk of SAH [45,55-57]. Some studies showed a statistically significant increased risk of SAH with OCP use, while others did not. A meta-analysis of 11 studies by Johnston et al. concluded that women taking OCPs have a significantly increased risk (RR, 1.42; 95% CI, 1.12 to 1.80; $p = .004$) of SAH [58]. When adjusted for smoking, this risk slightly increases. A small, but significant increase in mortality was also observed (RR, 1.54; 95% CI, 1.12 to 2.14). Estrogen dose was associated with a small, non-significant increase in risk of SAH. The authors conclude that the overall risk of SAH associated with OCP use is small, with only 5 new cases per 100,000 person-years directly attributable to OCP use.

Overall, there appears to be a small increased risk of hemorrhagic stroke--particularly SAH--with OCP use. This risk is increased in patients with hypertension or who smoke. Similar to ischemic stroke, the incidence of hemorrhagic stroke (excluding SAH) attributable to OCP use is small. Differences observed between developed nations and developing nations may be explained by a number of factors including differences in age, cardiovascular risk factors, screening practices (especially recognition of hypertension in young women), prescribing patterns, and possibly genetic variables. The influence of these factors require further characterization.

Table 2. Risk of cerebral venous thrombosis

Risk Factor	OR (95% confidence interval)
OCP*	5.59 (3.95-7.91
Hyperhomocysteinemia*	4.07 (2.54-6.52)
OCP + hyperhomocysteinemia†	19.5 (5.7-67.3)
Factor V Leiden mutation*	.38 (2.27-5.05)
OCP + factor V Leiden mutation†	30.0 (3.4-263.0)
Prothrombin mutation*	9.27 (5.85-14.67)
OCP + prothrombin mutation†	79.3 (10.0-629.4)

* Dentali et al. (2006); † Martinelli et al. (2003).

Cerebral Venous Thrombosis

Over the past 40 years, a number of studies have been undertaken to evaluate the risk of venous thromboembolic disease [19,20,29,30,59-62,]. Many of the older studies demonstrated relative risk estimates between 4 and 11 for OCP users versus non-users, but many of these studies were performed before reliable diagnostic testing was widely available [63]. Studies from the 1990's demonstrated a lower risk (ranging from 2- to 6-fold increased risk) [20,63]. Still, OCPs are felt to be responsible for most venous thromboses in young women [63].

Along with evidence for an increased risk of venous thromboembolic disease in general, many reports have suggested an increased risk of cerebral venous thrombosis (CVT) among users of OCPs [64-70]. Risk increases even more when patients have underlying thrombophilic disorders (see Table 2).

De Bruijn et al. reported an 18-fold increased risk among women age 18 to 49 [67]. Women with prothrombotic conditions had a 3-fold increased risk of CVT if also using OCPs. Martinelli et al. found that the presence of a prothrombin-gene mutation increased the risk of CVT 10-fold (OR 10.2; 95% CI, 2.3 to 31.0) [69]. Factor V Leiden mutation was also associated with increased risk of CVT (OR 7.8; 95% CI, 1.8 to 34.1). They also found that OCP use was more prevalent in women with cerebral venous thromboses than controls, regardless of the presence of prothrombotic conditions (OR 22.1; 95% CI, 5.9 to 84.2). The OR for combined presence of prothrombin-gene mutation and OCP use was 149.3 (95% CI, 31.0 to 711); and for combined factor V Leiden mutation and OCP use, 15.8 (95% CI, 4.3 to 57.2). A pooled analysis of 17 studies demonstrated an increased risk of cerebral sinus thrombosis in patients taking OCPs compared to controls (OR 5.59; 95% CI, 3.95 to 7.91; $p < .001$) [71]. They also noted a significantly increased risk in patients with factor V Leiden mutation, prothrombin gene mutation, and hyperhomocysteinemia (Table 2). Because few studies evaluated the risk of cerebral venous thrombosis in women using OCPs, they were unable to evaluate their interactions. Martinelli et al. found that OCP users with hyperhomocysteinemia, factor V Leiden mutation, or prothrombin-gene mutation had odds ratios of 19.5, 30.0, and 79.3, respectively [72]. Overall, the available data supports an increased risk of cerebral venous thrombosis in OCP users, which is amplified when a prothrombotic condition is also present.

Cervical Artery Dissection

A few studies have suggested a positive association between OCP use and cervical artery dissection. Rubinstein et al. performed a systematic review evaluating the risk factors for cervical artery dissection and was unable to identify any case-control studies that specifically evaluated the risk with OCP use [73]. However, one case-control study did find a significant, independent association between current OCP use and cervical artery dissection [74]. Another study evaluating the role of infection in cervical artery dissection reported that 40% of women with cervical artery dissection were taking OCPs [75]. This was not statistically significant when compared to controls ($p = .50$); but it should be noted that the control group in this study was comprised of patients who had also suffered ischemic strokes, and there is evidence that OCPs increase the risk of ischemic strokes as discussed above. A comparison to non-stroke patients may have yielded different results. The overall association between cervical artery dissection and OCP use remains unclear, but there is some evidence from small studies and case reports to suggest a slight risk. As with cerebral venous thrombosis, this risk may be increased by the presence of other comorbidities (for example, connective tissue disorders or smoking). Further studies are needed, although large-scale studies may be difficult given the relative rarity of strokes in OCP users, cervical artery dissection, and potentially comorbid risk factors.

Pathogenic Mechanisms of Stroke with Oral Contraceptives

Estrogens are neuroprotective in experimental animal studies of ischemic stroke [76-82]. Multiple mechanisms have been suggested, including enhanced neurogenesis [81], attenuation of oxidative damage due to free radicals [83], and maintenance of calcium homeostasis [84]. Progesterone has also been demonstrated to have post-ischemic neuroprotective properties [85-89], although at least one study demonstrated a worsening effect with progesterone [90]. The majority of the experimental studies were performed using physiologic or supraphysiologic doses of conjugated equine estrogens (CEEs) or 17-beta estradiol, the type of formulations prescribed to postmenopausal women for hormone replacement. There have been no experimental studies performed using synthetic formulations such as the types contained in OCPs; therefore it is unknown if these formulations are neuroprotective. In postmenopausal women, estrogen with or without progestins (CEEs or 17-beta estradiol) do not prevent stroke [91], and in fact may increase the risk, as shown in the Women's Health Initiative [92]. It is important to understand the mechanisms by which hormone therapy increases stroke risk, as these factors can influence screening and prescribing practices to reduce the risk of stroke in young women. There is evidence that OCPs promote stroke in a variety of ways, including mechanisms that disrupt hemostasis and promote platelet aggregation, endothelial damage, alterations in physiologic mechanisms that control hemodynamic and metabolic pathways, and immune mechanisms.

Overview of the Hemostatic System

In order to understand the mechanisms by which OCPs promote an increased risk of stroke, it is important to understand the basic pathophysiology of the hemostatic system and the role of the endothelium, platelets, and coagulation factors in that system. The endothelial lining of blood vessel walls serves, among other things, to prevent exposure of the subendothelial matrix to circulating platelets.

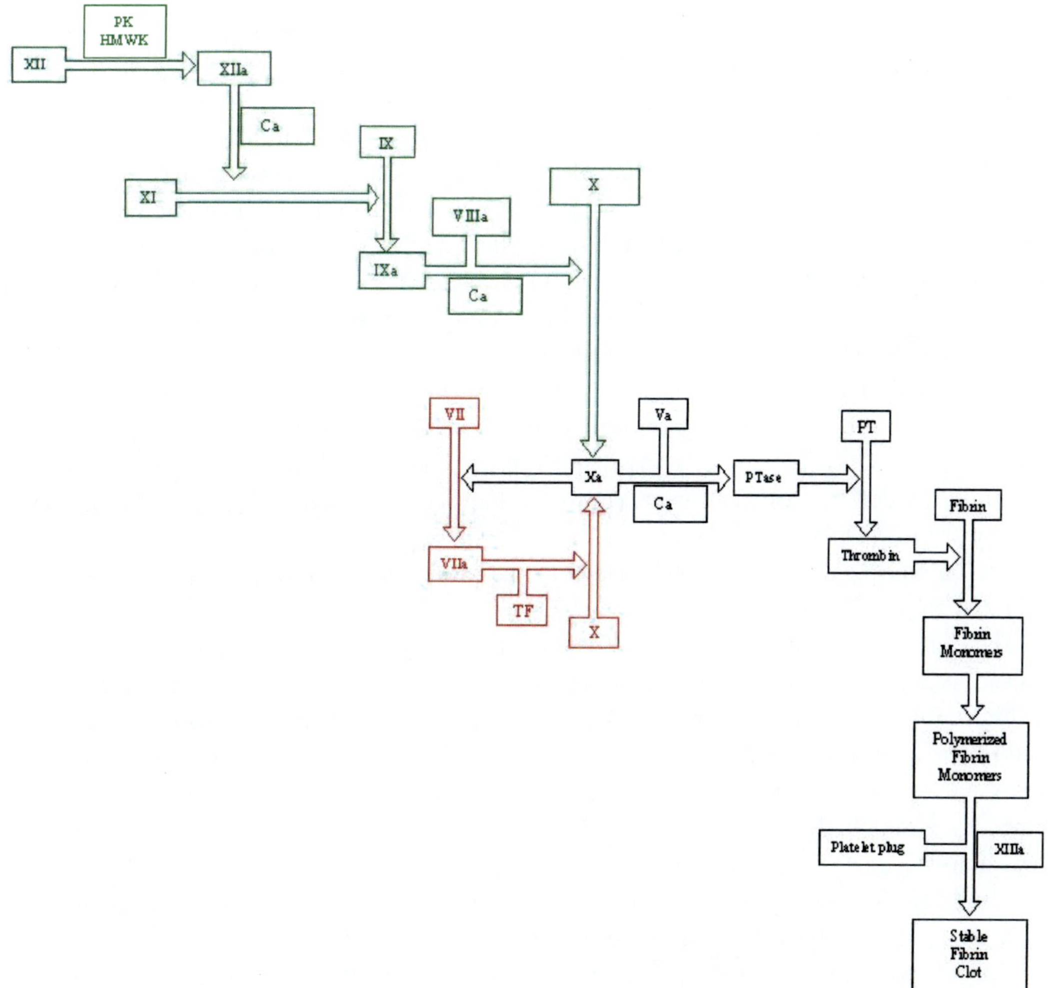

Figure 1. Overview of the coagulation cascade. The intrinsic (green) and extrinsic (red) pathways converge at factor Xa to progress through the common pathway (black), resulting in formation of a stable fibrin clot. Ca: calcium. HMWK: high molecular weight kininogen. PK: prekallekrein. PTase: prothrombinase. PT: prothrombin. TF: tissue factor.

Endothelial cells also secrete substances such as prostaglandins, prostacyclin, nitric oxide, and ADP-ases to inhibit platelet activation and thrombus formation [93]. Endothelial cells bind thrombin on their surfaces via thrombomodulin to inhibit coagulation by multiple mechanisms [94]. These mechanisms include preventing activation of factors V, VIII, and XIII, inactivation of protein S, preventing fibrin clot formation and platelet aggregation. The thrombin-thrombomodulin complex also promotes activation of protein C, which inactivates factors Va and VIIIa by cleaving them. The endothelium also synthesizes protein S, which serves as a cofactor of protein C but which can also act independently to inhibit coagulation [93]. Heparin sulfate proteoglycans are also secreted by endothelial cells and activate antithrombin to inactivate thrombin and other procoagulant factors [93]. Typically, the formation of a thrombus begins with disruption of the endothelial lining of the vascular system by one of several mechanisms, including shear forces, hypoxia, acidosis, traumatic injury, and inflammation, to name a few. When this occurs, platelets, which normally circulate in the serum as individual cells, are exposed to subendothelial proteins including collagens, von Willebrand factor, fibronectin, laminins and others. These subendothelial proteins promote platelet adhesion to the damaged vessel wall and aggregate to form a platelet plug. Once activated, platelets release the contents of internal granules (including some factor V and protein S) that further promote platelet activation and aggregation, as well as promote the coagulation cascade. Activated platelets also release thromboxane-A_2, which further promotes platelet activation. Thrombin is released from the endothelial surface after injury and plays a role in platelet activation. Along with these events, the anticoagulant properties of the endothelium are down-regulated.

Coagulation factors circulate in the serum as inactive proteins called zymogens. Once activated, these proteins possess protease activity and serve to activate the next step in the pathway. Several co-factors are involved in the coagulation cascade. The cascade is classically divided into two pathways (intrinsic and extrinsic) that converge and progress in the common pathway (see Figure 1).

The common pathway ultimately leads to the production of thrombin and subsequently fibrin, which stabilizes blood clots.

The intrinsic pathway is initiated when circulating factor XII (Hageman factor) is exposed to and binds the subendothelial matrix. Then, in the presence of prekallekrein (PK) and high molecular weight kininogen (HMWK), factor XII is cleaved to factor XIIa. Using calcium as a cofactor, factor XIIa cleaves factor XI to activated factor XIa, which then cleaves factor IX (Christmas factor) to IXa. Factor IXa then binds factor VIIIa (previously formed by thrombin activation of factor VIII) in the presence of calcium to form a complex which activates factor X to factor Xa.

The extrinsic pathway is initiated when endothelial damage exposes tissue factor (TF), which binds factor VIIa to form a tissue factor/VIIa complex that converts factor X to factor Xa. Via positive feedback, factor Xa promotes further conversion of factor VII to factor VIIa, which accelerates the coagulation cascade via the extrinsic pathway.

In the common pathway, factor Xa binds to factor Va (previously formed by thrombin activation of factor V on membrane surfaces) in the presence of calcium to form a complex known as prothrombinase. Prothrombinase converts prothrombin to thrombin. Thrombin then promotes formation of fibrin monomers from fibrinogen. These monomers then polymerize and become interwoven in the platelet plug to form a stable fibrin clot. This stabilization is promoted by factor XIIIa (previously formed by thrombin activation of factor XIII). The net effect of platelet activation and aggregation along with the coagulation cascade is the formation of a stable thrombus.

The fibrinolytic system acts to counterbalance the coagulation cascade. In this system, tissue-type plasminogen activator (tPA) or urokinase-type plasminogen activator (uPA) binds to fibrin. This complex increases activation of plasminogen to its active form, plasmin. This process is inhibited by plasminogen activator inhibitors (PAI's), α_1-antitrypsin, antithrombin III, α_2-macroglobulin, and other proteins [93]. When plasmin is present, it leads to breakdown of fibrin and dissolution of clots.

Disruption of Hemostasis

Alteration of multiple coagulation factors has been demonstrated in the presence of sex steroid hormones. Gordon et al. demonstrated an increase in factor XII in OCP users [95,96]. Increased factor XII production has also been demonstrated in estrogen-treated rats [97,98]. There is evidence for an increase in gene transcription for factor XII by estrogen [99]. Kluft and Lansink reviewed data from available studies in OCP users and noted significant changes in at least fifteen hemostatic variables [100]. These variables included Factors VII, X, XII, and XIII, as well as plasminogen, protein S activity, prothrombin, prokallikrein, and tPA, among others. Multiple other variables were affected to a lesser extent including total protein S, protein C, fibrinogen, antithrombin, von Willebrand factor, plasmin inhibitor, and factors VIIIc and IX. Most of these changes were due to the estrogen component of combined OCPs, with little effect from the progestin component [101,102]. There is, however, some evidence that third-generation OCPs may result in a greater increase of vitamin K-dependent factors such as factors VII and X and prothrombin [100].

Kluft and Lansink provide a thoughtful summary of the impact of OCP use on coagulation and fibrinolysis [100]. From the coagulation perspective, OCP use leads to decreases in protein S, antithrombin, and activated protein C ratio and increases in fibrinogen, prothrombin, and factors VII, XIII, IX, X, and XI. Factor V appears to be relatively unaffected. From the fibrinolytic perspective, plasminogen is increased, while tPA and uPA antigen are decreased. Factor XIII (which stabilizes the fibrin clot) is increased while plasminogen activator inhibitor activity is reduced.

Ultimately, while OCP use may impact factors that promote and inhibit both coagulation and fibrinolysis, there appears to be a net tendency in favor of coagulation and against fibrinolysis. There does appear to be a clearly increased risk with higher doses of estrogen. Studies have shown an increase in activated protein C resistance and a decrease in antithrombin III and protein S in patients taking combined OCPs with estrogen doses of 50 micrograms vs. lower dose formulations [100,102-104]. While these parameters remained altered in lower dose preparations, the changes were less significant.

The progestin component does not clearly correlate with prothrombotic risk. There has been much controversy regarding whether third-generation OCPs actually pose an increased risk of thromboembolism compared to second-generation OCPs. Multiple studies have been undertaken in an attempt to resolve the issue [105-107]. Factor VIIc is significantly increased in third-generation OCP users compared to second-generation users. In an analysis of 17 studies, fibrinogen was increased, while antithrombin III and factor V were decreased. However, these changes were not statistically significant. Activated protein C resistance does appear significantly increased (i.e. less sensitivity to activated protein C) in third-generation OCP users compared to second-generation users [108]. The Oral Contraceptive and Hemostasis Study Group demonstrated a significant increase in prothrombin fragment 1 + 2 (a by-product of thrombin activation) and factor VII, as well as increased activated protein C resistance in third-generation users compared to those using second-generation OCPs [103]. They also noted decreased protein S levels (both free and total) in the same group.

There is evidence that women with congenital coagulation abnormalities are at increased risk of thromboembolic disease when taking OCPs. Multiple studies have indicated an increased risk of thromboembolic disease in patients with factor V Leiden mutation who are taking OCPs [109-112]. Factor V is required for conversion of prothrombin to thrombin; and mutations in factor V increase resistance to cleavage by activated protein C. The risk of venous thromboembolism is 10 to 35 times higher for those with the mutation who use OCPs compared to those without the mutation and/or those who do not use OCPs [113]. Women with prothrombin G20210A mutations taking OCPs have significantly increased risk of thromboembolic disease compared to neither or either alone [114,110]. One study noted that women with the prothrombin gene mutation have a 150-fold increased risk of cerebral vein thrombosis compared to healthy controls [69]. Despite evidence of alteration in numerous hemostatic variables in women taking OCPs, the majority of women taking OCPs do not develop clinically significant thromboembolic disease. Increases in levels of hemostatic factors do not necessarily correlate with thrombus formation. It is not yet clear whether alterations in specific hemostatic factors in OCP users--or the magnitude of such alterations--directly cause thrombosis. There is some evidence that the prothrombotic effects of OCPs are at least partially counterbalanced by their pro-fibrinolytic effects [100]. It is likely that hemostatic alterations work in concert with other effects of OCPs, such as platelet aggregation or endothelial damage, and cumulatively increase the risk of thromboembolism. For most patients, it is not possible to predict whether thromboembolic disease will occur with OCP use.

Platelet Aggregation

The vascular endothelium secretes a number of molecules to inhibit platelet activation and aggregation. Among these are prostacyclins, nitric oxide, and ADP-ases [94]. Prostacyclin is produced by vascular endothelial and smooth muscle cells and acts to inhibit platelet activation and aggregation. Under adverse physiologic conditions, prostacyclin production normally increases [94]. Nitric oxide also plays a role in inhibiting platelet aggregation and acts synergistically with prostacyclin to reverse platelet aggregation [94]. Stimulation of prostacyclin and nitric oxide production can occur in the presence of thrombin and histamines, as well as shear stress and other mediators [94]. ADP-ases are produced by endothelial cells and work at the surface of endothelial cells. Activated platelets produce

ADP (adenosine diphosphate), which further activates other platelets and enhances platelet aggregation. ADP-ases help to limit platelet aggregation by processing ADP to AMP (adenosine monophosphate).

Von Willebrand Factor (vWF) plays an important role in platelet aggregation. Under conditions of shear stress, vWF binds to glycoprotein IIb/IIIa (GP IIb/IIIa) on the platelet surface to promote platelet activation and aggregation [94]. Activation of the GP IIb/IIIa receptor promotes a conformational change, allowing it to bind to soluble fibrinogen, promoting platelet aggregation and thrombus formation [115]. Deficient levels or the absence of vWF is associated with bleeding diatheses. Several studies in women and female animals have been undertaken to evaluate the effects of OCPs on platelet activity and aggregation. There is evidence for multiple mechanisms by which platelet aggregation may be enhanced in OCP users, resulting in a prothrombotic state. For example, OCP use was associated with increased platelet aggregation in response to ADP and thrombin administration [116,117], as well as increased production of 12-hydroxyeicosatetraenoic acid (12-HETE), which reduces prostacyclin synthesis [116,118]. In addition, there is an increase in arachidonic acid activity, which promotes thromboxane A_2 (TXA_2) synthesis, with concomitant increased platelet aggregation [116,119]. This mechanism is important because TXA_2 and its metabolite thromboxane B_2 (TXB_2) have been demonstrated to promote platelet hyperactivity in women taking OCPs [120,121]. Also, in vitro studies of platelets from OCP users treated with aspirin (a cyclooxygenase inhibitor) demonstrated reduced thromboxane activity [116]. This may provide evidence that women at risk of thromboembolism may benefit from concomitant aspirin therapy, although this approach has not been studied. Estrogens may increase free radical production, which is in turn associated with increased platelet activity [122]. Blache et al. have demonstrated that smoking increases lipid peroxides, resulting in platelet hyperactivity [123,124]. This phenomenon may help explain the increased risk of thromboembolic disease in smokers who use OCPs. Additionally, there is evidence that administration of vitamin E, which acts as a free radical scavenger, results in near-normalization of thromboxane production in OCP users [116,125]. There is also evidence that genetic factors play a role in platelet hyperactivity in OCP users. A polymorphism of GP IIIa, known as $P1^{A2}$, has been identified as a heritable risk factor for coronary thrombosis [126]. A study evaluating the effect of estrogen on platelet response to epinephrine, ADP, and aspirin in men and premenopausal women with the $P1^{A1/A1}$ and $P1^{A1/A2}$ polymorphisms demonstrated an enhanced inhibition of platelet aggregation in patients with the $P1^{A1/A2}$ polymorphism compared to those with the $P1^{A1/A1}$ polymorphism [127]. Other variants of platelet glycoprotein receptors have been associated with increased stroke risk in young women, but not all of these have been studied in relation to OCP use [128,129].

Alteration of Endothelial Function

Another mechanism by which OCPs may increase the risk of stroke is by altering endothelial function. Impaired endothelial function is an early sign of atherosclerotic disease and may precede formation of atherosclerotic plaques [130]. The endothelium plays an important role in vascular tone, largely by release of nitric oxide (NO) [131,132]. As noted above, it also plays a major role in coagulation and platelet aggregation. Endothelium-dependent vasodilatation has been studied in premenopausal and postmenopausal women and compared to that of men. A more robust vasodilatory response is seen in premenopausal women compared to other groups [133-135]. Premenopausal women have increased NO availability, as well as reduced oxidative stress, compared to the other groups. This differential response is felt to be due to differences in estrogen levels. It has been demonstrated that postmenopausal women exposed to estrogen have improved endothelial function [136-138]. Some have speculated that the progestin component of OCPs counteracts the apparent vasodilatory benefit of estrogen, while others reject this notion [139-141]. A study of 17-beta-estradiol plus norethisterone (used for hormone replacement therapy) found a decrease in nitric oxide levels in postmenopausal women [142]. Evidence from animal studies suggests that OCPs may promote hyperplasia of the endothelial and intimal layers of the vasculature. A study of the endothelium of ovariectomized rats exposed to ethinylestradiol demonstrated increased intimal thickening and increased vascular permeability [143]. Winegrove et al. demonstrated an increase in matrix metalloproteinases (MMPs) released by vascular smooth muscle cells exposed to 17-beta-estradiol [144]. MMPs break down intimal matrix components such as collagen and elastin [31]. This process may expose endothelial and subendothelial matrix components that activate the coagulation cascade and platelet aggregation.

Alteration in Blood Pressure

In the 1960's and 1970's, several cases of women with elevated blood pressures—many of which were markedly elevated—while using OCPs were published [145-147]. These reports prompted numerous studies during this period evaluating the risk of hypertension in OCP users [148-155]. In the Nurses' Health Study II, 68,297 women ages 25 to 42 taking OCPs were evaluated for risk of hypertension [156]. The study noted OCP users had an adjusted relative risk of 1.8 (95% CI, 1.5 to 2.3) for developing hypertension compared to never-users. The overall incidence of OCP-induced hypertension was 415 per 100,000 person-years. Similarly, the Royal College of General Practitioners Oral Contraceptive Study found OCP users to be 2 to 2.5 times more likely than nonusers to develop hypertension [152]. Onset of frank hypertension occurs in approximately 5 percent of women using high-dose ($\geq$ 50 mcg estrogen) OCPs [157-159]. Less severe blood pressure elevation has been demonstrated in women using lower-dose OCPs [160,161]. In one of the larger studies, systolic blood pressures rose by 5 to 6 mm Hg, while diastolic blood pressures rose by 1 to 2 mm Hg [151]. Most studies of progestin-only pills demonstrate no increase in blood pressure [149,161-163]. Fortunately, blood pressure often returns to normal when OCPs are discontinued [156,164]. Certain groups of women may be at greater risk of developing hypertension when taking OCPs. These groups include age greater than 35, history of hypertension during pregnancy, preexisting hypertension, family history of hypertension, and obesity [148,149,156,165,166]. Genetic factors may also play a role in development of hypertension in OCP users. Mulatero et al. demonstrated an increased prevalence of the 235T allele of the angiotensinogen gene (AGT) in patients with OCP-induced hypertension compared to normal controls and those with essential hypertension [165]. They also found a non-random distribution of angiotensin converting enzyme insertion/deletion (ACE I/D) polymorphisms in those with OCP-induced hypertension compared to other groups. The mechanism by which OCPs promote hypertension in a small percentage of users--and elevated blood pressures over baseline values in most users--remains unclear. Several studies have tried to understand the role of the renin-angiotensin-aldosterone pathway in this process. Increases in renin substrate [167,168], aldosterone excretion [8,167,169,170], and renin activity [8,167,170] have been reported in OCP users who develop hypertension. However, these changes are not significantly different from women taking OCPs who remain normotensive [31]. In the presence of increased renin substrate, most women taking OCPs are able to suppress additional renal release of renin [31]. It is possible that an inability to suppress renin release in some women may explain a susceptibility of some women to OCP-induced hypertension while others with similar changes in other renin-angiotension-aldosterone pathway factors remain normotensive [31]. Further studies on this issue are needed. There is additionally evidence of increased cardiac output and stroke volume in OCP users, which may contribute to systemic hypertension [31,171-174]. Hypertension is well-known to be a major risk factor for stroke and this may be one mechanism by which OCPs increase the risk of stroke. The dose-reduction of the estrogen component of OCPs over the years has likely reduced the incidence and degree of OCP-induced hypertension. However, a small percentage of women using the newest OCPs are at risk for hypertension. Therefore, periodic monitoring of blood pressure is recommended in all users. Gene-environment interactions may explain this effect in certain populations, but known risk factors should be carefully considered when prescribing OCPs.

Alteration in Lipid Metabolism

Another mechanism by which OCPs may influence stroke risk is by their effect on lipid metabolism. Godsland et al. note that when OCPs were first coming into widespread use, there was some evidence to suspect a beneficial effect of OCPs on cardiovascular disease [31,175]. First, premenopausal females had a lower incidence of myocardial infarction compared to males of the same age; and their plasma lipoprotein levels were generally lower than males. Additionally, postmenopausal women were noted to have lipid profiles similar to males and to have an increased risk of myocardial infarction. In 1966, a small study of women taking 50 mcg of ethinyl estradiol and 4 mg norethindrone noted significant increases in triglycerides, total cholesterol, and low-density lipoprotein, with significant decreases in high-density lipoprotein (HDL) [176]. Another group studied lipid profiles in women taking 100 mcg mestranol and 0.5 to 2.0 mg ethynodial diacetate and demonstrated significant increases in triglycerides, very low-density lipoprotein (VLDL), intermediate-density lipoprotein (IDL), and LDL [177,178]. The USA Lipid Research Clinics studied 424 OCP users and 1575 controls to evaluate lipid and lipoprotein level differences [179,180]. They found increased total cholesterol and triglyceride levels, as well as VLDL levels, among OCP users compared to controls. LDL was only elevated in patients under age 35 compared to controls. They additionally found that increases in total cholesterol, triglycerides, and VLDL were positively related to estrogen dose [179-181]. Bradley et al. evaluated the effect of estrogens, progestins, or combined OCPs on HDL [182]. They noted a roughly 6 to 15 mg/dL increase in HDL in estrogen users compared to nonusers and a roughly 16 mg/dL decrease in HDL for progestin users compared to nonusers. For combined preparations, the effect on HDL was dependent upon type and dose of steroid components. There is a general increase in HDL with increasing estrogen dose and variable effects with different progestins. Progestin-only OCPs have almost no effect on plasma lipoprotein levels [31].

Overall, estrogens appear to increase triglycerides and HDL while lowering LDL. The progestin component of OCPs typically has the opposite effect--particularly the more androgenic progestins [183]. OCPs with more androgenic progestins such as levonorgestrel and norgestrel typically have less favorable atherogenic profiles than those containing less androgenic progestins such as desogestrel, norgestimate, or gestodene [183,184]. Lower doses of progestins are associated with more favorable atherogenic profiles than higher doses. For example, lower-dose triphasic levonorgestrel preparations have only a small effect on LDL and HDL, whereas older levonorgestrel-containing OCPs are associated with significantly increased LDL and significantly reduced HDL levels [175]. There is evidence that even when LDL levels remain fairly stable, a shift in the overall LDL pattern to a pattern with more dense subfractions in OCP users may be associated with increased risk of cardiovascular disease [185,186]. Understanding the effects of OCPs on lipids in young women is important because elevated LDL and triglycerides, as well as decreased HDL, are clearly associated with increased risk of cardiovascular and cerebrovascular disease [187-191]. The overall effect of OCPs on lipid metabolism is mediated by a balance between the estrogen and progestin components. Combinations with lower estrogen doses and lower-dose, less androgenic progestin components have the most favorable profile regarding cardiac risk.

Altered Carbohydrate Metabolism

Diabetes is a well-known risk factor for stroke and cardiovascular disease. There is now evidence that the "metabolic syndrome," characterized by increased insulin resistance or impaired glucose tolerance among other features, is associated with increased stroke and cardiovascular risk [192,193]. Several studies have demonstrated impaired glucose tolerance or insulin resistance in users of virtually all types of OCPs [194]. Wynn and Doar demonstrated the presence of diabetic glucose levels in OCP users in 1966 [195]. Glucose levels have generally been lower after the reduction of estrogen dose [31]. There is some suggestion that estrogens increase corticosteroid activity, which would subsequently increase glucose levels [196]. Of interest, Godsland and Wynn noted more impaired glucose tolerance in OCP users compared to moderately overweight nonusers [31]. Hyperinsulinemia has been linked as an independent risk factor to coronary artery disease [31]. The mechanism by which this increased risk occurs is not completely clear. There is some evidence that insulin increases levels of plasminogen activator inhibitor-1, a protein that opposes fibrinolysis [192,197]. Although only a few small studies have investigated the impact of OCP use on insulin resistance, there is some evidence that insulin-resistance was increased in OCP users compared to controls. In addition, this increased resistance appeared to be primarily dependent upon the estrogen dose [31]. Though there is evidence of altered carbohydrate metabolism by various means in OCP users, the contribution of the alterations to stroke risk are uncertain. The Cochrane Collaboration study group concluded that the effect of altered carbohydrate metabolism from OCP use in nondiabetic women is small. It is likely, however, that women with diabetes and those at risk for diabetes (for example, obese women) who use OCPs may have a more substantial stroke risk related to altered carbohydrate metabolism than women without these risk factors.

Hyperhomocysteinemia

Homocysteine is an intermediate in the metabolism of methionine by demethylation. Subsequently, homocysteine may be metabolized by trans-sulfuration to cystathione (a process dependent upon vitamin B6) or remethylated to form methionine (dependent upon vitamin B12). In the latter process, 5-methyltetrahydrofolate is converted to tetrahydrofolate. Tetrahydrofolate can then be converted back to 5-methyltetrahydrofolate through a series of steps, one of which requires the 5,10-methyltetrahydrofolate reductase (MTHFR) enzyme (see Figure 2).

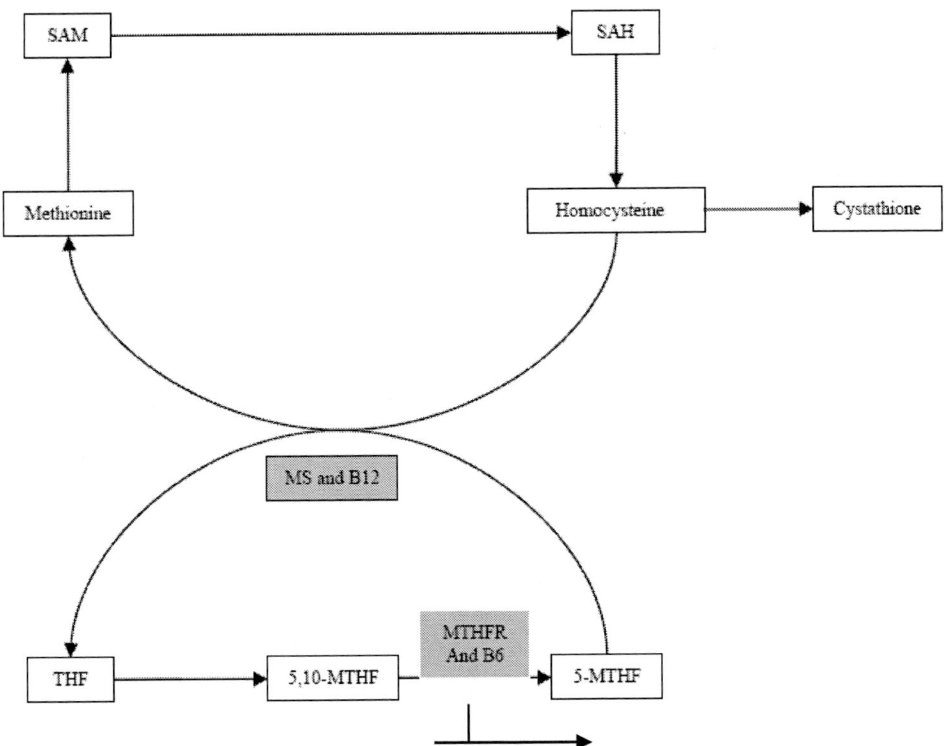

Figure 2. Homocysteine metabolism. A schematic of the conversion of homocysteine to methionine in a process involving the simultaneous converstion of 5-methyltetrahydrofolate (5-MTHF) to tetra-hydrofolate (THF). This process is mediated by the methionine synthase (MS) enzyme and vitamin B12. Mutation of the methyltetrahydrofolate reductase (MTHFR) enzyme blocks this process and leads to excess homocysteine. (SAM: S-adenosyl-methionine. SAH: S-adenosyl-homocysteine).

There is evidence that elevated homocysteine levels are associated with increased risk of stroke [198]. Mutation of the MTHFR gene has been associated with elevated homocysteine levels and with increased risk of thrombosis [49,199-201]. The role of hyperhomo cysteinemia as a stroke risk factor in OCP users is unclear. In fact, most studies show that OCPs are associated with either a decrease or no change in homocysteine levels [202-209]. On the other hand, a study of 200 regular users of OCPs reported elevated homocysteine levels among the 100 women with vascular occlusive disease compared to the 100 healthy controls [210]. Of interest, more than half of those with occlusive disease had occlusions in the cerebral vasculature. The study also noted those with occlusive disease were older and more frequently smokers than controls. Another study found a cyclical variation in homocysteine levels in low-dose OCP users [211]. OCP users were found to have elevated homocysteine levels compared to nonusers on Cycle Day 3. Levels were lower on Day 21 in OCP users and not different than nonusers. It appears that hyperhomocysteinemia may play only a minor role (if any) in strokes that occur in OCP users. OCPs have been associated with deficiencies of factors in the metabolism of homocysteine--namely vitamins B6 and B12 and folate [205,212]. Deficiencies of these vitamins have all been associated with stroke risk and may play a small role in stroke risk in OCP users [205,212,213]. Supplementation of these vitamins in OCP users is inexpensive and safe. Sub-groups of OCP users, such as those with MTHFR mutations, may be at slightly increased risk of stroke associated with hyperhomocysteinemia. However, this risk is likely to be small, and its validity requires further study.

Immune Activation

In 1976, Beaumont and colleagues published the first report suggesting an association between OCP-induced immune complex formation and thrombosis [214]. They followed this report with several other studies. In 1979, they noted that 11 of 12 OCP users had antiethinylestradiol antibody activity, whereas 3 never-users and a pool of normal human gamma-globulins showed no activity [215]. They noted in this study that women with a prior history of arterial thrombosis during OCP therapy had higher antibody levels than OCP users with no history of thrombosis. The preceding year, they demonstrated the presence of circulating immune complexes in roughly 30 percent of OCP users and none in non-users [216]. In that study, 90 percent of OCP users with thrombotic events had these antibodies. In a case-control study of 1,318 OCP users with thrombotic events (763 of whom had strokes), 124 healthy current OCP users, and 61 non-users, Beaumont and colleagues noted antiethinylestradiol antibodies in a third of healthy, current users and in 72 percent of those with thrombosis [217]. They noted the prevalence of concomitant smoking and antiethinylestradiol antibodies in those with thrombosis (47.6%) was greater than that of either risk factor alone (15.6 percent for smoking and 31.1 percent for antiethinylestradiol antibodies). In England, Plowright et al. evaluated 114 women with history of myocardial infarction, cerebral artery thrombosis, or pulmonary embolism and 224 women with no such history [218]. They found that in both current and past users of OCPs, levels of circulating immune complexes were significantly higher in stroke patients and pulmonary embolism patients compared to healthy controls. There was no significant difference between those with myocardial infarction and controls; however, they noted that those with myocardial infarction had other major risk factors for coronary artery disease. Two other groups have questioned the methodology of Beaumont and colleagues [219,220]. These groups found no difference in immune complex levels in sera from controls, users with thrombotic events, never-users with thrombotic events, and current and past users of OCPs. They argue that there is a lack of specificity with the isolation methods of the prior studies [219,220]. It is plausible that immune complexes may play a role in the risk of thrombotic stroke with OCP use, since these complexes have been demonstrated in other causes of stroke [221,222]. The mechanism by which immune complexes may lead to stroke in OCP users is unclear. Histological evaluations of OCP users who died of thrombotic events demonstrate no evidence of an inflammatory process in the vascular wall [31]. It is possible that these immune complexes damage the endothelium, leading to initiation of the coagulation cascade and platelet aggregation. Further research is needed to determine whether circulating immune complexes in OCP users are truly associated with increased risk of thrombotic disease and, if so, by what mechanism.

Special Considerations: Medical Comorbidities and Stroke Risk in Oral Contraceptive Users

While oral contraceptives may increase the overall stroke risk in healthy users, there are some medical conditions that are clearly associated with an accelerated risk. Awareness of these risk factors will allow patients and prescribers to make sound decisions when choosing a contraceptive method. There is evidence that screening for some of these risk factors before prescribing OCPs reduces the incidence of adverse outcomes such as venous thromboembolic disease, myocardial infarction, and stroke [35,223].

Hypertension

Hypertension is one of the most important risk factors for stroke in OCP users. Data from the WHO Collaborative Study [33], the Transnational Research Group [36], the RATIO study [37], the Danish Nurse Study [224] and others [4,35,87,223] found an increased risk of ischemic stroke among women using sex steroid hormones compared to nonusers. When blood pressure is screened before prescribing OCPs--and appropriately managed--the risk of ischemic stroke is reduced [35, 223]. While at least one study found no increased risk of stroke among hypertensive OCP users [44], most practitioners agree that the risk is increased. It is therefore recommended that blood pressure be screened before prescribing OCPs. The American College of Obstetricians and Gynecologists recommends that if women are under age 35 with well-controlled and monitored hypertension and do not smoke or have evidence of end-organ vascular disease, a trial of low-dose OCPs is acceptable [225].

Smoking

Like hypertension, cigarette smoking is a well-known risk factor for stroke. This risk is increased not only in the older population but also in young persons [32,38,41-43]. Evidence from multiple studies shows that women who smoke and use OCPs have a significantly increased risk of ischemic stroke, ranging from about 2-fold to 8-fold [33,34,36,37,39,44,52,87]. The WHO Collaborative Study also demonstrated an increased risk of hemorrhagic stroke with young women who smoke [45]. Some studies found that the additional risk of stroke due to smoking occurred only in current OCP users who smoked more than 20 cigarettes per day, while others found the risk to be increased with 10 or more cigarettes per day [36,44]. Some studies show former smokers who currently use OCPs to be at increased risk of stroke, while others show no increased risk [34,87]. It is recommended that women who plan to use OCPs avoid smoking while on these medications, particularly if over the age of 35. Smoking cessation, independent of the synergistically increased risk of stroke with the combination of smoking and OCP use, is a very important step in reducing overall stroke risk among young people.

Migraine Headache with Aura

Migraine headache--particularly classical migraine with aura--is an independent risk factor for ischemic stroke [226,227]. This risk appears to be greatest in young women [38,228]. One potential mechanism by which migraine headache may increase stroke risk is by causing vasospasm [229]. There is some supporting evidence for this concept as observed with increased risk of stroke in medications that cause vasoconstriction, such as ergotamines and triptans [229]. There is some evidence that patients with genetic factors that make them susceptible to thrombophilia are also at increased risk for migraine headache [230,231]. Other potential mechanisms may be endothelial dysfunction or abnormalities in the composition of the arterial wall that predispose both to migraine headaches and stroke [229]. OCP users who also have migraine headaches have an increased risk of stroke vs. women without migraine headaches. The WHO Collaborative Study showed that women with migraine headache who used OCPs were roughly eight times more likely to have ischemic stroke than those with either risk factor alone and more than 16 times as likely as those with neither risk factor [232]. When women with both risk factors also smoked, a greater than multiplicative effect was seen on stroke risk, with an OR of 34.4 compared to those with none of the risk factors. Another study found a nearly 14-fold increase in migraneurs who used OCPs compared to those with neither risk factor [233]. A pooled analysis of two studies from the United States found a lower, but still significant, risk of ischemic stroke in migraineurs who used OCPs [50]. Lidegaard and Kreiner also found a small significantly increased risk of stroke in those with both risk factors compared to controls [34]. Allais et al. recommend that women who have migraines without auras and no other stroke risk factors can safely take OCPs. Young women who have migraines with aura that are infrequent, of short duration (less than 30 minutes), and are limited to visual phenomena only may portend an acceptable risk. In this group, the progestin-only pill may be the safest choice. Women with frequent, prolonged, complicated auras should avoid OCPs [234]. The International Headache Society Task Force on Combined Oral Contraceptives and Hormone Replacement Therapy recommends consideration of progestin-only pills in those with stroke risk factors. They also suggest that further evaluation, and possibly cessation of OCPs, may be needed in users who develop new persisting headaches, new-onset migraine with aura, increased headache frequency or intensity, or unusual aura symptoms including prolonged aura [235].

Thrombophilia

As discussed earlier, OCP use alters a variety of coagulation factors; and this may play an important role in the increased risk of stroke in users. There is evidence that women with underlying thrombophilic disorders are at increased stroke risk when using OCPs. Slooter et al. found that OCP users with Factor V Leiden mutation were at a greater than 11-fold increased risk of stroke than nonusers without the mutation [185]. OCP users with the MTHFR 677TT mutation were at a rougly 5-fold increased risk compared to those without either risk factor. The risk of stroke with OCP use and MTHFR mutation is more than double that of either risk factor alone [236]. Other studies have yielded similar results [237]. OCP users with the prothrombin G20210A mutation have been reported to have up to a 150-fold greater risk of cerebral vein thrombosis compared to nonusers without the mutation [69]. Similarly, Martinelli et al. found a 30-fold increased risk of cerebral vein thrombosis in OCP users with factor V Leiden and a nearly 80-fold increased risk in users with prothrombin G20210A mutation [72]. The association between arterial stroke or cerebral vein thrombosis and concurrent OCP use in patients with other thrombophilic disorders is less well studied.

Obesity

Obesity is associated with an approximately 10- to 24-fold increased risk of venous thrombosis [238,239]. Obesity, as measured by body mass index and abdominal circumference, has also been associated with a small but significant increased risk of stroke [42]. Obesity in combination with OCP use has been demonstrated to further increase the risk of stroke in young women. The RATIO Study noted a four-fold increase in stroke risk in obese OCP users compared to non-obese women who do not use OCPs and a two-fold increased risk compared to non-obese women who use OCPs [37]. Although there have not been any large studies that have definitively addressed the risk of stroke in obese OCP users, there are several reasons why the association may exist. First, obese patients are known to be at risk for hypercoagulability. They are also at increased risk for insulin-resistance and diabetes, hypertension, and hyperlipidemia--all factors that increase the risk of stroke. The combined effect of obesity and OCP use on such risk factors--and its overall significance to stroke risk in young women--is yet to be determined.

Screening Patients before Prescribing Oral Contraceptives

It is evident that certain populations of women are at significantly increased risk of stroke and other vascular diseases while taking oral contraceptives. These include women over age 35, those with uncontrolled hypertension, and those who smoke. While other risk factors may play a role in stroke risk in OCP users, their overall contributions may be much smaller. It is prudent to take measures to reduce the risk of stroke in OCP users as with other at-risk populations. The recommendation that patients stop smoking before initiating OCP use is unquestionably important. In addition, controlling blood sugars in those with diabetes and lowering cholesterol are also valuable risk reduction strategies. Screening for hypertension prior to prescribing OCP use is recommended in women of all ages. As discussed earlier, a significant reduction of stroke risk occurs when hypertension is diagnosed and treated before OCPs are prescribed. Hypertension is not an absolute contraindication to OCP therapy, but elevated blood pressures should be treated appropriately if OCPs are to be used. Periodic blood pressure monitoring is recommended during the course of OCP therapy to ensure optimal risk reduction. As yet, there are no clear guidelines for screening of thrombophilic disorders in patients planning to use OCPs. Indeed, the risk of stroke is increased in the presence of thrombophilias, particularly in young people, and this risk is further increased by concomitant use of OCPs. However, the overall risk of stroke in OCP users is very low; the presence of thrombophilia in OCP users who have had a stroke is even less common. Andreassi et al. have proposed screening for prothrombotic disorders before prescribing OCPs in all women with prior history of venous or arterial thrombosis, asymptomatic women with a first-degree relative with an inherited venous thromboembolism, and women with recurrent pregnancy loss or unexplained intrauterine fetal growth retardation or stillbirth [113]. The Royal College of Obstetricians and Gynaecologists recommend against routine screening, but state that screening may be considered in women with a first-degree relative under age 45 with venous thromboembolism [240]. Cosmi et al. found a similar prevalence of thrombophilic defects in women with and without family history of venous thromboembolism and suggested that screening only in those with a family history would miss many women who are at-risk [241] It is probably prudent to screen--if not already done--for the more common thrombophilic disorders (e.g. factor V Leiden, MTHFR, and prothrombin G20210A mutations) in women with a prior personal history or a family history of thrombotic disease without another obvious cause should they still wish to use oral contraceptives.

Conclusion

Stroke is an uncommon occurrence in young women. Oral contraceptives impart a clinically and statistically significant increased risk of stroke in those who use them. However, the attributable risk of stroke is about 2 cases per 100,000 women-years for low-dose OCPs and 8 cases per 100,000 women-years for high-dose OCPs [45]. By contrast, the rate of stroke with pregnancy ranges between 11 and 26 cases per 100,000 deliveries [242].

The excess risk of stroke due specifically to pregnancy is about 8 cases per 100,000 deliveries [243]. Therefore, the risk of stroke with OCP use must be interpreted in the context of similar or greater stroke risk in pregnancy, as well as the many other noncontraceptive health benefits of OCPs discussed earlier. Nonetheless, it is necessary for providers to take appropriate steps to minimize stroke risk in OCP users. Such measures include screening for and appropriately treating hypertension before prescribing OCPs and discouraging smoking while taking OCPs. In addition, providers need to inform women about the increased risk associated with diabetes, hyperlipidemia, obesity, and migraine with aura. Providers should then take appropriate steps to reduce these risk factors, as well as consider screening for inherited thrombophilic disorders in selected patients. Further studies are needed--both clinical and basic science--to fully understand the mechanisms by which OCP use promotes stroke in order to guide medical practice.

References

[1] Tyrer L. Introduction of the pill and its impact. *Contraception* 1999;59:11S-16S.

[2] World Health Organization. Cardivascular disease and steroid hormone contraception. Report of a WHO scientific group. WHO Technical Report Series 877. Geneva: World Health Organization, 1998.

[3] Blackburn RD, Cunkelman JA, Zlidar VM. Oral contraceptives--an update. Population Reports. 2000 Spring;28(1),Series A-9, Oral Contraceptives: 1-40.

[4] Chan WS, Ray J, Wai EK, Ginsburg S, Hannah ME, Corey PN, Ginsberg JS. Risk of stroke in women exposed to low-dose oral contraceptives: a critical evaluation of the evidence. *Archives of Internal Medicine* 2004;164:741-747.

[5] Hannaford PC, Croft PR, Kay CR. Oral contraception and stroke: evidence from the Royal College of General Practitioners' Oral Contraception Study. *Stroke* 1994; 5(5):935-942.

[6] Frye CA. An overview of oral contraceptives: mechanism of action and clinical use. *Neurology* 2006; 6(Suppl 3):S29-S36.

[7] Kiley J, Hammond C. Combined oral contraceptives: a comprehensive review. *Clinical Obstetrics and Gynecology* 2007;50:868-877.

[8] Crane M, Harris J. Plasma renin activity and aldosterone excretion rate in normal subjects: II. Effect of oral contraceptive agents. *Journal of Clinical Endocrinology* 1969;29:558-562.

[9] Curtis KM, Chrisman CE, Mohllajee AP, Peterson HB. Effective use of hormonal contraceptives: part 1: combined oral contraceptive pills. *Contraception* 2006; 3:115-124.

[10] Vessey MP, Painter R. Endometrial and ovarian cancer and oral contraceptives--findings in a large cohort study. *British Journal of Cancer* 1995;71:1340-1342.

[11] Cerel-Suhl SL, Yeager BF. Update on oral contraceptive pills. *American Family Physician* 1999;60:2073-2084.

[12] Fraser IS. Forty years of combined oral contraception: the evolution of a revolution. *Medical Journal of Australia* 2000;173:541-544.

[13] Ross RK, Pike MC, Vessey MP, Bull D, Yeates D, Casagrande JT. Risk factors for uterine fibroids: reduced risk associated with oral contraceptives. *British Medical Journal* 1986;293:359-362.

[14] Vessey MP, Villard-Mackintosh L, Painter R. Epidemiology of endometriosis in women attending family planning clinics. *British Medical Journal* 1993;306:182-184.

[15] Kuohung W, Borgatta L, Stubblefield P. Low-dose oral contraceptives and bone mineral density: an evidence-based analysis. *Contraception* 2006;61:77-82.

[16] Family Practice Notebook. Progestin Androgenic Activity. http://www.fpnotebook. om/Gyn/Pharm/PrgstnAndrgncActvty.htm.

[17] Jick H, Jick SS, Gurewich V, Myers MW, Vasilakis C. Risk of idiopathic cardiovascular death and nonfatal venous thromboembolism in women using oral contraceptives with differing progestagen components. *Lancet* 1995;346:1589-1593.

[18] World Health Organization Collaborative Study of Cardiovascular Disease and Steroid Hormone Contraception. Effect of different progestagens in low estrogen oral contraceptives on venous thromboembolic disease. *Lancet* 1995;346:1582-1588.

[19] World Health Organization Collaborative Study of Cardiovascular Disease and steroid Hormone Contraception. Venous thromboembolic disease and combined oral contraceptives: results of international multicentre case-control study. *Lancet* 1995;346:1575-1582.

[20] Jick H, Kaye JA, Vasilakis-Scaramozza C, Jick SS. Risk of venous thromboembolism among users of third generation oral contraceptives compared with users of oral contraceptives with levonorgestrel before and after 1995: cohort and case-control analysis. *British Medical Journal* 2000;321:1190-1195.

[21] Kemmeren JM, Algra A, Grobbee DE. Third generation oral contraceptives and risk of venous thrombosis; meta-analysis. *British Medical Journal* 2001;323:131-134.

[22] Ball MJ, Ashwell E, Jackson M, Cillmer MDG. Comparison of two triphasiccontraceptives with different progestogens: effects on metabolism and coagulation proteins. *Contraception* 1990;41:363-376.

[23] Melis GB, Fruzzetti F, Nicoletti I, Ricci C, Lammers P, Atsma WJ, Fioretti P. A comparative study on the effects of a monophasic pill containing desogestrel 20 μg ethinylestradiol, a triphasic combination containing levonorgestrel and a monophasic combination containing gestodene on coagulatory factors. *Contraception* 1991;23-31.

[24] Heinemann LAJ. Emerging evidence on oral contraceptives and arterial disease. *Contraception* 2000;62:29S-36S.

[25] Jacobs BS, Boden-Albala B, Lin IF, Sacco RL. Stroke in the young in the Northern Manhattan Stroke Study. *Stroke* 2002;33(12):2789-2793.

[26] Lewis MA. Myocardial infarction and stroke in young women: what is the impact of oral contraceptives? *American Journal of Obstetrics and Gynecology* 1998;179:S68-S77.

[27] Naess H, Nyland HI, Thomassen L, Aarseth J, Nyland G, Myhr K-M. Incidence and short-term outcome of cerebral infarction in young adults in western Norway. *Stroke* 2002;33(8):2105-2108.

[28] Rosenthul-Sorokin N, Ronen R, Tamir A, Geva H, Eldar R. Stroke in the young in Israel: incidence and outcomes. *Stroke* 1996;27:838-841.

[29] Vessey MP, Doll R. Investigation of relation between use of oral contraceptives and thromboembolic disease. *British Medical Journal* 1968;2(5599):199-205.

[30] Vessey MP, Doll R. Investigation of relation between use of oral contraceptives and thromboembolic disease. *British Medical Journal* 1969;2(5658):651-657.

[31] Godsland IF, Winkler U, Lidegaard O, Crook D. Occlusive vascular diseases in oral contraceptive users: epidemiology, pathology, and mechanisms. *Drugs* 2000;60(4):721-869.

[32] Carolei A, Marini C, Ferranti E, Frontoni M, Prencipe M, Fieschi C, National Research Council Study Group. A prospective study of cerebral ischemia in the Young: analysis of pathogenic determinants. *Stroke* 1993;24(3):362-367.

[33] World Health Organization Collaborative Study of Cardiovascular Disease and Steroid Hormone Contraception. Ischemic stroke and combined oral contraceptives: results of an international, multicentre, case-control study. *Lancet* 1996;348:498-505.

[34] Lidegaard O, Kreiner S. Contraceptives and cerebral thrombosis: a five-year national case-control study. *Contraception* 2002;65:197-205.

[35] Heinemann LAJ, Lewis MA, Thorogood M, Spitzer WO, Guggenmoos-Holzmann I, Bruppacher R, the Transnational Research Group on Oral Contraceptives and The Health of Young Women. Case-control study of oral contraceptives and risk of thromboembolic stroke: results from international study on oral contraceptives and health of young women. *British Medical Journal* 1997;315:1502-1504.

[36] Heinemann LAJ, Lewis MA, Spitzer WO, Thorogood M, Guggenmoos-Holzmann I, Bruppacher R, the Transnational Research Group on Oral Contraceptives and The Health of Young Women. Thromboembolic stroke in young women: a European case-control study on oral contraceptives. *Contraception* 1998;57:29-37.

[37] Kemmeren JM, Tanis BC, van den Bosch MAAJ, Bollen ELEM, Helmerhorst FM, van der Graaf Y, Rosendaal FR, Algra A. Risk of Arterial Thrombosis in Relation to Oral Contraceptives (RATIO) Study: oral contraceptives and the risk of ischemic stroke. *Stroke* 2002;33(5):1202-1208.

[38] Barinagarrementeria F, Gonzalez-Duarte A, Miranda L, Cantu C. Cerebral infarction in young women: analysis of 130 cases. *European Neurology* 1998; 40:228-233.

[39] Kittner SJ, Stern BJ, Wozniak M, Buchholz DW, Earley CJ, Feeser BR, Johnson CJ, Macko RF, McCarter RJ, Price TR, Sherwin R, Sloan MA, Wityk RJ. Cerebral Infarction in young adults: the Baltimore-Washington Cooperative Young Stroke Study. *Neurology* 1998;50:890-894.

[40] Li Y, Zhou L, Coulter D, Gao E, Sun Z, Liu Y, Wang X. Prospective cohort study of the association between use of low-dose oral contraceptives and stroke in Chinese women. *Pharmacoepidemiology and Drug Safety* 2006;15:726-734.

[41] Mehndiratta MM, Agarwal P, Sen K, Sharma B. Stroke in young adults: a study from a university hospital in north India. *Medical Science Monitor* 2004;10(9):CR535-541.

[42] Nightingale AL, Farm RDT. Ischemic stroke in young women: a nested case-control study using the UK General Practice Research Database. *Stroke* 2004;35(7):1574-1578.

[43] Rasura M, Spalloni A, Ferrari M, De Castro S, Patella R, Di Lisi F, Beccia M. A case series of young stroke in Rome. *European Journal of Neurology* 2006;13:146-152.

[44] Siritho S, Thrift AG, McNeil JJ, You RX, Davis SM, Donnan GA. Risk of ischemic stroke among users of the oral contraceptive pill: the Melbourne Risk Factor Study (MERFS) Group. *Stroke* 2003;34(7):1575-1580.

[45] World Health Organization Collaborative Study of Cardiovascular Disease and Steroid Hormone Contraception. Hemorrhagic stroke, overall stroke risk, and Combined oral contraceptives: results of an international, multicentre, case-control study. *Lancet* 1996; 348:505-510.

[46] Hirvonen E, Idanpaan-Heikkila J. Cardiovascular death among women under 40 years of age using low-estrogen oral contraceptives and intrauterine devices in Finland from 1975 to 1984. *American Journal of Obstetrics and Gynecology* 1990;163:281-284.

[47] Mant J, Painter R, Vessey M. Risk of myocardial infarction, angina and stroke in users of oral contraceptives: an updated analysis of a cohort study. *British Journal of Obstetrics and Gynecology* 1998;105:890-896.

[48] Stampfer MJ, Willett WC, Colditz GA, Speizer FE, Hennekens CH. A prospective study of past use of oral contraceptive agents and risk of cardiovascular diseases. *New England Journal of Medicine* 1988;319:1313-1317.

[49] Brattstrom L, Wilcken DE, Ohrvik J, Brudin L. Common methylenetetrahydrofolate reductase gene mutation leads to yperhomocysteinemia but not to vascular disease: the result of a meta-analysis. *Circulation* 1998;98:2520-2526.

[50] Schwartz SM, Petitti DB, Siscovick DS, Longstreth WT Jr., Sidney S, Raghunathan TE, Quesenberry CP Jr., Kelaghan J. Stroke and the use of low-dose oral contraceptives in young women: a pooled analysis of two U.S. studies. *Stroke* 1998;29:2277-2284.

[51] Gillum LA, Mamidipudi SK, Johnston SC. Ischemic stroke risk with oral contraceptives: a meta-analysis. *Journal of the American Medical Association* 2000 July 5;284(1):72-78.

[52] Baillargeon J-P, McClish DK, Essah PA, Nestler JE. Association between the current use of low-dose oral contraceptives and cardiovascular arterial disease: a meta-analysis. *The Journal of Clinical Immunology and Metabolism* 2005;90:3863-3870.

[53] Petitti DB, Sidney S, Bernstein A, Wolf S, Quesenberry C, Ziel HK. Stroke in users of low-dose oral contraceptives. *The New England Journal of Medicine* 1996;335:8-15.

[54] Schwartz SM, Siscovick DS, Longstreth WT, Psaty BM, Beverly RK, Raghunathan TE, Lin D, Koepsell TD. Use of low-dose oral contraceptives and stroke in young women. *Annals of Internal Medicine* 1997;127(8, part 1):596-603.

[55] Inman WHW. Oral contraceptives and fatal subarachnoid hemorrhage. *British Medical Journal* 1979;2:1468-1470.

[56] Thorogood M, Adam SA, Mann JI. Fatal subarachnoid hemorrhage in young women: role of oral contraceptives. *British Medical Journal* 1981;283:762.

[57] Vessey MP, Lawless M, Yeates D. Oral contraceptives and stroke: findings in a large prospective study. *British Medical Journal* 1984;289:530-531.

[58] Johnston SC, Colford JM, Gress DR. Oral contraceptives and the risk of subarachnoid hemorrhage: a meta-analysis. *Neurology* 1998; 51:411-418.

[59] Royal College of General Practitioners' Oral Contraception Study. Oral contraceptives, venous thrombosis, and varicose veins. *Journal of the Royal College of General Practitioners* 1978;28:393-399.

[60] Sarwell PE, Masi AT, Arthes FG, Greene GR, Smith HE. Thromboembolism and oral contraceptives: an epidemiological case-control study. *American Journal of Epidemiology* 1969;90:365-380.

[61] Thorogood M, Mann J, Murphy M, Vessey M. Risk factors for fatal venous thromboembolism in young women: a case-control study. *International Journal of Epidemiology* 1992;21:48-52.

[62] Vessey M, Mant D, Smith A, Yeates D. Oral contraceptives and venous thromboembolism: findings in a large prospective study. *British Medical Journal* 1986; 292:526.

[63] Rosendaal FR, Helmerhorst FM, Vandenbroucke JP. Female hormones and thrombosis. *Arteriosclerosis, Thrombosis, and Vascular Biology* 2002;22:201-210.

[64] Atkinson EA, Fairburn B, Heathfield KWG. Intracranial venous thrombosis as complication of oral contraception. *Lancet* 1970;1:914-918.

[65] 65. Buccino G, Scoditti U, Pini M, Tagliaferri AR, Manotti C, Mancia D. Low-estrogen oral contraceptives as a major risk factor for cerebral venous and sinus thrombosis: evidence from a clinical series. *Italian Journal of Neurological Sciences* 1999;20:231-235.

[66] Buchanan DS, Brazinsky JH. Dural sinus and cerebral venous thrombosis. Incidence in young women receiving oral contraceptives. *Archives of Neurology* 1970;22:440-444.

[67] De Bruijn SF, Stam J, Koopman MM, Vandenbroucke JP. Case-control study of risk of cerebral sinus thrombosis in oral contraceptives users who are carriers of hereditary prothrombotic conditions. The Cerebral Venous Sinus Thrombosis Study Group. *British Medical Journal* 1998;316:589-592.

[68] Estanol B, Rodriguez A, Conte G, Aleman JM, Loyo M, Pizzuto J. Intracranial venous thrombosis in young women. *Stroke* 1979;10(6):680-684.

[69] Martinelli I, Sacchi E, Landi G, Taioli E, Duca F, Mannucci PM. High risk of cerebral-vein thrombosis in carriers of a prothrombin-gene mutation and in use of oral contraceptives. *The New England Journal of Medicine* 1998;338:1793-1797.

[70] Scoditti U, Buccino GP, Pini M, Pattacini C, Mancia D. Risk of acute cerebrovascular events related to low oestrogen oral contraceptives treatment. *Italian Journal of Neurological Sciences* 1998;19:15-19.

[71] Dentali F, Crowther M, Ageno W. Thrombophilic abnormalities, oral contraceptives, and risk of cerebral vein thrombosis: a meta-analysis. *Blood* 2006;107:2766-2773.

[72] Martinelli I, Bettaglioli T, Pedotti P, Cattaneo M, Mannucci PM. Hyperhomocysteinemia in cerebral vein thrombosis. *Blood* 2003;102:1363-1366.

[73] Rubinstein SM, Peerdeman SM, van Tulder MW, Riphagen I, Haldeman S. A systematic review of the risk factors for cervical artery dissection. *Stroke* 2005; 36:1575-1580.

[74] D-Anglejan-Chatillon J, Ribeiro V, Mas JL, Youl BD, Bousser MG. Migraine--a risk factor for dissection of cervical arteries. *Headache* 1989;29:560-561.

[75] Grau AJ, Brandt T, Buggle F, Orberk E, Mytilineos J, Werle E, Conradt C, Krause M, Winter R, Hacke W. Association of cervical artery dissection with recent infection. *Archives of Neurology* 1999;56:851-856.

[76] Alkayed NJ, Murphy SJ, Traystman RJ, Hurn PD. Neuroprotective effects of female gonadal steroids in reproductively senescent female rats. *Stroke* 2000;31:161-168.

[77] Bushnell C. Oestrogen and stroke in women: assessment of risk. *Lancet Neurology* 2005; 4:743-751.

[78] Littleton-Kearney MT, Klaus JA, Hurn PD. Effects of combined oral conjugated estrogens and medroxyprogesterone acetate on brain infarction size after experimental stroke in rat. *Journal of Cerebral Blood Flow and Metabolism* 2005;25:421-426.

[79] McCoullough LD, Alkayed NJ, Traystman RJ, Williams MJ, Hurn PD. Postischemic estrogen reduces hypoperfusion and secondary ischemia after Experimental stroke. *Stroke* 2001;32:796-802.

[80] Shi J, Bui JD, Yang S-H, He Z, Lucas TH, Buckley DL, Blackband SJ, King MA, Day AL, Simpkins JW. Estrogens decrease reperfusion-associated cortical ischemic damage: an MRI analysis in a transient focal ischemia model. *Stroke* 2001;32:987-992.

[81] Suzuki S, Gerhold LM, Bottner M, Rau S, Dela Cruz C, Yang E, Zhu H, Yu J, Cashion AB, Kindy MS, Merchenthaler I, Gage FH, Wise PM. Estradiol enhances neurogenesis following ischemic stroke through estrogen receptors α and β. *The Journal of Comparative Neurology* 2007;500:1064-1075.

[82] Yang S-H, Shi J, Day AL, Simpkins JW. Estradiol exerts neuroprotective effects when administered after ischemic insult. *Stroke* 2000;31:745-750.

[83] Behl C, Skutella T, Lezouale'h F, Post A, Widmann M, Newton CJ, Holsboer F. Neuroprotection against oxidative stress by estrogens: structure-activity Relationship. *Molecular Pharmacology* 1997;51:535-541.

[84] Mermelstein PG, Becker JB, Surmeier DJ. Estradiol reduces calcium currents in rat neostriatal neurons via a membrane receptor. *Journal of Neuroscience* 1996;16:595-604.

[85] Cervantes M, Gonzalez-Vidal MD, Ruelas R, Escobar A, Morali G. Neuroprotective effects of progesterone on damage elicited by acute global cerebral ischemia in neurons of the caudate nucleus. *Archives of Medical Research* 2002;33:6-14.

[86] Gibson CL, Constantin D, Prior MJW, Bath PMW, Murphy SP. Progesterone suppresses the inflammatory response and nitric oxide synthase-2 expression following cerebral ischemia. *Experimental Neurology* 2005;193:522-530.

[87] Gibson CL, Murphy SP. Progesterone enhances functional recovery after middle cerebral artery occlusion in male mice. *Journal of Cerebral Blood Flow and Metabolism* 2004; 24:805-813.

[88] Jiang N, Chopp M, Stein D, Feit H. Progesterone is neuroprotective after transient middle cerebral artery occlusion in male rats. *Brain Research* 1996;735:101-107.

[89] Kuman Y, Kim SC, Tompkins P, Stevens A, Sakaki S, Loftus CM. Neuroprotective effect of postischemic administration of progesterone in Spontaneously hypertensive rats with focal cerebral ischemia. *Journal of Neurosurgery* 2000;92:848-852.

[90] Murphy SJ, Traystman RJ, Hurn PD. Progesterone exacerbates striatal stroke injury in progesterone-deficient female animals. *Stroke* 2000;31:1173-1178.

[91] Viscoli CM, Brass LM, Kernan WN, Sarrel PM, Suissa S, Horwitz RI. A clinical trial of estrogen-replacement therapy after ischemic stroke. *The New England Journal of Medicine* 2001;345:1243-1249.

[92] Writing Group for the Women's Health Initiative Investigators. Risks and benefits of estrogen plus progestin in healthy postmenopausal women: principle results from the Women's Health Initiative randomized controlled trial. *Journal of the American Medical Association* 2002;288:321-333.

[93] Hoffman R, Benz EJ Jr., Shattil SJ, Furie B, Cohen HJ, Silberstein LE, McGlave P. Hematology: Basic Principles and Practice, 4th ed. Philadelphia: Churhill Livingstone, 2005.

[94] Wu KK, Thiagarajan P. Role of endothelium in thrombosis and hemostasis. *Annual Review of Medicine* 1996;47:315-331.

[95] Gordon EM, Douglas J, Ratnoff OD. Influence of augmented Hageman factor (factor XII) titers on the cryoactivation of plasma prorenin in women using oral contraceptive agents. *Journal of Clinical Investigation* 1983;72:1833-1838.

[96] Gordon EM, Ratnoff OD, Saito H, Donaldson VH, Pensky J, Jones PK. Rapid fibrinolysis, augmented Hageman factor (factor XII) titers and decreased C1 esterase inhibitor titers in women using oral contraceptives. *Journal of Laboratory and Clinical Medicine* 1980;96:762-769.

[97] Gordon EM, Douglas JG, Ratnoff OD, Arafah BM. The influence of estrogen and prolactin on Hageman factor (factor XII) titer in ovarectimized and hypophysectomized rats. *Blood* 1985;66:602-605.

[98] Gordon EM, Johnson TR, Ramos LP, Schmeidler-Sapiro KT. Enhanced expression of factor XII (Hageman factor) in isolated livers of estrogen- and prolactin-treated rats. *Journal of Laboratory and Clinical Medicine* 1991;117:353-358.

[99] Farsetti A, Misti S, Citarella F, Felici A, Andreoli M, Fantoni A, Sacchi A, Pontecorvi A. Molecular basis of estrogen regulation of Hageman factor XII gene Expression. *Endocrinology* 1995;136:5076-5083.

[100] Kluft C, Lansink M. Effect of oral contraceptives on haemostasis variables. *Thrombosis and Haemostasis* 1997;78:315-326.

[101] Kuhl H. Effects of progestogens on haemostasis. *Maturitas* 1996;24:1-19.

[102] Winkler UH. Blood coagulation and oral contraceptives: a critical review. *Contraception* 1998;57:203-209.

[103] The Oral Contraceptive and Hemostasis Study Group. The effects of seven monophasic oral contraceptive regimens on hemostatic variables: conclusions from a large randomized multicenter study. *Contraception* 2003;67:173-185(210-10).

[104] Sabra A, Bonnar J. Hemostatic changes induced by 50 μg and 30 μg estrogen/progestin oral contraceptives. Modification of estrogen effects by levonorgestrel. *Journal of Reproductive Medicine* 1983;28(Suppl):85-91.

[105] Kluft C. Effects on haemostasis variables by second and third generation combined oral contraceptives: a review of directly comparative studies. *Current Medicinal Chemistry* 2000;7:585-591.

[106]Middeldorp S, Meijers JCM, van den Ende AE, van Enk A, Bouma BN, Tans G, Rosing J, Prins MH, Buller HR. Effects on coagulation of levonorgestrel- and desogestrel-containing oral contraceptives: a cross-over study. *Thrombosis and Haemostasis* 2000;84:4-8.

[107]Tans G, Curvers J, Middeldorp S, Thomassen CLGD, Meijers JCM, Prins MH, Bouma BN, Buller HR, Rosing J. A randomized cross-over study on the effects of levonorgestrel- and desogestrel-containing oral contraceptives on the anticoagulant pathways. *Thrombosis and Haemostasis* 2000;84:15-21.

[108]Rosing J, Tans G, Nicolaes GA, Thomassen MC, van Oerle R, van der Ploeg PM, Heijnen P, Hamulyak K, Hemker HC. Oral contraceptives and venous Thrombosis: different sensitivities to activated protein C in women using second- and third-generation oral contraceptives. *British Journal of Haematology* 1997;98;491-492.

[109]Bloemenkamp KW, Rosendaal FR, Helmerhorst FM, Buller HR, Vandenbroucke JP. Enhancement by factor V Leiden mutation of risk of deep-vein thrombosis associated with oral contraceptives containing third-generation progestogen. *Lancet* 1995; 346: 1593-1596.

[110]Martinelli I, Taioli E, De Stefano V, Chiusolo P, Mannucci PM. Interaction between the G20210A mutation of the prothrombin gene and oral contraceptive use in deep vein thrombosis. *Arteriosclerosis, Thrombosis, and Vascular Biology* 1999;19:700-703.

[111]Spannagl M, Heinemann LA, Schramm W. Are factor V Leiden carriers who use oral contraceptives at extreme risk for venous thromboembolism? *The European Journal of Contraception and Reproductive Health Care* 2005;5:105-112.

[112]Vandenbroucke JP, Koster T, Briet E, Reitsma PH, Bertina RM, Rosendaal FR. Increased risk of venous thrombosis in oral-contraceptive users who are carriers of factor V Leiden mutation. *Lancet* 1994;344:1453-1457.

[113]Andreassi MG, Botto N, Maffei S. Factor V Leiden, prothrombin G20210A,substitution and hormone therapy: indications for molecular screening. *Clinical Chemistry and Laboratory Medicine* 2006;44:514-521.

[114]Legnani C, Palareti G, Guazzaloca G, Cosmi B, Lunghi B, Bernardi F, Coccheri S. Venous thromboembolism in young women; role of thrombophilic mutations and oral contraceptive use. *European Heart Journal* 2002;23:984-990.

[115]Shattil S, Hoxie J, Cunningham M, Brass L. Changes in the platelet membrane glycoprotein IIb/IIIIa complex during platelet activation. *Journal of Biological Chemistry* 1985;260:11107-11114.

[116]Durand P, Blache D. Enhanced platelet thromboxane synthesis and reduced macrophage-dependent fibrinolytic activity related to oxidative stress in oral contraceptive-treated female rats. *Atherosclerosis* 1996;121:205-216.

[117]Norris LA, Bonnar J. Effect of oestrogen dose on whole blood platelet activation in women taking new low dose oral contraceptives. *Thrombosis and Haemostasis* 1994; 72:926-930.

[118]Hadjiagapiou C, Spector AA. 12-hydroxyeicosatetraenoic acid reduces prostacyclin production by endothelial cells. *Prostaglandins* 1986;31:1135.

[119]Pan JQ, Hall ER, Wu KK. Alteration of platelet responses to metabolites or arachidonic acid by oral contraceptives. *British Journal of Haematology* 1984;58:317.

[120]Norris LA, Devitt M, Bonnar J. The role of thromboxane A2 in increased whole blood platelet aggregation in oral contraceptive users. *Thrombosis Research* 1996;81:407-417.

[121]Schlit AF, Grandjean P, Donnez J, Lavenne E. Large increase in plasmatic 11-dehydro-TXB_2 levels due to oral contraceptives. *Contraception* 1995;51:53-58.

[122]Liehr JG, Roy D. Free radical generation by redox cycling of estrogens. *Free Radical Biology and Medicine* 1990;8:415.

[123]Blache D. Involvement of hydrogen and lipid peroxidases in the acute tobacco smoking-induced platelet hyperactivity. *American Journal of Physiology* 1995; 268: H679.

[124]Blache D, Bouthillier D, Davignon J. Acute influence of smoking on platelet behaviour endothelium and plasma lipids and normalization by aspirin. *Atherosclerosis* 1992; 93: 179.

[125]Renaud S, Ciavatti M, Perrot L, Berthezene F, Dargent D, Condamin P. Influence of vitamin E administration on platelet functions in hormonal contraceptive users. *Contraception* 1987;36:347-358.

[126]Weiss EJ, Bray PF, Tayback M, Schulman SP, Kickler TS, Becker LC, Weiss JL, Gerstenblith G, Goldschmidt-Clermont PJ. A polymorphism of a plateletGlycoprotein receptor as an inherited risk factor for coronary thrombosis. *New England Journal of Medicine* 1996;334:1090-1094.

[127]Boudoulas KD, Cooke GE, Roos CM, Bray PF, Goldschmidt-Clermont PJ. The I^A polymorphism of glycoprotein IIIa functions as a modifier for the effect of Estrogen on platelet aggregation. *Archives of Pathology and Laboratory Medicine* 2001;125:112-115.

[128]Bushnell CD. Hormone replacement therapy and stroke: the current state of knowledge and directions for future research. *Seminars in Neurology* 2006;26:123-130.

[129]Reiner AP, Kumar PN, Schwartz SM, Longstreth WT Jr., Pearce RM, Rosendaal FR, Psaty BM, Siscovick DS. Genetic variants of platelet glycoprotein receptors and risk of stroke in young women. *Stroke* 2000;31:1628-1633.

[130]Celermajer DS, Sorensen KE, Gooch VM, Spiegelhalter DJ, Miller OI, Sullivan ID, Lloyd JK, Deanfield JE. Non-invasive detection of endothelial dysfunction in children and adults at risk of atherosclerosis. *Lancet* 1992;340:1111-1115.

[131]Buchner NJ, Rump LC. Oral contraceptives and endothelial function: harm or benefit? *Journal of Hypertension* 2003;21:2227-2230.

[132]John S, Jacobi J, Schlaich MP, Delles C, Schmieder RE. Effects of oral contraceptives on vascular endothelium in premenopausal women. *American Journal of Obstetrics and Gynecology* 2000;183:28-33.

[133]Taddei S, Virdis A, Ghiadoni L, Mattei P, Sudano I, Bernini G, Pinto S, Salvetti A. Menopause is associated with endothelial dysfunction in women. *Hypertension* 1996; 28: 576-582.

[134]Virdis A, Ghiadoni L, Pinto S, Lombardo M, Petraglia F, Gennazzani A, Buralli S, Taddei S, Salvetti A. Mechanisms for endothelial dysfunction associated with acute estrogen deprivation in normotensive women. *Circulation* 2000;101:2258-2263.

[135] Virdis A, Ghiadoni L, Sudano I, Buralli S, Salvetti G, Taddei S, Salvetti A. Endothelial function in hypertension: role of gender. *Journal of Hypertension* 2002; 20(suppl 2): S11-S16.

[136] Gilligan DM, Badar DM, Panza JA, Quyyumi AA, Cannon RO III. Acute vascular effects of estrogen in postmenopausal women. *Circulation* 1994;90:786-791.

[137] Herrington DM, Espeland MA, Crouse JR III, Robertson J, Riley WA, McBurnie MA, Burke GL. Estrogen replacement and brachial artery flow-mediated vasodilation in older women. *Arteriosclerosis, Thrombosis, and Vascular Biology* 2001;21:1955-1961.

[138] Lieberman EH, Gerhard MD, Uehata A, Walsh BW, Selwyn AP, Ganz P, Yeung AC, Creager MA. Estrogen improves endothelium-dependent, flow-mediated vasodilation in postmenopausal women. *Annals of Internal Medicine* 1994;121:936-941.

[139] Faludi AA, Aldright JM, Bertolami MC, Saleh MH, Silva RA, Nakamura Y, Pereira IR, Abdalla DS, Ramires JA, Sousa JE. Progesterone abolishes estrogen and/or atorvastatin endothelium dependent vasodilatory effects. *Atherosclerosis* 2004;177:89-96.

[140] Gerhard M, Walsh BW, Tawakol A, Haley EA, Creager SJ, Seely EW, Ganz P, Creager MA. Estradiol therapy combined with progesterone and endothelium-dependent vasodilation in postmenopausal women. *Circulation* 1998;98:1158-1163.

[141] Sorensen KE, Dorup I, Hermann AP, Mosekilde L. Combined hormone replacement therapy does not protect women against the age-related decline in endothelium-dependent vasomotor function. *Circulation* 1998;97:1234-1238.

[142] Christodoulakos G, Panoulis C, Kouskouni E, Chondros C, Dendrinos S, Creatsas G. Effects of estrogen-progestin and raloxifene therapy on nitric oxide, prostacyclin and endothelin-1 synthesis. *Gynecological Endocrinology* 2002;16:9-17.

[143] Gammal EB, Monture MC. Uptake of Evans blue-bound albumin in the aorta of estrogen-treated rats. *British Journal of Experimental Pathology* 1979;60:58-64.

[144] Wingrove C, Garr E, Godsland IF, Stevenson JC. 17 beta oestradiol enhances release of matrix metalloproteinase-2 from human vascular smooth muscle cells. *Biochemica et Biophysica Acta* 1998;1406:169-174.

[145] Dussek JE. Hypertension and the pill. *British Medical Journal* 1969;3:416-17.

[146] Laragh JH, Sealey JE, Ledingham JGG, Newton MA. Oral contraceptives. Renin, aldosterone, and high blood pressure. *Journal of the American Medical Association* 1967; 201:918-922.

[147] Woods JW. Oral contraceptives and hypertension. *Lancet* 1967;2:653-654.

[148] Clezy TM, Foy BN, Hodge RL, Lumbers ER. Oral contraceptives and hypertension. An epidemiological survey. *British Heart Journal* 1972;34:1238-1243.

[149] Dong W, Colhoun HM, Poulter NR. Blood pressure in women using oral contraceptives: results from the Health Survey for England 1994. *Journal of Hypertension* 1997;15:1063-1068.

[150] Fuchs Nora, Dusterberg B, Weber-Diehl F, Muhe B. The effect on blood pressure of a monophasic oral contraceptive containing ethinylestradiol and gestodene. *Contraception* 1995;51:335-339.

[151] Ramcharan S, Pellegrin FA, Hoag EJ. The occurrence and course of hypertensive disease in users and nonusers of oral contraceptive drugs. In: Ramcharan S, ed. The Walnut Creek Contraceptive Drug Study: a prospective study of the side effects of oral

contraceptives, vol 2. U.S. Department of Health, Education, and Welfare puplication no. (NIH)76-563. Washington, D.C.: Government Printing Office. 1976; 1-16.

[152]Report of the Royal College of General Practioners. Hypertension. In: Oral Contraceptives and Health. London: Pitmann, 1974; 34-42.

[153]Saruta T, Saade GA, Kaplan NM. A possible mechanism for hypertension induced by oral contraceptives. *Archives of Internal Medicine* 1970;126:621-626.

[154]Tyson JEA. Oral contraception and elevated blood pressure. *American Journal of Obstetrics and Gynecology* 1968; 100:875-876.

[155]Weir RJ, Briggs E, Mack A, Naismith L, Taylor L, Wilson E. Blood pressure in women taking oral contraceptives. *British Medical Journal* 1974;1:533-535.

[156]Chasan-Taber L, Willett WC, Manson JE, Spiegelman D, Hunter DJ, Curhan G, Colditz GA, Stampfer MJ. Prospective study of oral contraceptives and hypertension among women in the United States. *Circulation* 1996;94:483-489.

[157]Fisch IR, Frank J. Oral contraceptives and blood pressure. *Journal of the American Medical Association* 1977;237:2499-2503.

[158]Meade TW, Haines AP, North WRS, Chakrabarti R, Howarth DJ, Stirling Y. Haemostatic, lipid and blood-pressure profiles of women on oral contraceptives containing 50 μg or 30 μg oestrogen. *Lancet* 1977;2:948-951.

[159]Woods JW. Oral contraceptives and hypertension. *Hypertension* 1988; 11(3 Part 2): II11-15.

[160]Weir RJ. Effect on blood pressure of changing from high to low dose steroid preparations in women with oral contraceptive induced hypertension. *Scottish Medical Journal* 1982;27:212-215.

[161]Wilson ESB, Cruickshank J, McMaster M, Weir RJ. A prospective controlled study of the effect on blood pressure of contraceptive preparations containing different types and dosages of progestogen. *British Journal of Obstetrics and Gynaecology* 1984; 91:1254-1260.

[162]Hussain SF. Progestogen-only pills and high blood pressure: is there an association? A literature review. *Contraception* 2004;69:89-97.

[163]Spellacy WN, Birk BS. The effect of intrauterine devices, oral contraceptives, estrogens, and progestogens and blood pressure. *American Journal of Obstetrics and Gynecology* 1972;112:912-919.

[164]Lubianca JN, Moreira LB, Gus M, Fuchs FD. Stopping oral contraceptives: an effective blood pressure-lowering intervention in women with hypertension. *Journal of Human Hypertension* 2005;19:451-455.

[165]Mulatero P, Rabbia F, di Cella SM, Schiavone D, Plazzotta C, Pascoe L, Veglio F. Angiotensin-converting enzyme and angiotensinogen gene polymorphisms are non-randomly distributed in oral contraceptive-induced hypertension. *Journal of Hypertension* 2001; 19:713-719.

[166]Petitti DB, Klatzky AL. Malignant hypertension in women aged 15 to 44 years and its relation to cigarette smoking and oral contraceptives. *American Journal of Cardiology* 1983; 52:297-298.

[167] Crane M, Harris J. Plasma renin activity and aldosterone excretion rate in normal subjects: I. Effect of ethinylestradiol and medroxyprogesterone acetate. *Journal of Clinical Endocrinology* 1969; 29:550-557.

[168] Helmer OM, Griffith RS. Effect of the administration of estrogens on the renin-substrate (hypertensinogen) content of rat plasma. Endocrinology. 1952;51:421-426.

[169] Laidlaw J, Ruse J, Gornall A. The influence of estrogen and progesterone on aldosterone excretion. *Journal of Clinical Endocrinology* 1962;22:161-177.

[170] Wolfsen AR. Complications of systemic contraceptive agents: hypertension. *Western Journal of Medicine* 1975. 122(1):38-40.

[171] Lehtovirta P. Haemodynamic effects of combined oestrogen/progestogen oral contraceptives. *Journal of Obstetrics and Gynaecology of the British Commonwealth* 1974; 81:517-525.

[172] Littler WA, Bojorges-Bueno R, Banks J. Cardiovascular dynamics in women during the menstrual cycle and oral contraceptive therapy. *Thorax* 1974; 29:567-570.

[173] Walters W, Lim Y. Cardiovascular dynamics in women receiving oral contraceptive therapy. *Lancet* 1969; 2:879-881.

[174] Walters W, Lim Y. Haemodynamic changes in women taking oral contraceptives. *Journal of Obstetrics and Gynaecology of the British Commonwealth* 1970; 77:1007-1012.

[175] Crook D, Godsland I. Safety evaluation of modern oral contraceptives: effects on lipoprotein and carbohydrate metabolism. *Contraception* 1998;57:189-201.

[176] Aurell M, Craimer K, Rybo G. Serum lipids and lipoproteins during long-termadministration of an oral contraceptive. *Lancet* 1966;1:291-293.

[177] Wynn V, Doar JWH, Mills GL. Some effects of oral contraceptives on serum lipid and lipoprotein levels. *Lancet* 1966;2:720-723.

[178] Wynn V, Doar JWH, Mills GL, Stokes T. Fasting serum triglyceride, cholesterol, and lipoprotein levels during oral contraceptive therapy. *Lancet* 1969;2:756-760.

[179] Wallace RB, Hoover J, Barrett-Connor E, Rifkind BM, Hunningshake DB, Mackenthun A, Heiss G. Altered plasma lipid and lipoprotein levels associated with oral contraceptive and oestrogen use. *Lancet* 1979;1:111-115.

[180] Wallace RB, Hoover J, Sandler D, Rifkind BM, Tyroler HA. Altered plasma-lipids associated with oral contraceptive or oestrogen consumption. The Lipid Research Clinic Program. *Lancet* 1977;1:11-14.

[181] Wahl P, Walden C, Knopp R, Hoover J, Wallace R, Heiss G, Rifkind B. Effect of estrogen/progestin potency on lipid/lipoprotein cholesterol. *New England Journal of Medicine* 1983;308:862-867.

[182] Bradley DD, Wingerd J, Petitti DB, Krauss RM, Ramcharan S. Serum high-density-lipoprotein cholesterol in women using oral contraceptives, estrogens and progestins. *New England Journal of Medicine* 1978;299:17-20.

[183] Foulon T, Payen N, Laporte F, Bijaoui S, Dupont G, Roland F, Groslambert P. Effects of two low-dose oral contraceptives containing ethinylestradiol and either desogestrel or levonorgestrel on serum lipids and lipoproteins with particular regard to LDL size. *Contraception* 2001;64:11-16.

[184] Wiegartz I, Jung-Hoffmann C, Gross W, Kuhl H. Effect of two oral contraceptives containing ethinyl estradiol and gestodene or norgestimate on different lipid and lipoprotein parameters. *Contraception* 1998;58:83-91.

[185] De Graaf J, Swinkels DW, Demacker PNM, de Haan AFJ, Stalenhoef AFH. Differences in the low-density lipoprotein subfraction profile between oral contraceptive users and controls. *Journal of Clinical Endocrinology and Metabolism* 1993; 76:197-202.

[186] Dejager S, Turpin G. Atherogenicity of low-density lipoproteins (LDL). A problem of quantity or quality. *Presse Medicale* 1995; 24:1772-1776.

[187] Gordon DJ, Probstfield JL, Garrison RJ, Neaton JD, Castelli WP, Knoke JD, Jacobs DR Jr., Bangdiwala S, Tyroler HA. High-density lipoprotein cholesterol and cardiovascular disease. Four prospective American studies. *Circulation* 1989; 79:8-15.

[188] Hokanson JE, Austin MA. Plasma triglyceride is a risk factor for cardiovascular disease independent of high-density lipoprotein cholesterol level: a meta-analysis of population-based prospective studies. *Journal of Cardiovascular Risk* 1996;3:213-220.

[189] Miller GJ, Miller NE. Plasma high-density lipoprotein concentration and development of ischaemic heart-disease. *Lancet* 1975;1:16-19.

[190] Scandinavian Simvastatin Survival Study Group. Randomized trial of cholesterol lowering in 4444 patients with coronary heart disease. *Lancet* 1994;344:1383-1389.

[191] Yaari S, Goldbourt, Even-Zohar S, Neufeld HN. Associations of serum high density lipoprotein and total cholesterol with total cardiovascular and cancer mortality in a 7-year prospective study of 10,000 men. *Lancet* 1981;1:1011-1015.

[192] Boden-Albala B, Sacco RL, Lee H-S, Grahame-Clarke C, Rundek T, Elkind MV, Wright C, Giardina E-GV, DiTullio MR, Homma S, Paik MC. Metabolic syndrome and ischemic stroke risk; northern Manhattan study. *Stroke* 2008;39:30-35.

[193] Park K, Yasunda N, Toyonaga S, Tsubosaki E, Nakaabyashi H, Shimizu K. Significant associations of metabolic syndrome and its components with silent lacunar infarction in middle-aged subjects. *Journal of Neurology, Neurosurgery and Psychiatry* 2008;(Epub ahead of print).

[194] Lopez LM, Grimes DA, Schulz KF. Steroidal contraceptives: effect on carbohydrate metabolism in women without diabetes mellitus (review). Cochrane Database of Systematic Reviews (Online). 2007;2:CD006133.

[195] Wynn V, Doar J. Some effects of oral contraceptives on carbohydrate metabolism. *Lancet* 1966;2:715-719.

[196] Godsland IF. The influence of female sex steroids on glucose metabolism and insulin action. *Journal of Internal Medicine* 1996;738(Suppl):1-60.

[197] Kooistra T, Bosma P, Tons H, van den Berg AP, Meyer P, Princen HM. Plasminogen activator inhibitor 1: biosynthesis and mRNA level are increased by insulin in cultured human hepatocytes. *Thrombosis and Haemostasis* 1989;62:723-728.

[198] Madonna P, de Stefano V, Coppola A, Cirillo F, Cerbone AM, Orefice G, Di Minno G. Hyperhomocysteinemia and other inherited prothrombotic conditions in young adults with a history of ischemic stroke. *Stroke* 2002;33:51-56.

[199] Frosst P, Blom HJ, Milos R, Goyette P, Sheppard CA, Matthew RG, Boers GA, den Heijer M, Kluijtmans LA, van den Heuve LP, Rozen R. A candidate genetic risk factor for vascular disease: a common mutation in methylenetetrahydrofolate reductase. *Nature Genetics* 1995;10:111-113.

[200] Kim RJ, Becker RC. Association between factor V Leiden, prothrombin G20210A, and methylenetetrahydrofolate reductase C677T mutations and events of the arterial circulatory system: a meta-analysis of published studies. *American Heart Journal* 2003; 146:948-957.

[201] Perry DJ. Hyperhomocysteinaemia. *Bailliere's Clinical Haematology* 1999;12:451-477.

[202] Bruschi F, Dal Pino D, Fiore V, Parazzini F, Di Pace R, Cesana BM, Melotti D, Crosignani PG. Effect of oral or transdermal hormone replacement therapy on homocysteine levels: a randomized clinical trial. *Maturitas* 2004;48:33-38.

[203] Cagnacci A, Tirelli A, Renzi A, Paoletti AM, Volpe A. Effects of two different oral contraceptives on homocysteine metabolism in women with polycystic ovary syndrome. *Contraception* 2006;73:348-351.

[204] Evio S, Tiitinen A, Turpeinen U, Ylikorkala O. Failure of the combination of sequential oral and transdermal estradiol plus norethisterone acetate to affect plasma homocysteine levels. *Fertility and Sterility* 2000;74:1080-1083.

[205] Lussana F, Zighetti ML, Bucciarelli P, Cugno M, Cattaneo M. Blood levels of homocysteine, folate, vitamin B_6 and B_{12} in women using oral contraceptives compared to non-users. *Thrombosis Research* 2003;112:37-41.

[206] Machado RB, Baracat EC, Fernandes CE, Lakryc EM, De Lima GR. Effects of estrogen and estrogen-progestogen therapy on homocysteine levels and their correlation with carotid vascular resistance. *Gynecological Endocrinology* 2007;23:619-624.

[207] Merki-Feld GS, Imthurn B, Keller PJ. Effects of two oral contraceptives on plasma levels of nitric oxide, homocysteine, and lipid metabolism. *Metabolism* 2002;51:1216-1221.

[208] Morris MS, Jacques PF, Selhub J, Rosenberg IH. Total homocysteine and estrogen status indicators in the Third National Health and Nutrition Examination Survey. *American Journal of Epidemiology* 2000;152:140-148.

[209] Tanis BC, Blom HJ, Bloemenkamp DGM, van den Bosch MAAJ, Algra A, van der Graaf Y, Rosendaal FR. Folate, homocysteine levels, methylenetetrahydrofolate reductase (MTHFR) 677C→T variant, and the risk of myocardial infarction in young women: effect of female hormones on homocysteine levels. *Journal of Thrombosis and Haemostasis* 2004;2:35-41.

[210] Beaumont V, Malinow MR, Sexton G, Wilson D, Lemort N, Upson B, Beaumont JL. Hyperhomocysteinemia, anti-estrogen antibodies and other risk factors for thrombosis in women on oral contraceptives. *Atherosclerosis* 1992;94:147-52.

[211] Steegers-Theunissen RP, Boers GH, Steegers EA, Trijbels FJ, Thomas CM, Eskes TK. Effects of sub-50 oral contraceptives on homocysteine metabolism: a preliminary study. *Contraception* 1992;45:129-139.

[212] Shojania AM. Oral contraceptives: effects on folate and vitamin B_{12} metabolism. *Canadian Medical Association Journal* 1982;126:244-247.

[213]Schwammenthal Y, Tanne D. Homocysteine, B-vitamin supplementation, and stroke prevention: from observational to interventional trials. *Lancet Neurology* 2004;3:493-495.

[214]Beaumont JL, Lemort N. Oral contraceptive, pulmonary artery thrombosis and anti-ethinyl-estradiol monoclonal IgG. *Clinical and Experimental Immunology* 1976; 24:455-463.

[215]Beaumont JL, Lemort N, Lorenzelli-Edouard L, Delplanque B, Beaumont V. Antiethinyloestradiol antibody activities in oral contraceptive users. *Clinical and Experimental Immunology* 1979; 38:445-452.

[216]Beaumont V, Lemort N, Lorenzelli L, Mosser A, Beaumont JL. Hormone contraceptives, vascular risk and abnormal precipitation of serum gamma-globulins. *Pathologie-Biologie* 1978; 26:531-537.

[217]Beaumont V, Lemort N, Beaumont JL. Oral contraceptives, sex steroid-induced antibodies and vascular thrombosis: results from 1318 cases. *European Heart Journal* 1991;12:1219-1224.

[218]Plowright C, Adam SA, Thorogood M, Beaumont V, Beaumont JL, Mann JI. Immunogenicity and the vascular risk of oral contraceptives. *British Heart Journal* 1985;53:556-561.

[219]Huang NH, Li C, Goldzieher JW. Absence of antibodies to ethinyl estradiol in users of oral contraceptive steroids. *Fertility and Sterility* 1984;41:587-592.

[220]Van den Brule FA, Coibion M, Hendrick JC, Gaspard UJ. Antisteroid immune complexes and vascular thrombosis during steroid hormone therapy. *Contraception* 1994;49:571-577.

[221]Sturfelt G, Mousa F, Jonsson H, Nived O, Thysell H, Wollheim F. Recurrent cerebral infarction and the antiphospholipid syndrome: effect of intravenous gammaglobulin in a patient with systemic lupus erythematosus. *Annals of Rheumatologic Disease* 1990; 49:939-941.

[222]Tarnacka B, Gromadzka G, Czlonkowska A. Increased circulating immune complexes in acute stroke: the triggering role of Chlamydia pneumoniae and cytomegalovirus. *Stroke* 2002;33:936-940.

[223]Curtis KM, Mohllajee AP, Martins SL, Peterson HB. Combined oral contraceptive use among women with hypertension: a systematic review. *Contraception* 2006; 73:179-188.

[224]Lokkegaard E, Jovanovic Z, Heitmann BL, Keiding N, Ottesen B, Hundrup YA, Obel EB, Pedersen AT. Increased risk of stroke in hypertensive women using hormone therapy: analyses based on the Danish Nurse Study. *Archives of Neurology* 2003; 60:1379-1384.

[225]American College of Obstetricians and Gynecologists (ACOG). The use ofhormonal contraception in women with coexisting medical conditions. Washington, D.C.: American College of Obstetricians and Gynecologists (ACOG); 2006 June 20: ACOG practice bulletin, number 73.

[226]Carolei A, Marini C, De Matteis G. History of migraine and risk of cerebral ischaemia in young adults. *Lancet* 1996; 347:1503-1506.

[227]Henrich JB, Horwitz RI. A controlled study of ischemic stroke risk in migraine patients. *Journal of Clinical Epidemiology* 1989;42:773-780.

[228]Merikangas KR, Fenton BT, Cheng SH, Stolar MJ, Risch N. Association between migraine and stroke in a large-scale epidemiological study of the United States. *Archives of Neurology* 1997;54:362-268.

[229]Tietjen GE. Migraine and ischaemic heart disease and stroke: potential mechanisms and treatment implications. *Cephaallgia* 2007;27:981-987.

[230]D'Amico D, Moschiano F, Leone M, Ariano C, Ciusani E, Erba E, Bussone G. Genetic abnormalities of the protein C system: shared risk factors in young adults with migraine with aura and with ischemic stroke? *Cephalalgia* 1998;18:618-621.

[231]Lea RA, Ovcaric M, Sundholm J, MacMillian J, Griffiths LR. The methylenetetrahydrofolate reductase gene variant C677T influences susceptibility to migraine with aura. *BMC Medicine* 2004;12:2-3.

[232]Chang CL, Donaghy M, Poulter N, World Health Organization Collaborative Study of Cardiovascular Disease and Steroid Hormone Contraception. Migraine and stroke in young women: case-control study. *British Medical Journal* 1999;318:13-18.

[233]Tzourio C, Tehindrazanarivelo A, Iglesias S, Alperovitch A, Chedru F, d'Anglejan-Chatillon J, Bousser M-G. Case-control study of migraine and risk of ischaemic stroke in young women. *British Medical Journal* 1995;310:830-833.

[234]Allais G, De Lorenzo C, Mana O, Benedetto C. Oral contraceptives in women with migraine: balancing risks and benefits. *Neurological Sciences* 2004;25:S211-S214.

[235]Bousser M-G, Conard J, Kittner S, de Lignieres B, MacGregor EA, Massiou H, Silberstein SD, Tzourio C. The International Headache Society Task Force on Combined Oral Contraceptive and Hormone Replacement Therapy. Recommendations on the risk of ischaemic stroke associated with use of combined oral contraceptives and hormone replacement therapy in women with migraine. *Cephalalgia* 2000;20:155-156.

[236]Pezzini A, Grassi M, Iacoviello L, Del Zotto E, Archetti S, Giossi A, Padovani A. Inherited thrombophilia and stratification of ischaemic stroke risk among users of oral contraceptives. *Journal of Neurology, Neurosurgery and Psychiatry* 2007;78:271-276.

[237]Martinelli I, Battaglioli T, Burgo I, Di Domenico SD, Mannucci PM. Oral contraceptive use, thrombophilia and their interaction in young women with ischemic stroke. *Haematologica* 2006;91:844-847.

[238]Abdolahi M, Cushman M, Rosendaal FR. Obesity: risk of venous thrombosis and the interaction with coagulation factor levels and oral contraceptive use. *Thrombosis and Haemostasis* 2003;89:493-498.

[239]Pomp ER, le Cessie S, Rosendaal FR, Doggen CJM. Risk of venous thrombosis: obesity and its joint effect with oral contraceptive use and prothrombotic mutations. *British Journal of Haemotology* 2007;139:289-296.

[240]Royal College of Obstetricians and Gynaecologists--Medical Specialty. Venous thromboembolism and hormonal contraception. 2004 Oct. (Guideline; Number 40).

[241]Cosmi B, Legnani C, Bernardi F, Coccheri S, Palareti G. Value of family history in identifying women at risk of venous thromboembolism during oral contraception: observational study. *British Medical Journal* 2001;322:1024-1025.

[242]Davie CA, P'Brien P. Stroke and Pregnancy. *Journal of Neurology, Neurosurgery and Psychiatry* 2008;79:240-245.

[243]Kittner SJ, Stern BJ, Feeser BR, Hebel R, Nagey DA, Buchholz DW, Earley CJ, Johnson CJ, Macko RF, Sloan MA, Wityk RJ, Wozniak MA. Pregnancy and the risk of stroke. *New England Journal of Medicine* 1996;335:768-774.

In: Cerebral Ischemia in Young Adults
Editors: A. Pezzini and A. Padovani
ISBN 978-1-60741-627-2

Chapter 5

Drug Abuse and Stroke

Sean D Treadwell[1] and Bhomraj Thanvi
Department of Integrated Medicine, University Hospitals of Leicester NHS Trust,
Leicester Royal Infirmary, Leicester, UK

Abstract

The growing number of case reports describing illicit drug-related stroke, and the increasing evidence supporting this aetiological link, suggests that drug abuse should always be considered as a possible cause of cerebral ischemia, especially in younger patients and in patients who lack other known vascular risk factors. Actually, illicit drug use has been causally implicated in less than 10% of all cerebral infarctions in hospital series, and in up to 40% of infarctions in young patients. Toxicology screening should therefore be included alongside standard investigations in this group, or when a history of substance misuse is suspected. Of the illicit substances used, cocaine, opiates, amphetamines, phencyclidine, and marijuana have all been reported in association with ischemic stroke, and will be considered in the present chapter.

Introduction

Consumption of drugs for recreational purposes has been observed for thousands of years. The term 'drug abuse' is defined by the World Health Organization as 'persistent or sporadic excessive use inconsistent with or unrelated to medical practice' [1], and more recently the term 'harmful use' has been introduced to suggest a pattern of use which causes mental or physical harm. 'Drug misuse' is an alternative phrase, though suggests value judgements and carries implications according to the type of drug, social acceptability, illegality, or harmfulness. The term 'drug use' is often used, with an appropriate adjective to

[1] Correspondence: Sean D Treadwell, e-mail: seantreadwell@hotmail.com.

clarify the context in which a drug is taken, for example 'illegal', 'non-medical', or 'hazardous'.

As well as the desired psychotropic effects, drugs consumed for recreational purposes also exhibit a number of adverse effects relating to both acute toxicity and chronic use. Stroke associated with drug abuse has been reported frequently, and illicit drug use has been causally implicated in 6% of all cerebral infarctions in some hospital series [2], and in 15 to 40% of infarctions in young patients [3]. In the younger age group, thrombo-embolism and intracranial small vessel disease are unlikely, and so the less common causes of stroke including drug abuse become increasingly more important.

The involvement of a drug should be suspected whenever there is a temporal relationship between exposure and stroke onset, and support for an aetiological link has come primarily from case reports and cases series. In many cases, abuse of the alleged substance is the most likely cause of stroke but in some cases the association is somewhat less secure. The increased risk of stroke may be due to direct effects of the substance or adulterants used, or complications due to the method of administration and associated medical problems. Social and life-style factors associated with drug addiction may also play an indirect role in the increased risk. Pathophysiology remains incompletely understood and in individual cases it may be difficult to define an underlying mechanism, though multiple factors are likely to be involved. Stroke has been associated with abuse of several illicit and prescription drugs, but most commonly implicated substances include cocaine, amphetamines and opiates.

Cocaine

Background

In England and Wales cocaine is the most commonly used Class A drug. It is derived from the leaves of the Erythroxylon Coca plant found in South America, and its use dates back thousands of years. Coca leaves have been chewed by Peruvian Indians for centuries and remnants of chewed coca leaves have been found near gravestones as far back as 2500 BC.

In 1859 the purification of cocaine was achieved by a German chemist called Albert Niemann. It became widely available towards the end of the 19th century, with no laws restricting sale or consumption. Cocaine was sold in a number of forms including cigarettes, inhalers and cocaine crystals [4,5], and in 1884 Sigmund Freud published a paper advocating the therapeutic use of cocaine as a stimulant, an aphrodisiac, a local anaesthetic and a remedy for a number of disorders including asthma, wasting diseases and nervous exhaustion [6]. Angelo Mariani added cocaine to his own blend of wine, and at the end of the 19th century, John Styth Pemberton reformulated cocaine with caffeine which was advertised as a 'brain tonic', and eventually became known as 'Coca-cola'. Until 1903, this contained approximately 60mg of cocaine per serving. The increased availability led to misuse and subsequent addiction which resulted in the Harrison Narcotics Act of 1914, banning the distribution of cocaine except on prescription.

In the early 1970s cocaine was re-discovered as a recreational drug, and the perception at this time was that cocaine was safe and non-addictive. In fact, even the medical literature supported this idea stating that 'used no more than two or three times a week, cocaine creates no serious problems' [7]. The hydrochloride salt is taken by nasal inhalation, though in the 1980s a more potent alkaloidal form called 'crack' emerged which was relatively inexpensive and could be smoked.

Pharmocology

Cocaine (benzoylmethylecgonine) is a weak base extracted from Coca leaves of the Erythroxylon plant which is ground into a paste and contains 70% pure cocaine. It is usually treated with hydrochloric acid to form cocaine hydrochloride salt which is water soluble and can therefore be absorbed through the nasal mucosa. However, because of its high melting and boiling point it cannot be smoked. Cocaine alkaloid exists as freebase and crack which are chemically identical, though differ in their method of preparation. The melting point is 98 degrees centigrade, and heating converts cocaine to a stable vapour which can therefore be inhaled [4]. Crack is made by dissolving cocaine hydrochloride into water, mixing it with baking soda, and then heating which results in a hard precipitant [8].

Cocaine can be absorbed through any mucous membrane, smoked or injected [8]. In the 1970s the most common route of administration was nasal inhalation of cocaine hydrochloride resulting in peak levels at around 60 minutes. Using this method, uptake is limited by the small available surface area, and associated vasoconstriction of the nasal mucosa [8,9]. Crack cocaine which emerged in the 1980s can be smoked and is therefore more rapidly absorbed by the pulmonary vasculature reaching peak levels at 5-10 minutes.

Cocaine has a short half life of approximately 60 minutes, and is metabolized primarily by the liver into two products, benzoylecgonine and ecgonine methyl ester [8,9]. If taken with alcohol, a transesterification process leads to the production of cocaethylene which has similar pharmacological properties to cocaine [10], so prolonging the euphoria. The short half life of cocaine means that it is usually fully metabolized by the time it is excreted, and therefore not usually found in the urine. Its two main metabolites, benzoylecgonine and ecgonine methyl ester, can be detected in the urine for 6-14 days after cocaine use [11], and screening reagents are therefore designed to detect these.

Cocaine causes vasoconstriction, local anaesthesia and central nervous system stimulation, and sympathomimetic effects are achieved by blocking the re-uptake of catecholamines at the pre-synaptic sympathetic nerve terminals [10]. Cocaine induces euphoria and central nervous system stimulation by preventing the re-uptake of dopamine and serotonin into pre-synaptic neurones within the mesolimbic and mesocortical areas of the brain [10]. The anaesthetic effect of cocaine results from slowing of nerve conduction due to blockage of fast sodium channels [10]. Following chronic use, the body's reservoirs of neurotransmitters may deplete and therefore chronic users may experience features of tolerance and withdrawal [12].

Clinical Features

Cocaine is a potent central nervous stimulant, and initial euphoria is associated with restlessness, hyperactivity, increased sensory awareness, enhanced self confidence, and reduced appetite. Sexual pleasure may be amplified, and the euphoria is occasionally followed by feelings of discomfort and depression. Sympathomimetic effects result in elevated blood pressure and heart rate, and cause symptoms of sweating, palpitations, tremor and hyperthermia. Cocaine toxicity may manifest in a variety of ways [13-28], and often depend upon the dose and route of administration, the purity of the sample and the chronicity of use. The major medical complications associated with both acute and chronic cocaine use are outlined in Table 1.

The first report of stroke related to cocaine use was in 1977 by Brust and Richter [29]. Intramuscular administration in a male user was followed one hour later by aphasia and right sided hemiparesis. During the 1980s, increased production of alkaloidal 'crack', and the subsequent epidemic led to a significant increase in the number of case reports of cocaine-related stroke. The onset of symptoms is usually immediate or within 3 hours of cocaine use [30-33], and 73% of patients with cocaine-induced stroke have no prior cardiovascular risk factors [30].

Table 1. Medical complications of cocaine abuse

Cardiac	Neurology
• Cardiac arrest	• Stroke
• Myocardial infarction	• Seizures
• Arrhythmias	• Headache
• Myocarditis	• Cerebral atrophy
• Cardiomyopathy	• Cerebral vasculitis
Pulmonary	Head and neck
• Pneumothorax	• Enamel erosion
• Pneumomediastinum	• Gingival ulceration
• Pulmonary oedema	• Chronic rhinitis
• Pulmonary haemorrhage	• Osteolytic sinusitis
• Bronchiolitis obliterans	• Abnormal olfaction
Psychiartic	• Perforated nasal septum
• Anxiety and depression	• Midline granuloma
• Paranoia	Gastrointestinal
• Delirium	• Ischaemic colitis
• Psychosis	Other
Endocrine	• Rhabdomyolysis
• Gynaecomastia	• Optic neuropathy
• Galactorrhoea	• Arterial and venous thrombosis
• Sexual dysfunction	• Weight loss

Cocaine is associated with both ischaemic and haemorrhagic stroke and early studies suggested a higher proportion of haemorrhagic events related to cocaine use. Since then, reports of cocaine-induced stroke have demonstrated roughly equal proportions of ischaemic and haemorrhagic events. The differences noted are likely to be due to the type of cocaine used. 80% of strokes related the hydrochloride form are haemorrhagic, as compared to alkaloidal 'crack' which was developed later in the 1980s, and results in equal numbers of ischaemic and haemorrhagic stroke [34]. In 1994, Daras et al studied 54 patients over a 6 year period that developed either acute neurological deficit or headache with signs of meningeal irritation after cocaine use [30]. Ischaemic and haemorrhagic strokes occurred in roughly equal proportions with 25 infarcts and 29 haemorrhages.

Cocaine-induced strokes have been reported in both anterior and posterior arterial territories, and ischaemic events have included retinal infarction, spinal cord infarction and transient ischaemic attacks [30,33,35-39]. Haemorrhagic strokes have been intraparechymal, intraventricular and subarachnoid [30,33,37,40,41].

Mechanisms of Stroke

The underlying mechanism of cocaine related stroke remains unclear and is likely to be multi-factorial. There does not appear to be a direct neurotoxic action [42], and potential mechanisms involved in cocaine induced stroke include vasospasm, cerebral vasculitis, enhanced platelet aggregation, cardio-embolism, and hypertensive surges associated with altered cerebral autoregulation and cerebral blood flow.

Animal studies have demonstrated increased platelet activation in response to cocaine administration [43], and cocaine in vitro causes an enhanced response of platelets to arachadonic acid, leading to increased thromboxane production and platelet aggregation [44]. However, data regarding in-vitro studies have been conflicting, also demonstrating a decrease [45], and no change [46] in platelet aggregation in response to cocaine.

Acute platelet rich thrombi have been described in fatal cocaine related infarcts in both normal and atherosclerotic coronary vessels [47]. It has also been suggested that the repeated release of cell growth factors by cocaine activated platelets might promote atherosclerosis in the setting of chronic cocaine use [48]. Heesch et al demonstrated platelet activation, alpha granule release and platelet containing microaggregate formation with decreased bleeding time following in vivo cocaine administration to healthy volunteers, even at low doses [49]. Reduced regional cerebral blood flow has been demonstrated in association with increased platelet aggregation in cocaine dependant patients, with significant improvement of hypoperfusion after abstinence [50].

Cocaine prevents the re-uptake of noradrenaline, serotonin and dopamine at pre-synaptic nerve terminals and is therefore a potent vasoconstrictor due to its sympathomimetic action. It also has direct effects on calcium channels, promoting intracellular calcium release from the sarcoplasmic reticulum in cerebral vascular smooth muscle cells [51]. Animal studies have demonstrated significant increase in free calcium concentration in cultured canine cerebral vascular smooth muscle cells treated with cocaine [52]. Cocaine induced vasospasm has been suggested by cerebral angiography in several patients with cocaine related ischaemic strokes

[31,33,34,35,53], and this response has also been reported in several animal studies, where angiographic evidence of vasospasm severe enough to cause vascular occlusion was demonstrated [54-58]. Johnson et al [59] established that cocaine induced cerebral vasospasm was relatively specific to dopamine rich brain areas and hypothesized that dopamine pathways play a central role in controlling cerebral blood flow. Vasospasm and ischaemia in cocaine users may therefore be related to the increased availability of dopamine in these areas.

A decrease in cerebral glucose metabolism occurs following cocaine administration [60], and cocaine induced reductions in cerebral metabolism may therefore lead to feedback down regulation of blood flow [61]. Volkow et al found there to be more areas of decreased cerebral blood flow in chronic cocaine users compared to healthy volunteers [62], though the significance of abnormal patterns of cerebral blood flow in cocaine users in relation to stroke remains unclear.

The arteriosclerotic toxicity of cocaine has been demonstrated in animal studies [56], and advanced atherosclerosis has been observed in the renal arteries and aorta of cocaine users [63]. Cerebral vascular thrombosis may result secondary to vasospasm, and it has been suggested that vasospasm results in endothelial injury and platelet aggregation with subsequent release of smooth muscle growth factor and obstructive intimal hyperplasia [64]. The same pathophysiological process may also occur in intracerebral vessels of cocaine users leading to cocaine-induced infarction. Konzen et al reported 3 cases whose angiographic and pathological data suggested that vasospasm with secondary thrombus formation may be an important mechanism of cocaine induced cerebral infarction [65]. Histology in one of these cases demonstrated small calibre intracerebral arteries with markedly infolded and irregular internal elastica lamina in multiple territories, presumably related to cocaine induced vasoconstriction.

Cardio-embolism may provide another mechanism for cocaine related stroke. Petty et al reported a 39 year old female with onset of left hemiparesis due to embolic upper division middle cerebral artery branch occlusion 3 hours after smoking crack cocaine [66]. Cerebral emboli with subsequent infarction can originate from cardiac thrombi which form during cocaine induced myocardial infarction [67], and case reports have also documented embolic stroke secondary to cocaine related cardiomyopathy [66,68]. Experiments on isolated myocytes exposed to cocaine demonstrated prolongation of the transmembrane action potential, providing a possible mechanism for cocaine arrhythmogenesis [69]. Prolongation of the QT interval has also been noted in patients presenting with cocaine toxicity [70]. Contaminants mixed with cocaine may provide a further mechanism for cardio-embolism due to arrhythmia. As with any substance injected intravenously, cocaine administered by this route can predispose to endocarditis, resulting in embolic vessel occlusion [26,27] or haemorrhagic stroke following rupture of a septic aneurysm [71-73].

Cerebral vasculitis following cocaine use may result in ischaemic stroke. Vasculitis has previously been attributed to cocaine on the basis of typical findings of arterial beading on cerebral arteriography [32,74]. Angiographic arterial beading is a non specific sign of vascular injury and should not necessarily be attributed to vasculitis [75], though cases of histologically confirmed cerebral vasculitis associated with cocaine use have also been described [76]. Vasculitis has been demonstrated in other drug-induced strokes, especially those related to amphetamines [77]. These can cause an inflammatory vasculopathy with vessel wall necrosis potentially leading to vessel wall rupture [78]. Amphetamines have a similar mechanism of action to cocaine by increasing the availability of catecholamines at nerve terminals, and so there may be similarities in terms of the aetiology of the vasculitic changes. It should be noted that amphetamines may also be present as adulterants in cocaine preparations.

Cocaine use is associated with both intracerebral haemorrhage [79], and subarachnoid haemorrhage [80,81]. By blocking the re-uptake of catecholamines at pre-synaptic nerve endings, cocaine use results in tachycardia and marked transient increases in blood pressure [82,83]. Cerebral autoregulation maintains constant cerebral blood flow despite fluctuations in arterial blood pressure, although above this upper limit blood flow may increase resulting in a risk of arterial rupture [84,85]. Cocaine disturbs cerebral autoregulation by lowering this upper limit of blood pressure at which constant cerebral blood flow is maintained [86], therefore increasing flow and predisposing to vascular rupture. This disturbance of cerebral autoregulation may also result in re-perfusion injury and haemorrhagic transformation of an infarct [79,87].

78% of patients with cocaine-related subarachnoid haemorrhage, and 48% of patients with cocaine-related intracerebral haemorrhage have an underlying vascular abnormality [79], and post-mortem studies have also demonstrated a higher incidence of hypertensive cardiovascular disease in cocaine-induced haemorrhagic stroke [40,41]. Positive toxicology for cocaine was demonstrated in 59% of 17 non-traumatic haemorrhagic strokes, with no pathological evidence of an underlying vasculopathy [40]. Evidence suggests that cocaine-induced haemorrhagic stroke may result as a consequence of the haemodynamic effects of cocaine in a susceptible sub-group of individuals.

Amphetamines

Background

Amphetamine was first synthesized in 1887 by a German chemist called Lazar Edeleanu. The term amphetamine is derived from its chemical name alpha-methylphenethylamine, and is also used to refer to the compounds derived from amphetamine, the so-called substituted amphetamines. Its pharmacological use remained unknown until 1927 when Gordon Alles, a psychopharmacologist who was looking for an ephedrine substitute resynthesized it. Although originally used as a bronchodilator in 1930s, its central nervous system stimulant effects were soon recognized. During World War II, amphetamines were given to soldiers and pilots to fight off fatigue. Pharmacological uses of amphetamines included treatment of asthma, narcolepsy, and attention deficit disorders. Due to their stimulant effects, amphetamines soon became popular substances of abuse, leading to legal restriction on their use by the medicine regulatory agencies. In the United Kingdom, it is illegal to produce, supply or possess these drugs, and amphetamine is a Class B drug but carries Class A penalties if prepared for injection. In the United States, amphetamine and methamphetamine are Schedule II controlled drugs.

Table 2. Amphetamine compounds and common street names

Compound	Street names
• Amphetamine	hearts, black beauties
• Dextroamphetamine	dex
• Methamphetamine	meth, chalk, speed, crank
• Dextromethamphetamine	ice
• Methamphetamine hydrochloride	crystal, glass
• 3, 4-methylenedioxymethamphetamine (MDMA)	ecstasy
• Methamphetamine and heroin combined	speed balls

Despite legal restrictions, amphetamines continued to be popular substances of abuse. Data from Office of Applied Studies Substance Abuse and Mental Health Services Administration (OAS- SAMHS) in the United States showed that between 1995 and 2005 the percentage of substance abuse treatment admissions for primary abuse of amphetamine more than doubled from 4% to 9% [88]. Ecstasy is an amphetamine derivative that has gained significant popularity in recent years and has become the recreational drug of choice for many adolescents and young adults. Its use in the UK has dramatically increased over the past few years and it is suggested that ecstasy users are poised to overtake the combined number of heroin and cocaine users.

Pharmacology

Amphetamine is the parent compound of its own structural class with a basic phenylethylamine structure. Amphetamine-like compounds are derived from modifications of this basic structure, and the compounds most commonly used for recreational purposes along with their popular street names are outlined in Table 2. Other amphetamine-like drugs include methylphenidate (Ritalin), ephedrine, pseudoephedrine, phenylpropanolamine, and a large number of other agents marketed as nasal decongestants and appetite suppressants.

The structure of amphetamines is similar to that of the naturally occurring neurotransmitter molecules epinephrine and dopamine which are involved in a variety of physiological responses such as ‘fight-or-flight’ and feelings of pleasure. Amphetamines are weak bases that are easily absorbed through the airways, nasopharynx, gut, vagina, and placenta. The half-life in humans ranges from 10 to 30 hours depending on the drug, dosage, and urinary pH [89]. The duration of action is much longer than for cocaine and amphetamine-induced euphoria lasts four to eight times longer. Peak plasma levels occur 30 minutes after intravenous or intramuscular injection, and 2 to 3 hours after oral ingestion.

Amphetamines are indirect-acting sympathomimetics and increase the concentration of bioamines (dopamine, noradrenaline, and serotonin) in the synaptic cleft. This is done by several mechanisms: by binding to the pre-synaptic membrane of dopaminergic neurones promoting the release of dopamine from the nerve terminal; by binding to the dopamine re-uptake transporter causing it to act in reverse and transport free dopamine out of the nerve terminal; by binding to monoamine oxidase (MAO) in dopaminergic neurones preventing the degradation of dopamine; and by interacting with dopamine containing synaptic vesicles releasing free dopamine into the nerve terminal. Amphetamines also have a similar effect on noradrenergic and serotonergic neurones, though the main behavioural and stimulant effects are related to increased dopaminergic activity, primarily in the mesolimbic dopamine system.

Recently, the role of a novel mediator called trace amine-associated receptor 1 (TAAR1) has been proposed to explain some of the effects of amphetamines [90]. TAAR1 is a G protein-coupled receptor activated by a broad range of monoamines and amphetamine-related psychostimulants [91]. Recent studies have demonstrated a wide distribution of TAAR1 in the brain, coexpression of TAAR1 with dopamine transporter (DAT) in a subset of dopamine neurones in mouse and rhesus monkey substantia nigra, and monoamine transporter-modulated activation [91]. TAAR1 may be involved in functional regulation of DAT and hence may potentially serve as an important target for the treatment of methamphetamine addiction [91].

Clinical Features

Acute physiological effects of amphetamines include an increase in heart rate, blood pressure, stamina, alertness, and libido. Sweating, nausea, headaches, and decreased hunger are also features. Toxic and long term effects are outlined in Table 3, and fatalities have been reported after ingestion of even low doses of methamphetamine [92].

Table 3. Complications of amphetamine abuse

Cardiac	Neurological
• Cardiac arrest	• Stroke
• Myocardial infarction	• Cerebral vasculitis
• Arrhythmias	• Cerebral oedema
• Hypertension	• Headache
• Cardiomyopathy	• Seizures
Psychiatric	• Choreoathetoid movement
• Anxiety and depression	Other
• Paranoia	• Metabolic acidosis
• Psychosis	• Rhabdomyolysis
• Aggression	• Hyperpyrexia
• Suicidal ideation	• Acute renal failure
• Euphoria	• Disseminated intravascular coagulation
Respiratory	• Refractory hypotension
• Tachypnoea	• Dental problems
• Pulmonary oedema	
• Pulmonary hypertension	

Intracerebral haemorrhage associated with amphetamine abuse was first described in 1945 [93]. Since then several cases of amphetamine related stroke have been reported, with haemorrhagic stroke far more common than cerebral infarction. In fact, in a population-based study of patients hospitalized with substance abuse, multivariate logistic regression models demonstrated that amphetamines were strongly associated with haemorrhagic stroke, but not with ischaemic stroke [94]. The same data suggested that amphetamine abuse was associated with twice the risk of haemorrhagic stroke than cocaine abuse, and amphetamines, but not cocaine, were associated with a higher risk of death after haemorrhagic stroke. Phenylpropranolamine (PPA) and pseudoephedrine are sympathomimetic amines structurally similar to amphetamines which are present in many over-the-counter cough and cold preparations, and have also been associated with an increased risk of stroke, particularly PPA with haemorrhagic stroke [95].

Examples of reported cases of stroke related to amphetamine use include a 21-year old female who complained of headache and right arm parasthesia a couple of hours after taking ecstasy [96]. She awoke the next morning with aphasia and a right hemiparesis, and computerized tomography (CT) demonstrated a large left fronto-parietal haematoma with mass effect. At craniotomy, a small angioma was demonstrated which was thought to be the source of the bleed. A 54-year old male amphetamine user found dead had a massive central pontine haematoma at post-mortem [97], and methamphetamine was detected in blood samples. A young female presented with a left hemiparesis and right frontal intracranial haemorrhage (ICH) following the ingestion of just a small quantity of amphetamine [98]. An 18-year old man with a prior history of drug abuse presented with headache after taking amphetamine. CT and angiogram appearances were normal, though cerebrospinal fluid analysis confirmed the presence of a subarachnoid haemorrhage [99]. Seizures were the presenting feature in two young men following amphetamine use, and CT confirmed left parietal ICH in one [100], and subarachnoid haemorrhage in the other [101]. Right temporal ICH in association with an arteriovenous malformation (AVM) was demonstrated in a 28-year old man presenting with blurred vision and headache following intravenous amphetamine use [102]. Amphetamine-induced ischaemic stroke was reported in a young woman with acute left middle cerebral artery distribution infarction [103], and in a 16-year old boy presenting with generalized seizures [104]. Ischaemic stroke has also been reported in a young man following intranasal use of amphetamine combined with caffeine [105], and following recreational use of ecstasy [106].

ICH may follow amphetamines administration via any route, though oral ingestion and smoking have been most commonly reported in the published series. Severe headache is common within a few minutes of drug exposure, and blood pressure is often elevated. In a case series of amphetamine-induced cerebral haemorrhage, the characteristics of 45 patients reported between 1945 and 2000 were identified [107]. The mean age was 28 years (median 26, range 16-60), and most patients were repeat abusers. Of the 25 patients who underwent CT, 21 (84%) demonstrated ICH, 3 had subarachnoid haemorrhage, and 1 had a brainstem haemorrhage. In the 35 patients who underwent angiography, 20 were normal, 16 showed beading suggestive of vasculitis, and 1 showed AVM. In many cases of amphetamine-related stroke, the event has occurred on a background of chronic use, though has also been reported in some individuals after a single low dose exposure [108-110].

Mechanisms of Stroke

Mechanisms likely to play a major role in stroke related to amphetamine abuse include acute hypertension, cerebral vasculitis, or a combination of the two.

Complications are thought to be primarily mediated through excess catecholamines, and hypertension is commonly observed in patients with amphetamine-related ICH. The close temporal relationship between exposure and the onset of symptoms supports the role of drug-induced systemic hypertension as a contributory factor, though documented elevations in blood pressure may also be a consequence of the stroke itself. The presence of cerebral aneurysm [111] and AVM [102] identified following amphetamine-related ICH suggests the possibility of catecholamine-induced hypertensive surges in susceptible patients.

Cerebral vasculitis is thought to play a significant role in the pathogenesis of amphetamine-related stroke. This is based primarily on radiological studies, and characteristic angiographic findings associated with vasculitis include extensive irregular segmental narrowing or beading of small arteries [112]. Based on the temporal sequence of arterial stenosis with complete resolution by 3 months and a characteristic beaded appearance on angiography, vasculitis with local thrombus formation was presumed to be a possible mechanism of ischaemic stroke in a young lady who abused amphetamine [103]. The transcranial Doppler showed the presence of microembolic signals, suggesting an acute thrombosis at the site of vasculitis with distal embolism. In a case series of amphetamine-induced cerebral haemorrhage, of the 35 patients who underwent angiography, 16 showed a typical beading pattern suggestive of vasculitis [107]. In a radiographic study of 19 drug abusers admitted with either stroke or coma, widespread segmental constriction of large and medium sized cerebral arteries was noted. Most, but not all were taking intravenous methamphetamine, suggesting that these changes may also be associated with other substances. Angiographic arterial beading has in fact been reported with other substances including cocaine [74], though it should also be noted that this can be a non-specific sign of vascular injury and should not necessarily be attributed to vasculitis [75]. A similar angiographic appearance of segmental vasoconstriction may also occur following subarachnoid haemorrhage, though this tends to affect the trunks of major cerebral arteries with relative sparing of the distal branches.

Histological confirmation of cerebral vasculitis has been demonstrated in a 54-year amphetamine abuser who suffered a fatal pontine haemorrhage [97]. Necrotizing angiitis characterized by fibrinoid necrosis of the intima and media, and cell infiltration was observed. Necrotizing angiitis has also been demonstrated in 14 multi-drug abusers, all but two of whom had used intravenous methamphetamine [78], and hypersensitivity angiitis in an amphetamine abuser with mononeuritis multiplex has been demonstrated on sural nerve biopsy [113].

Animal studies have demonstrated changes in cerebral vasculature in response to amphetamines. Rhesus monkeys given intravenous methamphetamine demonstrated irregularity of small cerebral arteries within 10 minutes of administration, with a return to normal within 24 hours [114]. Pathological examination included subarachnoid haemorrhage, petechial haemorrhages, oedema, infarcts, and perivascular white cell infiltration. Electron microscopy studies in rats demonstrated abnormalities in the luminal walls of cerebral endothelial cells and vesicle formation within the cytoplasm following methamphetamine administration [115].

The pathogenesis of cerebral vasculitis in amphetamine abuse is unclear and may be the result of direct toxicity or hypersensitivity. A man with subarachnoid haemorrhage following ephedrine use and vasculitic beading pattern on cerebral angiography demonstrated IgM deposits and C3 complement in dermal vessels following a skin biopsy, suggesting an immune mediated reaction [116]. Particulate contaminants in injected solutes may also play a role in the pathogenesis of vasculitis, though this would not explain similar changes observed following other routes of administration.

Hyper-pyrexia is a recognized complication of amphetamine toxicity, and may be a factor contributing to the increased risk of ICH [117,118]. Heat stroke in humans may be complicated by coagulation abnormalities and ICH, and animal studies have demonstrated haemorrhagic changes in the brain following severe hyper-pyrexia associated with lethal doses of amphetamines [119].

Opiates

Background

Opium is the parent drug of this class, the name of which originates from the Greek name for juice. It is obtained from the opium poppy plant *Papaver somniferum*, which grows in large areas of South-East Asia and the Middle East. Exudate from the unripe seed capsules is dried and powdered, forming crude opium. The opium poppy was cultivated as long ago as 3400 BC in lower Mesopotamia, and in 330 BC Alexander the Great introduced opium to the people of Persia and India. In 1680 the English physician Thomas Sydenham introduced Sydenham's Laudanum, a compound of opium, sherry wine and herbs, which became a popular remedy for numerous ailments. The active ingredient of opium, morphine was discovered in 1803, and codeine was later extracted in 1832. Throughout the 1800s opium preparations were readily available without restriction. Heroin was first synthesized in 1874 by the English chemist C.R.Wright by boiling morphine with acetic anhydride over a stove. The Bayer Company of Elberfield, Germany, began production of diacetylmorphine in 1895, under the name of 'heroin', probably derived from the word 'heroisch', German for heroic. Heroin was marketed as a non-addictive morphine substitute, though at the beginning of the 1900s the associated side effects and withdrawal symptoms became more apparent, and heroin addiction rose to alarming rates. Passage of the Harrison Narcotics Act in 1914 aimed to control the distribution of heroin, and subsequent legislation banned the sale and manufacture of heroin in the United States, opening up a thriving black market throughout the 1900s. In the United Kingdom, heroin is a legal prescription drug under the name 'diamorphine'.

Table 4. Different opioid drugs

Naturally occurring	Synthetic
• Morphine	• Pethidine
• Codeine	• Methadone
Semi-synthetic	• Fentanyl
• Diamorphine	• Dextropropoxyphene
• Buprenorphine	• Dipipanone
• Dihydrocodeine	• Dextromoramide

Pharmacology

Opium contains two classes of natural alkaloids: phenanthrene (morphine and codeine) and benzylisoquinoline (papaverine and noscapine). Traditionally, these naturally occurring substances were referred to as 'opiates' while the synthetic drugs derived from them were called 'opioids', though these terms are now often used interchangeably. Examples of different opioid drugs are shown in Table 4.

Three major subtypes of opioid receptors are known, designated mu, kappa, and delta. These are present in all vertebrates, and endogenous opioid peptides idendified in humans include encephalins, beta-endorphin, and dynorphin. The analgesic properties of opioids appear to be mediated by supraspinal activation of mu receptors and activation of kappa receptors in the spinal cord.

Heroin (diacetylmorphine) is a semi-synthetic opioid first synthesized in 1874, and is derived from morphine by acetylation of the phenolic and alcoholic OH groups. In its pure form, heroin is a white powder with a bitter taste. Heroin is usually administered parenterally, though it may be taken orally, sublingually, subcutaneously, rectally, snorted or smoked. It is highly lipid membrane soluble and rapidly absorbed by the blood-brain barrier creating a sensation of intense pleasure within one minute when injected intravenously. The half-life of heroin is 15-30 minutes, and it is rapidly deacetylated to morphine and 6-monoacetylmorphine (MAM) by the liver, brain and kidneys. Heroin is eliminated in the urine as free morphine and a glucuronide product, and small amounts of unchanged MAM may be detected.

Clinical Features

In addition to the therapeutic analgesic effects, opioid use may result in a number of unwanted effects including drowsiness, respiratory depression, pupillary constriction, nausea and constipation due to reduced gastric motility, hypotension, cutaneous vasodilatation, urinary retention, and pruritis resulting from histamine release.

Continued use of opioids for either therapeutic or recreational purposes usually results in tolerance to many of the effects of the drug, requiring increased doses in order to obtain the same desired effect. Physical dependence may then occur if drug administration is regular, though may only become apparent if the drug is stopped or an opioid antagonist is used. This results in a typical withdrawal syndrome, the severity of which indicates the degree of physical dependence that had developed. The first signs of withdrawal include sweating, lacrimation and yawning, followed by muscle aches, anorexia, irritability, and goose flesh. Abdominal cramps, vomiting, insomnia, tachycardia, tachypnoea, and low grade fever then occur at 2-3 days. The syndrome can be immediately relieved by opioid administration, though untreated resolves after about one week.

Drug overdose and heroin toxicity may occur if there has been an increase in the usual administered dose, or heroin has been used again after a prolonged period of abstinence. Deaths from opioid overdose are usually caused by respiratory depression [120]. A number of complications involving all major systems are associated with both acute and long-term opioid abuse [71,121-141], the major ones outlined in Table 5.

Table 5. Medical complications of heroin abuse

Cardiac	Infections (in intravenous users)
• Cardiac arrest	• Bacterial endocarditis
• Myocardial infarction	• Intracranial abscess
• Arrhythmias	• Meningitis
• Hypotension	• HIV
Pulmonary	• Hepatitis B and C
• Non-cardiogenic pulmonary oedema	• Tetanus
• Respiratory depression/ arrest	• Osteomyelitis
• Bronchospasm	• Tuberculosis
Neurology	• Cellulitis
• Stroke	• Local abscess formation
• Myelopathy	Vascular injury (from injection sites)
• Seizures	• Pseudoaneurysms
• Post-anoxic encephalopathy	• Arterial dissection
• Guillain-Barre syndrome	Other
• Spongiform leukoencephalopathy	• Deafness
Gastrointestinal	• Vestibular dysfunction
• Constipation	• SIADH
• Anorexia	• Rhabdomyolysis
• Malnutrition	• Trauma/ violence
Renal	• Anaphylaxis
• Heroin associated nephropathy	• Compartment syndrome
• Nephrotic syndrome	• Reduced libido
• Glomerulonephritis	• Focal myopathy following injection
• Renal amyloid	

Stroke has been well documented as a complication of heroin abuse. In 1976, Brust and Richter reported a case series of nine heroin addicts between the ages 25 to 45 years presenting with stroke [142], and since then numerous similar cases have been described. Ischaemic stroke, intracerebral haemorrhage, and subarachnoid haemorrhage have all been reported in relation to heroin use, and stroke has occurred following both intravenous [143] and nasal [144] administration. Often, stroke occurs immediately following heroin administration, though if associated with overdose and coma may not become clinically apparent until recovery, when conscious level improves [145]. In this instance it may be difficult to determine the extent to which coma and respiratory depression have contributed to the neurological deficit. Stroke has also been reported several hours following heroin use [143], and may also occur unrelated to administration in chronic users [142]. Two of the patients reported by Brust and Richter [142] had a stroke following initiation of methadone maintenance treatment.

Examples of stroke reported in heroin abusers include that of a 30-year old man who developed right sided hemiparesis and aphasia due to a left anterior choroidal territory infarct 3 hours after sniffing a dose of heroin [146]. A 54-year old woman with a 35 years history of intravenous heroin abuse presented with a subarachnoid haemorrhage following cervical intra-arterial heroin injection [139]. A 20-year old man developed a left homonymous hemianopia immediately following his first intravenous injection of heroin in 8 months [147]. Infarction of the globus pallidus was reported in an adolescent who presented with respiratory failure and seizures after snorting an unknown quantity of heroin [148]. Left sided hemiballismus was reported in a 19-year old heroin addict following intravenous heroin overdose [145]. Magnetic resonance imaging (MRI) showed an infarct in the right striatum, and ballistic movements ceased after treatment with haloperidol. A man who injected heroin for the first time in two years developed quadriplegia, dysphagia, and sensory loss compatible with a pontine lesion following recovery from coma, though whether or not this represented a vascular aetiology remained undetermined [149]. Other presentations related to heroin administration which have been reported include oculogyric crisis and generalized dystonia [150], cortical blindness [151], mixed transcortical aphasia [152], and cerebellar ataxia [153].

Mechanisms of Stroke

Potential mechanisms of stroke occurring in opiate abusers include direct toxic effects relating either to the opiate or adulterants present in the preparations, associated medical problems, and complications specific to intravenous administration.

Although cerebral vasculitis has been more clearly demonstrated with other substances such as cocaine and amphetamines, vasculitis has also been suggested on angiographic findings as a cause for ischaemic stroke related to heroin use in a number of patients [142,143,147,154]. A 25-year old heroin user with bilateral borderzone infarctions attributed to vasculitis of the basal cerebral arteries was treated with corticosteroids with complete resolution of his neurological deficit [154]. Brust reported cerebral infarction in a heroin user which did not follow a recent injection, and angiography suggested widespread small vessel arteritis [142]. Similarly, vasculitis may also be responsible for some cases of heroin associated myelopathy, as small vessel vasculitis has been reported following cord biopsy in a heroin addict presenting with a suspected spinal cord tumour [155].

Stroke may occur in heroin users following re-exposure after a period of abstinence [147] suggesting a hypersensitivity reaction of the cerebral vessels to either opiate or adulterant. Opiates have been reported to cause acute allergic reactions including urticaria and anaphylaxis [156]. Laboratory findings which further support immunologic mechanisms in heroin users include the presence of hypergammaglobulinaemia [157,158], circulating immune complexes [158], and false positive serology [159]. Consistent with hypersensitivity, in a case series of nine heroin addicts with stroke [142], one patient had 10% eosinophilia, hypergammaglobulinaemia, and a positive direct Coombs test, and another had an elevated erythrocyte sedimentation rate.

Respiratory depression and hypotension are both complications of heroin overdose, and may result in a number of neurological manifestations. Single-photon emission tomography has demonstrated a reduction in global cerebral perfusion in chronic heroin users [160], and cortical haemoglobin deoxygenation has been shown in opioid dependent subjects following heroin injection [161], most likely a result of respiratory depression. A patient presenting with ballistic movements following heroin overdose showed bilateral ischaemic lesions of the globus pallidus on MRI suggestive of generalized cerebral hypoxia during the comatose state [145]. A 17-year old who developed respiratory failure following heroin overdose subsequently showed evidence of hypoxic-toxic encephalopathy on neuropsychologic examination, and MRI also revealed globus pallidus infarction [148]. Bilateral globus pallidus infarction is commonly observed at post-mortem examination in heroin users [162], and these changes are thought to be caused by recurrent hypoxic episodes due to respiratory depression following overdose rather than the direct effects of heroin. Similar lesions are seen following carbon monoxide poisoning [163]. Borderzone infarcts are also commonly observed in heroin addicts [154], and these are likely to reflect a decrease in cerebral perfusion pressure secondary to overdose. During coma, cerebral perfusion may be further compromised because of positional changes in the neck, resulting in localized vascular compression, reduced cerebral blood flow, and ischaemic stroke [164].

Since the AIDS epidemic, fear of infection through the parenteral route has led to increasing use of alternative methods of administration among drug abusers, and although heroin may be smoked or sniffed, the intravenous route is still commonly used. Intravenous administration of any abused substance carries the risk of numerous complications. Stroke may occur as a result of direct vascular injury associated with injection site complications, or more indirectly through associated conditions which predispose to stroke such as bacterial endocarditis and HIV infection.

Complications from intravenous injection sites in heroin users are usually related to infection. With repeated use over time vascular access of the superficial veins becomes more difficult and sometimes the user inadvertently punctures an artery. A 54-year old female heroin user presented with a subarachnoid haemorrhage following repeated cervical intra-arterial injections of heroin due to a lack of peripheral access [139]. Angiography revealed extensive intracranial and skull base vascular pathology including right internal carotid artery dissection and fusiform aneurysm, and focal dissection of the left vertebral artery with pseudoaneurysms consistent with a puncture injury.

Accidental arterial puncture during attempted injection into the jugular vein or paradoxical embolism of intravenous injected substances may result in embolization of foreign material to the brain. Occlusion of the posterior cerebral artery has been reported following intravenous injection of a melted hydromorphone suppository [165], possibly a result of paradoxical fat embolism of the cocoa butter content. Combinations of pentazocine (a synthetically prepared opioid analgesic) and tripelennamine (an antihistamine) were used for recreational use during the 1970s because of the euphoric effects similar to heroin, and both ischaemic and haemorrhagic strokes were reported in users [166]. Tablets were crushed and injected intravenously, and substances used to bind the drugs have been shown to cause pulmonary arteriolar occlusion at post-mortem examination [167]. This may result in increased pulmonary artery pressures, predisposing to opening of arterio-venous shunts and the associated risk of paradoxical embolism of thrombus or injected foreign material.

Infective endocarditis may complicate intravenous administration of any abused substances, and is common in heroin addicts [168]. Stroke complicating endocarditis may be ischaemic or haemorrhagic, and occurs in approximately 20% of cases [121]. Infarction may occur due to embolic vessel occlusion, and haemorrhagic stroke secondary to septic (mycotic) aneurysm rupture. In a case series reported by Hart et al, of 133 episodes involving native mitral or aortic valves, ischaemic stroke occurred in 19%, haemorrhagic stroke in 7%, and non-cerebral emboli in 11% [121]. In two of these episodes, ischaemic stroke was an isolated presenting feature, with endocarditis initially unsuspected. Emboli tended to occur early, with a relatively low risk once infection was controlled. Tricuspid infection has been reported in approximately a third of cases of endocarditis occurring in intravenous drug addicts [169]. Paradoxical embolism through a patent foramen ovale has been reported in patients with tricuspid valve endocarditis [170], though unrecognised associated mitral or aortic valve involvement may also underlie the mechanism of stroke in these patients.

The prevalence of human immunodeficiency virus (HIV) infection amongst intravenous drug users worldwide has been reported up to 20% [171]. A number of neurological manifestations may occur in patients with HIV relating to opportunistic infection, neoplasia, iatrogenic causes, or directly from HIV infection of the central nervous system [172]. There is an increased risk of cerebrovascular disease in patients with HIV infection, and a retrospective study performed by Engstrom et al [173] suggested that young patients with acquired immunodeficiency syndrome (AIDS) are 40 times more likely to develop stroke than the general population. Cerebral infarction is more common than ICH, occurring in 96% in one series [174]. Stroke may also be the first and only manifestation of HIV infection [175]. Neuropathological features described in a post-mortem series of patients with AIDS include hyaline small vessel thickening, perivascular space dilatation, rarefaction, and pigment deposition, though these changes had been largely asymptomatic and did not correlate with clinical stroke like syndromes [123].

There are a number of potential mechanisms contributing to the increased risk of stroke in patients with HIV. Non-bacterial thrombotic endocarditis and HIV myocarditis with thrombus formation may serve as potential cardioembolic sources. Associated cerebral opportunistic infection and cerebral neoplasia may predispose to cerebral infarction, and the occurrence of cerebrovascular disease related to HIV has in fact been reported mainly in association with these features. HIV associated vasculopathy has been shown to affect both the extracranial and intracranial vessels [123,174,176,177], and has been reported in HIV related stroke in the absence of any other causes [174]. The underlying mechanism is poorly understood, though may be related to direct HIV infection of vascular endothelial cells with immune activation as the initiating event [178,179]. Abnormalities of coagulation, including protein S deficiency [180] and the presence of antiphospholipid antibodies [181,182] are more common in patients with HIV. Anticardioloipin antibodies correlate well with the presence of perfusion defects on single positron emission computed tomography scanning in HIV patients [183]. The previously reported aetiological link between stroke and protein S deficiency in HIV patients [184,185] has recently been questioned, and a comparison between HIV infected men with and without stroke suggested that protein S deficiency may not be related to an increased risk [186]. Anti-retroviral agents may also play a part in the increased risk of stroke. Accelerated atherosclerosis due to dyslipidaemia and insulin resistance associated with these drugs may underlie the increased risk of cardiovascular disease observed in these patients [187,188].

Cannabis

Background

Cannabis is obtained from the plant Cannabis sativa, which is grown in many countries as a source of rope fibre. Its use for medicinal, religious, and recreational purposes date back thousands of years, though it wasn't until the 19th century that the medicinal use of cannabis became widely accepted by Western practitioners, predominantly for its analgesic effects. Since the 20th century most countries have enacted laws regarding the legality of cannabis use. Cultivation and use of cannabis was generally outlawed in the United Kingdom in 1928, and in 1937 the Roosevelt administration crafted the Marijuana Tax Act making cannabis possession illegal in the United States. Despite these measures the prevalence of recreational cannabis use has increased markedly over the last decade, and it is estimated that about 4% of the world's adult population use cannabis annually [189]. In 2004 cannabis was re-classified in the UK from Class B to Class C of the Misuse of Drugs Act 1971, though the health and social impact of cannabis use remains controversial.

Pharmacology

The Cannabis sativa plant produces psychoactive chemicals collectively known as cannabinoids, of which more than 60 have been identified. The most important of these in terms of biological activity and recreational use is delta-9-tetrahydrocannabinol (THC). The potency of different preparations of cannabis relates to the THC content, which is extremely variable and depends upon which part of the plant is used, and the climate where it is grown. The various preparations of cannabis and the approximate THC content are outlined in Table 6.

Table 6. Different cannabis preparations

• Marijuana	Dried leaves, flowering tops and stalks of uncultivated plants which are smoked (THC 1-2%)
• Ganja	Small upper leaves of cultivated female plants. Three time more potent than marijuana (THC 3-6%)
• Hashish / cannabis resin	Pure resin from flowering tops of female plants in the form of sticky cakes or bricks (THC 10-20%)
• Hashish oil	Extraction product using organic solvents (THC may be up to 60%)
• Bhang	Dried leaves of uncultivated plants which are infused and drunk

THC is absorbed quickly when smoked reaching peak plasma concentrations at 10-30 minutes, and is highly lipid soluble with a high volume of distribution. The plasma half-life of THC is approximately 56 hours in occasional users, and 28 hours in chronic users [190]. However, because of the high lipid solubility, cannabinoids accumulate in fatty tissues, and complete elimination of a single dose may take up to 30 days [191]. THC is metabolized by the liver to 11-hydroxy THC which also has psychoactive properties, along with a number of other inactive metabolites. Cannabinoids exert their effects at CB_1 and CB_2 receptors in the brain and periphery. The endogenous ligand for these receptors is a derivative of arachadonic acid called anandamine, though the physiological function of this endogenous cannabinoid system remains unclear.

Clinical Features

The desired effects associated with cannabis use are of euphoria, self-confidence, relaxation and a general sense of well being. The acute toxicity of cannabis is extremely low, though potential adverse effects relating to mood, sedation, psychomotor performance, memory, and psychosis are well described [192]. A cannabis withdrawal syndrome may occur on cessation following chronic use [193] suggesting that a degree of physical and psychological dependence to cannabis occurs. The possibility of long term cognitive impairment has been suggested following chronic heavy cannabis use [194].

Cannabis is the most widely used illicit drug worldwide, and so strokes occurring in cannabis users may be coincidental and unrelated to the drug. Establishing causality may be difficult, and this relationship is usually based on a temporal link between cannabis use and the occurrence of stroke in patients without any other obvious risk factors. The association between cannabis use and stroke is less well established than for other illicit drugs, and despite the widespread usage of cannabis, cases supporting an aetiological link have been reported only infrequently.

The first reported case of neurological deficit related to cannabis use was in 1964, whereby a young man developed a left gaze paresis, however there were no imaging studies available and an underlying aetiology remained undetermined [195]. In 1991, Zachariah reported two cases of focal neurological deficit following cannabis use. Both were young men presenting with dysarthria and hemiparesis, and in each case CT scan demonstrated basal nuclei infarctions [196]. There was no history of other illicit drug use, and all other investigations were normal. A 30-year old man presented with expressive dysphasia during cannabis use, and MRI demonstrated striatocapsular infarction [197]. A 22-year old man with a history of three previous transient ischaemic attacks presented with a left hemiparesis and internal capsule infarction following one week of heavy cannabis use. He had also taken LSD at this time, though two of the preceding TIAs were related to cannabis use alone [198]. Hemiparesis and receptive dysphasia occurred in a 23-year old man after using large amounts of cannabis, and CT showed a large subcortical infarction involving the striatum and internal capsule [199]. Another man suffered a posterior cerebral artery infarction during an episode of coital headache 30 minutes after smoking cannabis [200], and an 18-year old man with hemianopia due to an occipital infarct and posterior cerebral artery occlusion presented soon after smoking cannabis earlier that day [201].

Cerebellar hemispheric infarction occurred in a 15-year old who presented with nausea and incoordination following heavy cannabis use [202]. Cerebral angiography was normal, as were other investigations apart from the identification of a small patent foramen ovale. More recently two further cases of cerebellar infarction following cannabis use have been reported in adolescent males, both of whom died within 24 hours of admission [203]. Acute cerebellar infarcts involving multiple arterial territories were identified at post-mortem, in contrast to most other cerebellar strokes which typically occur in the distribution of a single vessel [204]. The authors suggested the possibility of a predilection to the posterior circulation in children who present with cannabis related stroke, however no underlying mechanism was identified in these cases.

In 2005, Mateo et al reported a case of recurrent stroke related to cannabis which perhaps carries the most convincing evidence with regards to an aetiological link [205]. A 36-year old man developed aphasia following heavy cannabis consumption, and MRI revealed left temporal lobe infarction. There was no history of any other illicit drug use, and no other vascular risk factors were identified. He suffered another episode of aphasia and hemiparesis one year later immediately after smoking cannabis for the first time since his first stroke, and MRI showed an acute left frontal infarct. After an 18 month abstinence period he suffered from auditory agnosia following further heavy intake of cannabis, and MRI revealed an acute right posterior temporal infarct. The clear-cut temporal relationship between drug intake and recurrent stroke in different arterial territories, and the absence of any other identifiable cause for stroke strongly suggested an aetiological role for cannabis in this case.

Mechanisms of Stroke

There is much uncertainty regarding the underlying mechanism involved in cannabis related stroke, and experimental data on the cerebrovascular effects of cannabis use are lacking. In cases theorizing pathogenesis, proposed mechanisms have usually involved vasospasm and hypotension. Cannabis can result in systemic hypotension, and can alter peripheral vasomotor reflexes and cerebral blood flow, though the significance of these changes in relation to stroke aetiology remains uncertain.

Hypotension has been considered as a possible cause of stroke related to cannabis use, and has been demonstrated in both human [206], and animal models [207] in experiments assessing the effects of cannabis on the cardiovascular system. Animal data suggest that cannabis may inhibit sympathetic activity via receptors on the pre-synaptic nerve terminals on post-ganglionic sympathetic fibres [208]. Other animal models have suggested variable effects on vasomotor activity [209], and this may reflect a dose dependent effect with low levels causing an increase in sympathetic activity, and higher doses inhibiting sympathetic activity. This may explain why the majority of reported cases follow episodes of heavy cannabis use. Despite this, none of the imaging studies in cases of cannabis related stroke demonstrated borderzone infarction compatible with hypoperfusion, and none of the patients were found to be hypotensive at presentation. In fact, many patients were found to be hypertensive, and as a possible explanation it has been proposed that observed elevations in systemic blood pressure may reflect a reaction to cerebral vasospasm preceded by hypotension [196].

Vasospasm has been commonly proposed as a mechanism for cannabis related stroke, and may explain the close timing of symptoms relating to drug use, and also the absence of vessel abnormalities on vascular imaging in the majority of cases. However, the majority of cases demonstrated striatocapsular infarction on imaging studies which is not typically associated with vasospasm. Mesec et al reported evidence of arterial spasm on transcranial ultrasound and MRI studies in a patient with cannabis related stroke [199], though in experimental human studies vasospasm has not been demonstrated.

Although the specific effects of cannabis on cerebral perfusion have not been fully elucidated, studies have suggested that cerebral blood flow is affected in relation to cannabis use. Xenon inhalation studies showed that cannabis users had overall lower regional cerebral blood flow measurements which then improved with abstinence [210]. Mathew et al used the same technique to analyse acute changes in cerebral blood flow associated with cannabis smoking, and found that experienced smokers showed an increase, and inexperienced smokers a decrease in cerebral flow after smoking cannabis [211]. The same authors later used transcranial ultrasound to demonstrate reduced middle cerebral artery velocities yet normal systemic pressures after smoking cannabis, suggesting the possibility of impaired cerebral autoregulation [212]. Another transcranial Doppler study demonstrated an increased pulsatility index in cannabis abusers suggesting that cerebral perfusion in these young patients was comparable to a normal 60-year old [213]. Carboxyhaemoglobin levels are also increased in cannabis users, therefore decreasing the oxygen transportation capacity [214].

Cannabis has been described in association with atrial flutter [215], atrial fibrillation [216], and myocardial infarction [217], serving as potential cardioembolic sources for stroke related to cannabis use. Cardioembolism can result in striatocapsular infarcts which were demonstrated in most cases of cannabis related stroke, and the predisposition to rapid dissolution observed with cardiogenic thrombi [218] may account for the absence of vessel abnormalities seen.

Cerebral vascular imaging studies are usually normal in cannabis related stroke, though in a patient reported by Mateo et al [205], MRI angiography revealed a persistent mild decrease in the distal branches of the left MCA. The authors suggested the possibility of an underlying toxic or immune inflammatory vasculopathy, though acknowledged that these changes may also represent partial emboli recanalisation following cardioembolism. Cerebral vasculitis has been observed in stroke related to other illicit drug users but has not been reported in relation to cannabis, though peripheral vessel arteritis has been described [219].

Other Drugs

Phencyclidine

Phencyclidine (phenylcyclohexylpiperiden) is also known as 'PCP' or 'angel dust', and was originally used as an anaesthesic agent but withdrawn due to its adverse effects. It acquired great popularity in the 1970s amongst drug abusers in the United States, and can be taken orally, smoked, or injected. In lower doses it produces euphoria and emotional lability, and at higher doses can lead to confusion, excitation, psychosis, seizures, and death due to cardio-respiratory collapse. PCP works primarily on N-methyl-D-Aspartate (NMDA) and dopamine receptors [220], and enhances catecholamine release [221].

PCP poisoning resulting in hypertensive crisis and death was reported in a 13-year old boy, and post-mortem examination revealed ICH [222]. In another case, fatal subarachnoid haemorrhage was reported in a young man after smoking PCP [223].

Lysergic Acid Diethylamide

Lysergic acid diethylamide (LSD) was first synthesized by the Swiss chemist Albert Hofmann at the Sandoz Laboratories. It is synthesized from lysergic acid which is derived from ergot, a fungus which typically grows on rye, and was initially introduced as a psychotropic drug but soon became popular for its recreational use. The effects on dopamine and NMDA receptors are presumed to be the underlying mechanisms for LSD-induced psychosis [224], the effects of which can be observed even at low doses. Severe hypertension, convulsions, and coma may occur at higher doses.

Seizures, left hemiplegia, and internal carotid artery occlusion were reported in a 14 year old boy after ingestion of LSD [225]. A young woman also presented with left hemiparesis following oral ingestion of LSD [226], and in another patient angiographic evidence of vasculitis was reported with LSD use [227].

References

[1] World Health Organization (1969). WHO Expert Committee on Drug Dependence. Sixteenth Report. (Technical report series 407). Geneva:WHO.

[2] Sloan M, Kittner S, Rigamonti D, et al. Occurrence of stroke associated with use/abuse of drugs. *Neurology* 1991;41:1358–1364.

[3] Sloan M. Toxicity/Substance Abuse. In: Welch K, Caplan L, Reis D, et al, eds. Primer on Cerebrovascular Diseases. San Diego: Academic Press 1997:413-416.

[4] Prakash A, Das G. Cocaine and the nervous system. *Int. J. Clin. Pharmacol. Ther. Toxicol.* 1993;31:575-81.

[5] Das G. Cocaine abuse in North America: a milestone in history. *J. Clin. Pharmacol.* 1993;33:296-310.

[6] Freud S. Uber Coca (On Cocaine). In: Byck R, ed. Cocaine papers. New York: Stonehill Publishing 1974:49-73.

[7] Grinspoon L, Bakalar JB. Drug dependence: non narcotic agents. In: Kaplan HI, Freedman AM, Sadock BJ, eds. Comprehensive textbook of psychiatry/III. Vol 2. Baltimore: Williams and Wilkins 1980:1621.

[8] Warner EA. Cocaine abuse. *Ann. Int. Med.* 1993;119:226-35.

[9] Flemming JA, Byck R, Barash PG. Pharmacology and therapeutic applications of cocaine. *Anaesthesiology* 1990;73:518-31.

[10] Benowitz NL. Clinical pharmacology and toxicology of cocaine. *Pharmacol. Toxicol.* 1993;72:3-12.

[11] Das G, Laddu A. Cocaine: friend or force? (Part1) *Int. J. Clin. Pharmacol. Ther. Toxicology* 1993;31:449-55.

[12] Gold MS, Vereby K. The psychopharmacology of cocaine. *Psychiatr Ann.* 1984;140: 714-723.

[13] Coleman DL, Ross TF, Naughton JL. Myocardial ischaemia and infarction related to recreational cocaine use. *West J. Med.* 1982;136:444-6.

[14] Chokshi SK, Moore R, Pandian NG, et al. Reversible cardiomyopathy associated with cocaine intoxication. *Ann. Intern. Med.* 1989;111:1039-40.

[15] Nanji AA, Filipenko JD. Asystole and ventricular fibrillation associated with cocaine intoxication. *Chest* 1984;85:132-3.

[16] Virmani R, Robinowitz M, Smialek JE, et al. Cardiovascular effects of cocaine: an autopsy study of 40 patients. *Am. Heart J.* 1988;115:1068-76.

[17] Ettinger NA, Albin RJ. A review of the respiratory effects of smoking cocaine. *Am. J. Med.* 1989;87:664-8.

[18] Krutchkoff DJ, Eisenberg E, O'Brien JE, et al. Cocaine-induced dental erosions (Letter). *N. Engl. J. Med.* 1990;320:408.

[19] Libby DM, Klein L, Altorki NK. Aspiration of the nasal septum: a new complication of cocaine abuse. *Ann. Intern. Med.* 1992;116:567-8.

[20] Becker GD, Hill S. Midline granuloma due to illicit cocaine use. *Arch Otolaryngol. Head Neck Surg.* 1988;114:90-1.

[21] Newman NM, DiLoreto DA, Ho JT, et al. Bilateral optic neuropathy and osteolytic sinusitis. Complications of cocaine abuse. *JAMA* 1988;259:72-4.

[22] Mendelson JH, Mello NK, Teoh SK, et al. Cocaine effects on pulsatile secretion of anterior pituitary, gonadal and adrenal hormones. *J. Clin. Endocrinol. Metab.* 1989;69: 1256-60.

[23] Yang RD, Han MW, McCarthy JH. Ischaemic colitis in a crack abuser. *Dig. Dis. Sci.* 1991;36:238-40.

[24] Gawin FH, Kleber HD. Abstinence symptomatology and psychiatric diagnosis in cocaine abusers. Clinical observations. *Arch Gen. Psychiatry* 1986;43:107-13.
[25] Roth D, Alarcon FJ, Fernandez JA, et al. Acute rhabdomyolysis associated with cocaine intoxication. *N. Engl. J. Med.* 1988;319:673-7.
[26] Devenvi P, McDonough MA. Cocaine abuse and endocarditis. *Ann. Int. Med.* 1988;109:82-3.
[27] Chambers HF, Morris DC, Tauber MG, et al. Cocaine use and the risk for endocarditis in intravenous drug users. *Ann. Int. Med.* 1987;106:833-6.
[28] Chaisson RE, Bacchetti P, Osmond D, et al. Cocaine use and HIV infection in intravenous drug users in San Francisco. *JAMA* 1989;261:561-5.
[29] Brust JCM, Richter RW. Stroke associated with cocaine abuse. *N. Y. State J. Med.* 1977;77:1473.
[30] Daras M, Tuchman AJ, Koppel BS, et al. Neurovascular complications of cocaine. *Acta Neurol. Scand.* 1994;90:124-9.
[31] Jacobs IG, Roszler MH, Kelly JK, et al. Cocaine abuse neurovascular complications. *Radiology* 1989;170:223-7.
[32] Klonoff DC, Andrews BT, Obana WG. Stroke associated with cocaine use. *Arch Neurol.* 1989:46:989-93.
[33] Levine SR, Brust JC, Futrell N, et al. Cerebrovascular complications of the use of the 'crack' form of alkaloidal cocaine. *N. Engl. J. Med.* 1990;323:699-704.
[34] Levine SR, Brust JC, Futrell N, et al. A comparative study of the cerebrovascular complications of cocaine; alkaloidal versus hydrochloride [review]. *Neurology* 1991;141:1173-7.
[35] Mody CK, Miller BL, McIntyre HB, et al. Neurologic complications of cocaine abuse. *Neurology* 1988;38:1189.
[36] Brown E, Prajer J, Lee HY, et al. CNS complications of cocaine abuse: Prevalence, pathophysiology, and neuroradiology. *AJR* 1992;159:137.
[37] Devenyi P, Schneiderman JF, Devenyi RG, et al. Cocaine induced central retinal artery occlusion. *CMAJ* 1988;138:129.
[38] Daras M, Tuchman AJ, Marks S. Central nervous system infarction related to cocaine abuse. *Stroke* 1991:22;1230.
[39] Sawaya GR, Kaminski MJ. Spinal cord infarction after cocaine use. *South Med. J.* 1990;83:601.
[40] Nolte KB, Brass LM, Fletterick CF. Intracranial haemorrhage associated with cocaine abuse: A prospective autopsy study. *Neurology* 1996;46:1291-1296.
[41] Kibayashi K, Mastri AR, Hirsch CS. Cocaine-induced intracerebral haemorrhage: Analysis of predisposing factors and mechanisms causing haemorrhagic strokes. *Hum. Pathol.* 1995;26:659-63.
[42] Bahar M, Cole G Rosen M, et al: Histopathology of the spinal cord after intrathecal cocaine, bupivacaine, lignocaine, and adrenaline in the rat. *Eur. J. Anaesthesiol.* 1984;1:293-297.
[43] Kugelmass AD, Shannon RP, Yeo EL, et al. Intravenous cocaine induces platelet activation in the conscious dog. *Circulation* 1995;91:1336-40.

[44] Tonga G, Tempesta E, Tonga AR, et al. Platelet responsiveness and biosynthesis of thromboxane and prostacyclin in response to in vitro cocaine treatment. *Haemostasis* 1985;15:100-107.

[45] Jennings LK, White MM, Sauer CM, et al. Cocaine-induced platelet defects. *Stroke* 1993;24:1352-9.

[46] Rinder HM, Ault KA, Jatlow PI, et al. Platelet alpha granule release in cocaine users. *Circulatio*n 1994;90:1162-7.

[47] Kolodgie FD, Farb A, Virmany R. Pathological determinants of cocaine-associated cardiovascular syndromes. *Hum. Pathol.* 1995;26:583-6.

[48] Kolodgie FD, Virmani R, Cornhill, et al. Increase in athero-sclerosis and adventitial mast cells in cocaine abusers: an alternative mechanism of cocaine-associated coronary vasospasm and thrombosis. *J. Am. Coll. Cardiol.* 1991;17:1553-60.

[49] Heesch CM, Wilhelm CR, Ristich J, et al. Cocaine activates platelets and increases the formation of circulating platelet containing microaggregates in humans. *Heart* 2000;83:688-695.

[50] Kosten-Thomas R, Tucker K, Gottschalk PC, et al. Platelet abnormalities associated with cerebral perfusion defects in cocaine dependence. *Biol. Psychiatry* 2004;55:91-7.

[51] He G-Q, Zhang A, Altura BT, et al. Cocaine-induced cerebrovasospasm and its possible mechanism of action. *J. Pharmacol. Exp. Ther.* 1994;268:1532-9.

[52] Zhang A, Cheng TP, Altura BT, et al. Acute cocaine results in rapid rises in intracellular free calcium concentration in canine cerebral vascular smooth muscle cells: possible relation to etiology of stroke. *Neurosci. Lett.* 1996;215:57-9.

[53] Lowenstein DH, Massa SM, Rowbotham MC, et al. Acute neurologic and psychiatric complications associated with cocaine abuse. *Am. J. Med.* 1987;83:841-846.

[54] Powers RH, Madden JA. Vasoconstrictive effects of cocaine, metabolites and structural analogs on cat cerebral arteries. *FASEB J.* 1990;4:A1095.

[55] Langner RO, Bement CL, Perry LE. Arteriosclerotic toxicity of cocaine. *NIDA Res. Monogr.* 1988;88:325-336.

[56] Bennet CL, Cohen L, Nielson SW, et al. Arterial injury in rabbits following alternate day injections of cocaine. *FASEB J.* 1989;3:A297.

[57] Wang A-M, Suojanen JN, Colucci VM. Cocaine and methamphetamine-induced acute cerebral vasospasm: an angiographic study in rabbits. *AJNR Am. J. Neuroradiol.* 1990;11:1141-1146.

[58] Huang QF, Gebrewold A, Altura BT, et al. Cocaine-induced cerebral vascular damage can be ameliorated by Mg+2 in rat brain. *Neurosci. Lett.* 1990;109:113-116.

[59] Johnson B, Lamki L, Fang B, et al. Demonstration of dose-dependent global and regional cocaine-induced reductions in brain blood flow using a novel approach to quantitative single photon emission computerized tomography. *Neuropsychopharmacology* 1998;18:377-384.

[60] London ED, Cascella NG, Wong DL, et al. Cocaine-induced reduction of glucose utilization in human brain: a study using positron emission tomography and [fluorine 18]-fluorodeoxy-glucose. *Arch Gen. Psychiatry* 1990;47:567-574.

[61] Rogers KJ, Nahorski KJ. Depression of cerebral metabolism by stimulant doses of cocaine. *Brain Res.* 1973;57:255-258.

[62] Volkow ND, Mullani N, Gould KL, et al. Cerebral blood flow in chronic cocaine users. *Br. J. Psychiatry* 1988;152:641-648.

[63] Fogo A, Superdock KR, Atkinson JB. Severe arteriosclerosis in the kidney of a cocaine addict. *Am. J. Kidney Dis*. 1992;20:513-515.

[64] Simpson RW, Edwards WD. Pathogenesis of cocaine-induced ischaemic heart disease. *Arch Pathol. Lab. Med*. 1986;110:479-484.

[65] Konzen JP, Levine SR, Garcia JH. Vasospasm and thrombus formation as possible mechanisms of stroke related to alkaloidal cocaine. *Stroke* 1995;26:1114-1118.

[66] Petty GW, Brust JCM, Tatemichi TK, et al. Embolic stroke after smoking 'crack' cocaine. *Stroke* 1990;21:1632-1635.

[67] Sloan MA, Mattioni TA. Concurrent myocardial and cerebral infarctions after intranasal cocaine use. *Stroke* 1992;23:427-430.

[68] Sauer CM. Recurrent embolic stroke and cocaine-related cardiomyopathy. *Stroke* 1991;22:1203-5.

[69] Kimura S, Bassett AL, Xi H, et al. Early afterdepolarisations and triggered activity induced by cocaine. A possible mechanism of cocaine arrhythmogenesis. *Circulation* 1992;85:2227-2235.

[70] Chakko S, Sepulveda S, Kessler KM, et al. Frequency and type of electrocardiographic abnormalities in cocaine abuse. *Am. J. Cardiol*. 1994;74:710-713.

[71] Amine AR. Neurosurgical complications of heroin addiction: brain abscess and mycotic aneurysm. *Surg. Neurol*. 1977;7:385-6.

[72] Gilroy J, Andaya L, Thomas VJ. Intracranial mycotic aneurysms and subacute bacterial endocarditis in heroin addiction. *Neurology* 1973;23:1193.

[73] Jara FM, Lewis JF, Magilligan DJ. Operative experience with infective endocarditis and intracerebral mycotic aneurysm. *J. Thorac. Cardiovasc. Surg*. 1980;80:28.

[74] Kaye BR, Fainstat M. Cerebral vasculitis associated with cocaine abuse. *JAMA* 1987;258:2104-2106.

[75] Nadeau SE. Intracerebral haemorrhage and vasculitis related to ephedrine abuse. *Ann. Neurol*. 1984;15:114-115.

[76] Krendel DA, Ditter SM, Frankel MR, et al. Biopsy-proven cerebral vasculitis associated with cocaine abuse. *Neurology* 1990;40:1092-1094.

[77] Bostwick DG. Amphetamine induced vasculitis. *Hum. Pathol*. 1981;12:1031-33.

[78] Citron BP, Halpern M, McCarron M, et al. Necrotizing angiitis associated with drug abuse. *N. Engl. J. Med*. 1970;283:1003-11.

[79] Green RM, Kelly KM, Gabrielsen T, et al. Multiple inracerebral haemorrhages after smoking "crack" cocaine. *Stroke* 1990;21:657-62.

[80] Schwartz KA, Cohen JA. Subarachnoid haemorrhage precipitated by cocaine snorting. *Arch Neurol*. 1984;41:705.

[81] Lichtenfeld PJ, Rubin DB, Feldman RS. Subarachnoid haemorrhage precipitated by cocaine snorting. *Arch Neurol*. 1984;41:223-4.

[82] Jenkel JF, Podlewski H, Dean-Paterson S, et al. Epidemic freebase cocaine abuse. *Lancet* 1986;1:459-462.

[83] Cregler LL, Mark H. Medical complications of cocaine abuse. *N. Engl. J. Med.* 1986;315:1495-1499.

[84] Bill A, Linder J. Sympathetic control of cerebral blood flow in acute arterial hypertension. *Acta Physiol. Scand.* 1976;96:114-121.

[85] MacKenzie ET, Strandgaard S, Graham DI, et al. Effects of acutely induced hypertension in cats on pial arteriolar caliber, local cerebral blood flow, and the blood brain barrier. *Circ. Res.* 1976;39:33-41.

[86] Kelly PA, Sharkey J, Philip R, et al. Acute cocaine alters cerebral autoregulation in the rat neocortex. *Brain Res. Bull.* 1993;31:581-5.

[87] Caplan L. Intracerebral haemorrhage revisited. *Neurology* 1988;38:624-7.

[88] Substance Abuse and Mental Health Services Administration, Office of Applied Studies. (February 7, 2008). The DASIS Report: Primary Methamphetamine/n Amphetamine Admissions to Substance Abuse Treatment: 2005. Rockville, MD.

[89] Beckett AH, Rowland M. Urinary excretion of methylamphetamine in man. *Nature* 1965;206:1260-1.

[90] Reese EA, Bunzow JR, Arttamangkul S, et al. Trace amine-associated receptor 1 displays species-dependent stereoselectivity for isomers of methamphetamine, amphetamine, and para-hydroxyamphetamine. *J. Pharmacol. Exp. Ther.* 2007;321:178-86.

[91] Xie Z, Miller GM. Trace amine-associated receptor 1 is a modulator of the dopamine transporter. *J. Pharmacol. Exp. Ther.* 2007;321:128-36.

[92] Kramer JC, Fischman VS, Littlefield DC. Amphetamine abuse. Pattern and effects of high doses taken intravenously. *JAMA* 1967;201:305-9.

[93] Gericke OL. Suicide by ingestion of amphetamine sulfate. *JAMA* 1945;28:1098-9. Series DH2 No 24. London: HMSO, 1997.

[94] Westover AN, McBride S, Haley RW. Stroke in young adults who abuse amphetamines or cocaine: a population-based study of hospitalized patients. *Arch Gen. Psychiatry* 2007;64:495-502.

[95] Cantu C, Arauz A, Murillo-Bonilla LM, et al. Stroke associated with sympathomimetics contained in over-the-counter cough and cold drugs. *Stroke* 2003; 34:1667-72.

[96] Hughes JC, McCabe M, Evans RJ. Intracranial haemorrhage associated with ingestion of 'Ecstasy'. *Arch Emerg. Med.* 1993;10:372-4.

[97] Miyashita T, Hayashi T, Ishida Y, et al. A fatal case of pontine hemorrhage related to methamphetamine abuse. *J. Forensic Leg. Med.* 2007;14:444-447.

[98] El-Omar MM, Ray K, Geary R. Intracerebral haemorrhage in a young adult: Consider amphetamine abuse. *Br. J. Clin. Pract.* 1996;50:115-16.

[99] Goodman SJ, Becker DP. Intracranial hemorrhage associated with amphetamine abuse. *JAMA* 1970;212:480.

[100] Yu YJ, Cooper DR, Wellenstein DE, et al. Cerebral angiitis and intracerebral hemorrhage associated with methamphetamine abuse. *J. Neurosurg.* 1983;58:109-11.

[101] Imanse J, Vanneste J. Intraventricular hemorrhage following amphetamine abuse. *Neurology* 1990;40:1318-19.

[102] Lukes SA. Intracerebral hemorrhage from an arteriovenous malformation after amphetamine injection. *Arch Neurol.* 1983;40:60-1.

[103]De-Silva DA, Wong MC, Lee MP, et al. Amphetamine-associated ischemic stroke: clinical presentation and proposed pathogenesis. *J. Stroke Cerebrovasc. Dis.* 2007;16:185-6.

[104]Roebroek RM, Korten JJ. Epileptic insults, cerebral infarction and rhabdomyolysis as complications of amphetamine abuse. *Ned. Tijdshr Geneeskd.* 1996;140:205-7.

[105]Lambrecht GL, Malbrain ML, Chew SL, et al. Intranasal caffeine and amphetamine causing stroke. *Acta Neurol. Belg*. 1993;93:146-149.

[106]Manchanda S, Connolly MJ. Cerebral infarction in association with Ecstasy abuse. *Postgrad. Med. J*. 1993;69:874-75.

[107]Buxton N, McConachie NS. Amphetamine abuse and intracranial haemorrhage. *J. R. Soc. Med*. 2000;93:472-7.

[108]Alban-Lloyd JT, Walker DRH. Death after combined dexamphetamine and phenelzine. *BMJ* 1965;ii:168-9.

[109]Conci R, D'Angelo V, Tampieri D, et al. Intracerebral haemorrhage and angiographic beading following amphetamine abuse. *Ital. J. Neurol. Sci*. 1988;9:77-81.

[110]D'Souza T, Shraberg D. Intracranial hemorrhage associated with amphetamine abuse. *Neurology* 1981;31:922-3.

[111]Auer J, Berent R, Weber T, et al. Subarachnoid haemorrhage with "Ecstasy" abuse in a young adult. *Neurol. Sci*. 2002;23:199-201.

[112]Matick H, Anderson D, Brumlik J. Cerebral vasculitis associated with oral amphetamine overdose. *Arch Neurol*. 1983;40:253-4.

[113]Stafford CR, Bogdanoff BM, Green L, et al. Mononeuropathy multiplex as a complication of amphetamine angiitis. *Neurology* 1975;25:570.

[114]Rumbaugh CL, Bergeron RT, Scanlan RL, et al. Cerebral vascular changes secondary to amphetamine abuse in the experimental animal. *Radiology* 1971;101:345-51.

[115]Rumbaugh CL, Fang HCH, Higgins RE, et al. Cerebral microvascular injury in experimental drug abuse. *Invest. Radiol*. 1976;11:282-294.

[116]Wooten MR, Khangure MS, Murphy MJ. Intracerebral haemorrhage and vasculitis related to ephedrine abuse. *Ann. Neurol*. 1983;13:337-340.

[117]Clowes GHA, O'Donnell TF. Heat stroke. *N. Engl. J. Med*. 1974;291:564-7.

[118]Ferris EB, Blankenhorn MA, Robinson HW, et al. Heat stroke: Clinical and chemical observations on 44 cases. *J. Clin. Invest*. 1938;17:249-262.

[119]Zalis EG, Lundberg GD, Knutson RA. The pathophysiology of acute amphetamine poisoning with pathologic correlation. *J. Pharmacol. Exp. Ther*. 1967;158:115-27.

[120]Lucas CE, Ledgerwood AM, Kline RA. Alcohol and drugs. In: Mattox KL, Feliciano DV, Moore EE, eds. Trauma. New York, NY:McGraw-Hill;2000:1059-1074.

[121]Hart RG, Foster JW, Luther MF, et al. Stroke in infective endocarditis. *Stroke* 1990;21:695-700.

[122]Brust JCM, Richter RW, Tetanus in the inner city. *NY State J. Med*. 1974;74:1735-42.

[123]Connor MD, Lammie GA, Bell JE, et al. Cerebral infarction in adult AIDS patients: observations from the Edinburgh HIV autopsy cohort. *Stroke* 2000;31:2117-2126.

[124]Wallace JR, Lucas CE, Ledgerwood AM. Social, economic, and surgical anatomy of drug-related abscess. *Am. Surg*. 1986;52:398-401.

[125]Ell JJ, Uttley D, Silver JR. Acute myelopathy in association with heroin addiction. *J. Neurol. Neurosurg. Psychiatr.* 1981;44:448-450.

[126]Celius EG, Andersson S. Leucoencephalopathy after inhalation of heroin: a case report. *J. Neurol. Neurosurg. Psychiatr.* 1996;60:694-695.

[127]Smith WR, Wilson AF. Guillain-Barre syndrome in heroin addiction. *J. Am. Med. Assoc.* 1975;231:1367-1368.

[128]Loizou LA, Boddie HG. Polyradiculopathy associated with heroin abuse. *J. Neurol. Neurosurg. Psychiatr.* 1978;41:855-857.

[129]Alldredge BK, Lowenstein DH, Simon RP. Seizures associated with recreational drug abuse. *Neurology* 1989;39:1037-1039.

[130]Dettmeyer R, Schmidt P, Musshoff F, et al. Pulmonary oedema in fatal heroin overdose: immunohistological investigations with IgE, collagen IV and laminin- no increase of defects of alveolar capillary membranes. *Forensic. Sci. Int.* 2000;110:87-96.

[131]Anderson K. Bronchospasm and intravenous street heroin. *Lancet* 1986;1:1208.

[132]Rice EK, Isbel NM, Becker GJ, et al. Heroin overdose and myoglobinuric acute renal failure. *Clin. Nephrol.* 2000;54:449-454.

[133]Dettmeyer R, Stojanovski G, Madea B. Pathogenesis of heroin-associated glomerulonehritis. Correlation between the inflammatory activity and renal deposits of immunoglobulin and complement? *Forensic. Sci. Int.* 2000;113:227-231.

[134]Llach F, Descoeudres C, Massry SG. Heroin associated nephropathy: clinical and histological studies in 19 patients. *Clin. Nephrol.* 1979;11:7-12.

[135]Weber M, Diener HC, Voit T, et al. Focal myopathy induced by heroin injection is reversible. *Muscle Nerve* 2000;23:274-277.

[136]Ishiyama A, Ishiyama G, Baloh RW, et al. Heroin-induced reversible profound deafness and vestibular dysfunction. *Addiction* 2001;96:1363-1364.

[137]Cooley S, Lalchandani S, Keane D. Heroin overdose in pregnancy: an unusual case report. *J. Obstet Gynaecol.* 2002;22:219-220.

[138]Silverman SH, Turner WW Jr. Intraarterial drug abuse: new treatment options. *J. Vasc. Surg.* 1991;14:111-16.

[139]DiLuna ML, Bydon M, Gunel M, et al. Complications from cervical inra-arterial heroin injection. *J. Neurol. Neurosurg. Psychiatr.* 2007;78:1198.

[140]Frishman WH, Del-Vecchio A, Sanal S, et al. Cardiovascular manifestations of substance abuse: part 2: alcohol, amphetamines, heroin, cannabis, and caffeine. *Heart Dis.* 2003;5:253-71.

[141]Steffen T, Blattler R, Gutzwiller F, et al. HIV and hepatitis virus infections among injecting drug users in a medically controlled heroin prescription programme. *Eur. J. Public Health* 2001;11:425-430.

[142]Brust JCM, Richter RW. Stroke associated with addiction to heroin. *J. Neurol. Neurosurg. Psychiatry* 1976;39:194-199.

[143]Woods BT, Strewler GJ. Hemiparesis occurring six hours after intravenous heroin injection. *Neurology* 1972;22:863-6.

[144]Herskowitz A, Gross E. Cerebral infarction associated with heroin sniffing. *South Med. J.* 1973;66:778-784.

[145] Vila N, Chamorro A. Ballistic movements due to ischaemic infarcts after intravenous heroin overdose: report of two cases. *Clin. Neurol. Neurosurg.* 1997;99:259-62.

[146] Bartolomei F, Nicoli F, Swiader L, et al. Ischaemic stroke after heroin sniffing. A new case. *Presse Med.* 1992;21:983-986.

[147] King J, Richards M, Tress B. Cerebral arteritis associated with heroin abuse. *Med. J. Aust.* 1978;2:444-5.

[148] Zuckerman GB, Ruiz DC, Keller IA, et al. Neurologic complications following intranasal administration of heroin in an adolescent. *Ann. Pharmacother.* 1996;30:778-781.

[149] Hall JH, Karp HR. Acute progressive ventral pontine disease in heroin abuse. *Neurology* 1973;23:6-7.

[150] Schoser BG, Groden C. Subacute onset of oculogyric crisis and generalized dystonia following intranasal administration of heroin. *Addiction* 1999;94:431-434.

[151] Brandli M, Otte A, Muller-Brand J. Cortical blindness after heroin intoxication. *Nucl. Med.* 2000;2:16-19.

[152] Chenery HJ, Murdoch BE. A case of mixed transcortical aphasia following drug overdose. *Br. J. Disord. Commun.* 1986;21:381-391.

[153] Celius EG. Neurologic complications in heroin abuse. Illustrated by two unusual cases. Tidsskr Nor Laegeforen 1997;117:356-7.

[154] Niehaus L, Meyer BU. Bilateral borderzone brain infarctions in association with heroin abuse. *J. Neurol. Sci.* 1998;2:180-182.

[155] Judice DJ, LeBlanc HJ, McGarry PA. Spinal cord vasculitis presenting as spinal cord tumour in a heroin addict. *J. Neurosurg.* 1978;48:131-4.

[156] Schoenfeld MR. Acute allergic reactions to morphine, codeine, meperidine hydrochloride, and opium alkaloids. *N. Y. State J. Med.* 1960;60:2591-3.

[157] Cushman P, Grieco MH. Hyperimmunoglobulinemia associated with narcotic addiction. Effects of methadone maintenance treatment. *Am. J. Med.* 1973;54:320-326.

[158] Ortona L, Laghi V, Cauda R. Immune function in heroin addicts. *N. Engl. J. Med.* 1979;300:45.

[159] Boak RA, Carpenter CM, Miller JN. Biologic false-positive reactions for syphilis among narcotic addicts. A report on the incidence of BFP reactions as measured by the TPI test. *JAMA* 1961;175:326.

[160] Botelho MF, Relvas, JS, Abrantes M, et al. Brain blood flow SPET imaging in heroin abusers. *Ann. N. Y. Acad. Sci.* 2006;1074:466-477.

[161] Stohler R, Dursteler KM, Stormer R, et al. Rapid cortical hemoglobin deoxygenation after heroin and methadone injection in humans: a preliminary report. *Drug Alcohol Depend* 1999;57:23-28.

[162] Andersen SN, Skullerud K. Hypoxic/ischaemic brain damage , especially pallidal lesions in heroin addicts. *Forensic. Sci. Int.* 1999;102:51-59.

[163] Ginsberg MD, Hedley-Whyte ET, Richardson EPJ. Hypoxic-ischemic leukoencephalopathy in man. *Arch Neurol.* 1976;33:5-14.

[164] Jensen R, Olsen TS, Winther BB. Severe non-occlusive ischemic stroke in young heroin addicts. *Acta Neurol. Scand.* 1990;81:354-7.

[165]Bitar S, Gomez CR. Stroke following injection of a melted suppository. *Stroke* 1993;24:741-743.

[166]Caplan LR, Thomas C, Banks G. Central nervous system complications of addiction to "T's and Blues". *Neurology* 1982;32:623-8.

[167]Szwed JJ. Pulmonary angiothrombosis caused by "blue velvet" addiction. *Ann. Intern. Med.* 1970;73:771-4.

[168]Banks T, Fletcher R, Ali N. Infective endocarditis in heroin addicts. *Am. J. Med.* 1973;55:444-51.

[169]Openshaw H. Neurological complications of endocarditis in persons taking drugs intravenously. *West J. Med.* 1976;124:276-281.

[170]Shenoy MM, Grief E, Friedman SA, et al. Paradoxical embolism secondary to tricuspid valve endocarditis. *Am. J. Cardiol.* 1987;54:1374-1375.

[171]Aceijas C, Stimson GV, Hickman M, et al. Global overview of injecting drug use and HIV infection among injecting drug users. *AIDS* 2004;17:2295-2303.

[172]Simpson DM, Berger JR. Neurologic manifestations of HIV infection. *Med. Clin. North Am.* 1996;80:1363-1395.

[173]Engstrom JW, Lowenstein DH, Bredesen DE. Cerebral infarction and transient neurologic deficits associated with acquired immunodeficiency syndrome. *Am. J. Med.* 1989;86:528-532.

[174]Tipping B, de Villiers L, Wainwright H, et al. Stroke in patients with human immunodeficiency virus infection. *J. Neurol. Neurosurg. Psychiatry* 2007;78:1320-1324.

[175]Casado Naranjo I, Toledo Santos JA, Antolin Rodriguez MA. Ischemic stroke as the sole manifestation of human immunodeficiency virus infection. *Stroke* 1992;23:117-118.

[176]Berkefeld J, Enzensberger W, Lanfermann H. MRI in human immunodeficiency virus-associated cerebral vasculitis. *Neuroradiology* 2000;42:526–8.

[177]Kossorotoff M, Touzé E, Godon-Hardy S, et al. Cerebral vasculopathy with aneurysm formation in HIV-infected young adults. *Neurology* 2006;66:1121–2.

[178]Wiley CA, Schrier RD, Nelson JA, et al. Cellular localization of human immunodeficiency virus infection within the brains of acquired immune deficiency syndrome patients. *Proc. Natl. Acad. Sci. USA* 1986;83:7089-7093.

[179]Mazzoni P, Chiriboga CA, Millar WS, et al. Intracerebral aneurysms in human immunodeficiency virus infection: case report and literature review. *Pediatr Neurol.* 2000;23:252–5.

[180]Bissuel F, Berruyer M, Causse X, et al. Acquired protein deficiency: correlation with advanced disease in HIV-1-infected patients. *J. Acquir. Immune Defic. Syndr.* 1992;5:484-489.

[181]MacLean C, Flegg PJ, Kilpatrick DC. Anti-cardiolipin antibodies and HIV infection. *Clin. Exp. Immunol.* 1990;81:263-266.

[182]Abuaf N, Laperche S, Rajoely B, et al. Autoantibodies to phospholipids and to the coagulation proteins in AIDS. *Thromb. Haemost* 1997;77:856-861.

[183]Bock AR, Schwab J, Marienhagen J, et al. Anticardiolipin antibodies in HIV infection: associated with cerebral perfusion defects as detected by 99mTc-HMPAO SPECT. *Clin. Exp. Immunol.* 1994;98:361–8.

[184]Qureshi AI, Janssen RC, Karon JM, et al. Human immunodeficiency virus infection and stroke in young patients. *Arch Neurol.* 1997;54:1150–3.

[185]Mochan A, Modi M, Modi G. Stroke in black South African HIV-positive patients. *Stroke* 2003;34:10–15.

[186]Mochan A, Modi M, Modi G. Protein S deficiency in HIV associated ischaemic stroke: an epiphenomenon of HIV infection. *J. Neurol. Neurosurg. Psychiatry* 2005;76:1455–6.

[187]Sklar P, Masur H. HIV infection and cardiovascular disease - is there really a link? *N. Engl. J. Med.* 2003;349:2065–7.

[188]Jericó C, Knobel H, Calvo N, et al. Subclinical Carotid Atherosclerosis in HIV-Infected Patients. *Stroke* 2006;37:812-817.

[189]United Nations Office on Drugs and Crime 2006. "Cannabis: Why we should care", World Drug Report 1, ISBN 9-2114-8214-3.

[190]Busto U, Bendayan R, Sellers EM. Clinical pharmokinetics of non-opiate abused drugs. *Clin. Pharmokinet.* 1989;16:1-26.

[191]Maykut MO. Health consequences of acute and chronic marijuana use. *Prog. Neuropsychopharmacol. Biol. Psychiatry* 1985;9:209-38.

[192]Ashton CH. Adverse effects of cannabis and cannabinoids. *Br. J. Anaesth.* 1999;83:637-49.

[193]Mendelson JH, Mello NK, Lex BW, et al. Marijuana withdrawal syndrome in a woman. *Am. J. Psychiatry* 1984;141:1289-90.

[194]Pope HG, Gruber AJ, Yurgelun-Todd D. The residual neuropsychological effects of cannabis: the current status of research. *Drug Alcohol Depend* 1995;38:25-34.

[195]Mohan H, Sood G. Conjugate deviation of the eyes after cannabis indica intoxication. *Br. J. Opthalmol.* 1964;48:160-161.

[196]Zachariah S. Stroke after heavy marijuana smoking. *Stroke* 1991;22:406-409.

[197]Barnes D, Palace J, O'Brien M. Stroke following Marijuana smoking. *Stroke* 1992;23:1381.

[198]Lawson T, Rees A. Stroke and transient ischemic attacks in association with substance abuse in a young man. *Postgrad. Med. J.* 1996;72:692-693.

[199]Mesec A, Rot U, Grad A. Cerebrovascular disease associated with marijuana abuse: a case report. *Cerebrovasc. Dis.* 2001;11:284-285.

[200]Alvaro L, Iriondo I, Villaverde F. Sexual headache and stroke in a heavy cannabis smoker. *Headache* 2002;42:224-226.

[201]Marinella M. Stroke after marijuana smoking in a teenager with factor V mutation. *South Med. J.* 2001;94:1217-1218.

[202]White D, Martin D, Geller T, et al. Stroke associated with marijuana abuse. *Pediat. Neurosurg.* 2000;32:92-4.

[203]Geller T, Loftis L, Brink DS. Cerebellar infarction in adolescent males associated with acute marijuana use. *Pediatrics* 2004;113:e365-e370.

[204]Amarenco P, Hauw JJ, Gautier JC. Arterial pathology in cerebellar infarction. *Stroke* 1990;21:1299-1305.

[205]Mateo I, Pinedo A, Gomez-Beldarrain M, et al. Recurrent stroke associated with cannabis use. *J. Neurol. Neurosurg. Psychiatry* 2005;76:435-437.

[206]Clark S. Marijuana and the cardiovascular system. *Pharmacol. Biochem. Behav.* 1974;3:299-306.

[207]Varga K, Lake K, Martin B, et al. Novel antagonist implicates the CB1 cannabinoid receptor in the hypotensive action of anandamide. *Eur. J. Pharmacol.* 1995;278:279-283.

[208]Kunos G, Jarai Z, Batkai S, et al. Endocannabinoids as cardiovascular modulators. *Chem. Phys. Lipids* 2000;108:159-168.

[209]Adams M, Earnhardt J, Dewy W, et al. Vasoconstrictor actions of tetrahydrocannabinol in the rat. *J. Pharmacol. Exp. Ther.* 1976;196:649-656.

[210]Tunving K, Thulin O, Risberg J, et al. Regional cerebral blood flow in long term heavy cannabis use. *Psychiatry Res.* 1986;17:15-21.

[211]Mathew RJ, Wilson WH, Tant SR. Acute changes in cerebral blood flow associated with marijuana smoking. *Acta Psychiatry Scand.* 1989;79:118-128.

[212]Mathew R, Wilson W, Humphreys D, et al. Middle cerebral artery velocity during upright posture after marijuana smoking, *Acta Psychiatry Scand.* 1992;86:173-178.

[213]Herning RI, Better WE, Tate K, et al. Marijuana users are at increased risk for stroke. *An. N.Y. Acad. Sci.* 2001;413-414.

[214]Aronow WS, Cassidy J. Effect of marihuana and placebo-marihuana smoking on angina pectoris. *N. Engl. J. Med.* 1974;291:65-7.

[215]Fisher BAC, Ghuran A, Vadamalai V, et al. Cardiovascular complications induced by cannabis smoking: a case report and review of the literature. *Emerg. Med. J.* 2005;22:679-680.

[216]Singh GK. Atrial fibrillation associated with marijuana use. *Pediatr. Cardiol.* 2000;21:284.

[217]Bachs L, Morland H. Acute cardiovascular fatalities following cannabis use. *Forensic. Sci. Int.* 2001;124:200-203.

[218]Sergura T, Sergura J, Castellanos M, et al. Embolism in acute middle cerebral artery stenosis. *Neurology* 2001;56:497-501.

[219]Disdier P, GranelB, Serratrice J, et al. Cannabis arteritis revisited- ten new case reports. *Angiology* 2001;52:1-5.

[220]Kapur S, Seeman P NMDA receptor antagonists ketamine and PCP have direct effects on the dopamine D (2) receptors-implications for models of schizophrenia. *Mol. Psychiatry* 2002;7:837-44.

[221]Ilett KF, Jarrott B, O'Donnell SR, Wanstall JC. Mechanism of cardiovascular actions of 1-(1-phenylcyclohexy) piperidine hydrochloride (phencyclidine). *Br. J. Pharmacol. Chemother.* 1966;28:73-83.

[222]Eastman JW, Cohen SN. Hypertensive crisis and death associated with phencyclidine poisoning. *JAMA* 1975;231:1270-1.

[223]Bessen HA. Intracranial hemorrhage associated with phencyclidine abuse. *JAMA.* 1982;248:585-6.

[224] Seeman P, Ko F, Tallerico T. Dopamine receptor contribution to the action of PCP, LSD and ketamine psychotomimetics. *Mol. Psychiatry* 2005;10:877-83.

[225] Sobel J, Espinas OE, Friedman SA.Carotid artery obstruction following LSD capsule ingestion. *Arch Intern. Med.* 1971;127:290-1.

[226] Lieberman AN, Bloom W, Kishore PS, Lin JP. Carotid artery occlusion following ingestion of LSD. *Stroke* 1974;5:213-5.

[227] Rumbaugh CL, Bergeron RT, Fang HC, McCormick R. Cerebral angiographic changes in the drug abuse patient. *Radiology* 1971;101:335-44.

In: Cerebral Ischemia in Young Adults
Editors: A. Pezzini and A. Padovani
ISBN 978-1-60741-627-2

Chapter 6

The Relationship between Alcohol Consumption and Cerebrovascular Risk: From Epidemiological Evidence to Biological Plausibility

Simona Costanzo, Augusto Di Castelnuovo, Maria Benedetta Donati, Giovanni de Gaetano and Licia Iacoviello*
Research Laboratories, John Paul II Center for High Technology Research, Care and Education in Biomedical Sciences, Catholic University, Campobasso, Italy

Abstract

Several epidemiological studies have consistently shown an inverse association between light to moderate *alcohol* consumption (1-2 drinks/day) and cardiovascular disease morbidity and mortality.

While the benefit of moderate alcohol consumption on overall cardiovascular disease is well established, the specific relationship with cerebrovascular disease, mainly stroke, is still controversial. Risk factors differ for the two major stroke types (hemorrhagic and ischemic) and several subtypes of each. Alcohol appears to have different associations with these various types.

The overall evidence suggests a reduced risk of ischemic stroke in light-moderate drinkers, but little or no protection against hemorrhagic stroke. All cerebrovascular events substantially increase in heavy alcohol and binge consumers: moreover, heavy alcohol consumption is a risk factor for both hemorrhagic and ischemic stroke in young adults.

---

* Correspondence: Licia Iacoviello, Laboratory of Genetic and Environmental Epidemiology, Largo Gemelli, 1, 86100 Campobasso, Italy. Phone: +39-0874-312274, Fax: +39-0874-312710. E-mail: licia.iacoviello@rm.unicatt.it.

Numerous mechanisms have been proposed that mediate the protective effect of alcohol in cardiovascular disease (e.g., increased levels of high-density lipoprotein cholesterol, decreased levels of low-density lipoprotein cholesterol, reduction in platelet aggregation, beneficial effects on inflammation). On the other hand anti-atherogenic and anti-thrombotic effects and regulation of endothelial function (e.g., enhanced release of nitric oxide) were mainly ascribed to (red) wine polyphenols.

Introduction

Studies on alcohol and its effects on health have a long history, starting from anecdotal accounts in biblical times to more recent rigorous studies of populations.

Many epidemiological studies have consistently shown an inverse association between light to moderate *alcohol* consumption (1-2 drinks/day) and cardiovascular disease morbidity and mortality, independently from age, sex, and major cardiovascular risk factors, such as smoking [1-3]. The beneficial effect of alcohol also applies to total mortality [4-6]. The dose-response relationship between alcohol intake and rate of cardiovascular events or of all-cause mortality has been depicted as a U- or J-shaped curve (Figure 1), in relation to different populations or subgroups (gender, age classes) or reference groups (abstainers *vs* occasional drinkers) [4-7]. The U- or J-shaped relationship between alcohol consumption and clinical events reflects non drinkers or occasional drinkers having higher incidence and mortality rates than light or moderate drinkers, but similar or lower rates than heavy drinkers.

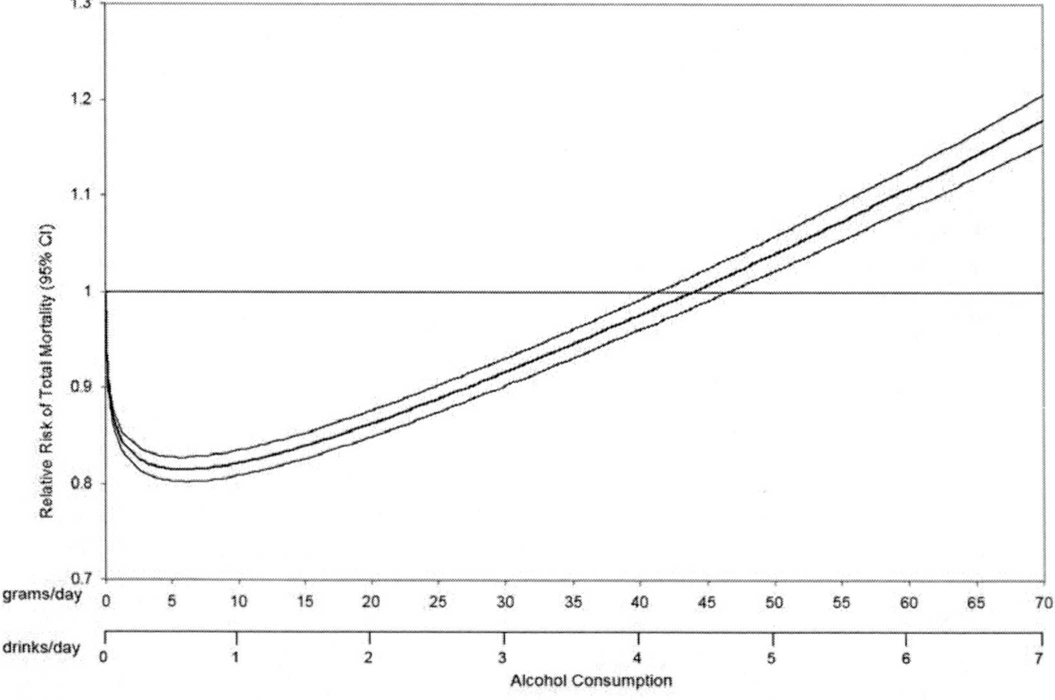

Figure 1. Relative risk of total mortality (95% confidence interval) and alcohol intake. From figure 1, Di Castelnuovo and Coll. 2006, with permission.

Renaud and de Lorgeril [8] proposed that wine intake was one possible explanation for the lower than expected coronary heart disease mortality rates in France, despite the high prevalence of risk factors (the "French Paradox"). Subsequently, many ecological and observational studies have dealt with the question whether different alcoholic beverages were equivalent in their ability to protect against cardiovascular disease, or a specific beverage, wine in particular, might offer a greater protection [2,3,9] most likely related to its non-alcoholic components.

While the benefit of moderate alcohol consumption on overall cardiovascular disease (CVD) is well established, the specific relationship with cerebrovascular disease, mainly stroke, is controversial.

Earlier studies on relationships of alcohol drinking with stroke were made difficult by imprecise diagnosis of stroke types, before modern imaging techniques improved diagnostic accuracy.

Risk factors differ somewhat for the two major stroke types (hemorrhagic and ischemic stroke) and several subtypes of each (e.g., atherothrombotic, lacunar, embolic, subarachnoid hemorrhage, intracerebral hemorrhage). Hemorrhagic stroke is consequent to ruptured blood vessels on the brain surface and within the brain substance, while ischemic stroke is the result of vascular occlusion of an intracerebral artery (clot formation in the brain blood vessels, blood clot emboli to the brain from the heart or elsewhere, or blockage of blood vessels (carotid arteries) outside the brain) [10].

Alcohol appears to have clearly different associations with various stroke types. Moreover, studies on alcohol and stroke are also made complicated by the different relationships of stroke and alcohol with other cardiovascular conditions. Age and hypertension are major risk factors for all stroke types, and most cardiovascular conditions have differing relations to various types of stroke. In particular two of the strongest chronic risk factors for ischemic stroke, hypertension and atrial fibrillation [11], have been associated to heavy drinking.

In the first part of this report we shall discuss recent major epidemiological studies reporting specific data on alcohol consumption and cerebrovascular disease, in the second part we will focus on younger subjects. Finally, possible pathogenetic mechanisms explaining the alcohol effect on cerebrovascular disease will be discussed.

Epidemiological Evidence

Alcohol Consumption and Cerebrovascular Disease. Total, Ischemic and Hemorrhagic Stroke

Several reports suggest that alcohol use, especially heavy drinking, is associated with higher risk of stroke. Some studies examined only binge drinking, some others did not differentiate between hemorrhagic and ischemic strokes.

The overall evidence suggests a reduced risk of ischemic stroke, but little or no protection against hemorrhagic stroke in light-moderate drinkers. All cerebrovascular events substantially increase in heavy alcohol consumers.

The Nurse's Health Study (more than 87,000 women, aged 34-59 years) [12] suggests that among middle-aged women, moderate alcohol consumption decreases the risks of ischemic stroke but may increase the risk of subarachnoid hemorrhage, although in the latter, the number of cases was small. The relative risks (RR) of *ischemic stroke* were 0.3 (95% confidence interval (95% CI), 0.1 to 0.7) for alcohol intake of 5-14 grams/day and 0.5 (95% CI, 0.2 to 1.1) for intake ≥15 grams/day. In contrast, the consumption of 5-14 grams/day was associated with increased risk of subarachnoid hemorrhage (RR, 3.7 (95% CI, 1.0 to 13.8)).

In The Kaiser Permanente Study, alcohol consumption was associated with lower hospitalization rates for ischemic stroke, an inverse relation present in both genders, in whites and blacks, for both extracranial and intracerebral occlusive lesions [13]. Later, analysing a longer follow-up of the same study, Klatsky and Coll. reported a U-shaped association between alcohol intake and hospitalization for ischemic stroke. Relative risks were 0.8 (95%CI, 0.7 to 1.0) among those who consumed between one drink a month and one drink a day and 1.0 (95% CI, 0.8 to 1.2) among those who consumed 3 or more drinks/day [13,14]. In a supplementary Kaiser Permanente study analysis [15], the Authors showed that heavier drinkers, but not lighter drinkers, were at increased risk of hemorrhagic stroke. Higher blood pressure in heavier drinkers appeared to be a partial mediator of this relationship.

Another recent report from a large study in Americans (38,156 men who were free of known CVD or cancer at baseline, The Health Professionals Follow-Up Study) [16], concluded that light-moderate alcohol intake (<30 grams/day) was generally not associated with an increased risk for ischemic stroke, but intake of more than 2 drinks/day may be associated with a higher risk. As the heterogeneity of ischemic stroke may influence its association with alcohol intake, Mukamal and Coll. examined the risks for thrombotic and embolic stroke according to alcohol consumption. Although their analyses were limited by the small number of each stroke subtype, risk for embolic stroke appeared to have a positive association with alcohol use. In contrast, alcohol consumption was not associated with the risk for thrombotic stroke. However, this recent large study did not evidence an effective protection by alcohol consumption on ischemic cerebrovascular events.

Djoussé and Coll. [17] used data collected on participants in the Framingham Study to evaluate the association between total alcohol intake, type of alcoholic beverage and development of ischemic stroke, overall and according to age. Overall, compared with never drinkers in a multivariate Cox regression, current alcohol consumption was not significantly related to ischemic stroke in either sex. Former drinking of ≥12 grams/day of alcohol was associated with a 2.4 times higher risk of ischemic stroke among men but not among women. After stratification by age, alcohol intake was associated with lower risk of ischemic stroke among subjects aged 60-69 years. However, the results of this study were limited by the insufficient statistical power for analyses, even if the Authors used a "pooling method": In other words, each subject contributed to 1 (n = 1,110), 2 (n = 1,203) or 3 (n = 1,885) observations in the analyses, if he/she was free of stroke at the beginning of the three 10 year periods of observation. In this way, a "virtual cohort" was obtained and the final data set consisted of 9,171 person-observations, against 4,198 enrolled subjects.

The limitations of these last two studies [16,17] show as it would be important to design large studies with effective and powered classification of ischemic stroke subtypes.

Several and specific meta-analyses on the relation between alcohol consumption and total, ischemic and/or hemorrhagic stroke risk report statistical synthesis of the data from recent and previously published studies and yield a quantitative summary of the pooled results about this topic.

In a first systematic review of the relationship between alcohol consumption and stroke, Mazzaglia and Coll. [18] concluded that there was not sufficient evidence that high-to-moderate alcohol or wine intake had beneficial effects on stroke, while the risk of stroke in binge drinkers was reportedly higher than in regular drinkers.

In 2003, Reynolds and Coll. [19] performed an original meta-analysis on alcohol consumption and risk of stroke. They selected 35 observational studies (cohort or case-control, with more than 10,000 events divided into total stroke, ischemic (15 studies), or hemorrhagic (12 studies) stroke. They suggested, that, compared with abstention, consumption of less than 12 grams/day was associated with a reduced relative risk of total stroke (RR, 0.83; 95% CI, 0.75 to 0.91) and ischemic stroke (RR, 0.80; 95% CI, 0.67 to 0.96); consumption of 12-24 grams/day was associated with a reduced relative risk of ischemic stroke (RR, 0.72; 95% CI, 0.57 to 0.91); while consumption of more than 60 grams/day was associated with an increased risk of total stroke (RR, 1.64, 95% CI, 1.39 to 1.93); ischemic stroke (RR, 1.69; 95% CI, 1.34 to 2.15) and hemorrhagic stroke (RR, 2.18; 95% CI, 1.48 to 3.20). Performing a meta-regression analysis, they revealed a significant non-linear relationship (J-shape curve) between alcohol consumption and both total ($p = 0.002$) and ischemic stroke ($p = 0.004$) and a linear relationship between alcohol consumption and hemorrhagic stroke ($p = 0.004$) (Figure 2). Their main conclusion was that heavy alcohol consumption increased the relative risk of stroke while light to moderate alcohol consumption might be protective against total and ischemic stroke.

Corrao and Coll. [20], while confirming the protective action of low dose of alcohol on the risk of coronary heart disease, could not find any association between ischemic and hemorrhagic stroke, and moderate alcohol intake. For ischemic (893 cases, 6 studies) and hemorrhagic stroke (1,192 cases, 9 studies), the nadirs (the maximum protection) were reached at 15 and 3 grams/day, respectively, but no evidence of significant protective effect was observed. Significantly increased risks were obtained starting from 53 to 28 grams/day, respectively.

In a meta-analysis of longitudinal and case-control studies on subarachnoid hemorrhage, Feigin and Coll. [21] found an increased risk restricted to heavier intake (>150 grams/week). For heavy drinkers, the pooled relative risk was 2.1 (95% CI, 1.5 to 2.8) in the meta-analysis of cohort studies, and 1.5 (95% CI, 1.3 to 1.8), in case-control studies, with greater hazards effects in women in both meta-analyses. In a similar meta-analysis of 8 case-control studies of intracerebral hemorrhage, Ariesen and Coll. [22] found a overall odds ratios (OR) of 2.05 (95% CI, 1.35 to 3.11) for "moderate intake" (≤56 grams/day) and 4.11 (95% CI, 2.54 to 6.65) for higher intake (>56 grams/day). In the meta-analysis of 3 cohort studies (average alcohol intake 36 grams/day), they could not find any strong association between alcohol consumption and intracerebral hemorrhage. The difference in strength of association might be that the alcohol intake in the cohort studies was lower (about 36 grams/day) than in the case-control studies (average 56 grams/day).

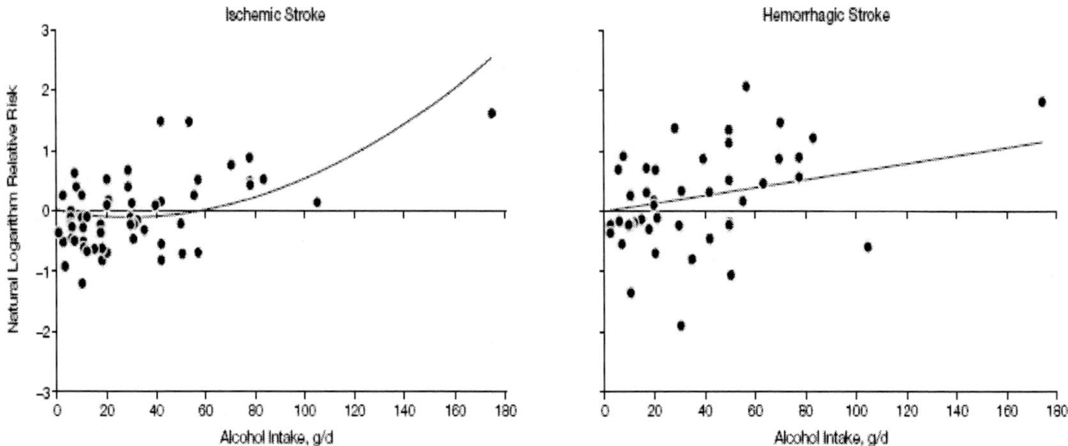

Figure 2. Meta-regression curve of stroke associated with alcohol consumption by subtype stroke. From figure 1; Reynolds and Coll, 2003, with permission.

Wine and Beer Consumption and Cerebrovascular Disease

Only a small number of studies have evaluated whether the beneficial or harmful effects of alcohol on the risk of stroke depends on the type of beverage consumed.

The Copenhagen City Heart Study [23] prospectively examined a cohort of 13,329 subjects for 16 years and showed that the effect of drinking beer, wine, and spirits on risk of total stroke varied among the 3 types of alcoholic beverages. Weekly wine consumption (compared with subjects who never/hardly ever drank wine) was significantly associated to a reduced risk of stroke (ischemic and hemorrhagic) and the association for daily wine consumption was statistically borderline ($p = 0.06$). Intake of either beer or spirits was not associated with reduced risk of stroke; on the other hand subjects who drunk ≥42 units *per* week had a 1.5 fold, significant, increase in risk.The Northern Manhattan Stroke Study [24] found that, among 667 cases and 1,139 controls, drinking up to 2 drinks/day of any type of alcoholic beverages was significantly associated with a lower risk of a first ischemic stroke, in a elderly multiethnic population. However, those who were predominantly wine drinkers had the lowest risk (RR, 0.40; 95% CI, 0.23 to 0.70) and consumed, on average, less alcohol than those who drank beer or spirits or were drinkers of all types of alcoholic beverages. Intake of 7 or more drinks of alcohol *per* day was significantly associated to an almost 3 fold increased risk.

From an Australian study [25] among 331 matched case-control pairs, wine, beer, and spirit consumption were associated with a lower intracerebral hemorrhage risk, but the relation was statistically significant only for wine drinkers; in a separate analysis by gender,

Table 1. Subgroup analysis using studies included in a" Wine or Beer drinkers *versus* non-drinkers" meta-analysis

	WINE			BEER		
	N	RR	99% CI	N	RR	99% CI
Vascular Events	13	0.68	0.59-0.77*	15	0.78	0.70-0.86*
Type of event						
Coronary heart disease	11	0.71	0.59-0.85	13	0.79	0.68-0.91
Cerebrovascular disease	2	0.43	0.24-0.78	2	0.67	0.41-1.10
Non-fatal vascular events	8	0.71	0.56-0.90	7	0.74	0.57-0.96
Cardiovascular mortality	2	0.49	0.34-0.70	3	0.76	0.55-1.05

N: number of studies; RR: relative risk; 99% CI: 99% confidence interval, from Table 2, Di Castelnuovo and Coll. 2002, with permission). *95% CI.

both wine and spirits were associated to a lower intracerebral hemorrhage risk in men (OR_{wine}, 0.3; 95% CI, 0.1 to 0.9; OR_{spirit}, 0.3; 95% CI, 0.1 to 0.8); while for women wine only was protective, although not significantly. This study too confirmed that heavy drinking of alcohol (more than 6 units/day) was significantly associated to a 3.4 fold increased risk of stroke.

In the Framingham Study population Djoussé and Coll. [17] assessed the effects of beer, wine, and spirits on the risk of ischemic stroke and observed a borderline association of current wine drinking with ischemic stroke (HR, 0.8; 95% CI, 0.6 to 1.0) but no effects for beer (HR, 1.0; 95% CI, 0.8 to 1.4) or spirits (HR, 0.9; 95% CI, 0.7 to 1.2). Mukamal and Coll. [16], with a semi-quantitative food-frequency questionnaire, ascertained regular and light consumption of beer, red and white wine, and liquor in a large prospective cohort study of male health professionals. Red wine consumption was inversely associated with risk of ischemic stroke in a graded manner ($p = 0.02$ for trend), while the other beverages were not.

The most important difference between wine and beer consumption was observed by our group in a meta-analysis of studies reporting wine and beer consumption in relation to vascular risk [9]. Pooling data from 13 prospective and case-control studies reporting relative risk of moderate (1-2 drinks *per* day, 150-300 ml *per* day) *versus* no wine consumption, the overall effect was a significant risk reduction of 32% (RR, 0.68; 99% CI, 0.59 to 0.77); in a subgroup analysis where the main endpoint was cerebrovascular disease the pooled relative risk was 0.43 (99% CI, 0.24 to 0.78) for wine intake, and 0.67 (95% CI, 0.41 to 1.10) for beer intake (Table 1).

Overall these reports suggest a benefit on the risk of stroke for wine intake only; however at the present, a rigorous estimation of the ischemic and hemorrhagic stroke risk associated with any specific alcoholic beverage is lacking.

Ischemic Stroke in Young Subjects: is alcohol consumption a real risk factor?

More than 10% of patients with stroke due to cerebral infarction are aged 55 years or less [26]. Stroke in the young is particularly detrimental for the lifetime disablement and requires a deeper evaluation in terms of risk. Indeed, an effective stroke prevention in the young cannot be attempted until the risk factors are clearly documented

While a number of studies have addressed the issue of stroke mechanism in the young, quantitation of major risk factors for stroke has rarely been undertaken and has not been systematically studied. Reasons for this probably include difficulties in making precise diagnoses before modern imaging techniques, selection of appropriate controls, and availability of sufficient sample size.

Heavy alcohol consumption as a risk factor for stroke in young adults has been observed in both hemorrhagic and ischemic subtypes studies. In young women light-moderate alcohol consumption had protective effect on ischemic stroke.

In The Melbourne Risk Factor Study [27], a total of 201 consecutive patients with first-onset stroke due to cerebral infarction, aged 15 to 55 years (mean, 45.5 years) were recruited from four teaching hospitals during 1985 to 1992 and compared with age- and sex-matched neighbourhood controls. Significantly increased risk of stroke was found among those with diabetes, hypertension, heart disease, current cigarette smoking and long-term heavy alcohol consumption (more than 60 grams/day) (odds ratio (OR), 15.3; 95% CI, 1.0 to 232.0). However, heavy alcohol ingestion within 24 hours preceding stroke onset was not a risk factor (OR, 0.9; 95% CI, 0.3 to 3.4).

The Hemorrhagic Stroke Project is a case-control study of hemorrhagic stroke among men and women aged 18 to 49 years, with the main purpose of identifying risk factors for intracerebral hemorrhage [28]. A total of 1,714 patients with hemorrhagic stroke were identified. Out of them, 217 cases met the criteria for primary intracerebral hemorrhage and were matched to 419 controls. Independent risk factors for intracerebral hemorrhage included hypertension, diabetes, current cigarette smoking, caffeinated drinks> 5/day and more than 2 alcoholic drinks for day (OR, 2.23; 95% CI, 1.16 to 4.32).

The incidence of ischemic stroke in young women ranges from 4.3 to 8.9/100 000 per year in the United States and continental Europe [29,30]. In a recent study, Nightingale and Coll. [31] determined the incidence and risk factors for ischemic stroke in young women (aged 15-49 years) in the UK. The incidence of ischemic stroke was 3.56/100 000 per year. Among factors associated with an increased risk they found heavy alcohol consumption (more than 168 grams/week of alcohol; OR, 8.5; 95% CI, 3.6 to 20.0), however light alcohol consumption was found to be protective (<72 grams/week of alcohol; OR, 0.17; 95% CI, 0.09 to 0.34).

In The Stroke Prevention in Young Women Study [32], a population-based case-control study on stroke in young women, light to moderate alcohol consumption appeared to be associated with a reduced risk of ischemic stroke in young women. Alcohol consumption, up to 24 grams/day, during the past year was associated with fewer ischemic strokes (<12 grams/day: OR, 0.57, 95% CI, 0.38 to 0.86; 12 to 24 grams/day: OR, 0.38; 95% CI, 0.17 to 0.86; >24 grams/day: OR, 0.95; 95% CI, 0.43 to 2.10) in comparison to never drinking.

Analysis of beverage type (beer, wine, liquor) indicated a protective effect for light wine consumption in the previous year (<12 grams/week: OR, 0.58; 95% CI, 0.35 to 0.97).

The majority of the cerebrovascular risk factors identified in these studies are modifiable. Thus, appropriate prevention strategies should have the potential to reduce the occurrence of stroke. In particular primary prevention initiatives addressed to heavy and binge drinkers in young population should be launched and supported.

Biological Mechanisms of the Protective Effects of Alcohol and Wine-derived Products

Anti-atherogenic Effects

Alterations in plasma lipoproteins, particularly increase in high density lipoprotein (HDL) cholesterol, was considered as the most plausible mechanism of the protective effect of alcohol consumption from coronary heart disease (CHD) [33-35]. Commonly referred to as "good" cholesterol, HDL bind to cholesterol into the bloodstream and bring it back to the liver for elimination or reprocessing, lowering total cholesterol levels in body tissues and reducing the cholesterol build-up on the arterial wall.

However, the mechanisms through which wine might exert anti-atherogenic effects appear to be distinct from those of alcohol, and mainly attributable to the biological activities of its non-alcoholic constituents.

Reactive oxygen species (ROS), generated by redox reaction pathways in aerobic cells are considered important mediators that regulate cell signalling and response. Excessive ROS production, at the site of vascular injury or inflammation, overwhelming the antioxidant defence of the organism, may be pathogenic for a variety of human diseases [36], including cardiovascular disease. Epidemiologic and laboratory studies have linked the intake of antioxidants to the reduction of CHD risk [37]. According to the oxidative hypothesis of atherosclerosis, low density lipoproteins (LDL) initially accumulating in the extracellular subendothelial space of arteries, are mildly oxidized by local generation of ROS [38,39]. This minimally modified LDL are per se potent inducers of inflammatory molecules and therefore can stimulate vascular cells to produce monocyte-chemotactic and granulocyte- and macrophage–colony stimulating factors, leading to monocyte recruitment and differentiation in arterial wall. The accumulating monocytes and macrophages stimulate further LDL peroxidation and, simultaneously the protein component of LDL becomes more negatively charged. These highly modified LDL are avidly recognized by scavenger receptors on macrophages and internalized to form so-called foam cells, a very early event in the pathogenesis of atheroma. Furthermore oxidized LDL also play a role in thrombus development, since they stimulate procoagulant activities in endothelial cells and in monocytes, and inhibit vasodilation by down regulating the expression of endothelial nitric oxide (NO)-synthase [40].

Some of the observed effects of polyphenols on cellular systems involved in the pathogenesis of CVD can be therefore reconducted to their recognized antioxidant and radical scavenging properties [41], which may delay the onset of atherogenesis by reducing chemically and enzimatically mediated peroxidative reactions.

The potential in vivo antioxidant properties of wine and its derived product have been evaluated in terms of their ability to enhance plasma antioxidant status, considered as an index of the capacity of the organism to generally counteract oxidative processes, as well as to reduce specific oxidative processes, those related to atherogenic LDL modifications in particular.

Studies in human volunteers showed increased plasma antioxidant capacity or protection of LDL from oxidation after consumption of red wine [42,43]; marked suppression of plasma post-prandial hydroperoxide increase was found in volunteers when a fatty meal was consumed with wine, instead of water [44]. Other relevant antiatherogenic modifications concern the reported ability of red wine to increase plasma levels of HDL at levels above that obtained after alcohol consumption [45], or to reduce lipid deposition, in animal models, independently of their effects on lipid peroxidation [46]. As inflammation is a crucial component of the atherosclerotic process, it is of interest that resveratrol, a wine-derived polyphenol, significantly reduces the degree of colon injury, neutrophil infiltration, the levels of cytokines and the COX-2 expression in an animal model of experimentally induced colitis [47].

Anti-thrombotic Effects

Other potential mechanisms contributing to the cardio-protective effect of moderate alcohol consumption include alterations of blood platelet function, coagulation and fibrinolysis. Alcohol seems to affect several factors involved in maintaining the delicate equilibrium between clot formation (to protect against bleeding) and clot dissolution (to prevent blood clots from forming in arteries), which have been implicated in the risk for myocardial infarction [48].

Alcohol consumption has been associated with increased levels of tissue plasminogen activator (tPA), the clot dissolving enzyme, and lower levels of fibrinogen and antithrombin III [49-52]; reduced susceptibility of platelets to aggregation has also been reported after alcohol consumption [53,54].

Polyphenols have been shown to be able to modulate the function of the different cellular components involved in the process of thrombosis in several systems. Interference with the arachidonic acid metabolism in both platelets and leukocytes have been reported, which resulted in inhibition of platelet aggregation and reduced synthesis of pro-thrombotic and pro-inflammatory mediators [55-57].

Polyphenols can also down-regulate the expression of adhesive molecules and tissue factor activity, induced by several agonists, such as cytokines or chemotactic agents, in both endothelial cells and leukocytes, resulting in functional modulation of cell-cell interactions and procoagulant activities [58-60].

Nitric Oxide

Hypertension is associated with increased risk for atherosclerotic diseases such as stroke, and heart and kidney disease. Essential hypertension involves endothelial dysfunction with alterations in nitric oxide (NO) bioavailability and calcium handling, smooth muscle cell proliferation, thickening of the vessel walls, and increased peripheral vascular resistance and blood pressure [61,62].

Preserving normal endothelial function is crucial to blood pressure homeostasis and vessel integrity. One of the major factors involved in regulation of endothelial function is NO. Endothelium-derived NO is not only a potent vasodilator but inhibits platelet aggregation, vascular smooth muscle cell proliferation and intimal migration, and monocyte adhesion, thus regulating blood pressure and protecting vascular function [62]. Abnormalities in NO have been demonstrated in both hypertension and atherosclerosis.

The vasodilator effect of alcohol is related to a higher expression of the endothelial nitric oxide synthase (eNOS) and NO production [63]. Wine polyphenols were also shown to modulate NO-mediated responses. Fitzpatrick and Coll. [64] first showed that certain wine extracts were able to relax pre-contracted smooth muscle of intact aortic ring, and Andriambeloson and Coll. [65] demonstrated that the endothelium-dependent vaso-relaxation of rat aorta was mediated by an increase of NO aortic content. In addition, incubation of endothelial cells with red wines up regulated NO synthase mRNA and protein expression, and produced up to three times more bioactive NO than did control cells [66]. Wallerath and Coll. [67] provides evidence that a blend of polyphenolic compounds in red wine likely stimulate the expression of the eNOS gene (and preserve eNOS activity), thus leading to an enhanced production of vascular NO. Martin and Coll. [68] showed that both delphinidin and anthocyanidin (two polyphenols from red wine), inhibit endothelial cell apoptosis via NO pathway and regulation of calcium homeostasis. Wine itself may ameliorate endothelial dysfunction. A work of Wollny and Coll. [69] provides evidence that red wine rather than white wine or alcohol by itself modulates primary haemostasis and prevents experimental thrombosis in rats, independently of its alcohol content, by a NO-mediated mechanism.

The different acute and chronic responses of vascular endothelium to alcohol may reflect an enhanced release of NO with low intakes of alcohol, but endothelial injury with acute heavier intake.

Alcohol Consumption and Omega-3 Polyunsaturated Fatty Acids

More recently an original mechanism to explain the protective effect of alcohol has been proposed by de Lorgeril and Coll.: the "fish-like effect of moderate wine drinking" hypothesis [70].

Omega-3 fatty acids (ω3 FA) consumption reduces risk of sudden cardiac death in humans [71,72] and induces myocardial protection in animal experiments [73]. The Lyon Diet Heart Study (a cross-sectional study on French male patients with CHD), showed that moderate wine consumption was associated with higher levels of "marine" ω3 FA in plasma [70] independently from the dietary intake of specific plant and marine ω3. The Authors concluded that the protection resulting from moderate alcohol drinking may be mediated through increased ω3 FA. These results were confirmed in a recent animal study of the same research group [74]. They showed that moderate alcohol consumption was associated with increased levels of ω3 FA both in plasma and in red blood cell membranes.

The association of alcohol consumption with ω3 FA in both plasma and red blood cells was also separately studied in women and in men enrolled in Italy, Belgium and England, in the framework of the IMMIDIET study [75] Eicosapentanoic acid (EPA), docosahexanoic acid (DHA) and EPA+DHA in plasma, and EPA and EPA+DHA in red blood cells were all positively associated with alcohol intake. The association was stronger in women than in men. In whole population the association between different beverages (wine or beer) and levels of ω3 FA was also investigated in wine drinkers, the association was confirmed both in plasma and red cell, while in beer and spirits drinkers only a weak association with DHA in plasma was found [76].

Conclusions

The relationship between alcohol consumption and cerebrovascular disease, and in particular stroke, is complex, in part reflecting the heterogeneity of vascular diseases.

Evidence suggests a J-shaped relationship between alcohol consumption and ischemic stroke, with lower risk for moderate alcohol consumers (1-2 drinks/day). Heavy alcohol consumption increases the relative risk of total stroke (both ischemic and hemorrhagic).

Up to now, the relationship between alcohol consumption and the different subtypes of ischemic and hemorrhagic stroke (i.e. atherothrombotic, lacunar, embolic, subarachnoid hemorrhage, intracerebral hemorrhage) has not been extensively investigated. Today, the modern imaging techniques, by improving diagnostic accuracy of stroke subtypes, might allow a rightly designed epidemiologic study and hopefully bring robust results.

Alcohol consumption should not be encouraged for those who do not already drink because of the harm associated with potential heavy use. Further research is needed to determine whether moderate alcohol consumption has a beneficial effect for specific subtypes of ischemic and hemorrhagic stroke.

An intensive programme is barely needed to reduce the gap between effective preventive strategies on the risk of stroke associated with irregular or heavy alcohol consumption and the joint effects with other risk factors, especially in young population.

Acknowledgments

The support of European Research Advisory Board (ERAB) grants (EA 05 20 and EA 08 27) is gratefully acknowledged.

References

[1] Maclure M. Demonstration of deductive meta-analysis: ethanol intake and risk of myocardial infarction. *Epidemiol. Rev.* 1993;15:328-51.

[2] Rimm EB, Klatsky A, Grobbee D, Stampfer MJ. Review of moderate alcohol consumption and reduced risk of coronary heart disease: is the effect due to beer, wine, or spirits. *BMJ* 1996;312:731-6.

[3] Cleophas TJ. Wine, beer and spirits and the risk of myocardial infarction: a systematic review. *Biomed Pharmacother*. 1999;53:417-23.

[4] Di Castelnuovo A, Costanzo S, Bagnardi V, Donati MB, Iacoviello L, de Gaetano G. Alcohol dosing and total mortality in men and women: an updated meta-analysis of 34 prospective studies. *Arch Intern. Med.* 2006;166(22):2437-45.

[5] Thun MJ, Peto R, Lopez AD, Monaco JH, Henley SJ, Heath CW Jr, Doll R. Alcohol consumption and mortality among middle-aged and elderly U.S. adults. *N. Engl. J. Med.* 1997;337:1705-14.

[6] White IR, Altmann DR, Nanchahal K. Alcohol consumption and mortality: modelling risks for men and women at different ages. *BMJ* 2002;325:191.

[7] Corrao G, Bagnardi V, Zambon A, Arico S. Exploring the dose-response relationship between alcohol consumption and the risk of several alcohol-related conditions: a meta-analysis. *Addiction* 1999; 94:1551:73.

[8] Renaud S, De Lorgeril M. Wine, alcohol, platelets, and the French paradox for coronary heart disease. *Lancet* 1992;339:1523-6.

[9] Di Castelnuovo A, Rotondo S, Iacoviello L, Donati MB, de Gaetano G. Meta-analysis of wine and beer consumption in relation to vascular risk. *Circulation* 2002;105:2836-2844.

[10] Donnan GA, Fisher M, Macleod M, Davis SM. Stroke. *Lancet* 2008;371:1612-23.

[11] Mukamal KJ, Tolstrup JS, Friberg J, Jensen G, Grønbaek M. Alcohol Consumption and risk of atrial fibrillation in men and women: the Copenhagen City Heart Study. *Circulation* 2005; 112:1736-1742.

[12] Stampfer MJ, Colditz GA, Willett WC, Speizer FE, Hennekens CH. Prospective study of moderate alcohol consumption and the risk of coronary disease and stroke in women. *N. Engl. J. Med.* 1988;319:267–73.

[13] Klatsky AL, Armstrong MA, Friedman GD. Alcohol use and subsequent cerebrovascular disease hospitalizations. *Stroke* 1989;20:741–6.

[14] Klatsky AL, Armstrong MA, Sidney S, Friedman GD. Alcohol drinking and risk of ischemic stroke. *Am. J. Cardiol.* 2001;88:703–6.

[15] Klatsky AL, Armstrong MA, Friedman GD, Sidney S. Alcohol and risk of hemorrhagic stroke. *Neuroepidemiology* 2002;21:115–22.

[16] Mukamal KJ, Ascherio A, Mittleman MA, Conigrave KM, Camargo CA Jr, Kawachi I, Stampfer MJ, Willett WC, Rimm EB. Alcohol and risk for ischemic stroke in men: the role of drinking patterns and usual beverage. *Ann. Intern. Med.* 2005;142:11–9.

[17] Djoussé L, Ellison RC, Beiser A, Scaramucci A, D'Agostino R, Wolf PA. Alcohol consumption and risk of ischemic stroke: the Framingham Study. *Stroke* 2002;33:907–912.

[18] Mazzaglia G, Britton Annie R, Altmann DR, Chenet L. Exploring the relationship between alcohol consumption and non-fatal stroke: a systematic review. *Addiction* 2001; 96:1743-56.

[19] Reynolds K, Lewis B, Nolen JD, Kinney GL, Sathya B, He J. Alcohol consumption and risk of stroke: a meta-analysis. *JAMA* 2003;289:579-588.

[20] Corrao G, Bagnardi V, Zambon A, La Vecchia C. A meta-analysis of alcohol consumption and the risk of 15 diseases. *Prev. Med.* 2004;38:613-619.

[21] Feigin VL, Rinkel GJ, Lawes CM, Algra A, Bennett DA, van Gijn J, Anderson CS.Risk factors for subarachnoid hemorrhage: an updated systematic review of epidemiological studies. *Stroke* 2005; 36: 2773–2780.

[22] Ariesen MJ, Claus SP, Rinkel GJ, Algra A. Risk factors for intracerebral hemorrhage in the general population: a systematic review. *Stroke* 2003;34:2060–2065.

[23] Truelsen T, Grønbaek M, Schnohr P, Boysen G. Intake of beer, wine, and spirits and risk of stroke. The Copenhagen city heart study. *Stroke* 1998;29:2467-72.

[24] Sacco RL, Elkind M, Boden-Albala B, Lin IF, Kargman DE, Hauser WA, Shea S,Paik MC. The protective effect of moderate alcohol consumption on ischemic stroke. *JAMA* 1999;281:53-60.

[25] Thrift AG, Donnan GA, McNeil JJ. Heavy drinking, but not moderate or intermediate drinking, increases the risk of intracerebral hemorrhage. *Epidemiology* 1999;10:307-12.

[26] Gunzerath L, Faden V, Zakhari S, Warren K. National Institute on Alcohol Abuse and Alcoholism report on moderate drinking. *Alcohol. Clin. Exp. Res.* 2004; 28(6):829-47.

[27] You RX, McNeil JJ, O'Malley HM, Davis SM, Thrift AG, Donnan GA. Risk Factors for Stroke Due to Cerebral Infarction in Young Adults. *Stroke* 1997 28(10):1913-8.

[28] Feldmann E, Broderick JP, Kernan WN, Viscoli CM, Brass LM, Brott T,Morgenstern LB, Wilterdink JL, Horwitz RI. Major risk factors for intracerebral hemorrhage in the young are modifiable.Stroke 2005;36(9):1881-5.

[29] Schwartz SM, Siscovick DS, Longstreth WT Jr, Psaty BM, Beverly RK, Raghunathan TE, Lin D, Koepsell TD. Use of low-dose oral contraceptives and stroke in young women. *Ann. Intern. Med.* 1997;127(8 Pt 1):596-603.

[30] Kristensen B, Malm J, Carlberg B, Stegmayr B, Backman C, Fagerlund M, Olsson T. Epidemiology and etiology of ischemic stroke in young adults aged 18–44 years in northern Sweden. *Stroke* 1997;28:1702–9.

[31] Nightingale AL, Farmer R. Ischemic Stroke in Young Women A Nested Case–Control Study Using the UK General Practice Research Database Stroke. 2004;35:1574-1578.

[32] Malarcher AM, Giles WH, Croft JB, Wozniak MA, Wityk RJ, Stolley PD, Stern BJ, Sloan MA, Sherwin R, Price TR, Macko RF, Johnson CJ, Earley CJ, Buchholz DW, Kittner SJ. Alcohol intake, type of beverage, and the risk of cerebral infarction in young women. *Stroke* 2001;32(1):77-83.

[33] Gaziano JM, Buring JE, Breslow JL, Goldhaber SZ, Rosner B, VanDenburgh M, Willett W, Hennekens CH. Moderate alcohol intake, increased levels of high-density lipoprotein and its subfractions, and decreased risk of myocardial infarction. *N. Engl. J. Med.* 1993; 329:1829-1834.

[34] Langer RD, Criqui MH, Reed DM. Lipoproteins and blood pressure as biological pathways for effect of moderate alcohol consumption on coronary heart disease. *Circulation* 1992;85:910-915.

[35] Suh I, Shaten BJ, Cutler JA, Kuller LH. Alcohol use and mortality from coronary heart disease: the role of high- density lipoprotein cholesterol. The Multiple Risk Factor Intervention Trial Research Group. *Ann. Intern. Med.* 1992;116:881-887.

[36] Halliwell B. Free radicals, antioxidants, and human disease: curiosity, cause, or consequence? *Lancet* 1994;344:721-724.

[37] Diaz MN, Frei B, Vita JA, Keaney JF Jr. Antioxidants and atherosclerotic heart disease. *N. Engl. J. Med.* 1997;337:408-416.

[38] Steinberg D. Arterial metabolism of lipoproteins in relation to atherogenesis. *Ann. N. Y. Acad. Sci.* 1990;598:125-135.

[39] Ross R. The pathogenesis of atherosclerosis: a perspective for the 1990s. *Nature* 1993; 362:801-809.

[40] Ballantyne CM. Low-density lipoproteins and risk for coronary artery disease. *Am. J. Cardiol.* 1998;82:3Q-12Q.

[41] Rice-Evans C, Miller NJ, Paganga G. Antioxidant properties of phenolic compounds. *Trends Plant Sci.* 1997;2:152-159.

[42] Serafini M, Maiani G, Ferro-Luzzi A. Alcohol-free red wine enhances plasma antioxidant capacity in humans. *J. Nutr.* 1998;128(6):1003-7.

[43] Cao G, Russell RM, Lischner N, Prior RL. Serum antioxidant capacity is increased by consumption of strawberries, spinach, red wine or vitamin C in elderly women. *J. Nutr.* 1998;128(12):2383-90.

[44] Ursini F, Zamburlini A, Cazzolato G, Maiorino M, Bon GB, Sevanian A. Postprandial plasma lipid hydroperoxides: a possible link between diet and atherosclerosis. *Free Radic. Biol. Med.* 1998;25(2):250-2.

[45] de Gaetano G, De Curtis A, di Castelnuovo A, Donati MB, Iacoviello L, Rotondo S. Antithrombotic effect of polyphenols in experimental models: a mechanism of reduced vascular risk by moderate wine consumption. *Ann. N. Y. Acad. Sci.* 2002;957:174-88.

[46] Waddington E, Puddey IB, Croft KD. Red wine polyphenolic compounds inhibit atherosclerosis in apolipoprotein E-deficient mice independently of effects on lipid peroxidation. *Am. J. Clin. Nutr.* 2004;79(1):54-61.

[47] Martín AR, Villegas I, La Casa C, de la Lastra CA. Resveratrol, a polyphenol found in grapes, suppresses oxidative damage and stimulates apoptosis during early colonic inflammation in rats. *Biochem. Pharmacol.* 2004;67(7):1399-410.

[48] Rimm EB, Williams P, Fosher K, Criqui M, Stampfer MJ. Moderate alcohol intake and lower risk of coronary heart disease: meta-analysis of effects on lipids and haemostatic factors. *BMJ* 1999;319(7224):1523-8.

[49] Hendriks HF, Veenstra J, Velthuis-te Wierik EJ, Schaafsma G, Kluft C: Effect of moderate dose of alcohol with evening meal on fibrinolytic factors. *BMJ* 1994;308:1003-1006.

[50] Ridker PM, Vaughan DE, Stampfer MJ, Glynn RJ, Hennekens CH. Association of moderate alcohol consumption and plasma concentration of endogenous tissue-type plasminogen. *JAMA* 1994;272:929-933.

[51] Bijnen FC, Feskens EJ, Giampaoli S, Menotti A, Fidanza F, Hornstra G, Caspersen CJ, Mosterd WL, Kromhout D. Haemostatic parameters and lifestyle factors in elderly men in Italy and The Netherlands. *Thromb. Haemost.* 1996;76:411-416.

[52] Woodward M, Lowe GDO, Rumley A, Tunstall-Pedoe H, Philippou H, Lane DA, Morrison CE. Epidemiology of coagulation factors, inhibitors and activation markers: The Third Glasgow MONICA Survey II. Relationships to cardiovascular risk factors and prevalent cardiovascular disease. *Br. J. Haematol.* 1997;97:785-797.

[53] Renaud SC, Ruf JC. Effects of alcohol on platelet functions. *Clin. Chim. Acta* 1996; 246:77-89.

[54] Elwood PC, Beswick AD, O'Brien JR, Yarnell JWG, Layzell JC, Limb ES. Inter-relationships between haemostatic tests and the effects of some dietary determinants in the Caerphilly cohort of older men. *Blood Coagul. Fibrinolysis* 1993;4:529-536.

[55] Pace-Asciak CR, Rounova O, Hahn SE, Diamandis EP, Goldberg DM. Wines and grape juices as modulators of platelet aggregation in healthy human subjects. *Clin. Chem.* 1996;246:163-182.

[56] Polette A, Lemaitre D, Lagarde M, Véricel E. N-3 fatty acid-induced lipid peroxidation in human platelets is prevented by catechins. *Thromb. Haemost* 1996;75:945-949.

[57] Rotondo S, Rajtar G, Manarini S, Celardo A, Rotilio D, de Gaetano G, Evangelista V, Cerletti C. Effect of trans-resveratrol, a natural polyphenolic compound, on human polymorphonuclear leukocyte function. *Br. J. Pharmacol.* 1998;123:1691-1699.

[58] Pendurthi UR, Williams JT, Rao LV. Resveratrol, a polyphenolic compound found in wine, inhibits tissue factor expression in vascular cells : A possible mechanism for the cardiovascular benefits associated with moderate consumption of wine. *Arterioscler. Thromb. Vasc. Biol.* 1999;19:419-426.

[59] Di Santo A, Mezzetti A, Napoleone E, Di Tommaso R, Donati MB, de Gaetano G, Lorenzet R. Resveratrol and quercetin down-regulate tissue factor expression by human stimulated vascular cells. *J. Thromb. Haemost.* 2003;1(5):1089-95.

[60] Gerritsen ME, Carley WW, Ranges GE, Shen CP, Phan SA, Ligon GF, Perry CA: Flavonoids inhibit cytokine-induced endothelial cell adhesion protein gene expression. *Am. J. Pathol.* 1995;147:278-292.

[61] Portaluppi F, Boari B, Manfredini R. Oxidative stress in essential hypertension. *Curr. Pharm. Des.* 2004;10:1695-8.

[62] Taddei S, Ghiadoni L, Virdis A, Versari D, Salvetti A. Mechanisms of endothelial dysfunction: Clinical significance and preventative non-pharmacological therapeutic strategies. *Curr. Pharm. Des.* 2003;9:2385-402.

[63] Venkov CD, Myers PR, Tanner MA, Su M, Vaughan DE. Ethanol increases endothelial nitric oxide production through modulation of nitric oxide synthase expression. *Thromb. Haemost.* 1999;81, 638–642.

[64] Fitzpatrick DF, Hirschfield SL, Coffey RG. Endothelium-dependent vasorelaxing activity of wine and other grape products. *Am. J. Physiol.* 1993;265(2 Pt 2):H774-8.

[65] Andriambeloson E, Kleschyov AL, Muller B, Beretz A, Stoclet JC,Andriantsitohaina R. Nitric oxide production and endothelium-dependent vasorelaxation induced by wine polyphenols in rat aorta.*Br. J. Pharmacol.* 1997;120(6):1053-8.

[66] Wallerath T, Poleo D, Li H, Förstermann U. Red wine increases the expression of human endothelial nitric oxide synthase: a mechanism that may contribute to its beneficial cardiovascular effects. *J. Am. Coll. Cardiol.* 2003;41(3):471-8.

[67] Wallerath T, Li H, Gödtel-Ambrust U, Schwarz PM, Förstermann U. A blend of polyphenolic compounds explains the stimulatory effect of red wine on human endothelial NO synthase. *Nitric. Oxide* 2005;12(2):97-104.

[68] Martin S, Giannone G, Andriantsitohaina R, . Martinez MC. Delphinidin, an active compound of red wine, inhibits endothelial cell apoptosis via nitric oxide pathway and regulation of calcium homeostasis. *Br. J. Pharmacol.* 2003,139:1095-1102.

[69] Wollny T, Aiello L, Di Tommaso D, Bellavia V, Rotilio D, Donati MB, de Gaetano G, Iacoviello L. Modulation of haemostatic function and prevention of experimental thrombosis by red wine in rats: a role for increased nitric oxide production. *Br. J. Pharmacol.* 1999;127(3):747-55.

[70] de Lorgeril M, Salen P, Martin JL, Boucher F, de Leiris J. Interactions of wine drinking with omega-3 fatty acids in coronary heart disease patients. A fish-like effect of moderate wine drinking. *Am. Heart J.* 2008;155:175-81.

[71] Albert CM, Campos H, Stampfer MJ, Ridker PM, Manson JE, Willett WC, Ma J. Blood levels of long-chain n-3 fatty acids and the risk of sudden death. *N. Engl. J. Med.* 2002; 346:1113-8.

[72] GISSI-Prevenzione Investigators. Dietary supplementation with n-3 polyunsaturated fatty acids and vitamin E after myocardial infarction: results of the GISSI-Prevenzione trial. *Lancet* 1999;354:447-55.

[73] Oskarsson HJ, Godwin J, Gunnar RM, Thomas JX Jr. Dietary fish oil supplementation reduces myocardial infarct size in a canine model of ischaemia and reperfusion. *J. Am. Coll. Cardiol.* 1993;21:1280-5.

[74] Guiraud A, de Lorgeril M, Zeghichi S, Laporte F, Salen P, Saks V, Berraud N,Boucher F, de Leiris J. Interactions of alcohol drinking with n-3 fatty acids in rats: potential consequences for the cardiovascular system. *Br. J. Nutr.* 2008;29:1-8.

[75] Iacoviello L, Arnout J, Buntinx F, Cappuccio FP, Dagnelie PC, de Lorgeril M, Dirckx C, Donati MB, Krogh V, Siani A; European Collaborative Group of the IMMIDIET Project. Dietary habit profile in European Communities with different risk of myocardial infarction: the impact of migration as a model of gene-environment interaction-the IMMIDIET study. *Nutr. Metab. Cardiovasc. Dis.* (suppl.) 2001; 11: 122-6.

[76] di Giuseppe R, de Lorgeril M, Salen P, Laporte F, Di Castelnuovo A, Krogh V, Siani A, Arnout J, Cappuccio FP, van Dongen M, Donati MB, de Gaetano G, Iacoviello L; European Collaborative Group of the IMMIDIET Project. Alcohol consumption and n-3 polyunsaturated fatty acids in healthy men and women from 3 European populations. *Am J Clin Nutr.* 2009;89(1):354-62.

In: Cerebral Ischemia in Young Adults
Editors: A. Pezzini and A. Padovani

ISBN 978-1-60741-627-2

Chapter 7

Infections and Ischemic Stroke in Young Adults

Armin J. Grau **[*]** ***and Frederik Palm***
Department of Neurology,
Klinikum Ludwigshafen, Germany

Abstract

There is increasing evidence that, in addition to conventional risk factors, acute and chronic infectious diseases increase the risk of ischemic stroke. Acute infection, mainly respiratory, and both bacterial and viral infection, represent temporarily active trigger factors for cerebral ischemia. Chronic infectious diseases that may increase the risk of cerebral ischemia include periodontitis, chronic bronchitis and infections with microbial antigens, such as *Helicobacter pylori* and *Chlamydia pneumoniae*. Infection as a risk factor appears to be most important in young age groups. As acute and chronic infectious diseases are treatable and partly preventable conditions, their recognition as risk factors for brain ischemia could be important for stroke prevention.

This chapter summarizes current epidemiologic, clinical and experimental data regarding the interactions between infection and ischemic stroke and outlines possible targets for therapeutic intervention.

Introduction

In young adults with stroke, traditional vascular risk factors are frequently lacking. Not uncommonly, the most important stroke etiologies in older age groups such as cardioembolism, large artery atherosclerosis or cerebral microangiopathy, can not be

[*] Correspondence: Armin J Grau, Klinikum der Stadt Ludwigshafen am Rhein, Bremserstrasse, 67, 67063 Ludwigshafen am Rhein, Germany. e-mail: graua@klilu.de.

identified in young adults. This underscores the requirement to identify other risk factors in younger age groups that may be less important or less obviously present in older adults.

An association between acute infections and cerebrovascular disorders was primarily identified in children at the end of the 19th century. The famous French neurologist Pierre Marie [1] and the later founder of psychoanalysis, Sigmund Freud, were among the first who showed that infections frequently precede stroke in young subjects. In his monography „Die infantile Cerebrallähmung“ published in 1897, Freud wrote that „in almost one third of all cases with acquired hemiplegic cerebral palsy..., paresis occurred simultaneously or shortly after one of the common infectious diseases of childhood“. He further stated that diseases with and without accompanying infection do not differ clinically and that there is almost no infectious disease that may not be followed by hemiplegia. Certainly, in some cases hemiplegia was the sequel of meningoencephalitis or of other diseases, however, Freud quoted that in the majority of cases, the initial lesion was of vascular origin similar to adult patients [2]. During the 20th century there has been a number of case series mostly of children but also of younger adults indicating that stroke was frequently preceded by infections. However, the topic was systematically evaluated only during the last 20 years.

Another important finding was the observation that epidemics of influenza infection and other infectious diseases (mainly respiratory infection) were often followed by an increased mortality of stroke and other vascular diseases [3,4]. Epidemiological surveys showed similar temporal patterns of the mortality of infectious respiratory diseases such as pneumonia and stroke with stroke death rate peaking with some slight delay after infectious diseases [5]. Most [5-8] although not all respective epidemiological studies [9] found an increased stroke incidence during winter months when respiratory infections are also more preponderant. However, these epidemiological findings were not reported exclusively for younger subjects.

Stroke occurs suddenly at a given point of time that is hardly defined by variations of the traditional vascular risk factors. Recent infection is among the potential trigger factors that may contribute to the occurrence of stroke at a given time point.

Besides acute infections, during recent years several chronic infections were discussed to be emerging risk factors for stroke. These mainly include infections by microbial agents such as *Chlamydia pneumoniae* and *Helicobacter pylori* and periodontal disease. The potential role that these diseases may play in the pathogenesis of stroke in the young will be discussed in a short form at the end of the chapter.

Pathogenesis

Special infectious diseases and stroke

It is generally accepted that several defined infectious diseases can cause stroke. Among these diseases are:

- Infective endocarditis
- Bacterial and fungal meningitis
- Neurosyphillis

- Neuroborrelliosis
- Acquired immunodeficiency syndrome
- Varizella zoster infection of head and neck

There are also some rather rare infectious diseases that have been linked with stroke such as cat-scratch disease [10] or Rickettsial diseases such as Rocky Mountain spotted fever [11]. Furthermore, tropical diseases such as Chagas disease, helminthic diseases and others are known to cause stroke, a topic that is not dealt with here in further detail.

In these diseases, specific pathogenetic mechanisms are active. In infective endocarditis infective or non-infective emboli from affected and frequently destructed cardiac valves reach the brain and lead to cerebral ischemia or hemorrhage but also to brain abscess or meningitis. Ischemic stroke occurs in about 20% of patients mostly early before antibiotic therapy starts to be effective [12, 13]. In adolescents and young adults, intravenous drug abuse plays an important role in the pathogenesis of endocarditis.

In bacterial including tuberculotic and fungal meningitis, meningeal inflammation can lead to vasculitis, vasospasm, intravascular thrombosis and disturbance of cerebrovascular autoregulation [14].

Cerebral ischemia can occur in the secondary (about 6 weeks to 2 years after infection) but mainly in the tertiary stage of syphilis. *Treponema pallidum* can affect the adventitia, the vasa vasorum or the intima layer of cerebral arteries and cause pathological changes in small, medium-sized and large brain arteries. Furthermore, neurosyphillis can lead to a progress of atherosclerotic vessel changes in brain arteries in young adults [15]. Neuroborreliosis, another Treponema infection, rarely leads to stroke that is caused by vasculitis of arteries of different size. Subcortical and vertebrobasilar infarcts appear to dominate, however, it is unclear whether direct infection of the vessel wall or immunological mechanisms cause vasculitic changes [16].

HIV infection is dealt with in another chapter of this book.

Days to months after Herpes zoster infection at head, neck but possibly also at the trunk, cerebral ischemia can occur that is mostly located ipsilateral to the Zoster infection and is caused by a granulomatous and necrotizing vasculitis that leads to stenoses and occlusions of intracranial arteries [17]. The reactivated Zoster virus appears to propagate from the ganglia via neural pathways to vessel walls; possibly autoimmunological mechanisms also play a role [18]. In most cases both large and small intracerebral arteries are affected [19]. A rash or CSF pleocytosis are not required to diagnose varicella zoster virus (VZV) vasculopathy. Detection of anti-VZV IgG antibody in CSF is a more sensitive indicator for this diagnosis than detection of VZV DNA [19]. In immunosupprimized patients cytomegalovirus infection can also lead to cerebral vasculitis [20].

In a case reports on children and young adults with stroke, local affection of brain supplying arteries by infectious foci at the neck and face had also been reported. Bickerstaff [21] reported on several children with ischemic stroke after infections of tonsils, neck and throat, in whom angiography detected vessel wall irregularities of the internal carotid artery and of intracerebral arteries, a finding that was interpreted as inflammation of the arterial wall caused by local infections. However, such direct involvement of arterial vasculature leading to cerebral ischemia certainly represents a rare situation nowadays and in adults.

General Infections and Stroke

Procoagulant State Induced by Infections

Inflammatory mechanisms such as in acute infections are frequently followed by an activation of procoagulant pathways and an inhibition of anticoagulant mechanisms that together lead to a procoagulant state. Such activation of coagulation after acute infectious diseases is probably the most important link between infections and cerebral ischemia. It was described not only in septicaemia and very severe infectious diseases but also in mild infection [22].

Among the pathways that link inflammation and coagulation are the following:

- Proinflamatory cytokines (e.g. interleukin-1 and tumor necrosis factor (TNF)-α) that are produced during inflammation can render the vascular endothelium from an anticoagulant to a procoagulant cell-layer by

1) promoting the expression of tissue-factor, a membrane-bound glycoprotein that initiates the extrinsic pathway of coagulation
2) stimulating the expression of plasminogen-activator inhibitor (PAI)-1 and reducing the expression of tissue-plasminogen activator (t-PA) thus lowering thrombolytic activity
3) reducing the expression of thrombomodulin, an important anticoagulant protein [23].

- Proinflammatory cytokines and C-reactive protein (CRP) that is commonly increased in bacterial infections can induce tissue-factor expression by monocytes and macrophages thus rendering these cells to procoagulant players [24].
- The anticoagulant proteinC /protein S system can be impaired, e.g. by raised concentrations of C4b-binding protein, an acute phase reactant and the main binding protein of protein S [25].
- Procoagulant factors such as fibrinogen are elevated as part of the acute phase response after infections. Seasonal variations of fibrinogen and factor VIIc concentrations have been observed with higher concentrations during winter months associated with respiratory infections [26], a finding that could contribute to the understanding of the seasonal variation of stroke incidence.
- Platelets can be activated during viral and bacterial infective diseases by microbial agents themselves [27] or via leukocyte activation or other mechanisms [28].

Some of the above mechanisms potentially linking infection and thrombosis and stroke have been investigated in stroke patients:

- A decreased level of circulating activated protein C was found in stroke patients and levels were lowest in those patients with a preceding infection. In addition, levels of C4b-binding protein were increased in patients with infection-associated stroke [29]. This indicates a disturbance of anticoagulant mechanisms in infection-associated stroke.

- Stroke patients with a recent infection had a distinctively lower ratio of active tissue plasminogen activator to PAI-1 [29] indicating disturbed thrombolytic activity.
- Levels of CRP were higher in stroke patients with compared to patients without recent infection [30] although this finding was not replicated in another study [31].
- Fibrinogen and fibrin D-Dimer concentrations were increased in infection-associated stroke [32].
- Platelet activation was increased in stroke patients with a history of an infection within the preceding week [28].

Infection, Atherosclerotic Plaques and Damage to the Vasculature in General

Another potential mechanism linking acute infection and stroke refers to the biology of atherosclerotic plaques. Atherosclerosis is nowadays viewed as a chronic inflammatory disease and plaques contain varying amounts of macrophages, T cells and mast cells. Those plaques that are prone to complications such as plaque rupture and consecutive thrombosis and embolism (vulnerable plaque) contain particularly large numbers of inflammatory cells [33]. Unstable but not stable coronary atherosclerotic lesions were found to contain oligoclonal populations of T lymphocytes [34]. This indicates that antigen-driven activation and proliferation of effector T cells typically occur in unstable plaques. Several antigens have been identified that are responsible for the activation of T cells in atherosclerotic plaques including extracellular matrix proteins and lipids but also heat shock proteins and antigens of microbial origin including *Chlamydia pneumoniae*, the periodontal pathogen *Porphyromonas gingivalis* and viruses such as Epstein-Barr virus. Most recently influenza A virus specific T-cells were identified in human atherosclerotic plaques and Influenza virus-derived antigens may thus also be potential candidates for triggering or sustaining plaque inflammation eventually leading to plaque complications such as stroke [35]. These findings suggest that systemic infection may be able to activate immune cells within plaques and may thus contribute to plaque rupture and organ ischemia including stroke [36].

Furthermore, it could be demonstrated that infection of apolipoprotein E-deficient mice with influenza A leads to a marked increase in arterial smooth muscle cell proliferation, inflammation and thrombosis in arterial walls with atherosclerotic plaques [37].

These very recent findings add to postmortem studies in the older literature that had shown severe and multifocal damage in larger arteries of patients dying soon after infectious diseases of various origin [38]. French pathologists had formed the term "Artériite grippale" in order to describe the injury to the arterial vessel system in patients dying after influenza-like diseases [39]. To summarize, acute severe infection may be able to activate inflammation in atherosclerotic plaques and may thus increase the risk for ischemic complications and it may lead to inflammatory damage in previously healthy vasculature predisposing to thrombosis and ischemia.

Infection, Traditional Vascular Risk Factors and Genetic Predisposition

Animal experiments hint to the possibility that traditional vascular risk factors and acute infection cooperate in increasing stroke risk. Systemic application of bacterial lipopolysaccharide (endotoxin) to rats induced ischemic stroke and cerebral hemorrhages in older animals, animals with hypertension or diabetes mellitus and in stroke-prone rats but not in young and healthy animals [40]. This indicates differences in the responsiveness of the cerebral vasculature to inflammatory stimuli in association with age and vascular risk factors. In hypertensive rats, LPS induced a stronger increase of tumor necrosis-factor alpha in serum than in normotensive rats. Hypertensive rats hosted more macrophages in the arterial wall of the cerebral vasculature than normotensive animals [41,42]. It is possible that a higher number of inflammatory cells and an increased formation of proinflammatory cytokines by such cells is an important link between traditional risk factors and short-lived inflammatory trigger factors that both together increase stroke risk.

As stated above, not the infections by different microbial agents themselves but rather severity and type of the host immune response may influence stroke risk to an important degree. The inflammatory response to infectious stimuli is under strong genetic control and it is an interesting hypothesis that a genetically determined strong response to inflammatory stimuli may be associated with increased risk of atherogenesis, stroke and other vascular diseases. Several studies investigated single genetic polymorphisms that modulate the inflammatory response. Polymorphisms of the P-selectin glycoprotein ligand-1 that are associated with lower capacity of neutrophils to bind activated platelets were linked to a reduced risk of cerebral ischemia [43]. Polymorphisms of the cathepsin G gene and plasma platelet-activating factor acetylhydrolase were also associated with increased stroke risk [44,45]. A common polymorphism in the promoter of the monocytic LPS receptor CD14 gene showed to be associated with atherothrombotic and lacunar stroke in a German population [46]. Even more interesting than studies investigating single polymorphisms are those reports that tested the hypothesis that the number of proinflammatory polymorphisms in multiple genes is associated with risk of stroke or carotid atherosclerosis. Flex and coworkers studied polymorphisms in 7 inflammatory genes (CRP, IL-6, MIF, MCP-1, ICAM-1, E-selectin, MMP-3) in 237 stroke patients and in 223 control persons. Five of these polymorphisms were associated with stroke risk and stroke risk steadily increased along the number of proinflammatory polymorphisms (n = 1: OR, 3.3 (95% KI 1,6 - 6,9); n = 2: OR, 21.0 (95% KI 7,6 - 57,5); n = 3: 50,3 (95% KI, 10,2 - 248,1) [47]. In a study based on the Bruneck study, Markus et al. [48] found an association between proinflammatory variants in 3 genes (IL-6, IL-1RA, CD14) and intima-media thickness; furthermore, there were synergistic effects between smoking, chronic infections and obesity and a score based on proinflammatory genetic variants. These results support the hypothesis of synergistic effects between proinflammatory polymorphisms, inflammatory and traditional vascular risk factors. However, studies on the interaction between recent acute infection and proinflammatory genotypes have not been performed in stroke patients so far.

Clinical and Therapeutic Aspects

Infection and Stroke

As mentioned in the introduction, the association between stroke and infection was first described in children and a large number of case reports and case series has been published on this topic.

Riikonen and coworkers [49] found infections (mainly respiratory tract infections) within the preceding 3 weeks in 15 of 44 children (34 %) with ischemic stroke.

Table 1. Acute infection and stroke – Case-control studies

Study	Age of patients/ Control group	Patients n (infection rate)	Controls n (infection rate)	Adjusted OR (95% CI)	Prestroke interval	Type of relevant infection
Syrjänen et al. 1988	<50 y/ Population	54 (35.2%)	54 (5.6%)	14.5 (1.5-112)	1w	Mainly respiratory infection
Grau et al. 1995	< 80 y/ Population	197 (19.3%)	197 (5.1 %)	4.5 (2.1-9.7)	1w	Bacterial infection Mainly respir. infection
Grau et al. 1998	< 85 y/ Hospital	166 (22.3%)	166 (8.4%)	3.1 (1.6-6.1)	1w	Bacterial/viral infection
Bova et al. 1996	Ø73 y / Stroke	182 (24.2%)	194 (9.7%)	2.9 (1.6-5.3)	2m	-
Macko et al. 1996	Ø59y/ Population+Hospital	37 (35.1 %)	81 (11.1%)	p<0.02 (no OR)	1w	Febrile/nonfebrile infections and other inflammatory syndromes
Nencini et al. 2003	Population+Hospital	93 (18.3%)	200 (8.0%)	2.5 (1.1-5.4)	1w	-
Paganini-H. et al. 2003	<89y./Outpatients	233 (43%)	362 (56%)	n.s.*	1m	-

*Significant for subgroups without risk factors Ø mean.
y year; m month; w week; OR Odds Ratio.
CI confidence interval.

In another report, six out of eleven children with ischemic stroke had suffered from infections within up to three weeks before ischemia [50]. Within 6 weeks, 8 children in Minneapolis suffered from ischemic stroke following infections of unknown etiology with fever, nausea, vomiting and sore throat [51]. Infections in children with stroke were caused by a wide variety of microbial agents including several viruses and bacteriae. Several reports mentioned *Mycoplasma pneumoniae*, a microbe that is known to induce disturbances in the coagulation system as causative agent [52,53].

Hindfelt and Nilson [54] were among the first who reported on infection preceding stroke in young adults. In a retrospective study with 64 ischemic stroke patients aged 16 to 40 years, they found evidence for recent infection in 27 (42%) of the subjects studied. Infections most often preceded stroke with unknown origin that mainly occurred during the winter season (October to March). Syrjänen and coworkers were the first to perform prospective studies on infection and stroke in young adults. They found increased serum antimicrobial antibody levels in 44% of patients with stroke under the age of 45 as compared to 9% of controls. Streptococci, staphylococci and enterobacteriae were the most common agents detected, whereas no association between viral antibodies and stroke was found [55].

In a first case-control study the same Finnish group investigated 54 consecutive stroke patients under the age of 50 and 54 age- and sex-matched control subjects from the general population. Patients had significantly more often suffered from febrile (>37.5 °C) infection during the preceding month than control subjects (35% vs. 6%; odds ratio (OR) 9.0, 95% confidence interval (CI) 2.2 - 80.0; results for the preceding week: OR 7.0, 95% CI 1.6 - 63.4). Infections mostly affected the respiratory tract and were predominantly of bacterial origin. In multivariate analysis with hypertriglyceridemia, hypertension, smoking and previous alcohol intoxication, recent infection was an independent risk factor (OR 14.5, 95% CI 1.9 - 112.3). Recent febrile infection was the most important risk factor in this study. It was associated with a higher risk elevation than hypertension or other conventional risk factors [56]. In a further Finnish study, 10 out of 150 (7%) patients with definite bacteraemia developed a stroke within one month, mostly within one week after the first positive culture. Endocarditis was present only in a minority of these patients [57].

Thereafter, several other case-control studies also included older subjects and all but one of them reported an increased risk of stroke after recent infection. Comparisons of these studies are limited due to different definitions of infections, choice of different control groups and other important differences. Estimates of the relative risk of stroke after infection in the preceding month ranged between 1.8 (95% CI 0.6 – 3.6) and 9.0 (95% CI 2.2 – 80). The prevalence of infection in the previous month was between 18 and 40 % and in the previous week between 10 and 35% (see Table 1). In most studies, respiratory tract infections dominated among patients and some of the studies found evidence that both bacterial and viral infections contributed to stroke risk [31] whereas others found an association only for bacterial infections [57,58].

In some of the studies the effect of age on infection as a risk factor was investigated. In one case-control study, a significant risk increase by infection was only detected for patients aged 51 – 60 and 61 – 70 years but not for younger or older subjects. This effect is partly explained by the low number of young patients with stroke (n=24) in this study [58]. A significant inverse relation between age and acute infection as a risk factor ($p= 0.018$) independent from other risk factors could be found in another study [31]. This result and the fact that the highest increase in stroke risk was found in the study by Syrjänen et al. who only included subjects under the age of 50 support the idea that infection may be a risk or trigger factor particularly in younger age groups. However, present data do not yet allow definite conclusions in this question.

There are some principle limitations inherent to case-control studies investigating infection as a risk factor of stroke:

1) Infections are ascertained retrospectively, possibly leading to an ascertainment bias.
2) The selection of controls can represent a relevant bias, e.g. by underrepresentation of subjects with recent severe infection.

3) Information can be incomplete in the most severely affected patients possibly leading to a misclassification bias.
4) The sample size was rather small in all studies.

In 2004, Smeeth et al. published a study based on the UK General Practice Research Database (GPRD) that so far gives the most robust evidence for recent infection as a stroke risk factor. This large study that was based on within person comparisons using the case-series method, a design that avoids the necessity to select external control groups. The authors investigated patients who had both stroke (or myocardial infarction) and an infection (or vaccination). They tested the null hypothesis that vascular event rates remain constant within 90 days after exposure to vaccination or acute infection. The study included 20486 patients with first myocardial infarction and 19063 patients with first stroke and showed that both respiratory tract infections (incidence ratio (IR) 3.19; 95% CI 2.81 - 3.62) and urinary tract infections (IR 2.72; 95% CI 2.32 – 3.2) increase stroke risk within 3 days after diagnosis. Ischemic and hemorrhagic stroke could not be differentiated in this study. In comparison, the IR for myocardial infarction during the first 3 days after respiratory infection was 5.0 (95% CI 4.4 – 5.5) and 1.7 (95% CI 1.3 – 2.1) after urinary tract infection. Risk of stroke steadily declined during the following weeks after infection although the risk remained significantly elevated for 3 months. Regarding respiratory tract infections, the IR fell to 2.3 (95% CI 2.1 – 2.7) 4-7 days after diagnosis of infection, to 2.1 (95% CI 1.9 – 2.3) after 8 – 14 days, to 1.7 (95% CI 1.5 – 1.8) 15 – 28 days thereafter and to 1.3 (95% CI 1.3 – 1.4) after 29 – 91 days. Respective values for urinary tract infections were 2.1 (95% CI 1.8 – 2.5), 1.9 (95% CI 1.7 – 2.1), 1.7 (95% CI 1.6 – 1.9), and 1.2 (95% CI 1.2 – 1.3). The rates of recurrent stroke after systemic respiratory infection followed similar patterns to the rates for first-ever stroke, however with slightly smaller effect estimates. There were slightly more patients with a stroke during winter than during summer in this study; however, the significant graded effect of respiratory infection remained significant when the analysis was restricted to events occurring during summer. Vaccinations did not produce a detectable increase in vascular risk during the following days and months; in contrast, there was a small reduction of risk by vaccinations within 3 days that may be attributed to the fact that people are vaccinated at a time when they are in good health [59]. The results of this study provide strong support for the concept that acute infections temporarily increase stroke risk and particularly the association between time and effect size supports a causal role of infections.

Using a separate UK primary care database (IMS Disease Analyzer Mediplus database) a recently published study again supports the association between recent infection and stroke. The study used a case-control design und was based on 9208 patients with first stroke. Within 7 days following infection, the adjusted odds ratio for stroke was 1.92 (95% CI 1.24 – 2.97). The strength of the association fell over time. Urinary tract infection within the preceding month also increased stroke risk (OR 2.67; 95% CI 1.3 – 5.5). The existence of extensive data on cardiovascular risk factors allowed the authors to infer that the mechansism linking infection and stroke risk operate across different levels of prior stroke risk [60].

Infection and Stroke Subtypes

Subtypes of Ischemic Stroke

Some of the case-control studies had investigated the association between etiologic subgroups of cerebral ischemia and recent infection. In a case-control study with 197 patients, infection within one week was significantly associated with cardioembolism and with stroke due to cervical artery dissection but not with other stroke etiologies [30]. In a second case-control study from the same group, recent infection was again independently associated with cardioembolism (OR 3.25; 95% CI 1.06 – 10.0) and tended to be associated with large artery atherothrombotic stroke (OR 7.0; 95% CI 0.86 – 57). Furthermore, cryptogenic stroke tended to be more common among patients with than those without recent infection [31].

A study from the USA that did not identify recent infection as a general stroke risk factor (Table 1), reported that patients with a recent respiratory infection tended to suffer more often from large-vessel atherthromboembolic or cardioembolic stroke than patients without recent infection ($p = 0.07$) [61]. Similarly, an Italian case-control study with 93 stroke patients found that (infectious and non-infectious) inflammatory events within 30 days increased the risk of atherothrombotic (OR 5.72; 95% CI 2.14 – 15.25) and cardioembolic stroke (OR 3.02; 95% CI 1.20 - 7.63) whereas no association existed with lacunar or undetermined etiology [62].

None of these studies was large enough to possess the statistical power for subgroup analyses. However, if all studies are viewed together they unanimously report an association between recent infection and cardioembolic stroke and the lack of an association between infection and lacunar stroke. Furthermore, at least some of the studies detected a significant association between infection and large artery atherothrombotic stroke. The studies did not report an increased prevalence of endocarditis that could explain the link between infection and cardioembolic stroke. Results regarding cardioembolism and infection could be biazed as physicians may ask more readily for transesophageal echocardiography in patients with recent infection. However, there were no differences in the diagnostic work-up between patients with and without infection in one study that addressed this issue [30]. Atrial fibrillation tended to be more common in patients with than in those without infection [30]. Most likely, the prothrombotic state that is found in atrial fibrillation and other sources of cardioembolism [63] may be temporarily enhanced by acute infections leading to thrombosis and embolism.

As discussed above it is possible that systemic infection activates inflammatory mechanisms in atherosclerotic plaques thus increasing the risk of plaque rupture, thrombosis and embolism. This could explain an association between infection and large artery atherothrombotic stroke although such association was not reported by all studies.

Regarding young subjects with stroke it is of interest to note that there is a subgroup of mostly younger patients with recent infection in whom the etiology of stroke could not be determined although the association between infections and cryptogenic stroke did not reach statistical significance probably due to low numbers of subjects. The fact that many of these patients had suffered from previous respiratory infection and several of them had a cortical infarct suggestive of an embolic source fostered the hypothesis that local pulmonal infection may have led to thrombogenesis in pulmonal venes and subsequently to embolism to the brain via the left atrium. Such embolic pathway had been described in patients after lung transplantation [64] and systemic embolism can be derived from pulmonary venous thrombosis as shown in a post-mortem study [65]. However, a study investigating 18 young patients with cryptogenic stroke and TIA using MRA of the pulmonary venes did not detect evidence for pulmonary venous thrombosis in any of these subjects [66].

In some of the younger stroke patients with recent infections special stroke etiologies were reported. A post-mortem examination of a 53 year old male patients with febrile gastrointestinal infection shortly before extensive brainstem and cerebellar stroke revealed wide-spread vasculitis and intravascular coagulation in brain-supplying arteries. A 25 year old patient with recent bronchitis had a right-sided cortical MCA infarct and a right carotid siphon stenosis without evidence of atherosclerotic vessel changes or dissection. Laboratory parameters indicated an acute inflammatory and allergic reaction (e.g. very high IgE) [30]. During the terminal incubation period of severe mumps infection, a 40 year old patient suffered from proximal internal carotid artery occlusion and ipsilateral large middle cerebral artery infarction. Computed tomography of the neck detected a hemorrhage located ventromedial to the right common carotid artery. Four months later the right ICA was partly recanalized. Carotid surgery revealed an atherosclerotic plaque and a vessel wall, which was fragile and less compact than usually. A strong inflammatory reaction to mumps infection may have contributed to the pathogenesis of the cervical hemorrhage and to acute thrombosis and occlusion of the ICA in this patient [67].

The examples of these patients suggest that there may be rare pathogenetic mechanisms linking infections and stroke particularly among younger subjects and that vasculitis is one of these pathogenetic links. Such mechanisms may not be detected by large studies including subgroup analyses but only by meticulous analysis of single patients a fact that stresses the need for well-written case reports.

Infection and Cervical Artery Dissection

Cervical artery dissection (CAD) is among the most important etiologies of ischemic stroke in younger subjects. The pathogenesis of CAD is not established, however, there is profound evidence that alterations in the extracellular matrix that can be detected in skin biopsies by electron microscopy may contribute to the disease [68]. Furthermore, CAD shows some familial aggregation and analyses of healthy relatives of CAD patients suggested that the connective tissue phenotype is familial with an autosomal dominant inheritance [69].

One of the early case-control studies on infection and stroke had found that 3 out of 5 patients with CAD had a history of a recent infection [30]. In a case series three patients were reported one of whom suffered from simultaneous four-vessel dissection after acute respiratory infection and two had recurrent CAD after upper respiratory tract infections [70]. These observations prompted a prospective systematic evaluation of the association between infection and CAD. In a case-control study with 43 consecutive patients with acute non-traumatic CAD [age 43.2 ± 8.8 (mean $\pm$ SD)] and 58 consecutive patients under the age of 50 with acute cerebral ischemia from other etiologies (control patients; age 41.4 ± 7.2 years) infection within one week was more common in CAD patients (25/43, 58.1 %) as compared to control patients (19/58, 32.8%; $p = 0.011$). Respiratory tract infection dominated in both groups. Cough, vomiting or sneezing were more common among CAD patients than controls, however, in multivariate analysis recent infection but not the above mechanical factors were independently associated with CAD. CAD was more often diagnosed between November and April than between May and October ($p < 0.05$), a seasonal distribution that was not found among control patients. A number of biochemical and immunological studies (α1-antitrypsin and serum antibodies against *Chlamydia pneumoniae*, smooth muscle cells, collagen type I-IV and heat shock protein 65) did not contribute to the understanding of the pathogenesis of infection-associated CAD [71].

A second case-control study with 47 non-traumatic CAD patients and 52 patients with ischemic stroke from other origin also detected recent infections (within one month) more often in CAD patients (31.9%) than in the control group (13.5%; OR 3.0, 95% CI 1.1 – 8.2) although the prevalence of previous infection was lower than in the above study. The association with infections was stronger in patients with multiple (OR 6.4) than with single artery (OR 2.1) dissection. These two studies indicate that recent infection is a relevant trigger factor for CAD together with other factors such as minor trauma. However, mechanical factors themselves such as coughing or vomiting appear not to explain the association between infection and CAD.

Two observational studies also showed that there is a seasonal variability in the occurrence of non-traumatic CAD showing a peak in October [72] and during winter months [73], respectively. The cause of such seasonal patterns is not clear, however, infections besides other environmental factors could contribute to this phenomenon. C-reactive protein (CRP) and leukocyte counts were higher in patients with non-traumatic CAD as compared to patients with trauma-related CAD, a result supporting the hypothesis of inflammatory mechanisms contributing to non-traumatic CAD although there was no association with an elevated infection-rate in this retrospective study [74]. Another study found elevated CRP months after CAD, a finding that was independent from conventional risk factors and that was not detected in other stroke etiologies [75]. These results further support the hypothesis that inflammatory mechanisms contribute to the pathogenesis of CAD.

In conclusion, acute infection and inflammatory mechanisms appear to play a role in the etiology of CAD although the precise nature of the pathogenetic link remains unclear.

Histological studies only exceptionally detected slight adventitial inflammation in the vessel wall in CAD [76] and commonly CAD is not regarded as inflammatory arteriopathy. However, investigations in intracranial [77,78] and coronary artery dissection [79,80] often showed inflammatory infiltrates in the arterial wall and as these diseases more often lead to rapid death post-mortem studies are more numerous as in CAD. Therefore, it is possible that inflammatory mechanisms in CAD have been overlooked so far. As mentioned above, inflammatory mechanisms during infection and microbial agents themselves can cause substantial damage to the vascular wall, mainly to the tunica media [38,81] and such mechanisms may play a role in the pathogenesis of CAD.

Infection and Intracerebral and Subarachnoid Hemorrhage

Most studies on infection and stroke concentrated on ischemic stroke. One small case-control study investigated 44 patients with subarachnoid hemorrhage (SAH; age 55 ± 14 years) and 56 patients with intracerebral hemorrhage (age 65 ± 12 years) and the same number of age and sex-matched control subjects, respectively. After adjustment for other risk factors, there was a borderline significant association between the risk of subarachnoid hemorrhage and infection within 4 weeks (Odds ratio 6.0; 1.1 –31.8) but no association with intracerebral hemorrhage (odds ratio 1.1; 0.08 – 14.8) [82]. In another small study, Jones and coworkers found increased antibody titers against influenza virus in patients with SAH as compared to a control group [83]. This finding may also support the hypothesis of infection as a risk or trigger factor for SAH.

During sepsis and endocarditis cerebral aneurysms, so called mycotic aneurysms, can develop and cause SAH. Mycotic aneurysms can derive from septic cerebral embolism resulting in inflammatory destruction of the arterial wall, beginning at the endothelial surface. Alternatively, infected embolic material may reach the adventitial layer of the artery via the vasa vasorum, with inflammation disrupting the adventitia and tunica muscularis and thus resulting in aneurysmal dilatation [13]. In the above case-study, none of the patients had a recent sepsis or endocarditis and in addition severe infection in the past was not more common in patients with SAH than in the control group. But even in less severe infection, endothelial activation and increased adhesion of leukocytes to the endothelium may create a microenvironment where a release of proteases – insufficiently counterbalanced by antiproteases – or increased free radical formation by leukocytes may lead to substantial damage to the arterial wall. Particularly proteolytic processes by leukocytes invading the arterial wall may cause degradation of the extracellular matrix and may thus predispose to the formation or to the rupture of preformed aneurysms [84]. Complement factors C3c and C9, immunoglobulin G and M, the adhesion receptor VCAM-1, macrophages and T-lymphocytes are all frequently detected in – mostly unruptured – aneurysms but rarely in control basilar arteries [85]. This indicates that extensive inflammatory and immunological reactions are common in cerebral aneurysms and supports the hypothesis of a role of inflammatory processes – possibly triggered by infection – in formation and rupture of aneurysms.

In order to summarize, several case-control studies and a large study based on the case-series method unanimously identified recent infections as independent stroke risk factors. The decline of the risk elevation over time after infection is in strong favour of a causal relationship between infection and stroke. It is very unlikely that there exists a common precipitant for both acute infection and stroke. The strength of the association is considerable. Therefore, the benefits of reducing infection and mainly respiratory infection either through immunization or treating or preventing infection may therefore be substantial. There is a wide range of infection types (e.g. respiratory and urinary tract infections) and causative organisms (e.g. viral and bacterial) in association with stroke. This supports the idea that stroke risk associated with preceding infection is generic rather than linked to specific types of infections or organisms. Most likely, the inflammatory response to acute infection triggers a procoagulant state that temporarily increases the risk of stroke.

Preceding Infection, Post-stroke Infection, Stroke Severity and Outcome

It is well accepted that body temperature on admission after stroke is inversely correlated with stroke severity and outcome [86]. As stated above, recent infection is associated with cardioembolic stroke that leads to rather severe strokes. It is not associated with lacunar stroke that has a relatively good prognosis. For these reasons, it can be expected that infection preceding stroke may lead to more severe neurological deficits and worse outcome after stroke.

Patients with recent infection had a more severe neurological deficit on admission than those without infection in one of the first case-control studies, a finding that was associated with a higher rate of cortical MCA infarcts in the infection group and remained significant together with age, blood glucose and leukocyte count on admission after adjustment for other covariables [30]. However, in a second study from the same group recent infection was not associated with more severe neurological deficit on admission [31]. Greater stroke severity in patients with recent infection was reported in three [29,30,61] but was not detected in three other studies [31,32,87]. Altogether, results are at variance and it is insufficiently clear whether recent infection may lead to more severe strokes and worse outcome.

Experimental stroke models give interesting but also contradictory results regarding the association between acute inflammatory stimuli and stroke outcome. In a middle cerebral artery occlusion model, the application of lipopolysaccharide (LPS) exacerbated brain damage and neurological deficit by mechanisms that depended on interleukin-1 and the presence of neutrophilic leukocytes [88]. This study is in accordance with several previous ones that had shown that proinflammatory cytokines can exacerbate ischemic brain damage. On the other hand, bacterial LPS can protect the brain against subsequent ischemic damage when it is applied before in a dosage below an injurious threshold. Such LPS preconditioning appears to work similar to ischemic preconditioning, a term that refers to protection conferred by a subthreshold ischemic insult that activates endogenous protective mechanisms. LPS preconditioning led to smaller infarcts and reduced inflammatory cell activation and transmigration into the brain in animal models [89]. These results indicate that preceding infectious and inflammatory stimuli can both protect from ischemic injury and can exacerbate such injury probably dependent on timing and dosage of these stimuli. This may explain why clinical studies did not show clear associations between recent infections and stroke severity and outcome.

The time-course of peripheral blood inflammatory parameters after stroke does not follow the paradigm of an acute phase response [90]. However, there is evidence of a very early increase of inflammatory markers including CRP after ischemic stroke [91]. It is undefined whether such response is caused by stroke itself or whether a pre-existing inflammatory condition including previous infection may contribute to this finding.

Numerous studies investigated the role of infections after stroke [92]. Respiratory tract and urinary tract infections after stroke are very common although studies dealing with this topic reported widely varying results. Most studies found increased mortality and worse functional outcome in association with post-stroke infection and particularly pneumonia after stroke is among the most important factors that contribute to stroke mortality. Numerous mechanisms are relevant in post-stroke infections including initial stroke severity and immobility, dysphagia, iatrogenic factors such as urinary catheter and intravenous lines. Most interestingly, there is increasing evidence that stroke itself leads to immunodepression and thus increases the risk for systemic infection [92]. Furthermore, a considerable number of patients that develop infections after stroke had first signs and symptoms of such infection already prior to stroke [93]. Therefore it is likely, that previous infections are also responsible for a relevant proportion of post-stroke infections in addition to all other above mentioned mechanisms.

Therapeutic Implications of Infections as Stroke Risk Factors

Given the evidence that vulnerable individuals have an increased risk of stroke during episodes of infection prevention and early adequate treatment of infections could have important impact on stroke in the future. At present, no antiinfective therapy has proven to be effective in stroke prevention as randomized controlled trials have not been performed in this field. Interventional strategies could include early antiinfective therapy in high risk patients or vaccinations.

Recent observational studies support the idea that influenza vaccination may contribute to reduce stroke risk. During an average influenza season, about 5% of adults develop symptomatic influenza infection each year [94]. Influenza infection can take an asymptomatic course, but frequently it leads to various respiratory syndromes and to disorders affecting the heart, the brain and other organs. Fulminant primary viral and secondary bacterial pneumonia can develop. As stated above, influenza and other infections can cause considerable damage to the systemic vasculature and can therefore increase the risk of stroke. Epidemiological surveys showed that hospitalizations for stroke and cardiac diseases significantly increase during influenza epidemics [95, 96].

The association between influenza vaccination and stroke risk was investigated in two case-control and in one large cohort study. Lavallée et al. [97] studied 90 ischemic stroke patients and 180 community control subjects and observed an independent association between influenza vaccination and stroke (OR 0.5; 95% CI 0.26-0.94). A larger case-control study from Germany investigated 370 stroke/TIA patients and 370 age- and sex-matched community controls during two winter and one summer season; 19.2% of stroke patients and 31.4% of controls had an influenza vaccination during the last vaccination campaign ($p<0.0001$). In multivariate analysis with vascular risk factors and diseases, socioeconomic variables and factors reflecting health-related behaviour, influenza vaccination was associated with significantly reduced odds for stroke/TIA (0.46; 95% CI 0.28-0.77). Subgroup analyses showed significant associations between vaccination and a reduced risk of stroke/TIA in men, subjects at least 65 years of age, those with an indication for influenza vaccination according to German guidelines, and those with previous vascular diseases. Risk reduction by influenza vaccination was confined to one winter season in which the effect was so large that there remained an overall significant result when both winter and the summer season were combined. Interestingly, other vaccinations were not associated with reduced stroke risk in this study [98].

The most robust evidence for a protective role of influenza vaccination stems from a large cohort study that included data from more than 140.000 subjects aged ≥65 years that were followed for two influenza seasons (1998-2000). Influenza vaccination was associated with a significant reduction in the risk of hospitalization for cerebrovascular disease (hazard ratio (HR) 0.84; 95% CI 0.72-0.97), cardiac disease, influenza or pneumonia [99]. Although this study is less prone to misclassification of vaccination status and other study data than above case-control studies, residual confounding can not be completely excluded neither in the case-control studies nor in this large observational study. Therefore, interventional studies are desirable, however, it is doubtful whether randomized studies will ever be performed in patients with increased risk of stroke given the fact that current guidelines e.g. in Germany recommend influenza vaccinations in the elderly and in all individuals with chronic diseases comprising most subjects with increased risk of stroke.

Vaccinations cause an inflammatory response and can mimic acute infectious diseases. Therefore, the question is of interest whether vaccinations increase the short-term risk of stroke. The study on infection and stroke that was based on the UK GPRD data bank investigated this issue and did not find an increased rate of stroke or myocardial infarction shortly after vaccinations. In contrast, influenza vaccination (but not all other vaccinations) was associated with a short-term risk reduction, however, this may be explained by the fact that vaccinations are usually performed at times of good health conditions of the subjects [59].

Chronic Infections and Stroke Risk

In addition to acute infections several chronic infectious diseases have been discussed as stroke risk factors during recent years. This research line was stimulated by the discussion on the possible role of microbial agents in the pathogenesis of atherosclerosis. As mentioned above atherosclerosis is nowadays viewed as an inflammatory disease [33]. The inflammatory response to an injury to the vessel wall is supposed to be an essential component of atherogenesis. Several seroepidemiological studies and tissue analyses tried to find microbial agents as triggers for this inflammatory process. However, at present, it is still an unsolved issue whether microbial agents play a causal role in atherogenesis or whether they are mere bystanders.

Regarding stroke risk mainly infectious agents like *Chlamydia pneumoniae*, *Helicobacter pylori* and agents causing chronic dental infection have been investigated. Infections with these agents share several features. They cause chronic or persistent latent infection and reinfections are common.

Chlamydia Pneumoniae

During the last decades most studies on the association between infectious agents and stroke focused on *Chlamydia pneumoniae*, an obligate intracellular organism first identified as a cause of human illness in the 1980ies [100]. Within most populations *C. pneumoniae* is highly prevalent and serological evidence is estimated to be 50% throughout the world [101]. Saikku and colleagues first demonstrated an association between serological evidence of *C.*

pneumoniae infection and myocardial infarction [102]. Several seroepidemiological studies, tissue analyses and animal experiments dealing with atherogenesis, myocardial infarction and stroke followed [103]. Results from seroepidemiological studies on the association between stroke and *C. pneumoniae* infection vary widely although most studies found a positive correlation. The first of a series of studies was restricted to young patients (age 18 – 50 years) with stroke or TIA and reported an independent association between cerebral ischemia and elevated IgA titers against *C. pneumoniae* and specific IgG antibodies in circulating immuncomplexes [104]. In the Northern Manhattan Stroke Study, there was an association between antichlamydial IgA and stroke risk in both younger and older age groups [105].

The value of seroepidemiological studies of *C. pneumoniae* is limited by the fact that it is still unclear which classes and titres of antibodies represent acute first or acute reinfection, persistent but inactive or chronically active infection [106]. *C. pneumoniae* could be identified in atherosclerotic plaques using electron microscopy, PCR and immunocyto-chemistry. Again detection rates varied widely between 0 and 100% [103]. It is another limiting factor for seroepidemiological studies that serology and endovascular detection do not correlate well [107]. Poor repeatability was shown to complicate PCR, and detection of *C. pneumoniae* by in situ hybridization possess several technical problems, however, new methods may become available that are more robust in the assessment of *C. pneumonia* [108].

Several antibiotic trials that were directed towards eradication of *C. pneumonia* were performed in patients with coronary heart disease. In a metaanalysis with eleven studies antibiotic anti-chlamydial therapy was not associated with a reduction of mortality or any coronary event [109]. Sander and colleagues performed a randomized trial and observed the effect of a 30-day-roxithromycin treatment on progression of intima-media thickness (IMT) in *Cp*-positive patients. Compared with progression of IMT in the three years before antibiotic drug therapy, progression in treated subjects decreased in the following two years (0.07 vs. 0.12 mm/year $p<0.01$). Among *Cp*-positive patients, treatment with roxithromycin led to reduced IMT-progression within 2 years as compared to non-treated patients. However, progression again returned to pre-treatment values during the next two years. No influence on cerebrovascular events could be observed [110,111].

Altogether the role of *C. pneumoniae* in the pathogenesis of stroke and coronary heart disease remains doubtful at present. The failure of antibiotic trials does not prove that *C. pneumoniae* is not involved in these disease as it is possible that antibiotic treatment might have started too late in the course of *C. pneumoniae* infection in order to be effective and as it may be very difficult to eradicate *C. pneumoniae*. However, at present there are more arguments against than for a causal involvement in stroke pathogenesis.

Helicobacter Pylori

Infection with *H. pylori*, a gram negative spiral bacterium, mostly occurs during childhood and infection rates are influenced by socioeconomic factors [112]. Infection can cause gastritis, peptic ulcer and gastric cancer, but it often remains asymptomatic. As *C. pneumoniae H. pylori* could be detected in carotid plaques [113]. Results of studies investigating the relationship between *H. pylori* seropositivity and cardiovascular diseases are at variance, but the majority of studies and especially larger studies and those that adjusted for potential confounders showed no significant correlation [114]. Regarding cerebrovascular disease, several studies demonstrated a positive correlation between seropositivity to *H. pylori* and the risk of atherothrombotic or lacunar stroke [115-118]. In contrast, one study could not find a positive relation between *H. pylori* seropositivity and stroke in middle aged men [119]. Among *H. pylori* strains, those carrying the cytotoxin-associated gene A (CagA) are particulary virulent and associated with increased inflammation. Two case-control studies found a positive relationship between stroke and seroprevalence of CagA positive *H. pylori* strains but not with *H. pylori* in general after adjustment for other risk factors. In one of these studies increased titers of antibodies against CagA strains were only associated with large artery atherothrombotic but not with cardioembolic stroke [120]. In the other study, CagA seropositivity was a risk factor for ischemic stroke in general without differences between etiologic stroke subtypes [121]. Furthermore, CagA seropositivity (but not *H. pylori* seropositivity in general) was associated with an increased risk of carotid atherosclerosis in one study [122] but not with increased intima-media thickness in another report [123].

In a meta-analysis of seven studies Cremonini and colleagues [124] found an odds ratio of 1.49 (95% CI: 1.24 - 1.81) for the correlation between seroprevalence of *H. pylori* and stroke. The odds ratio for seropositivity of CagA strains and stroke was 2.23 (95% CI 1.49 - 3.36). Especially large vessel disease appeared to be associated with *H. pylori* seroprevalence. Age does not appear to influence the association between *H. pylori* infection and stroke and *H. pylori* may not play a more important role in younger than older subjects with stroke.

Although several studies found a correlation between *H. pylori* seropositivity and stroke residual confounding (e.g. by socioeconomic factors) can not be excluded. In the absence of interventional studies a causal association between stroke and *H. pylori* infection is not proven yet.

Periodontal Disease

Periodontal disease is among the most common human infectious diseases. In the National Health and Nutrition Examination Survey prevalence of periodontal disease in the US population was estimated to be 4.2% [125]. In periodontitis, a complex interplay between bacterial infection and host response leads to a destruction of tooth supporting tissue and finally often to tooth loss. Periodontal pathogens such as *Porphyromonas gingivalis* or *Prevotella intermedia* could be detected in carotid plaques together with other microbial antigens [126]. Chronic inoculation of *P. gingivalis* led to an increase of lipid profiles and enhanced atherogenesis in an animal model [127]. However, the question whether such bacteria contribute causally to the pathogenesis of atherosclerosis is not sufficiently clear at present.

Post hoc analyses of prospective studies and smaller case-control studies detected an association between periodontitis and stroke [57,103,128]. A larger case-control study confirmed an association between severity of periodontitis and risk of stroke or transient ischemic attack independent from traditional risk factors, socioeconomic factors and health behaviour. Defined as an average periodontal attachment loss of more than 6 mm, severe periodontitis was associated with a 4.3 times higher risk of stroke (95% CI 1.85 – 10.2) as compared to subjects without periodontitis. Such risk increase was even greater in subjects under the age of 60 (OR 6.13, 95% CI 1.62 – 23.2) but not significant in older subjects (OR 1.78, 95% CI 0.60 – 5.3) [129]. Periodontitis was particularly associated with stroke due to large artery atherosclerosis, cardioembolism and cryptogenic etiology.

An association between tooth loss, periodontitis and carotid artery plaque prevalence was observed in a cross-sectional study by Desvarieux and co-workers [130]. In a prospective study, seroepidemiological evidence for infection with two periodontal agents, *Porphyromonas gingivalis* and *Actinobacillus actinomycetemcomitans*, increased the risk of stroke [131]. This result was recently confirmed for *Porphyromonas gingivalis* in a further study [132].

The association between periodontitis and stroke could have important therapeutic implications. In interventional studies, D´Aiuto and colleagues [133,134] demonstrated a reduction of serum inflammatory markers such as CRP and IL-6, of blood pressure and an improvement in lipid profiles after standard and intensive periodontal therapy. In a randomised study with 120 patients with severe periodontitis intensive periodontal therapy resulted in improved endothelial function after 60 and 180 days [135]. In a double blind, placebo controlled study in patients with unstable coronary heart disease therapy with clarithromycin showed a protective effect only in patients without but not in those with periodontitis; this could mean that periodontal infection may reduce the antimicrobial effect of antibiotics directed against *C. pneumoniae* and other atypical respiratory bacteria [136]. Previous interventional studies on periodontitis used surrogate parameters as an endpoint, whereas studies with clinical endpoints are still lacking.

In conclusion, there is ample evidence from several studies that periodontitis is a risk factor for stroke and some evidence suggests that its role may be particularly important in younger age groups. As periodontitis is a common disease and treatment is easily available, additional interventional studies are required to investigate whether the association between stroke and periodontitis is a causal one.

Infectious Burden Concept

Multiple infectious agents that cause chronic and persistent infection have been discussed to play a role in stroke pathogenesis. Moreover, multiple microbial agents could be identified in single atherosclerotic plaques [126]. The existence of a single "atherosclerotic pathogen" is unlikely. Therefore, the concept was developed that the risk of an individuum for atherosclerosis and ischemic diseases increases with the number of pathogens to which the subject has been exposed to throughout life and that are chronically persistent [137]. Several results support this hypothesis. In a seroepidemiological study with 572 patients the AtheroGene Investigators demonstrated a graded relationship between seropositivity to one or more of eight pathogens and the risk of advanced atherosclerosis [138]. A significant relationship between evidence of infection with atypical pulmonary pathogens and the risk of stroke/TIA was demonstrated in a recent case-control study [139]. Using data from the Brunneck study (a prospective population-based survey on the pathogenesis of atherosclerosis) Kiechl et al. [140] found that chronic infections amplified the risk of carotid atherosclerosis. Although sufficient data on stroke as an endpoint are still lacking the forementioned results support the hypothesis that the aggregate burden of microbial agents rather than a single pathogen might be relevant for the risk of stroke.

Conclusion

In conclusion, there is sufficient evidence that acute infection transiently increases the risk of stroke and induction of a procoagulant state by infections is probably the most important mechanism linking infection and stroke. Influenza vaccination may be among the preventive strategies that could lower the burden of infection-associated stroke. The association between stroke and chronic infections is less clear and definite preventive strategies have not been developed in this field so far. Most likely, not one single microbial pathogen but rather the burden of chronic infections in single subjects may codetermine the risk of stroke. Besides these infectious components, the genetically determined inflammatory host response may play an important role regarding the risk of stroke. Whether acute or chronic infections are particularly important as a stroke risk factor in young subjects is not clearly defined. Some preliminary and indirect evidence supports the idea that at least acute infection is of relatively greater importance in younger age groups.

References

[1] Marie S. Hémiplégie cérébrale infantile et maladies infectieuses. *Le progrès médical* 1885;13:167-169.

[2] Freud S. Die infantile Cerebrallähmung. Nothnagel H: Specielle Pathologie 9,Teil 3 (I. Hälfte). Holder; Wien, 1897:1-327.

[3] Collins SD, Lehmann J. Excess deaths from influenza and pneumonia and from important chronic diseases during epidemic periods, 1918-51. *Public Health Monogr.* 1953;10:1-21.

[4] Gordon T, Thom T. The recent decrease in CHD mortality. *Prev. Med.* 1975;4:115-125.

[5] Haberman S, Capildeo R, Rose FC. The seasonal variation in mortality from cerebrovascular disease. *J. Neurol. Sci.* 1981;52:25-36.

[6] Shinkawa A, Ueda K, Hasuo Y, Kiyohara Y, Fujishima M. Seasonal variation in stroke incidence in Hisayama, Japan. *Stroke* 1990;21:1262-1267.

[7] Kelly-Hayes M, Wolf PA, Kase CS, Brand FN, McGuirk JM, d´Agostino RB. Temporal patterns of stroke onset. The Framingham study. *Stroke* 1995;26:1343-1347.

[8] Jakovljevic D, Salomaa V, Sivenius J, Tamminen M, Sarti C, Salmi K, Kaarsolo E, Narva V, Immonen-Räihä P, Torppa J, Tuomilehto J. Seasonal variation in the occurrence of stroke in a Finnish adult population. The Finmonica Stroke Register. *Stroke* 1996;27:1774-1779.

[9] Rothwell PM, Wroe SJ, Slattery J, Warlow CP, on behalf of the Oxforshire Community Stroke Project. Is stroke incidence related to season or temperature? *Lancet* 1996; 347:934-936.

[10] Selby G, Walker GL. Cerebral arteritis in cat-scratch disease. *Neurology* 1979; 29: 1413-1418.

[11] Miller JQ, Price TR. Tick-borne typhus including Rocky Mountain spotted fever. In: Vinken PJ, Bruyn GW, Klawans HL (eds) *Handbook of Neurology* Vol. 34: Infections

of the nervous system. Part II. North Holland; Amsterdam, New York, Oxford, 1978, pp 651-658.

[12] Hart RG, Foster JW, Luther MF, Kanter MC. Stroke in infective endocarditis. *Stroke* 1990;21:695-700.

[13] Pruitt AA, Rubin RH, Karchmer AW, Duncan GW. Neurologic complications of bacterial endocarditis. *Medicine* 1978;57:329-343.

[14] Pfister HW, Borasio GD, Dirnagl U, Bauer M, Einhäupl KM. Cerebrovascular complications of bacterial meningitis in adults. *Neurology* 1992;142:1497-1504.

[15] Prange H. Neurosyphilis. In: Neundörfer B, Schimrigk K, Soyka D (Hrsg) *Praktische Neurologie*, Band 4. edition medizin VCH, Weinheim 1987.

[16] May EF, Jabbari B. Stroke in neuroborreliosis. *Stroke* 1990;21:1232-1235.

[17] Patrick JT, Russell E, Meyer J, Biller J, Saver JL. Cervical (C2) herpes zoster infection followed by pontine infarction. *J. Neuroimaging.* 1995; 5: 192-193.

[18] Martin JR, Mtchell WJ, Henken DB. Neurotropic herpesviruses, neural mechanisms and arteritis. *Brain Pathol.* 1990;1:6-10.

[19] Nagel MA, Cohrs RJ, Mahalingam R, Wellish MC, Forghani B, Schiller A, Safdieh JE, Kamenkovich E, Ostrow LW, Levy M, Greenberg B, Russman AN, Katzan I, Gardner CJ, Häusler M, Nau R, Saraya T, Wada H, Goto H, de Martino M, Ueno M, Brown WD, Terborg C, Gilden DH. The varicella zoster virus vasculopathies: clinical, CSF, imaging, and virologic features. *Neurology* 2008;70:853-60.

[20] Koeppen AH, Lansing LS, Peng SK, Smith RS. Central nervous system vasculitis in cytomegalovirus infection. *J. Neurol. Sci.* 1981;51:395-410.

[21] Bickerstaff ER. Aetiology of acute hemiplegia in childhood. *BMJ* 1964; ii:82-87.

[22] Ogata K, Yagawa K, Hayashi S, Ogino H, Miyagawa Y, Masayuki M, Ichinose Y, Koga T. Thrombosis-inducing activity in plasma of patients with acute respiratory tract infection disappears after treatment. *Respiration* 1991;58:176-180.

[23] Van der Poll T, Büller HR, ten Gate H, Wortel CH, Bauer KA, van Deventer SJH, Hack CE, Sauerwein HP, Rosenberg RD, ten Gate JW. Activation of coagulation after administration of tumor necrosis factor to normal subjects. *N. Engl. J. Med.* 1990;322:1622-1627.

[24] Cermak J, Key NS, Bach RR, Balla J, Jacob HS, Vercellotti GM. C-reactive protein induces human peripheral blood monocytes to synthesize tissue factor. *Blood* 1993;82:513-520.

[25] Esmon CT, Taylor FB, Snow TR. Inflammation and coagulation: Linked processes potentially regulated through a common pathway mediated by protein C. *Thromb Haemost.* 1991;66:160-165.

[26] Woodhouse PR, Khaw KT, Plummer M, Foley A, Meade TW. Seasonal variations of plasma fibrinogen and factor VII activity in the elderly: winter infections and death from cardiovascular disease. *Lancet* 1994;343:435-439.

[27] Lourbakos A, Yuan YP, Jenkins AL, Travis J, Andrade-Gordon P, Santulli R, Potemba J, Pike RN. Activation of protease-activated receptors by gingipains from *porphyromonas gingivalis* leads to platelet aggregation: A new trait in microbial pathogenicity. *Blood* 2001;97:3790-3797.

[28] Zeller JA, Lenz A, Eschenfelder CC, Zunker P, Deuschl G. Platelet-leukocyte interaction and platelet-activation in acute stroke with and without preceding infection. *Arterioscler. Thromb Vasc. Biol.* 2005;25:1519-23.

[29] Macko RF, Ameriso SF, Barndt R, Clough W, Weiner JM, Fisher M. Precipitants of brain infarction. Roles of preceding infection/inflammation and recent psychological stress. *Stroke* 1996;27:1999-2004.

[30] Grau AJ, Buggle F, Steichen-Wiehn C, Heindl S, Banerjee T, Seitz R, Winter R, Forsting M, Werle E, Nawroth P, Becher H, Hacke W: Clinical and biochemical analysis in infection-associated stroke. *Stroke* 1995;26:1520-1526.

[31] Grau AJ, Buggle F, Becher H, Zimmermann E, Spiel M, Fent T, Maiwald M, Werle E, Zorn M, Hengel H, Hacke W. Recent bacterial and viral infection is a risk factor for cerebral ischemia: Clinical and biochemical studies. *Neurology*. 1998;50:196-203.

[32] Ameriso SF, Wong VLY, Quismorio Jr. FP, Fisher M. Immunohematologic characteristics of infection-associated cerebral infarction. *Stroke* 1991;22:1004-9.

[33] Ross R. Atherosclerosis is an inflammatory disease. *N. Engl. J. Med*. 1999;340:115-26.

[34] De Palma R, Del Galdo F, Abbate G, Chiariello M, Calabró R, Forte L, Cimmino G, Papa MF, Russo MG, Ambrosio G, Giombolini C, Tritto I, Notaristefano S, Berrino L, Rossi F, Golino P. Patients with acute coronary syndrome show oligoclonal T-cell recruitment within unstable plaque: evidence for a local, intracoronary immunologic mechanism. *Circulation* 2006;113:640-6.

[35] Keller TT, van der Meer JJ, Teeling P, van der Sluijs K, Idu MM, Rimmelzwaan GF, Levi M, van der Wal AC, de Boer OJ. Selective expansion of influenza A virus-specific T cells in symptomatic human carotid artery atherosclerotic plaques. *Stroke* 2008;39:174-9.

[36] Niessner A, Sato K, Chaikof EL, Colmegna I, Goronzy JJ, Weyand CM. Pathogen-sensing plasmacytoid dendritic cells stimulate cytotoxic T-cell function in the atherosclerotic plaque through interferon-alpha. *Circulation* 2006;114:2482-2489.

[37] Naghavi M, Wyde P, Litovsky S, Madjid M, Akhtar A, Naguib S, Siadaty MS, Sanati S, Casscells W. Influenza infection exerts prominent inflammatory and thrombotic effects on the atherosclerotic plaques of apolipoprotein E-deficient mice. *Circulation* 2003;107:762-8.

[38] Wiesel J. Die Erkrankungen arterieller Gefäße im Verlaufe akuter Infektionen. II. Teil. *Zeitschr f Heilkunde*. 1906;27:262-294.

[39] Fränkel A. Ueber einige Complicationen und Ausgänge der Influenza. Nebst Bemerkungen über putride und interlobäre Pleuritis. Berliner Klinische Wochenschrift 1897;34:338-341.

[40] Hallenbeck JM, Dutka AJ, Kochanek PM, Siren A, Pezeshkpour GH, Feuerstein G. Stroke risk factors prepare rat brainstem tissues for modified local Shwartzman reaction. *Stroke* 1988;19:863-869.

[41] Hallenbeck JM, Dutka AJ, Vogel SN, Heldman E, Doron DA, Feuerstein G. Lipopolysaccharide-induced production of tumor necrosis factor activity in rats with and without risk factors for stroke. *Brain Res*. 1991;541:115-120.

[42] Sirén AL, Heldman E, Doron D, Lysko PG, Yue TL, Liu Y, Feuerstein G, Hallenbeck JM Release of proinflammatory and prothrombotic mediators in the brain and

peripheral circulation in spontaneously hypertensive and normotensive Wistar-Kyoto rats. *Stroke* 1992;23:1643-1651.

[43] Lozano ML, González-Conejero R, Corral J, Rivera J, Iniesta JA, Martinez C, Vicente V. Polymorphisms of P-selectin glycoprotein ligand-1 are associated with neutrophil-platelct adhesion and with ischaemic cerebrovascular disease. *Br. J. Haematol.* 2001; 115:969-76.

[44] Hiramoto M, Yoshida H, Imaizumi T, Yoshimizu N, Satoh K. A mutation in plasma platelet-activating factor acetylhydrolase (Val279-->Phe) is a genetic risk factor for stroke. *Stroke* 1997;28:2417-20.

[45] Herrmann SM, Funke-Kaiser H, Schmidt-Petersen K, Nicaud V, Gautier-Bertrand M, Evans A, Kee F, Arveiler D, Morrison C, Orzechowski HD, Elbaz A, Amarenco P, Cambien F, Paul M. Characterization of polymorphic structure of cathepsin G gene: role in cardiovascular and cerebrovascular diseases. *Arterioscler. Thromb Vasc. Biol.* 2001;21:1538-43.

[46] Lichy C, Meiser H, Grond-Ginsbach C, Buggle F, Dörfer C, Grau A. Lipopolysaccharide receptor CD14 polymorphism and risk of stroke in a South-German population. *J. Neurol.* 2002;249:821-3.

[47] Flex A, Gaetani E, Papaleo P, Straface G, Proia AS, Pecorini G, Tondi P, Pola P, Pola R. Proinflammatory genetic profiles in subjects with history of ischemic stroke. *Stroke* 2004;35:2270-5.

[48] Markus HS, Labrum R, Bevan S, Reindl M, Egger G, Wiedermann CJ, Xu Q, Kiechl S, Willeit J. Genetic and acquired inflammatory conditions are synergistically associated with early carotid atherosclerosis. *Stroke* 2006;37:2253-2259.

[49] Riikonen R, Santavuori P. Hereditary and acquired risk factors for childhood stroke. *Neuropediatrics* 1994;25:227-233.

[50] Eeg-Olofsson O, Ringheim Y. Stroke in children. Clinical characteristics and prognosis. *Acta Paediatr. Scand.* 1983;72:391-395.

[51] Moran A, MacDonald J. Eight cases of childhood stroke. *Minnesota Med.* 1985; 68:675-677.

[52] Powell FC, Hanigan WC, McCluney KW. Subcortical infarction in children. *Stroke* 1994;25:117-121.

[53] Ode B, Cronberg S. Infection and intracranial arterial thrombosis. *Lancet* 1976;II: 863-864.

[54] Hindfelt B, Nilsson O. Brain infarction in young adults with particular reference to pathogenesis. *Acta Neurol. Scand.* 1977;55:145-157.

[55] Syrjänen J, Valtonen VV, Iivanainen M, Hovi T, Malkamäki M, Mäkelä PH. Association between cerebral infarction and increased serum bacterial antibody levels in young adults. *Acta Neurol. Scand.* 1986;73:273-278.

[56] Syrjänen J, Valtonen VV, Iivanainen M, Kaste M, Huttunen JK. Preceding infection as an important risk factor for ischaemic brain infarction in young and middle aged patients. *Br. Med. J.* 1988;296:1156-60.

[57] Syrjänen J. Central nervous system complications in patients with bacteraemia. *Scand. J. Infect. Dis.* 1989;21:285-296.

[58] Grau AJ, Buggle F, Heindl S, Steichen-Wiehn C, Banerjee T, Maiwald M, Rohlfs M, Suhr H, Fiehn W, Becher H, et al. Recent infection as a risk factor for cerebrovascular ischemia. *Stroke* 1995;26:373-379.

[59] Smeeth L, Thomas SL, Hall AJ, Hubbard R, Farrington P, Vallance P. Risk of myocardial infarction and stroke after acute infection or vaccination. *N. Engl. J. Med.* 2004;16;351:2611-8.

[60] Clayton TC, Thompson M, Meade TW. Recent respiratory infection and risk of cardiovascular disease: case-control study through a general practice database. *Eur. Heart J.* 2008;29:96-103.

[61] Paganini-Hill A, Lozano E, Fischberg G, Perez Barreto M, Rajamani K, Ameriso SF, Heseltine PN, Fisher M. Infection and risk of ischemic stroke: differences among stroke subtypes. *Stroke* 2003;34:452-7.

[62] Nencini P, Sarti C, Innocenti R, Pracucci G, Inzitari D. Acute inflammatory events and ischemic stroke subtypes. *Cerebrovasc. Dis*. 2003;15:215-21.

[63] Gustafsson C, Blombäck M, Britton M, Hamsten A, Svensson J. Coagulation factors and the increased risk of stroke in nonvalvular atrial fibrillation. *Stroke* 1990;21:47-51.

[64] Reilly MP, Plappert TJ, Wiegers SE. Cerebrovascular emboli related to pulmonary venous thrombosis after lung transplantation. *J. Am. Soc. Echocardiogr.* 1998;11:299-302.

[65] Sloop RD, Lium JH. Systemic arterial embolism arising from pulmonary thrombophlebitis. *Am. Surg*. 1971;37:503-505.

[66] Grau AJ, Schoenberg SO , Lichy C, Buggle F, Bock M, Hacke W. Lack of evidence for pulmonary venous thrombosis in cryptogenic stroke. A magnetic resonance angiography study. *Stroke* 2002;33:1416-1419.

[67] Grau AJ, Eckstein HH, Schäfer B, Schnabel PA, Brandt T, Hacke W: Stroke from internal carotid artery occlusion during mumps infection. *J. Neurol. Sci.* 1998;155:215-217.

[68] Brandt T, Hausser I, Orberk E, Grau A, Hartschuh W, Anton-Lamprecht I, Hacke W: Ultrastructural connective tissue abnormalities in patients with spontaneous cervico-cerebral artery dissections. *Ann. Neurol.* 1998;44:281-285.

[69] Wiest T, Hyrenbach S, Bambul P, Erker B, Pezzini A, Hausser I, Arnold ML, Martin JJ, Engelter S, Lyrer P, Busse O, Brandt T, Grond-Ginsbach C. Genetic analysis of familial connective tissue alterations associated with cervical artery dissections suggests locus heterogeneity. *Stroke* 2006;37:1697-702.

[70] Grau AJ, Brandt T, Forsting M, Winter R, Hacke W: Infection-associated cervical artery dissection. 3 cases. *Stroke* 1997;28:453-455.

[71] Grau AJ, Brand T, Buggle F, Orberk E, Mytilineos J, Werle E, Conradt C, Krause M, Winter R , Hacke W: Association of cervical artery dissection with recent infection. *Arch Neurol*. 1999;56:851-856.

[72] Schievink WI, Wijdicks EF, Kuiper JD. Seasonal pattern of spontaneous cervical artery dissection. *J. Neurosurg.* 1998;89:101-3.

[73] Paciaroni M, Georgiadis D, Arnold M, Gandjour J, Keseru B, Fahrni G, Caso V, Baumgartner RW. Seasonal variability in spontaneous cervical artery dissection. *J. Neurol. Neurosurg. Psychiatry*. 2006;77:677-9.

[74] Forster K, Poppert H, Conrad B, Sander D. Elevated inflammatory laboratory parameters in spontaneous cervical artery dissection as compared to traumatic dissection: a retrospective case-control study. *J. Neurol.* 2006;253:741-5.

[75] Genius J, Dong-Si T, Grau AJ, Lichy C. Postacute C-reactive protein levels are elevated in cervical artery dissection. *Stroke* 2005;36:2-4.

[76] Luken MG, Ascherl GF, Correll JW, Hilal SK. Spontaneous dissecting aneurysms of the extracranial internal carotid artery. *Clin. Neurosurg.* 1975; 26:353-375.

[77] Chang V, Rewcastle NB, Harwood-Nash DCF, Norman MG. Bilateral dissecting aneurysms of the intracranial internal carotid arteries in an 8-year-old boy. *Neurology.* 1975;25:573-579.

[78] Eskenasy-Cottier AC, Leu HJ, Bassetti C, Bogousslavsky J, Regli F, Janzer RC. A case of dissection of intracranial cerebral arteries with segmental mediolytic „arteritis". *Clin. Neuropathol.* 1994;13:329-337.

[79] Robinowitz M, Virmani R, McAllister HA. Spontaneous coronary artery dissection and eosinophilic inflammation: A cause and effect relationship? *Am. J. Med.* 1982;72:923-928.

[80] Dowling GP, Buja LM. Spontaneous coronary artery dissection occurs with and without periadventitial inflammation. *Arch Pathol. Lab. Med.* 1987;111:470-472.

[81] Somer T, Finegold SM. Vasculitides associated with infections, immunization, and antimicrobial drugs. *Clin. Infect. Dis.* 1995;20:1010-1036.

[82] Kunze A, Annecke A, Wigger F, Lichy C, Buggle F, Schnippering H, Schnitzler P, Grau AJ. Recent infection as a risk factor for intracerebral and subarachnoid hemorrhage. *Cerebrovasc. Dis.* 2000;10:352-358.

[83] Jones DB: An association between subarachnoid hemorrhage and influenza A infection. *Postgrad. Med. J.* 1979;55:853-855.

[84] Siebenmann RP, Turina M: Diagnose des inflammatorischen Bauchaortenaneurysmas. *Dtsch med Wschr.* 1989;114:1079-1081.

[85] Chyatte D, Bruno G, Desai S, Todor DR. Inflammation and intracranial aneurysms. *Neurosurgery* 1999;45:1137-46.

[86] Reith J, Jørgensen HS, Pedersen PM, Nakayama H, Raaschou HO, Jeppesen LL, Olsen TS. Body temperature in acute stroke: relation to stroke severity, infarct size, mortality, and outcome. *Lancet* 1996;347:422-5.

[87] Bova IY, Bornstein NM, Korczyn AD. Acute infection as a risk factor for ischemic stroke. *Stroke* 1996;27:2204-2206.

[88] McColl BW, Rothwell NJ, Allan SM. Systemic inflammatory stimulus potentiates the acute phase and CXC chemokine responses to experimental stroke and exacerbates brain damage via interleukin-1- and neutrophil-dependent mechanisms. *J. Neurosci.* 2007;27:4403-4412.

[89] Rosenzweig HL, Lessov NS, Henshall DC, Minami N, Simon RP, Stenzel-Poore MP. Endotoxin preconditioning prevents cellular inflammatory response during ischemic neuroprotection in mice. *Stroke* 2004;35:2576-81.

[90] Marquardt L, Ruf A, Mansmann U, Winter R, Buggle F, Kallenberg K, Grau AJ. Inflammatory response after acute ischemic stroke. *J. Neurol. Sci.*2005;236:65-71.

[91] Emsley HC, Smith CJ, Gavin CM, Georgiou RF, Vail A, Barberan EM, Hallenbeck JM, del Zoppo GJ, Rothwell NJ, Tyrrell PJ, Hopkins SJ. An early and sustained peripheral inflammatory response in acute ischaemic stroke: relationships with infection and atherosclerosis. *J. Neuroimmunol.* 2003;139:93-101.

[92] Emsley HC, Hopkins SJ. Acute ischaemic stroke and infection: recent and emerging concepts. *Lancet Neurology* 2008;7:341-353.

[93] Grau AJ, Buggle F, Schnitzler P, Spiel M, Lichy C, Hacke W. Fever and Infection Early After Ischemic Stroke. *J. Neurol. Sci.* 1999;171:115-120.

[94] Nicholson KG, Wood JM, Zambon M. Influenza. *N. Engl. J. Med.* 2003;362:1733-45.

[95] Housworth J, Langmuir AD. Excess mortality from epidemic influenza, 1957-1966. *Am. J. Epidemiol.*1974;100:40-48.

[96] Alling DW, Blackwelder WC, Stuart-Harris CH. A study of excess mortality during influenza epidemics in the United States 1968-1976. *Am. J. Epidemiol.* 1981;113:30-43.

[97] Lavallée P, Perchaud V, Gautier-Bertrand M, Grabli D, Amarenco P. Association between influenza vaccination and reduced risk of brain infarction. *Stroke* 2002; 33:513-8.

[98] Grau AJ, Fischer B, Barth C, Ling P, Lichy C, Buggle F. Influenza Vaccination Is Associated With a Reduced Risk of Stroke. *Stroke* 2005;36:1501-6.

[99] Nichol KL, Nordin J, Mullooly J, Lask R, Fillbrandt K, Iwane M. Influenza vaccination and reduction in hospitalizations for cardiac disease and stroke among the elderly. *N. Engl. J. Med.* 2003;348:1322-1332.

[100] Grayston JT, Kuo CC, Wang SP, Altman J. A new Chlamydia psittaci strain, TWAR, isolated in acute respiratory tract infections. *N. Engl. J. Med.* 1986;315:161-8.

[101] Kuo CC, Jackson LA, Campbell LA, Grayston JT. Chlamydia pneumoniae (TWAR). *Clin. Microbiol. Rev.* 1995;8:451-61.

[102] Saikku P, Leinonen M, Mattila K, Ekman M-R, Nieminen MS, Mäkelä PH, Huttunen JK, Valtonen V. Serological evidence of an association of a novel Chlamydia, TWAR, with chronic coronary heart disease and acute myocardial infarction. *Lancet* 1988; 2:983-985.

[103] Lindsberg P, Grau AJ. Inflammation and infections as risk factors for ischemic stroke. *Stroke* 2003;34:2518-2532.

[104] Wimmer ML, Sandmann-Strupp R, Saikku P, Haberl RL. Association of chlamydial infection with cerebrovascular disease. *Stroke* 1996;27:2207-2210.

[105] Elkind MS, Lin IF, Grayston JT, Sacco RL. Chlamydia pneumoniae and the risk of first ischemic stroke: The Northern Manhattan Stroke Study. *Stroke* 2000;31:1521-1525.

[106] Apfalter P. *Chlamydia pneumoniae*, stroke, and serological associations: anything learned from the atherosclerosis-cardiovascular literature or do we have to start over again? *Stroke* 2006;37:756-8.

[107] Maass M, Gieffers J, Krause E, Engel PM, Bartels C, Solbach W. Poor correlation between microimmunofluorescence serology and polymerase chain reaction for detection of vascular Chlamydia pneumoniae infection in coronary artery disease patients. *Med. Microbiol. Immunol.* 1998;187:103-6.

[108]Lajunen T, Vikatmaa P, Ikonen T, Lepäntalo M, Lounatmaa K, Sormunen R, Rantala A, Leinonen M, Saikku P. Comparison of polymerase chain reaction methods, in situ hybridization, and enzyme immunoassay for detection of Chlamydia pneumoniae in atherosclerotic carotid plaques. *Diagn. Microbiol. Infect. Dis.* 2008;6:156-64.

[109]Andraws R, Berger JS, Brown DL. Effects of antibiotic therapy on outcomes of patients with coronary artery disease: a meta-analysis of randomized controlled trials. *JAMA* 2005; 293:2641-7.

[110]Sander D, Winbeck K, Klingelhöfer J, Etgen T, Conrad B. Reduced progression of early carotid atherosclerosis after antibiotic treatment and Chlamydia pneumoniae seropositivity. *Circulation* 2002;106:2428-2433.

[111]Sander D, Winbeck K, Klingelhöfer J, Etgen T, Conrad B. Progression of early carotid atherosclerosis is only temporarily reduced after antibiotic treatment of Chlamydia pneumoniae seropositivity. *Circulation* 2004;109:1010-5.

[112]Mendall MA, Goggin PM, Molineaux N, Levy J, Toosy T, Strachan D, Northfield TC Childhood living conditions and *Helicobacter pylori* seropositivity in adult life. *Lancet* 1992;339:896-7.

[113]Ameriso SF, Fridman EA, Leiguarda RC, Sevlever GE. Detection of Helicobacter pylori in human carotid atherosclerotic plaques. *Stroke* 2001;32:385-91.

[114]Danesh J, Appleby P. Coronary heart disease and iron status: meta-analyses of prospective studies. *Circulation* 1999;99:852-4.

[115]Markus HS, Mendall MA. *Helicobacter pylori* infection: a risk factor for ischaemic cerebrovascular disease and carotid atheroma. *J. Neurol. Neurosurg. Psychiatry* 1998; 64:104-7.

[116]Heuschmann PU, Neureiter D, Gesslein M, Craiovan B, Maass M, Faller G, Beck G, Neundörfer B, Kolominsky-Rabas PL. Association between infection with Helicobacter pylori and Chlamydia pneumoniae and risk of ischemic stroke subtypes: Results from a population-based case-control study. *Stroke* 2001;32:2253-2258.

[117]Grau AJ, Buggle F, Lichy C, Brandt T, Becher H, Rudi J. Helicobacter pylori infection as an independent risk factor for cerebral ischemia of atherothrombotic origin. *J. Neurol. Sci.* 2001;186:1-5.

[118]Ponzetto A, Marchet A, Pellicano R, Lovera N, Chianale G, Nobili M, Rizzetto M, Cerrato P. Association of Helicobacter pylori infection with ischemic stroke of non-cardiac origin: the BAT.MA.N. project study. *Hepatogastroenterology* 2002;49:631-634.

[119]Whincup PH, Mendall, MA, Perry IJ, Strachan DP, Walker M. Prospective relations between Helicobacter pylori infection, coronary heart disease and stroke in middle-aged men. *Heart* 1996;75:568-72.

[120]Pietroiusti A, Diomedi M, Silvestrini M, Cupini LM, Luzzi I, Gomez-Miguel MJ, Bergamaschi A, Magrini A, Carrabs T, Vellini M, Galante A. Cytotoxin-associated gene-A-positive Helicobacter pylori strains are associated with atherosclerotic stroke. *Circulation* 2002;106:580-4.

[121]Preusch MR, Grau AJ, Buggle F, Lichy C, Bartel J, Black C, Rudi J. Association between cerebral ischemia and cytotoxin-associated gene-A-bearing strains of Helicobacter pylori. *Stroke* 2004;35(8):1800-4.

[122]Mayr M, Kiechl S, Mendall MA, Willeit J, Wick G, Xu Q. Increased risk of atherosclerosis is confined to CagA-positive Helicobacter pylori strains: prospective results from the Bruneck study. *Stroke* 2003;34:610-615.

[123]Markus HS, Risley P, Mendall MA, Steinmetz H, Sitzer M. *Helicobacter pylori* infection, the cytotoxin gene A strain, and carotid artery intima-media thickness. *J. Cardiovasc. Risk* 2002;9:1-6.

[124]Cremonini F, Gabrielli M, Gasbarrini G, Pola P, Gasbarrini A. The relationship between chronic H. pylori infection, CagA seropositivity and stroke: meta-analysis. *Atherosclerosis* 2004;173:253-9.

[125]Borrell LN, Burt BA, Taylor GW. Prevalence and trends in periodontitis in the USA: the [corrected] NHANES, 1988 to 2000. *J. Dent. Res.* 2005;84:924-30.

[126]Chiu B. Multiple infections in carotid atherosclerotic plaques. *Am. Heart J.* 1999; 138:S534-6.

[127]Li L, Messas E, Batista EL Jr, Levine RA, Amar S. Porphyromonas gingivalis infection accelerates the progression of atherosclerosis in a heterozygous apolipoprotein E-deficient murine model. *Circulation* 2002;105:861-7.

[128]Grau AJ, Buggle F, Ziegler C, Schwarz W, Meuser J, Tasman AJ, Bühler A, Benesch C, Becher H, Hacke W: Association between acute cerebrovascular ischemia and chronic and recurrent infection. *Stroke* 1997;28:1724-1729.

[129]Grau AJ, Becher H, Ziegler CM, Lichy C, Buggle F, Kaiser C, Lutz R, Bültmann S, Preusch M, Dörfer CE. Periodontal Disease as a Risk Factor for Ischemic Stroke. *Stroke* 2004;35:496-501.

[130]Desvarieux M, Schwahn C, Völzke H, Demmer RT, Lüdemann J, Kessler C, Jacobs DR Jr, John U, Kocher T. Gender differences in the relationship between periodontal disease, tooth loss, and atherosclerosis. *Stroke* 2004;35:2029-35.

[131]Pussinen PJ, Alfthan G, Rissanen H, Reunanen A, Asikainen S, Knekt P. Antibodies to periodontal pathogens and stroke risk. *Stroke* 2004;35:2020-23.

[132]Pussinen PJ, Alfthan G, Jousilahti P, Paju S, Tuomilehto J. Systemic exposure to Porphyromonas gingivalis predicts incident stroke. *Atherosclerosis* 2007;193:222-228.

[133]D'Aiuto F, Parkar M, Andreou G, Suvan J, Brett PM, Ready D, Tonetti MS. Periodontitis and systemic inflammation: control of the local infection is associated with a reduction in serum inflammatory markers. *J. Dent. Res.* 2004;83:156-60.

[134]D'Aiuto F, Parkar M, Nibali L, Suvan J, Lessem J, Tonetti MS. Periodontal infections cause changes in traditional and novel cardiovascular risk factors: results from a randomized controlled clinical trial. *Am. Heart J.* 2006;151:977-84.

[135]Tonetti MS, D´Aiuto F, Nibali L, Donald A, Storry C, Parkar M, Suvan J, Hingorani AD, Vallance P, Deanfield J. Treatment of periodontitis and endothelial function. *New Engl. J. Med.* 2007;356:911-920.

[136]Paju S, Pussinen PJ, Sinisalo J, Mattila K, Dogan B, Ahlberg J, Valtonen V, Nieminen MS, Asikainen S. Clarithromycin reduces recurrent cardiovascular events in subjects without periodontitis. *Atherosclerosis* 2006;188:412-9.

[137]Epstein SE, Zhou YF, Zhu J. Infection and atherosclerosis: emerging mechanistic paradigms. *Circulation* 1999;100: e20-8.

[138] Espinola-Klein C, Rupprecht HJ, Blankenberg S, Bickel C, Kopp H, Victor A, Hafner G, Prellwitz W, Schlumberger W, Meyer J. Impact of infectious burden on progression of carotid atherosclerosis. *Stroke* 2002;33:2581-6.

[139] Ngeh J, Goodbourn C. Chlamydia pneumoniae, Mycoplasma pneumoniae, and Legionella pneumophila in elderly patients with stroke (C-PEPS, M-PEPS, L-PEPS): a case-control study on the infectious burden of atypical respiratory pathogens in elderly patients with acute cerebrovascular disease. *Stroke* 2005;36:259-65.

[140] Kiechl S, Egger G, Mayr M, Wiedermann CJ, Bonora E, Oberhollenzer F, Muggeo M, Xu Q, Wick G, Poewe W, Willeit J Chronic infections and the risk of carotid atherosclerosis: prospective results from a large population study. *Circulation* 2001; 103:1064-70.

In: Cerebral Ischemia in Young Adults
Editors: A. Pezzini and A. Padovani

ISBN 978-1-60741-627-2

Chapter 8

HIV Infection and Ischemic Stroke

***Gustavo A. Ortiz*[1] *and Alejandro A. Rabinstein*[2*]**

1. Department of Neurology, University of Miami Miller School of Medicine, Miami, Florida, USA
2. Department of Neurology, Mayo Clinic College of Medicine, Rochester, Minnesota, USA

Abstract

The relationship of HIV infection with stroke, once thought to be of rather marginal clinical relevance, is undergoing remarkable changes and robust epidemiological evidence now support the notion that HIV infection is a risk factor for cerebral ischemia. The mechanisms underlying this relation are numerous and include cardioembolism, an accelerated process of atherosclerosis, the effect of antiretroviral drugs, the induction of a prothrombotic state, opportunistic vasculitis and a specific HIV-vasculopathy, as well as exposure to drug abuse, among others. In this chapter available data on the relation between HIV infection and ischemic stroke will be summarized, and clinical/pathogenic aspects of such a link will be highlighted with a particular focus on potential therapeutic implication.

Introduction

Cerebrovascular disease was formerly thought to be rather infrequent in patients with acquired immunodeficiency syndrome (AIDS), in an era when these patients were commonly affected by opportunistic infections and tumors. Even more, advanced immunodeficiency appeared to be the main cause of a possible increased risk of ischemic stroke. Thus, in the setting of advanced immunosuppression, many of the potential causes of stroke identified

* Correspondence: Alejandro A. Rabinstein, 200 First Street SW, Mayo W8, Mayo Clinic Rochester Neurology, Rochester, MN 55905 USA. E-mail: Rabinstein.Alejandro@mayo.edu.

included opportunistic infections, marantic endocarditis, cachexia, and coagulation abnormalities.

However, with the introduction of highly active antiretroviral therapy (HAART), a steep reduction in morbidity and mortality has been observed in HIV-infected patients in the United States and other western countries [1]. As a consequence of the increased life expectancy, chronic conditions have become more prevalent in these patients, including cardiovascular disease (CVD). Cardiovascular disease has been recognized as an important cause of morbidity and mortality among patients with HIV, due to several mechanisms, but probably mostly in relation to the antiretroviral therapy [2-6]. Along with this increased cardiovascular risk, increased stroke risk has been proposed through common pathophysiological mechanisms of disease with coronary atherosclerosis. However, this issue remains still controversial.

Many questions arise when we analyze the current knowledge on HIV and stroke: Does HIV infection constitute an independent risk factor for cerebrovascular disease? Do factors that increase cardiovascular risk also affect stroke-risk in HIV-patients? Are these patients more exposed to other environmental factors that increase stroke risk? Are opportunistic infections and malignancies still an important risk factor for stroke in HIV-patients?

In this chapter, we summarize current information on ischemic stroke in HIV infected patients from a clinical perspective. First, we will describe the prevalence of cerebrovascular complications in HIV-patients, with analysis of case-series studies and correlation to the general population. Then, we will discuss the possible mechanisms of stroke in HIV patients (cardioembolism, accelerated atherosclerosis, classic vascular risk factors, pro-thrombotic states, opportunistic vasculitis - HIV vasculopathy, and exposure to drug abuse). Finally, we will analyze the frequency of the different mechanisms of stroke in the HIV population, according to case series and cohort studies.

Prevalence of Cerebrovascular Disease in HIV-Infected Patients: Is HIV Infection Actually a Risk Factor for Ischemic Stroke?

Since the vast majority of HIV-infected patients are younger than 45 years of age, the incidence and prevalence of cerebrovascular events in this cohort should be compared to our knowledge on juvenile stroke. Studies in young population without HIV infection have shown annual incidence rates for cerebrovascular disorders between 10 and 34 per 100,000 [7]. In these non-HIV patients, premature atherosclerosis, cardioembolism, hereditary coagulopathies, inflammatory arterial disease (infectious and systemic vasculitis) and non-inflammatory arterial disease (dissection, subarachnoid hemorrhage with vasospasm) are the most common causes of ischemic stroke. In HIV-infected patients, autopsy studies have revealed a prevalence of cerebral infarction or hemorrhage, ranging from 6% to 34% [8-13]. However, this may be an overestimation biased by the fact that autopsies are done only in selected cases.

Histopathological evidence of cerebral infarction was found in only 10 cases out of 183 autopsies of adult HIV patients (7% if only considering AIDS patients) from the Edinburgh

HIV Cohort Study, after patients with cerebral opportunistic infections, lymphoma, non-HIV infections or other sources of emboli were excluded. The authors suggested that in AIDS patients presenting with a stroke or a transient ischemic attack (TIA), potentially treatable causes (such as cerebral co-infection or tumor) should be excluded before assuming that the cause is HIV itself, as a result of a vasculopathy or some as yet unrecognized pathogenic mechanism. None of these patients had received treatment with HAART [14].

In a retrospective study, 12 cases of ischemic stroke were identified among 1,600 AIDS patients followed for a 5-year period [15]. The calculated annual risk of stroke for these patients (0.75%) was substantially higher than that expected in the general population less than 45 years of age (0.025%). But in a comprehensive review of 6 clinical series of patients studied between 1979 and 1987[13] (in which most of the patients had AIDS and only a few asymptomatic HIV-patients were included), all types of stroke were frequently associated to opportunistic infections and tumors, thought to be responsible for the stroke. Given the limitations of the data, it was not clear whether there was an association between AIDS and stroke.

Another retrospective case-control study evaluated 236 young patients (aged 19-44), admitted with diagnosis of stroke between 1990 and 1994. Serologic HIV status was known in 113 patients and 25 were seropositive (10 had AIDS). Control cases were age and sex-matched patients with known HIV status, admitted with diagnosis of status epilepticus. After adjustment for several cerebrovascular risk factors, HIV-infection was associated with increased risk of stroke (odds ratio (OR) of 2.3; 95% confidence interval (CI) 1.0-5.3; $p = 0.05$) and particularly with cerebral infarction (OR, 3.4). Among patients with stroke, cerebral infarction was more frequent in those who were seropositive (80 vs 56%). In addition, seropositive patients had a higher frequency of cerebral infarction associated with meningitis ($p<0.001$) and protein S deficiency ($p = 0.06$, nonsignificant) compared with the seronegative group. The association between HIV-infection and cerebral infarction was not statistically significant when all cases with meningitis and protein S deficiency were excluded, suggesting that most of the excess risk of stroke in HIV patients could be mediated by these two mechanisms. Strokes of an undetermined cause were not more common in the HIV-infected patients, in contrast to the findings of previous studies. The authors did not provide information regarding serum lipid levels, antiretroviral regimens used, or subtypes of ischemic stroke, although no cardioembolic strokes were observed in HIV-infected patients.

HIV infection seems to impose a particularly increased risk of stroke in young patients. In a population-based study of 557 young patients with stroke, from the Baltimore-Washington Coperative Young Stroke Study [16], AIDS conferred an adjusted relative risk of 13.7 for ischemic stroke and 25.5 for intracerebral hemorrhage. After exclusion of cases in which other potential causes were identified, AIDS patients continued to have an increased risk of stroke with an adjusted relative risk of 9.1 for ischemic stroke and 12.7 for intracerebral hemorrhage. However, patients with HIV-infection who did not fulfill the diagnostic criteria for AIDS were also included in the non-AIDS group. In a prospective clinical cohort of patients admitted with diagnosis of stroke to a tertiary stroke unit in South Africa, 1087 patients were admitted with diagnosis of stroke, of which 67 (6.2%) were identified as HIV infected. The mean age of HIV infected stroke patients was 33.4 years (range 19-76), while the mean age of non-HIV patients was 64.0 years (range 17-96). Only

24% of all patients in the cohort were less than 46 years of age, but among the HIV infected patients, 61 were less than 46 years (91%), making the HIV positive stroke patients a predominantly young stroke population [17]. Finally, in a retrospective analysis of 82 patients with diagnosis of HIV and stroke admitted to a large metropolitan hospital in Miami, Florida, United States [18], the mean age was 42 years (range 3 to 72), 57% of the patients were 45 years old or younger (47/82) and 43% were 46 and older (35/82). The mean age in the younger group was 34 years, and in the older group 53 years (Table 1). In this series, patients with atherothrombotic strokes were older than patients with non-atherothrombotic strokes (45.3 ± 3 vs $40.1 \pm 1,6$; $p = 0.04$).

In a descriptive study of a population with high-prevalence of HIV infection in Malawi, Africa, 98 consecutive patients with acute neurological deficits were evaluated. HIV was diagnosed in 48% of the cases and in this particular group of HIV-positive patients stroke was the cause of the acute deficits in 58% of the cases. The authors identified 2 different clinical entities: 1) A young age group (20 to 40 years), in which ischemic stroke was common and occurred in absence of risk factors or previous evidence of vascular disease; this group had a high HIV positivity rate and 23% had evidence of brain infection; 2) An older age group (>50 years) in which ischemic strokes and intracerebral hemorrhages were both common, and there was evidence of vascular disease related to hypertension (e.g. left ventricular hypertrophy and carotid disease); in this group, there was a low HIV positivity rate and infections were not found [19].

The pronounced lengthening of disease-free survival achieved with HAART along with the growing number of new HIV infections in individuals who are of middle age or older has created a new population of HIV-infected patients whose age may put them at a higher risk for cerebrovascular disease.

In a cohort study of 772 HIV-infected patients (639 under the age of 46) followed up over 9 years, 15 patients were identified to have a cerebrovascular event, representing a prevalence rate of 1.9%. Six patients had a TIA and 9 had stroke. Ten patients were under 46 years of age (1.6% prevalence for this age group). The average annual incidence rate of TIA or stroke in this cohort was 216 per 100,000, about five times higher than the incidence of stroke in the non-HIV infected working population of the same age and region in Germany. The authors divided the sample into stroke occurring before and after 1997, when HAART was introduced, and there was no difference in the incidence rate of stroke. However, it was postulated that the sample was too small to elucidate the impact of HAART on this population [20].

Table 1. Age distribution in patients with HIV and stroke in Miami, Florida

	Frequency	Percent	Mean age
Group 1	47	57.3	34.17
Group 2	35	42.7	53.06
Total	82	100	42.23

Group 1: 45-year-old, or younger. Group 2: 46-year-old, or older.

Mechanisms of Stroke in HIV Infected Patients

In this section we will first analyze the pathogenesis linked to each possible mechanism of stroke in HIV patients, and then we will review the frequency of those mechanisms, according to results from case series and cohort studies.

Cardioembolism

Cardiac disease is common in HIV-infected patients and usually has been regarded as the main cause of embolic stroke in this population. In a pathology study of 54 patients who died of AIDS, cardiovascular pathology was seen in 30 patients (55%). Changes were seen in the endocardium (17%), myocardium (83%), and epicardium (3%). The most frequent finding was lymphocytic myocarditis [21]. A prospective case-control study evaluated the left ventricular function of 98 consecutive HIV-infected patients by echocardiography [22] and found diastolic dysfunction in 63% of the seropositive patients and depressed ejection fraction in 32%, with an 8% rate of symptomatic congestive heart failure. Echocardiographic abnormalities were significantly more frequent in HIV-infected patients compared with controls and the difference could not be explained by any other coexistent factor. Cardiac dysfunction was more common in later stages of the infection, but was also present in patients with asymptomatic HIV infection.

Non-bacterial thrombotic (marantic) endocarditis and bacterial endocarditis (with and without history of intravenous drug abuse) have been reported as causes of ischemic stroke in HIV-infected patients. Other cardiac conditions related to stroke in HIV patients include dilated cardiomyopathy, mural thrombi, myxoid degeneration of valves and, more questionably, HIV myocarditis [9, 15, 23, 24]. Aortic root dilatation associated with left ventricular dilation, increased viral load, and lower CD4 cell count has been documented in HIV-infected children [25].

Accelerated Atherosclerosis

As patients live longer with HIV, the emergence of metabolic disorders and premature atherosclerosis has caused alarm. Before HAART was available, obstructive coronary atherosclerosis was reported in young patients with HIV, in the absence of apparent coronary risk factors [26]. Later, premature coronary artery disease was associated with the use of protease inhibitors (PI) [27]. The absolute rates of atherosclerosis in the HIV population remain low, but this is likely to change as HAART continues to prolong survival.

Atherosclerosis was formerly considered to be a "lipid storage" disease. However, over the last decade inflammation has been recognized as a unifying link for the pathophysiological steps of atherogenesis, mediating all stages of the disease, from the early vascular lesions to the final events associated to thrombotic complications. Signs of inflammation, with leukocyte infiltration, are seen in the earliest lesions of atherosclerosis, both in experimental animals and in humans. Cellular adhesion molecules (CAM), like vascular cell adhesion molecule 1 (VCAM-1) and intercellular adhesion molecule 1 (ICAM-1), are expressed early in the atherogenic process and facilitate leukocyte adhesion to the endothelial surface. Some CAM are endothelial-specific, like E-selectin, but VCAM-1 and ICAM-1 are also produced by other cell types, like lymphocytes, epithelial cells, monocytes and smooth muscle cells. P-selectin is also found in platelet a-granules. Once the leukocytes are adherent to the endothelium, chemoattractant molecules induce their transmigration into the intima, followed by increased production of chemo-attractive molecules, inflammatory cytokines and growth factors. Lymphotoxin (tumor necrosis factor [TNF]–ß), γ-interferon, tissue plasminogen activator (TPA), plasminogen activator inhibitor-1 (PAI-1), von Willebrand factor (vWF), nitric oxide (NO) and C-reactive protein are some of the many molecules involved in this process. Eventually, activated macrophages ingest lipid particles and become foam cells, proliferation and migration of arterial smooth muscle cells (SMCs) is promoted, and extracellular matrix is degraded. Once the weakened plaque ruptures, macrophage-derived tissue factor promotes local thrombosis.

Inflammatory stimulation has also been found responsible for many mechanisms through which traditional cardiovascular risk factors, like dyslipidemia, hypertension, diabetes, and obesity are associated to atherogenesis. Chronic extravascular infection (e.g. gingivitis, prostatitis, bronchitis) has been associated to increased production of cytokines and accelerated evolution of remote atherosclerotic lesion. In HIV-infected patients, depletion of CD4+ T-cells in the gastrointestinal tract can lead to translocation of bacteria through the impaired intestinal mucosal barrier into the circulation, leading to chronic exposure to numerous microorganisms [28]. It has been postulated that a chronic bacterial endotoxemia could, by this mechanism, facilitate accelerated atherosclerosis in this population [29].

Several studies have shown that HIV can activate the endothelium either directly or by a leukocyte-mediated inflammatory cascade [30-32]. Many inflammatory markers related to atherogenesis are increased in patients with HIV-infection, specially at advanced stages of the disease [33-35], suggesting a clear association between endothelial injury and progression of HIV-infection.

Particularly in the immunosuppressed transplant population, cytomegalovirus (CMV) infection has been associated with accelerated atherosclerosis, and anti-CMV therapy has been reported to delay this process [36]. In the HIV population, increased CMV specific T-cell responsiveness has been correlated with the extent of atherosclerosis, measured by carotid artery intima-media thickness (IMT) [37]. However, it is still unknown whether anti-CMV therapy could impact the atherosclerotic process in HIV patients, the way it does in immunosuppressed transplant patients.

Antiretroviral Drugs

Various studies support the hypothesis that HAART induce activation of endothelial function. Ritonavir induced direct endothelial mitochondrial DNA damage and cell death in vitro [38], and Indinavir, another HIV-1 protease inhibitor, induced significant endothelial dysfunction in HIV-negative healthy males, after four weeks of exposure [39]. The interpretation was based on blood flow responses to intra-arterial infusions of vasoactive agents, particularly in relation to nitric oxide-dependent tone. These results were independent of the lipid profiles.

When comparing HIV patients on treatment with antiretroviral therapy versus HIV patients on no-treatment, impaired flow-mediated vasodilatation of the brachial artery (measured with high-resolution ultrasound) was found in the treatment group. This was also associated with significantly higher levels of total cholesterol, triglycerides and LDL in the treatment group. In this study, the conclusion was that the use of protease inhibitors was associated with atherogenic lipoprotein changes and endothelial dysfunction [40].

The prevalence of premature carotid stenosis has been found to be higher than expected in HIV patients treated with PI for at least 12 months. In one study, either atherosclerotic plaque or intima-media thickness >1mm were found in 53% of the group treated with PI, compared with 15% of PI-naïve HIV-infected patients and less than 7% of healthy non-HIV infected controls. However, this study failed to reveal significant differences in hemodynamic variables, such as pulsatility index, resistance index and peak, minimal and mean velocities [41].

The same authors compared PI-treated patients (group A) with PI-naïve patients treated with a regimen including non-nucleoside reverse transcriptase inhibitor (group B) and with patients treated with two nucleoside reverse transcriptase inhibitors or naïve to antiretroviral therapy (group C). All patients were treated for at least 12 months and evaluated for a familial history of cardiovascular disease, sedentary life, cigarette smoking, alcohol abuse, active drug addiction and fasting levels for glycemia, cholesterolemia and triglyceridemia. Intima characteristics, pulsation and resistance indexes and speed were assessed. Acquired lesions of the vascular wall were found in 57% of patients in group A, 16% group B and 14% in group C. Even though cigarette smoking, triglyceridemia and stage of HIV infection significantly increased the risk of vascular lesions, the highest significance was found in relation to the use of PI [42].

It is possible that the structure of the arterial lesions in HIV patients could present different characteristics with respect to the classical atheroma. Extensive inflammatory infiltration of the vascular wall has been found in the histology of young HIV patients with severe carotid stenosis [43] and ultrasonographic studies also have shown a different structure of the carotid lesions in HIV patients, resembling those of arteritis [44]. Maggi et al, have hypothesized that the atherosclerotic lesions in HIV patients may develop in two distinct phases.: initial inflammation of the vascular wall and subsequent evolution towards the classic features of atheroma [45]. The lesions in the first phase are probably determined by immunodeficiency, immune reconstitution and the effects of HAART. The second phase could be driven by the classic vascular risk factors.

Classic Vascular Risk Factors

Antiretroviral therapy and the HIV itself have both been implicated in the development of diabetes, insulin resistance, loss of peripheral fat (lipodystrophy), low high-density lipoprotein (HDL)-cholesterol, high triglycerides and chronic renal insufficiency with proteinuria, which are common in HIV patients [46-49].

At this time, the cardiovascular risk in HIV patients is calculated with conventional risk evaluation tools, like the Framingham risk score [50, 51]. This assessment tool takes into account age, sex, blood pressure, total cholesterol, HDL-cholesterol, smoking and diabetes to calculate a 10-year risk of coronary heart disease. However, as it was previously discussed, many other factors can influence the progression of atherogenesis in HIV patients, including heightened inflammation, altered immunity and antiretroviral treatments. Some of these HIV-specific factors influence the traditional Framingham risk factors as well. The risk prediction model should probably be modified for this particular population, for better accuracy of the assessment [51, 52]. For example, it is still unclear whether the assessment of C-reactive protein, coronary calcium score and carotid IMT are accurate means to evaluate cardiovascular risk in the HIV population.

Atherosclerosis prevention and pharmacologic treatment of vascular risk factors in HIV patients is based mostly on the recommendations from the treatment guidelines resulting from large-scale clinical trials. However, these trials did not include HIV-infected patients. Thus, it is unclear whether the application of these guidelines is really effective for the HIV population. Interaction between antiretroviral agents and cardiovascular therapies need to be considered. Smoking cessation, while always important in the general population, appears to have higher impact in HIV patients, with over 50% prevalence of tobacco abuse [53-55].

Pro-thrombotic States

A possible underlying pro-thrombotic state is commonly suspected to be the underlying cause of increased risk of stroke in the HIV population [56]. Various hemostatic abnormalities have been documented in HIV-patients with ischemic stroke, but perhaps the most consistently reported pro-thrombotic state has been protein S deficiency [57-62]. Antiphospholipid antibodies also have been found in various series [59, 63]. However, it is unclear whether the presence of these hemostatic abnormalities produces an actual increase in the risk of stroke. In a 3-year prospective study of 27 patients free of opportunistic disease who presented with transient neurologic deficits, a high prevalence of IgG anticardiolipin antibodies (70%) and protein S deficiency (53%) was found, but notably only 2 of these patients had documented strokes [64]. Furthermore, protein S deficiency has been proposed to be just an “epiphenomenon” of HIV infection [65] and there is no consensus on its relationship with ischemic stroke.

In terminally ill patients, stroke can be precipitated by disseminated intravascular coagulation or cerebral venous thrombosis as a consequence of dehydration and cachexia [8, 9]. Hyperviscosity has been reported at least once in AIDS and could represent a potential cause of cerebral infarction [66]. In trans-sexual men, use of estrogens can promote thrombotic strokes [67].

Unrecognized prothrombotic states have been suspected responsible for the high incidence of “cryptogenic” strokes, but no proof has been offered to support this hypothesis. Other forms of hypercoagulability also have been seen in HIV patients, but whether their frequency is higher than that in the normal population has not been assessed [68].

Opportunistic Vasculitis and HIV-Vasculopathy

Several opportunistic infections have been implicated in the development of vascular disease associated with ischemic strokes. They include tuberculosis, cytomegalovirus, herpes simplex virus, syphilis, cryptococcosis, candidiasis and lymphoma. Other potential causes in this category are toxoplasmosis, mucormycosis, aspergillosis and, more questionably, coccidioidomycosis and trypanosomiasis.

Varicella zoster virus (VZV) re-activation is a recognized but unusual cause of neurological disease in HIV-infected patients. A study from the Netherlands of 142 episodes of VZV reactivation in 113 HIV-positive patients revealed no complications among patients with unidermatomal zoster in a non-trigeminal distribution [69]. In a study of 15 patients with VZV-associated neurological disease, only 6 patients had a CSF pleocytosis [70]. CSF pleocytosis in the context of HIV infection must be interpreted with caution, as studies have attributed pleocytosis to HIV itself [71]. In our experience, VZV has been related to subcortical stroke without angiographic evidence of vasculitis (Figure 1) and also to multifocal intracerebral vasculitis, with more intense involvement of the basilar artery and subsequent pontine strokes, following herpes zoster oticus (Ramsay Hunt syndrome) (Figures 2A and 2B) [72]. Multiple small ischemic lesions were seen in a severely immuno compromised patient in whom herpes simplex virus was detected in the CSF (positive PCR), but there was no angiographic evidence of large artery vasculitis (Figure 3). Probably,the small lesions represented areas of focal encephalitis with ischemia. In another case withprogressive radiological signs of basilar arteritis associated to pontine strokes, extensive and dense perivascular lymphoplasmacytic infiltrates were found in the pons (Figure 4). Gram positive cocci were detected in pathological studies, most likely representing staphylococcus aureus.

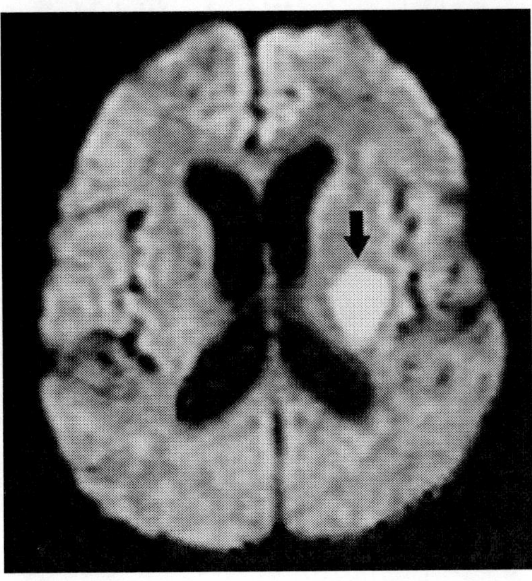

Figure 1. Large left subcortical stroke associated to VZV in the CSF, but no signs of vasculitis on cerebral angiography.

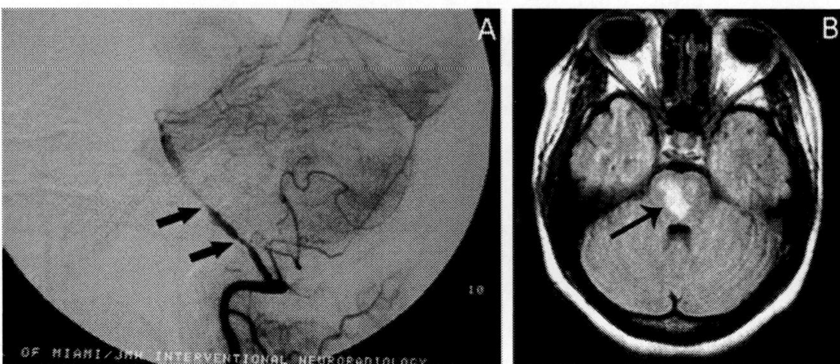

Figure 2. Basilar arteritis and pontine strokes after herpes zoster oticus (Ramsay Hunt syndrome), with VZV detected in the CSF. This patient has been reported elsewhere [72]. A: Basilar arteritis (arrows). B: Pontine stroke (arrow).

Primary angiitis of the CNS, with recurrent subcortical strokes, negative viral studies in the CSF and pathologic findings of multinucleated cells, lymphoplasmocytic infiltrates and focal fibrinoid degeneration has been reported, as well [73]. Table 2 summarizes the cases with acute ischemic stroke attributed to vasculitis in our population study from Miami, Florida.

The actual incidence of stroke in HIV-infected patients with these opportunistic diseases involving the central nervous system is unknown, but most likely low. These causes should generally be considered when the cerebral infarction occurs in an HIV-infected patient with advanced immunodeficiency. Fortunately, the current use of HAART has dramatically decreased the frequency of these conditions.

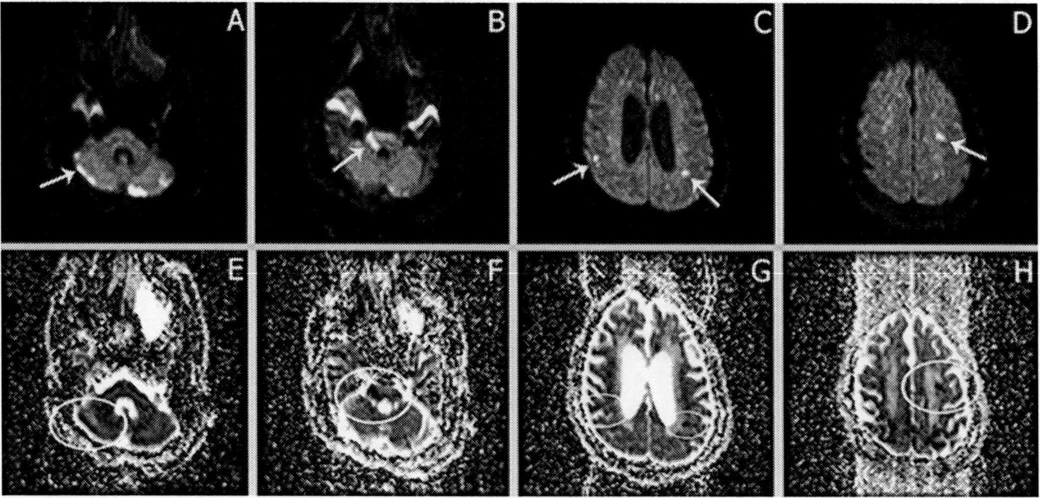

Figure 3. Multiple small acute ischemic lesions, seen as hyperintense (bright) lesions in diffusion weighted images (arrows in upper panels) and corresponding hypo-intensity in apparent diffusion coefficient (dark lesions within ovals in lower panels), over Cerebellum (A), Pons (B) and bilateral cerebral hemispheres (C and D) in a patient with HSV detected in the CSF. No signs of vasculitis in the cerebral angiography.

HIV-related Vasculopathy

The association between HIV and the occurrence of aneurysms was first reported in 1989 [74, 75]. Since then, there have been isolated case reports with a few case series on aneurysms in HIV infected patients. In these reports, the documented aneurysms have involved mostly the extracranial arteries, including the common carotid ant its branches, the subclavian arteries, aorta, femoral artery and its branches, and the popliteal arteries.

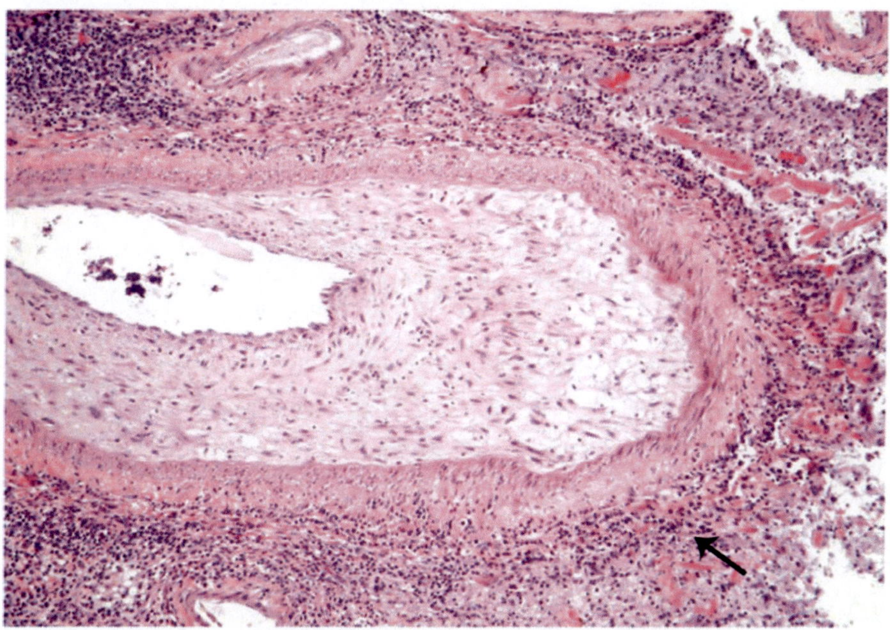

Figure 4. Dense perivascular lymphoplasmacytic infiltrate (arrow) in an HIV-patient with basilar arteritis and pontine strokes.

In the most extensive study to date on extracranial aneurysms in HIV positive patients, reported from KwaZuluNatal, South Africa, it was found that the patients were young, with no risk factors for degenerative arterial disease, multiple vessel involvement was common and atypical sites were involved [76]. In further reports from this region, the histology showed fragmentation with loss of the internal elastic lamina, medial and adventitial fibrosis with chronic inflammation, leukocytoclastic vasculitis and proliferation of slit-like vascular channels in the adventitia [77-79].

Intracranial aneurysms have been described more frequently in children (predominantly fusiform), with a reported incidence up to 1.9% in a large study of 426 HIV-positive children [80]. In adults, saccular aneurysms, as well as fusiform aneurysms have been reported, presenting clinically with headache and subarachnoid hemorrhage. Extracranial aneurysms in HIV positive patients are due to vasculitis of the vasa vasora, which are absent in the intracranial arteries, implying that the pathogenesis is different.

The exact mechanism of aneurysm formation in HIV is not known. Damage to the vessel wall by HIV itself, an immune reaction in the vessel wall, and infective processes akin to those described for mycotic aneurysms have been proposed. Direct involvement of HIV in aneurysm formation was suggested by monoclonal anti-gp41 antibody staining in the aneurysmal arterial walls at postmortem examination of a 6 year old boy with AIDS who had diffuse aneurysmal dilatations of the circle of Willis [81]. Immune activation in response to transendothelial migration of HIV strains with tropism for cerebral mononuclear cells has been postulated to be implicated in the pathogenesis of these aneurysms.

Table 2. Summary of cases with acute ischemic stroke attributed to vasculitis in the study from Miami, Florida

Case	Associated condition	Age (Years)	CD4 count (cells/mm3)	Supportive evidence	Diagnostic certainty
1	Ramsay Hunt syndrome	24	15	Angiography CSF (PCR for VZV)	Confirmed
2	Neurosyphilis	34	169	Angiography CSF (VDRL)	Confirmed
3	Bacterial endocarditis	51	70	Angiography CSF	Confirmed
4	TB meningitis, Cryptococcal meningitis	40	165	CSF culture (Cryptococcus) Biopsy proven systemic vasculitis	Confirmed
5	VZV radiculitis	46	76	CSF (PCR for VZV) MRA	Confirmed
6	Neurosyphilis	29	153	CSF (VDRL)	Confirmed
7	Sepsis with Candida	49	102	MRA	Probable
8	Orbital celullitis	66	267	MRA Candida isolated from orbital tissue biopsy	Probable
9	Aspergillus sinusitis	25	11	MRA	Probable
10	Systemic MAI	26	Not available	Multiple strokes without alternative cause Transverse myelitis	Possible

Subsequent alteration of dynamic vascular responsiveness to pulsatile blood flow regulated by alterations in circulating cytokines and growth factors may lead to vascular remodeling. Impaired cerebrovascular reactivity has been documented both with Nuclear Medicine studies and with Transcranial Doppler ultrasound in HIV infected patients, suggesting compromise of the small cerebral arterioles [82, 83]. Other opportunistic infections associated with HIV may contribute to the production of these cytokines and growth factors; whereas recurrent infections may contribute to an increase in elastases, leading to the fragmentation and thinning of the internal elastic lamina, an early histololgical finding in the development of fusiform aneurysms [84-86].

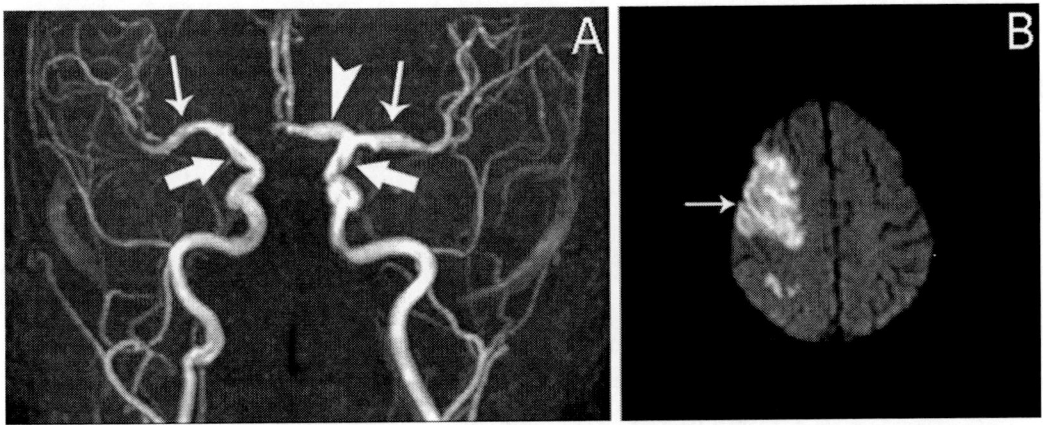

Figure 5. HIV vasculopathy in a 35-year-old woman. A: MR angiography, showing fusiform dilatation of both distal ICAs (thick arrows), both MCAs (thin arrows) and A1 segment of left ACA (arrow-head). B: Right MCA stroke associated to this HIV vasculopathy (arrow).

Figures 5 and 6 show a couple of cases of HIV vasculopathy in young patients, both of them with unremarkable CSF studies and large ischemic strokes.

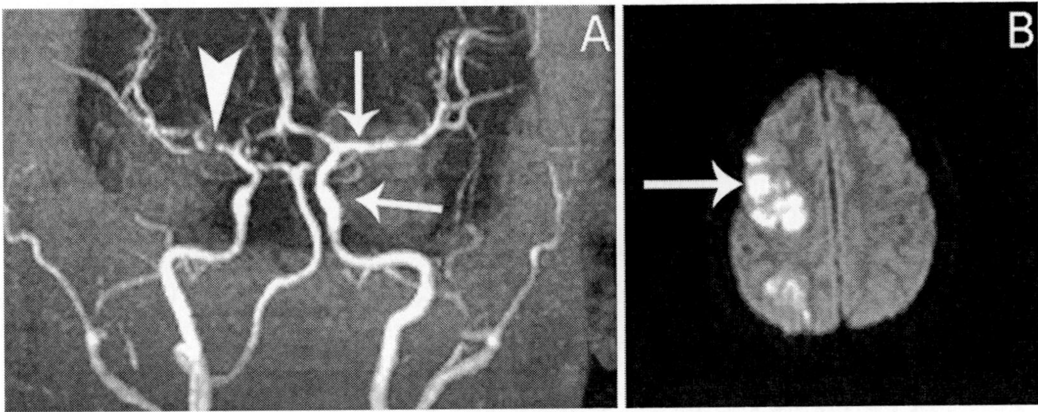

Figure 6. HIV vasculopathy in a 14-year-old boy. A: MR angiography, showing fusiform dilatation of the distal left ICA and left MCA, with "beading" of the right MCA (arrow-head). B: Brain MRI, showing a right MCA stroke (arrow) associated to the HIV vasculopathy.

The natural history of HIV associated intracranial aneurysms has not been well documented, yet. Before HAART, once a diagnosis of aneurysmal arteriopathy was made, progression of the disease seemed to be fast, with patients deteriorating rapidly and death occurring in less than 6 months [87]. However, antiretrovirals may have a remarkable impact, as it was reported in the cases of an 8-year-old girl with multiple intracranial aneurysms who showed stabilization of the disease after being started on treatment with HAART [88] and a 12-year-old girl with aneurysmal dilatations of the right carotid artery in whom resolution of the aneurysms was shown in radiologic studies 15 months after the initiation of HAART [89]. It remains to be seen if HAART may decrease the progression or promote resolution of intracranial aneurysms in adult HIV-infected patients.

Drug Abuse

Although infrequently reported as causes of cerebral infarction in HIV-infected patients, active use of cocaine and heroin increase the risk of stroke and their potential role should be investigated in each case. The mechanism of ischemia in cocaine-induced stroke is unclear. Vasoconstriction, increased platelet aggregation and apparent vasculitis have been postulated.

Table 3. Comparison of distribution of variables between HIV-infected patients with atherothrombotic and non-atherothrombotic ischemic strokes

Variables	Atherothromboti c	Non-atherothrombotic	P value
Age (years)	45.3 ± 3	40.1 ± 1.6	0.04
History of cocaine use n (%)	20 (37)	10 (19)	0.66
Recent cocaine use n (%)	0	13 (52)	0.02

In heroin users, strokes usually occurred following reintroduction of the drug after a period of abstinence, suggesting that the underlying mechanism could be immunologic [90]. In the series of cases from Miami, Florida, patients with non-atherothrombotic strokes were younger (40.1 ± 1.6 vs 45.3 ± 3) and more exposed to cocaine, compared to patients with athero-thrombotic strokes. History of cocaine use was present in 53 patients, 10 with atherothrombotic strokes (19%) and 20 with non-atherothrombotic strokes (37%) ($p = 0.66$). However, when toxicology screening was performed (in 31 patients with ischemic strokes), cocaine was not detected in any patient with atherothrombotic stroke (0/6), but was present in 13/25 tested patients (52%) with non-atherothrombotic strokes ($p=0.02$) (Table 3).

Evaluation of Frequency of Mechanisms of Stroke in HIV Patients

Three series of cases have evaluated the frequency of the different mechanisms of stroke in HIV-infected patients. In a case series of 35 South-African HIV-positive patients with stroke [91], more than one underlying cause of stroke was found in 10 patients. Eight patients (25%) had meningitis, 3 (9%) had a cardioembolic source, 2 had hypertension and 17 (49%) had coagulopathies: protein S deficiency in 11 patients, protein C deficiency in 1 patient and antiphospholipid antibodies in 5 patients. Vasculopathy/vasculitis was diagnosed in 4 patients, one patient had a spontaneous extracranial internal carotid artery dissection (with a middle cerebral artery stroke), 2 patients had HIV-vasculopathy, and 1 patient had herpes zoster vasculitis. Protein S co-existed with tuberculous meningitis in 2 patients, with antiphospholipid syndrome in 2 patients, with viral meningitis in 1 patient, with herpes zoster vasculitis in 1 patient, with hypertension in 1 patient and with protein C deficiency in 1 patient. No potential cause was identified in 5 patients (14%).

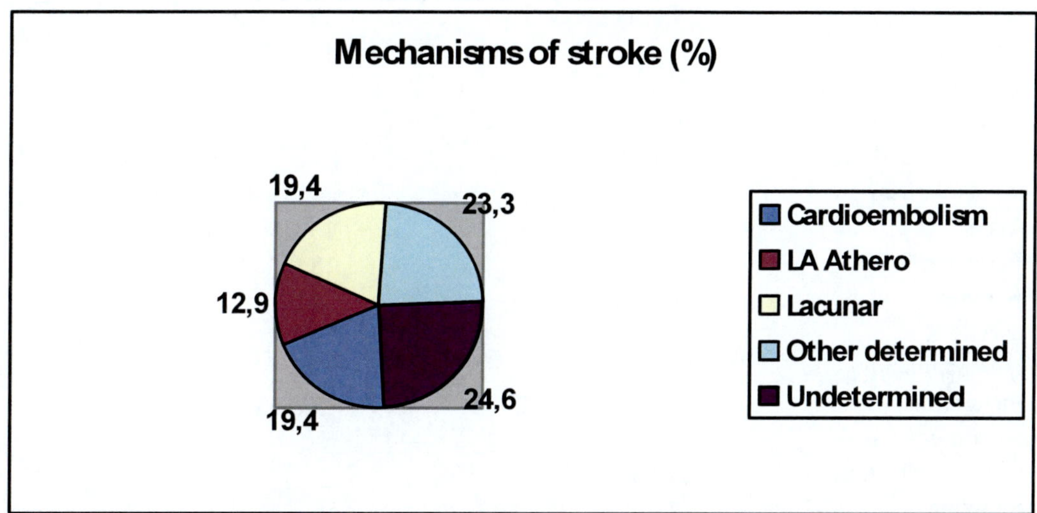

LA Athero: Large artery athesclerosis.

Figure 7. Mechanisms of stroke according to TOAST criteria in HIV-stroke patients from Miami, Florida.

Among the 64 patients with ischemic infarcts in the Cape Town cohort study [17], opportunistic infections were present en 18 (28%), HIV-vasculopathy in 13 (20%) (Including intracranial and extracranial aneurysms), coagulopathy in 12 (19%), cardioembolism in 9 (14%) and the mechanism was considered unknown in 12 (19%). Cardioembolism was less common in HIV positive young stroke patients (10%), compared with HIV negative young stroke cases (23%) ($p = 0.028$). Conversely, anticardiolipin antibodies were significantly more elevated in the young HIV stroke group, compared to young, non-HIV patients ($p = 0.002$). In the analysis from Miami, Florida [18], 77 patients were included with diagnosis of ischemic stroke and the mechanisms of stroke were classified according to TOAST criteria [92]: Large artery atherosclerosis was found in 10 patients (13%), including 4 with extracranial internal carotid artery stenosis (5%), 5 with middle cerebral artery stenosis (6.5%) and 1 with vertebrobasilar stenosis (1.3%). In 15 patients, the mechanism was cardioembolic (19%), 15 had lacunar strokes (19%) and 18 were classified as "other determined etiology", with 10 cases of vasculitis (13%), 1 vertebral artery dissection (1.3%) and 7 cases of hypercoagulability (9%). There were 19 cases of stroke of undetermined etiology, including 3 with negative evaluation, 3 with two or more causes identified and 13 with incomplete evaluation (17%) (Figure 7).

Anticardiolipin antibodies were found in 29% and protein S deficiency was found in 45% of the tested cases. In these patients, neither antiretroviral treatment at any time nor current use of HAART correlated with the type of ischemic stroke. Table 4 describes the distribution of the different mechanisms of stroke in these patients.

Table 4. Mechanisms of stroke in HIV patients, Miami, Florida (n = 77)

	N of Patients (%)	Total N (%)
LA athero		10 (12.9)
ICA stenosis	4 (5)	
IC athero	5 (6.5)	
VB athero	1 (1.3)	
Cardioembolism		15 (19.4)
Lacunar		15 (19.4)
Other determined		18 (23.3)
Vasculitis	10 (13)	
Dissection	1 (1.3)	
Hypercoagulability	7 (9)	
Undetermined etiology		19 (24.6)
Two or more causes	3 (3.8)	
Negative evaluation	3 (3.8)	
Incomplete evaluation	13 (16.8)	

Conclusion

The relationship of HIV infection with stroke, once thought to be of rather marginal clinical relevance, is undergoing remarkable changes. These changes parallel those observed in the management and prognosis of HIV infection itself and relate to the increased survival of HIV-infected patients and the metabolic effects of the drugs used for the treatment. While strokes associated with opportunistic infections or tumors may be showing a declining incidence, clinicians should remain alert to the possibility of a growing overall incidence of stroke in the HIV infected population due to the emergence of new mechanisms such as possible accelerated atherosclerosis in patients treated with HAART and a form of HIV related vasculopathy. Studies supporting the role of these novel mechanisms are available but information on their clinical impact is still lacking. Therefore, although concerning, the potential for new antiretroviral regimens to favor premature vascular events remains to be defined. Epidemiological studies focusing on the incidence of vascular disease in general and stroke in particular should be conducted on aging HIV-infected patients to help delineate the true magnitude of the problem and the relative contribution of the various mechanisms at play.

References

[1] Palella FJ Jr, Delaney KM, Moorman AC, Loveless MO, Fuhrer J, Satten GA, Aschman DJ, Holmberg SD. Declining morbidity and mortality among patients with advanced human immunodeficiency virus infection. HIV Outpatient Study Investigators. *N. Engl. J. Med.* 1998;338(13):853-60.

[2] DAD Study Group, Friis-Møller N, Reiss P, Sabin CA, Weber R, Monforte A, El-Sadr W, Thiébaut R, De Wit S, Kirk O, Fontas E, Law MG, Phillips A, Lundgren JD. Class of antiretroviral drugs and the risk of myocardial infarction. *N. Engl. J. Med.* 2007; 356(17): 1723-35.

[3] Friis-Møller N, Sabin CA, Weber R, d'Arminio Monforte A, El-Sadr WM, Reiss P, Thiébaut R, Morfeldt L, De Wit S, Pradier C, Calvo G, Law MG, Kirk O, Phillips AN, Lundgren JD; DAD Study Group. Combination antiretroviral therapy and the risk of myocardial infarction. *N. Engl. J. Med.* 2003;349(21):1993-2003.

[4] Obel N, Thomsen HF, Kronborg G, Larsen CS, Hildebrandt PR, Sørensen HT, Gerstoft J. Ischemic heart disease in HIV-infected and HIV-uninfected individuals: a population-based cohort study. *Clin. Infect. Dis*, 2007;44(12):1625-31.

[5] Sackoff JE, Hanna DB, Pfeiffer MR, Torian LV. Causes of death among persons with AIDS in the era of highly active antiretroviral therapy: New York City. *Ann. Intern. Med.* 2006;145(6):397-406.

[6] Triant VA, Lee H, Hadigan C, Grinspoon SK. Increased acute myocardial infarction rates and cardiovascular risk factors among patients with human immunodeficiency virus disease. *J. Clin. Endocrinol. Metab*, 2007;92(7):2506-12.

[7] Kristensen B, Malm J, Carlberg B, Stegmayr B, Backman C, Fagerlund M, Olsson T. Epidemiology and etiology of ischemic stroke in young adults aged 18 to 44 years in northern Sweden. *Stroke,* 1997;28(9):1702-9.

[8] Anders KH, Guerra WF, Tomiyasu U, Verity MA, Vinters HV. The neuropathology of AIDS. UCLA experience and review. *Am. J. Pathol.* 1986;124(3):537-58.

[9] Berger JR, Harris JO, Gregorios J, Norenberg M. Cerebrovascular disease in AIDS: a case-control study. *Aids* 1990;4(3):239-44.

[10] Kieburtz KD, Eskin TA, Ketonen L, Tuite MJ. Opportunistic cerebral vasculopathy and stroke in patients with the acquired immunodeficiency syndrome. *Arch Neurol.* 993; 0(4): 30-2.

[11] Mizusawa H, Hirano A, Llena JF, Shintaku M. Cerebrovascular lesions in acquired immune deficiency syndrome (AIDS). *Acta Neuropathol.*1988;76(5):451-7.

[12] Moskowitz LB, Hensley GT, Chan JC, Gregorios J, Conley FK. The neuropathology of acquired immune deficiency syndrome. *Arch Pathol. Lab. Med.* 1984;108(11):867-72.

[13] Pinto AN. AIDS and cerebrovascular disease. *Stroke* 1996;27(3):538-43.

[14] Connor MD, Lammie GA, Bell JE, Warlow CP, Simmonds P, Brettle RD. Cerebral infarction in adult AIDS patients: observations from the Edinburgh HIV Autopsy Cohort. *Stroke* 2000;31(9):2117-26.

[15] Engstrom JW, Lowenstein DH, Bredesen DE. Cerebral infarctions and transient neurologic deficits associated with acquired immunodeficiency syndrome. *Am. J. Med.* 1989; 86(5):528-32.

[16] Cole JW, Pinto AN, Hebel JR, Buchholz DW, Earley CJ, Johnson CJ, Macko RF, Price TR, Sloan MA, Stern BJ, Wityk RJ, Wozniak MA, Kittner SJ. Acquired immunodeficiency syndrome and the risk of stroke. *Stroke* 2004;35(1):51-6.

[17] Tipping B, de Villiers L, Wainwright H, Candy S, Bryer A. Stroke in patients with human immunodeficiency virus infection. *J. Neurol. Neurosurg. Psychiatry* 2007;78(12): 1320-4.

[18] Ortiz G, Koch S, Romano JG, Forteza AM, Rabinstein AA. Mechanisms of ischemic stroke in HIV-infected patients. *Neurology* 2007;68(16):1257-61.

[19] Kumwenda JJ, Mateyu G, Kampondeni S, van Dam AP, van Lieshout L, Zijlstra EE. Differential diagnosis of stroke in a setting of high HIV prevalence in Blantyre, Malawi. *Stroke* 2005;36(5):960-4.

[20] Evers S, Nabavi D, Rahmann A, Heese C, Reichelt D, Husstedt IW. Ischaemic cerebrovascular events in HIV infection: a cohort study. *Cerebrovasc. Dis.* 2003;15(3): 199-205.

[21] Roldan EO, Moskowitz L, Hensley GT. Pathology of the heart in acquired immunodeficiency syndrome. *Arch Pathol. Lab. Med.* 1987;111(10):943-6.

[22] Cardoso JS, Moura B, Martins L, Mota-Miranda A, Rocha Gonçalves F, Lecour H. Left ventricular dysfunction in human immunodeficiency virus (HIV)-infected patients. *Int. J. Cardiol.* 1998;63(1):37-45.

[23] Mesquita ET, Ramos RG, Ferrari AH, Martins Wde A, da Cruz GG. Rheumatic heart disease and infective endocarditis in a patient with acquired immunodeficiency syndrome. *Arq. Bras. Cardiol.* 1996;67(4):255-7.

[24] Snider WD, Simpson DM, Nielsen S, Gold JW, Metroka CE, Posner JB. Neurological complications of acquired immune deficiency syndrome: analysis of 50 patients. *Ann. Neurol.* 1983,14(4):403-18.

[25] Lai WW, Colan SD, Easley KA, Lipshultz SE, Starc TJ, Bricker JT, Kaplan S; P2C2 HIV Study Group, National Heart, Lung, and Blood Institute. Dilation of the aortic root in children infected with human immunodeficiency virus type 1: The Prospective P2C2 HIV Multicenter Study. *Am. Heart J.* 2001;141(4):661-70.

[26] Paton P, Tabib A, Loire R, Tete R. Coronary artery lesions and human immunodeficiency virus infection. *Res. Virol.* 1993;144(3):225-31.

[27] Henry K, Melroe H, Huebsch J, Hermundson J, Levine C, Swensen L, Daley J. Severe premature coronary artery disease with protease inhibitors. *Lancet* 1998; 351(9112): 1328.

[28] Kotler DP. HIV infection and the gastrointestinal tract. *Aids* 2005;19(2):107-17.

[29] Brenchley JM, Price DA, Schacker TW, Asher TE, Silvestri G, Rao S, Kazzaz Z, Bornstein E, Lambotte O, Altmann D, Blazar BR, Rodriguez B, Teixeira-Johnson L, Landay A, Martin JN, Hecht FM, Picker LJ, Lederman MM, Deeks SG, Douek DC. Microbial translocation is a cause of systemic immune activation in chronic HIV infection. *Nat. Med.* 2006;12(12):1365-71.

[30] Lifson JD, Reyes GR, McGrath MS, Stein BS, Engleman EG. AIDS retrovirus induced cytopathology: giant cell formation and involvement of CD4 antigen. *Science* 1986; 232(4754):1123-7.

[31] Ren Z, Yao Q, Chen C. HIV-1 envelope glycoprotein 120 increases intercellular adhesion molecule-1 expression by human endothelial cells. *Lab. Invest.* 2002;82(3):245-55.

[32] Stefano GB, Salzet M, Bilfinger TV. Long-term exposure of human blood vessels to HIV gp120, morphine, and anandamide increases endothelial adhesion of monocytes: uncoupling of nitric oxide release. *J. Cardiovasc. Pharmacol.* 1998;31(6):862-8.

[33] Hansson GK. Inflammation, atherosclerosis, and coronary artery disease. *N. Engl. J. Med.* 2005;352(16):1685-95.

[34] Hsue PY, Lo JC, Franklin A, Bolger AF, Martin JN, Deeks SG, Waters DD. Progression of atherosclerosis as assessed by carotid intima-media thickness in patients with HIV infection. *Circulation* 2004;109(13):1603-8.

[35] Sipsas NV, Sfikakis PP, Touloumi G, Pantazis N, Choremi H, Kordossis T. Elevated serum levels of soluble immune activation markers are associated with increased risk for death in HAART-naive HIV-1-infected patients. *AIDS Patient Care STDS* 2003;17(4): 147-53.

[36] Valantine HA, Gao SZ, Menon SG, Renlund DG, Hunt SA, Oyer P, Stinson EB, Brown BW Jr, Merigan TC, Schroeder JS. Impact of prophylactic immediate posttransplant ganciclovir on development of transplant atherosclerosis: a post hoc analysis of a randomized, placebo-controlled study. *Circulation* 1999;100(1):61-6.

[37] Hsue PY, Hunt PW, Sinclair E, Bredt B, Franklin A, Killian M, Hoh R, Martin JN, McCune JM, Waters DD, Deeks SG. Increased carotid intima-media thickness in HIV patients is associated with increased cytomegalovirus-specific T-cell responses. *Aids* 2006; 20(18):2275-83.

[38] Zhong DS, Lu XH, Conklin BS, Lin PH, Lumsden AB, Yao Q, Chen C. HIV protease inhibitor ritonavir induces cytotoxicity of human endothelial cells. *Arterioscler. Thromb. Vasc. Biol.* 2002;22(10):1560-6.

[39] Shankar SS, Dubé MP, Gorski JC, Klaunig JE, Steinberg HO. Indinavir impairs endothelial function in healthy HIV-negative men. *Am. Heart J.* 2005;150(5):933.

[40] Stein JH, Klein MA, Bellehumeur JL, McBride PE, Wiebe DA, Otvos JD, Sosman JM. Use of human immunodeficiency virus-1 protease inhibitors is associated with atherogenic lipoprotein changes and endothelial dysfunction. *Circulation* 2001;104(3):257-62.

[41] Maggi P, Serio G, Epifani G, Fiorentino G, Saracino A, Fico C, Perilli F, Lillo A, Ferraro S, Gargiulo M, Chirianni A, Angarano G, Regina G, Pastore G. Premature lesions of the carotid vessels in HIV-1-infected patients treated with protease inhibitors. *Aids* 2000; 14(16):F123-8.

[42] Maggi P, Fiorentino G, Epifani G, Ladisa N, Lillo A, Perilli F, Impedovo G, Ferraro S, Gargiulo M, Angarano G, Chirianni A, Pastore G. Premature vascular lesions in HIV-positive patients: a clockwork bomb that will explode? *Aids* 2002;16(6):947-8.

[43] Regina G, Impedovo G, Angiletta D, Martiradonna F, Lillo A, Perilli F, Marotta V, Marzullo A, Epifani G, Fiore JR, Maggi P. Surgical experience with carotid stenosis in young HIV-1 positive patients under antiretroviral therapy: an emerging problem? *Eur. J. Vasc. Endovasc. Surg.* 2005;29(2):167-70.

[44] Maggi P, Perilli F, Lillo A, Carito V, Epifani G, Bellacosa C, Pastore G, Regina G. An ultrasound-based comparative study on carotid plaques in HIV-positive patients vs. atherosclerotic and arteritis patients: atherosclerotic or inflammatory lesions? *Coron. Artery Dis.* 2007;18(1):23-9.

[45] Maggi P, Maserati R, Antonelli G. Atherosclerosis in HIV patients: a new face for an old disease? *AIDS Rev.* 2006;8(4):204-9.

[46] Lafeuillade A, Alessi MC, Poizot-Martin I, Boyer-Neumann C, Zandotti C, Quilichini R, Aubert L, Tamalet C, Juhan-Vague I, Gastaut JA. Endothelial cell dysfunction in HIV infection. *J. Acquir. Immune Defic. Syndr.* 1992;5(2):127-31.

[47] Puppo F, Brenci S, Scudeletti M, Lanza L, Bosco O, Indiveri F. Elevated serum levels of circulating intercellular adhesion molecule-1 in HIV infection. *Aids* 1993;7(4):593-4.

[48] Sipsas N, Sfikakis PP, Sfikakis P, Choremi H, Kordossis T. Serum concentrations of soluble intercellular adhesion molecule-1 and progress towards disease in patients infected with HIV. *J. Infect.* 1994;29(3):271-82.

[49] Zietz C, Hotz B, Stürzl M, Rauch E, Penning R, Löhrs U. Aortic endothelium in HIV-1 infection: chronic injury, activation, and increased leukocyte adherence. *Am. J. Pathol.* 1996;149(6):1887-98.

[50] Carr A, Samaras K, Chisholm DJ, Cooper DA. Pathogenesis of HIV-1-protease inhibitor-associated peripheral lipodystrophy, hyperlipidaemia, and insulin resistance. *Lancet* 1998;351(9119):1881-3.

[51] Hsue PY, Waters DD. What a cardiologist needs to know about patients with human immunodeficiency virus infection. *Circulation* 2005;112(25):3947-57.

[52] Friis-Møller N, Worm SW. Can the risk of cardiovascular disease in HIV-infected patients be estimated from conventional risk prediction tools? *Clin. Infect. Dis.* 2007; 45(8): 1082-4.

[53] Gritz ER, Vidrine DJ, Lazev AB, Amick BC 3rd, Arduino RC. Smoking behavior in a low-income multiethnic HIV/AIDS population. *Nicotine Tob. Res.* 2004;6(1):71-7.

[54] Savès M, Chêne G, Ducimetière P, Leport C, Le Moal G, Amouyel P, Arveiler D, Ruidavets JB, Reynes J, Bingham A, Raffi F; French WHO MONICA Project and the APROCO (ANRS EP11) Study Group. Risk factors for coronary heart disease in patients treated for human immunodeficiency virus infection compared with the general population. *Clin. Infect. Dis.* 2003;37(2):292-8.

[55] Stein JH, Hadigan CM, Brown TT, Chadwick E, Feinberg J, Friis-Møller N, Ganesan A, Glesby MJ, Hardy D, Kaplan RC, Kim P, Lo J, Martinez E, Sosman JM; Working Group 6. Prevention strategies for cardiovascular disease in HIV-infected patients. *Circulation* 2008;118(2):e54-60.

[56] Hoffmann M, Berger JR, Nath A, Rayens M. Cerebrovascular disease in young, HIV-infected, black Africans in the KwaZulu Natal province of South Africa. J Neurovirol 2000;6(3):229-36.

[57] Bissuel F, Berruyer M, Causse X, Dechavanne M, Trepo C. Acquired protein S deficiency: correlation with advanced disease in HIV-1-infected patients. *J. Acquir. Immune Defic. Syndr.* 1992;5(5):484-9.

[58] Erbe M, Rickerts V, Bauersachs RM, Lindhoff-Last E. Acquired protein C and protein S deficiency in HIV-infected patients. *Clin. Appl. Thromb Hemost* 2003;9(4):325-31.

[59] Hassell KL, Kressin DC, Neumann A, Ellison R, Marlar RA. Correlation of antiphospholipid antibodies and protein S deficiency with thrombosis in HIV-infected men. *Blood Coagul. Fibrinolysis* 1994;5(4):455-62.

[60] Sorice M, Griggi T, Arcieri P, Circella A, d'Agostino F, Ranieri M, Modrzewska R, Lenti L, Mariani G. Protein S and HIV infection. The role of anticardiolipin and anti-protein S antibodies. *Thromb Res*. 1994;73(3-4):165-75.

[61] Stahl CP, Wideman CS, Spira TJ, Haff EC, Hixon GJ, Evatt BL. Protein S deficiency in men with long-term human immunodeficiency virus infection. *Blood* 1993; 81(7):1801-7.

[62] Sugerman RW, Church JA, Goldsmith JC, Ens GE. Acquired protein S deficiency in children infected with human immunodeficiency virus. *Pediatr. Infect. Dis. J.* 1996; 15(2): 106-11.

[63] Abuaf N, Laperche S, Rajoely B, Carsique R, Deschamps A, Rouquette AM, Barthet C, Khaled Z, Marbot C, Saab N, Rozen J, Girard PM, Rozenbaum W. Autoantibodies to phospholipids and to the coagulation proteins in AIDS. *Thromb Haemost* 1997;77(5):856-61.

[64] Brew BJ, Miller J. Human immunodeficiency virus type 1-related transient neurological deficits. *Am. J. Med.* 1996;101(3):257-61.

[65] Mochan A, Modi M, Modi G. Protein S deficiency in HIV associated ischaemic stroke: an epiphenomenon of HIV infection. *J. Neurol. Neurosurg. Psychiatry*, 2005;76(10): 1455-6.

[66] Martin CM, Matlow AG, Chew E, Sutton D, Pruzanski W. Hyperviscosity syndrome in a patient with acquired immunodeficiency syndrome. *Arch Intern. Med.* 1989;149(6):1435-6.

[67] deMarinis M, Arnett EN. Cerebrovascular occlusion in a transsexual man taking mestranol. *Arch Intern. Med.* 1978;138(11):1732-3.

[68] Saif MW, Greenberg B. Greenberg, HIV and thrombosis: a review. *AIDS Patient Care STDS* 2001;15(1):15-24.

[69] Veenstra J, van Praag RM, Krol A, Wertheim van Dillen PM, Weigel HM, Schellekens PT, Lange JM, Coutinho RA, van der Meer JT. Complications of varicella zoster virus reactivation in HIV-infected homosexual men. *Aids* 1996;10(4):393-9.

[70] Brown M, Scarborough M, Brink N, Manji H, Miller R. Varicella zoster virus-associated neurological disease in HIV-infected patients. *Int. J. STD AIDS* 2001;12(2):79-83.

[71] Marshall DW, Brey RL, Cahill WT, Houk RW, Zajac RA, Boswell RN. Spectrum of cerebrospinal fluid findings in various stages of human immunodeficiency virus infection. *Arch Neurol.* 1988;45(9):954-8.

[72] Ortiz GA, Koch S, Forteza A, Romano J. Ramsay hunt syndrome followed by multifocal vasculopathy and posterior circulation strokes. *Neurology* 2008;70(13):1049-51.

[73] Nogueras C, Sala M, Sasal M, Viñas J, Garcia N, Bella MR, Cervantes M, Segura F. Recurrent stroke as a manifestation of primary angiitis of the central nervous system in a patient infected with human immunodeficiency virus. *Arch Neurol.* 2002;59(3):468-73.

[74] Dupont JR, Bonavita JA, DiGiovanni RJ, Spector HB, Nelson SC. Acquired immunodeficiency syndrome and mycotic abdominal aortic aneurysms: a new challenge? Report of a case. *J. Vasc. Surg.* 1989;10(3):254-7.

[75] Sinzobahamvya N, Kalangu K, Hämel-Kalinowski W. Arterial aneurysms associated with human immunodeficiency virus (HIV) infection. *Acta Chir. Bel*g, 1989. 89(4): p. 185-8.

[76] Nair R, Robbs JV, Naidoo NG, Woolgar J. Clinical profile of HIV-related aneurysms. *Eur. J. Vasc. Endovasc. Surg,* 2000. 20(3): p. 235-40.

[77] Chetty R. Vasculitides associated with HIV infection. *J. Clin. Pathol,* 2001. 54(4): p. 275-8.

[78] Chetty R, Batitang S, Nair R. Large artery vasculopathy in HIV-positive patients: another vasculitic enigma. *Hum. Pathol*, 2000. 31(3): p. 374-9.

[79] Nair R, Abdool-Carrim A, Chetty R, Robbs J. Arterial aneurysms in patients infected with human immunodeficiency virus: a distinct clinicopathology entity? *J. Vasc. Surg.* 1999; 29(4):600-7.

[80] Patsalides AD, Wood LV, Atac GK, Sandifer E, Butman JA, Patronas NJ. Cerebrovascular disease in HIV-infected pediatric patients: neuroimaging findings. *AJR Am. J. Roentgenol.* 2002;179(4):999-1003.

[81] Kure K, Park YD, Kim TS, Lyman WD, Lantos G, Lee S, Cho S, Belman AL, Weidenheim KM, Dickson DW. Immunohistochemical localization of an HIV epitope in cerebral aneurysmal arteriopathy in pediatric acquired immunodeficiency syndrome (AIDS). *Pediatr Pathol.* 1989;9(6):655-67.

[82] Brilla R, Nabavi DG, Schulte-Altedorneburg G, Kemény V, Reichelt D, Evers S, Schiemann U, Husstedt IW. Cerebral vasculopathy in HIV infection revealed by transcranial Doppler: A pilot study. *Stroke* 1999;30(4):811-3.

[83] Tran Dinh YR, Mamo H, Cervoni J, Caulin C, Saimot AC. Disturbances in the cerebral perfusion of human immune deficiency virus-1 seropositive asymptomatic subjects: a quantitative tomography study of 18 cases. *J. Nucl. Med.* 1990;31(10):1601-7.

[84] Bulsara KR, Raja A, Owen J. HIV and cerebral aneurysms. *Neurosurg. Rev.* 2005; 28(2): 92-5.

[85] Shah SS, Zimmerman RA, Rorke LB, Vezina LG. Cerebrovascular complications of HIV in children. *AJNR Am. J. Neuroradiol.* 1996;17(10):1913-7.

[86] Tipping B, de Villiers L, Candy S, Wainwright H. Stroke caused by human immunodeficiency virus-associated intracranial large-vessel aneurysmal vasculopathy. *Arch Neurol.* 2006;63(11):1640-2.

[87] Dubrovsky T, Curless R, Scott G, Chaneles M, Post MJ, Altman N, Petito CK, Start D, Wood C. Cerebral aneurysmal arteriopathy in childhood AIDS. *Neurology* 1998; 51(2):560-5.

[88] Mazzoni P, Chiriboga CA, Millar WS, Rogers A. Intracerebral aneurysms in human immunodeficiency virus infection: case report and literature review. *Pediatr Neurol.* 2000; 23(3):252-5.

[89] Martínez-Longoria CA, Morales-Aguirre JJ, Villalobos-Acosta CP, Gómez-Barreto D, Cashat-Cruz M. Occurrence of intracerebral aneurysm in an HIV-infected child: a case report. *Pediatr Neurol.* 2004;31(2):130-2.

[90] Caplan LR, Hier DB, Banks G. Current concepts of cerebrovascular disease--stroke: stroke and drug abuse. *Stroke* 1982;13(6):869-72.

[91] Mochan A, Modi M, Modi G. Stroke in black South African HIV-positive patients: a prospective analysis. *Stroke* 2003;34(1):10-5.

[92] Adams HP Jr, Bendixen BH, Kappelle LJ, Biller J, Love BB, Gordon DL, Marsh EE 3rd. Classification of subtype of acute ischemic stroke. Definitions for use in a multicenter clinical trial. TOAST. Trial of Org 10172 in Acute Stroke Treatment. *Stroke* 1993;24(1):35-41.

In: Cerebral Ischemia in Young Adults
Editors: A. Pezzini and A. Padovani
ISBN 978-1-60741-627-2

Chapter 9

Ischemic Stroke in Pregnancy and Puerperium

Elisabetta Del Zotto[1,2]*, Alessandro Pezzini[2], Alessia Giossi[2] Irene Volonghi[2], Paolo Costa[2] and Alessandro Padovani[2]

1. Dipartimento di Scienze Biomediche e Biotecnologie, Università degli Studi di Brescia, Brescia, Italia
2. Dipartimento di Scienze Mediche e Chirurgiche, Clinica Neurologica, Università degli Studi di Brescia, Brescia, Italia

Abstract

Ischemic stroke during pregnancy and puerperium represents a rare event. However, whenever it does occur, many concerns arise about the safety of the mother and the fetus in relation to common diagnostic tests and therapies leading to a more conservative approach. The physiological adaptations in the cardiovascular system and in the coagulability that accompany the pregnant state and result to be quite significant around delivery and in the postpartum period, likely contribute to increase the risk of an ischemic stroke.

Most of the underlying causes of ischemic stroke in the young have been also described in pregnant patients. Despite this, there are specific conditions related to pregnancy which may be considered when assessing this particular group of patients. With the exception of preeclampsia-eclampsia, these causes are rare and include choriocarcinoma, peripartum cardiomiopathy, amniotic fluid embolization and postpartum cerebral angiopathy.

In the last two decades particular interest has been raised surrounding the use of treatments and procedures of assisted reproductive technology to establish a pregnancy. Along with their use, cerebral thromboembolic complications have been also described.

This chapter will consider several questions related to pregnancy-associated ischemic stroke dwelling on epidemiological and specific etiological aspects, diagnostic

---

* Correspondence: Elisabetta Del Zotto, P.le Spedali Civili, 1, 25100 Brescia, Italia. Tel: +39.030.399 5631 – 5632, Fax: +39.030.399 5027, e-mail: betty.delzotto@tin.it.

issues concerning the use of neuroimaging and the related potential risks to the embryo and fetus. Therapeutic issues surrounding the use of anticoagulant and antiplatelets agents will be discussed and the few available reports regarding the use of thrombolytic therapy during pregnancy will be review. Finally, the attention will be focused on arterial ischemic stroke developing after the procedures of the assisted reproductive technology.

Introduction

Ischemic stroke between the age of 15 and 35 years is more common in women than in men [1] and women have a poorer outcome in terms of dependency and disability [2].

Use of oral contraceptives and postmenopausal hormone therapy represent risk factors for stroke and particular interest has been raised about the role of estrogens in ischemic stroke. These aspects are covered in Chapter 4.

Further conditions that may partly contribute to an increased incidence of ischemic stroke in young women include pregnancy and puerperium. Ischemic and hemorrhagic strokes associated with pregnancy and puerperium have long been recognized as uncommon events, but when they occur, they represent a potentially devastating event for a young woman.

Stroke is a significant cause of maternal mortality contributing to more than 12% of all maternal deaths [3] and survivors may suffer profound and permanent disability [4]. A conservative approach is frequently adopted because there is fear of any adverse effects of treatment and etiological investigations on the mother and the unborn fetus. Moreover, since pregnancy represents a delicate moment for a woman and also for her family, the psychological consequences of an acute event, like a stroke, should also be taken into account.

Ischemic stroke during pregnancy recognizes the same causes as in young patients, but the combination of physiological changes in hemodynamic and haemostatic system during pregnancy and puerperium may expose young women to increased risk of cerebral complications.

In the present chapter we will describe the physiological changes occurring in pregnancy that may have a role in increasing the risk of cerebrovascular events, review epidemiological studies, specific pregnancy-related conditions leading to an ischemic stroke, and focus on diagnostic and treatment options. Finally, the issue of arterial thrombotic complications associated with the assisted reproductive technology (ART) used to achieve pregnancy will be discussed.

Maternal Physiological Changes during Pregnancy Predisposing to Ischemic Stroke

During pregnancy the human female organism is subject to a complex physiological adaptation necessary for the normal course of pregnancy. Modifications of the hemodinamics and the haemostatic systems are part of these physiological changes and consequence of the variations of the hormonal status. These major changes in cardiovascular system, vascular tissue structure and coagulation profile may increase the risk of stroke, although this relationship is likely complex and the effects of such changes on stroke risk not completely understood.

Hemodynamic and Connective Tissue Changes during Pregnancy

During pregnancy retention of water is a physiological adaptation due an increase in the level of aldosterone and renin activity; by consequence serum sodium concentration and osmolarity slightly decrease. In the first 10 weeks of pregnancy there is an increased of total body water; it then remains stably increased by almost 50% above prepregnancy levels until 1 to 2 weeks after delivery, after which it gradually returns to normal. A physiological dilutional anemia of pregnancy is a consequence of the increase of plasma volume, which starts after 6 to 8 weeks of gestation and reaches a peak at 32 weeks.

Increasing circulatory demands of fetus and placenta, combined with the hypervolemia of the pregnant state, result in an increase of 30 to 50% of cardiac output, stroke volume and heart rate. Half of this change occurs during the first 8 weeks of pregnancy; a peak is reached at 25 to 30 weeks and then measures of cardiac function remain stable until delivery. Cardiac output may increase to 50% more than prepregnancy levels as a consequence of pain and apprehension of labor and delivery, and by another 20 to 30% in the first 30 minutes after delivery. Cardiac output gradually decreases to 50% above prepregnancy levels within 2 weeks after delivery and returns to normal by 6 to 12 weeks.

Blood pressure as a consequence of decrease in systemic vascular resistance starts to lower around the seventh week, hits the lowest levels at 24 to 32 weeks and then increases progressively to pre-pregnancy levels at term. Venous compliance increases throughout pregnancy, leading to decreased blood flow, increased stasis and a tendency toward orthostatic pressure drops. Data from both animals and humans suggest that reduced vasomotor tone and remodeling of resistance-sized arteries participate in the pregnancy-associated fall of cardiac afterload [5, 6]. With pregnancy there are changes of arterial composition with a reduction in collagen and elastin content and a loss of distensibility that partially normalizes near term [7]. Moreover data from animals models of cerebral arteries indicate also consequences on contractility and endothelial reactivity of arterial vessels [8]. Thus, the maternal cardiovascular system undergoes remarkable and complex adaptive changes to accommodate increases in both blood volume and cardiac output while maintaining normal or slightly reduced blood pressure. However, what role such changes may have in increasing the risk of stroke is not clear.

Haemostatic Changes during Pregnancy

Pregnancy is normally associated with significant changes in venous flow and the molecular mediators of haemostasis, to the extent that the procoagulant effect becomes dominant [9].

The process of haemostasis is a dynamic and delicate equilibrium between the coagulation and the fibrinolytic systems. However, during pregnancy the overall balance shifts towards a hypercoagulable state which is more marked around term and in the immediate post-partum period, returning to that of the non-pregnant state at approximately 4 weeks after delivery [10]. These effects may be augmented by the acute phase response to acute blood loss and iron deficiency anemia immediately after delivery and for several weeks postpartum.

Regarding the coagulation factor changes that occur during pregnancy, levels of fibrinogen (factor I) and factor VII, VIII, IX, X and XII increase, whereas concentrations of factor V and XIII increase in the early stages of pregnancy, followed by a decrease and stabilization. Also levels of von Willebrand factor (VWF) antigen increase significantly. By contrast, conflicting results have been reported for factor XI and prothrombin (factor II) [11].

Table 1. Modifications of haemostatic factors during pregnancy

Procoagulant factors	
Fibrinogen (factor I)	↑
von Willebrand factor	↑
Factors VII, VIII, IX, X, XII	↑
Fcators V, XIII	↑ ↓
Factor XI	C
Factor II	C
Coagulation inhibitors	
Protein S	↓
Protein C, antithrombin III	=
Fibrinolytic factors	
Tissue plasminogen activator	↓
Plasminogen activator inhibitor 1 and 2 (PAI-1, PAI-2)	↑
Thrombin activable fibrynolysis inhibitor (TAFI)	↑
Others	
Platelet count	↓
Prothrombin fragment 1+2	↑
Thrombin-antithrombin complex	↑
D-dimer, fibrinopeptide-A	↑

↑: increase; ↓: decrease; =: no change; ↑↓: early increase followed by decrease; C: controversial data.

In contrast to a comprehensive elevation of procoagulant factors the levels of some coagulation inhibitors fall during pregnancy. Total and free levels of protein S are significantly decreased during the first and second trimesters. Protein C activity and antithrombin appear to be unaffected by gestation while there is a progressive increase in activated protein C resistance in pregnancy [11].

Finally, several studies have demonstrated a gradual decrease in fibrinolysis during normal pregnancy, characterized by a decrease in tissue plasminogen activator (t-PA) activity and an increase in endothelial-derived plasminogen activator inhibitor-1 (PAI-1), placenta-derived plasminogen activator inhibitor-2 (PAI-2) and thrombin activable fibrinolysis inhibitor (TAFI) levels [11]. Other indicators of hypercoagulation in normal pregnancy include increased levels of D-dimer, thrombin-antithrombin (TAT) complexes, prothrombin fragments 1 + 2 (F1+2) and fibrinopeptide A (FPA), which are sensitive markers of coagulation activation [11] (Table 1).

The increase in clotting activity culminates at the time of delivery and is presumably related to the expulsion of the placenta and release of thromboplastic substances at the site of separation. Three weeks after delivery blood coagulation and fibrinolysis have generally normalized. In association with a venous stasis condition, this resulting hypercoagulable state likely accounts for an increased risk of thromboembolic complications, in particular during the third trimester and the puerperium.

Epidemiology

Since stroke is a relatively uncommon event in pregnancy, it is difficult to establish the exact risk and to compare it with the risk among non-pregnant women. The reported incidence of stroke associated with pregnancy and puerperium is widely variable. According to previous hospital-based and community-based reports, the incidence rates for ischemic strokes associated with pregnancy or puerperium vary from 4.3 to 210 per 100,000 deliveries [12]. A reliable estimation requires very large population; the wide variability reflects small sample sizes of most studies, inadequate consideration of referral bias, different study designs (e.g., not all were population based), and the incorporation of different subgroups of patients. Moreover, another limitation regards studies reported before CT scan became widely available [13, 14]. Therefore, comparisons of available retrospective data are limited because authors used different methods to define and capture their populations and different definitions of strokes and stroke subtypes.

However, data published since 1985 shows an incidence of ischemic stroke ranging from 4 to 41 per 100,000 pregnancies [3, 12, 14-20]. Data from the three population-based studies, indicates a lower incidence varying from 4 to 11 cases per 100,000 deliveries [12, 14, 16]. This difference may be partly explain by the presence of a referral bias in the hospital-based studies; a further explanation may be found in a lack of a consistent definitions of duration of the postpartum period in the three population-based studies since Kittner et al included six postpartum weeks, Sharshar et al two weeks, and Wiebers and Whisnant did not include any postpartum period (Table 2).

Table 2. Studies of pregnancy related stroke since 1985

Author, year	Methodology	Period	Postpartum period	N° deliveries	Total stroke N°	Ischemic stroke N°	Hemorrhagic stroke N°	Mortality N° (%)	Ischemic stroke mortality N°
Wiebers and Whisnant, 1985 [14]	Retrospective population based study	1955-1979	NR	26099 a	1	1	0	NR	NR
Awada et al, 1995 [15]	Retrospective hospital based	1983-1993	15 days	NR	12	9	3	4 (33)	1
Sharshar et al, 1995 [12]	Retrospective and prospective population based study	1989-1992	2 weeks	348295	31	15	16	4 (13)	0
Kittner et al, 1996 [16]	Retrospective population based study	1988-1991	6 weeks	141243	31	17 b	14	NR	NR
Witlin et al, 1997 [17]	Retrospective hospital based	1985-1995	NR	79301	24 c	5	6	7 (29,2)	
Jiagobin and Silver, 2000 [18]	Retrospective hospital based	1980-1997	6 weeks	50711	34	13	13	3 (9)	0
Skidmore et al, 2001 [19]	Retrospective hospital-based	1992-1999	12 weeks	58429	36	21	11	1 (2,7)	1
Jeng et al, 2004 [20]	Retrospective hospital based	1984-2002	6 weeks	49796	23	13	10	NR	NR
Liang et al, 2006 [3]	Retrospective hospital based	1992-2004	6 weeks	66781	26	11 b	17	5 (19)	1

a: live births; b: includes arterial ischemic stroke and cerebral venous thrombosis; c: includes 3 patients with hypertensive encephalopathy; NR: not reported.

Recently, in the United States a large population study based on data from the Nationwide Inpatient Sample has found a rate of pregnancy-related stroke of 34,2 per 100,000 deliveries for the period from 2000 to 2001 [4]. Although in this study the incidence of stroke for women who were not pregnant was not computed, comparing data with those of other studies, the authors found a 3-fold increased incidence of stroke during pregnancy than outside pregnancy in childbearing age women. However, as these data were limited to information derived from discharge record abstractions, detailed and precise information on diagnosis are not available and different subtypes of stroke were considered at the same time.

Further studies analyzed the association of pregnancy with the risk of stroke according to a woman's status with respect to pregnancy. In the study of Wiebers and Wisnant a 13-fold increased risk was calculated [14]. In the study by Kittner et al. the relative risk of cerebral infarction was 0.7 (95% CI, 0.3 to 1.6) during pregnancy, but it increased to 8.7 (95% CI, 4.6 to 16.7) during the six weeks after pregnancy (after a live birth or stillbirth) [16], suggesting that the postpartum period is associated with the greatest risk of ischemic stroke.

With regard to the timing of stroke associated with pregnancy, in a hospital-based series of patients with ischemic events related to pregnancy 81% of the events occurred after the onset of the third trimester, with a peak in the first postpartum week [19]. Similarly, Jaigobin and Silver showed that most of the arterial strokes presented in the third trimester and puerperium [18]. More specifically, in a large Swedish cohort of over 650,000 women with over 1 million deliveries in an eight-year time period the greatest risk of ischemic and hemorrhagic stroke was around the delivery [33,8 (95% CI 10.5 to 84.0), two days before and one day after] with an increased but declining risk over the subsequent six week [8.3 (95% CI, 4.4 to 14.8] [21]. The clustering of events in the third trimester and postpartum period implies a possible link between the physiological changes of pregnancy and stroke; in particular with delivery there is a rapid normalization in hemodynamic and coagulation profile that potentially may increase the risk in susceptible patients and may explain the increased risk found in several studies in the postpartum period.

Risk Factors and Associated Conditions

Ethnic background and age influence the risk of cerebral ischemic events in pregnancy and puerperium. African American women have significantly higher risk than Caucasians [4]. Stroke subtypes may also be different according to race. Recently, a meta-analysis of Taiwan studies showed that hemorrhagic stroke is slightly more common than ischemic subtype, which is different from that reported in most Western countries, suggesting the role of genetic background in increasing the risk of specific subtypes of stroke [3].

Women over the age of 35 have an increased risk of pregnancy related stroke [4]. In the study based on data from the Nationwide Inpatient Sample in United States for the period from 2000 to 2001, several medical conditions, identified as risk factors among non-pregnant women of childbearing age, resulted associated with stroke in pregnancy such as hypertension, diabetes, smoking, heart disease, and sickle cell disease [4]. Other risk factors found in case series and reports include alcohol abuse and illicit drug use, particularly cocaine [4; 22]. Migraine headaches also resulted strongly associated to stroke [4]. However, it is difficult to distinguish among migraine headaches associated with pregnancy-related stroke, preeclampsia as a symptom of an impending stroke or as a consequence of this, and migraine as an independent risk factor.

Thrombophilia is a well recognized risk factor in pregnancy and an association with stroke and transient ischemic events has been reported [4, 23].

Other factors associated with pregnancy related stroke include complications of pregnancy such as infection, hyperemesis, fluid and electrolyte imbalance [4, 24]. Multiple gestation and greater parity may also predispose to stroke [25].

Caesarean delivery has been shown to be associated with a 3-12 times increased risk of peripartum and postpartum stroke [24, 26]. However, a possible explanation for this association may be found in an increased number of caesarean delivery among patients with previous stroke or with conditions that can increase the risk of stroke such as preeclampsia-eclampsia. Despite this, the association of postpartum stroke with cesarean delivery suggests that cesarean delivery may increase the risk of these events.

Etiology of Ischemic Stroke in Pregnancy

Several known etiologies of ischemic stroke in the young have been reported in pregnancy and the puerperium [27]. Therefore, in most cases it is quite difficult to distinguish whether pregnancy is coincidental or plays a role in the occurrence of the cerebral infarction.

However, there are specific conditions associated with pregnancy that warrant special consideration when assessing this group of patients, including preeclampsia and eclampsia, choriocarcinoma, amniotic fluid embolism, peripartum cardiomyopathy and postpartum cerebral angiopathy. Except for preeclampsia, these conditions represent rare complications of pregnancy. Peripartum cardiomyopathy and postpartum cerebral angiopathy were described sometimes in non-pregnant patients.

Since most studies included small numbers of patients and authors defined strokes and stroke etiologies differently, a comparison of the conditions that contribute to ischemic stroke is limited. However, summarizing the results of these studies, preeclampsia-eclampsia and cardioembolic causes are the leading conditions that contribute to ischemic stroke (Table 3). In line with data from series of non-pregnant young patients, a high proportion of cases, raging from 28% to 46%, are diagnosed as of undetermined cause.

Specific causes of ischemic stroke will be discussed in the next section of the present Chapter, while a comprehensive discussion of non-specific conditions is reported elsewhere.

Table 3. Etiologies of ischemic stroke complicating pregnancy and the puerperium

Author, year	N° case	Cardiac	Coagulopathy	Large artery	Preeclampsia eclampsia	Other causes	Other pregnancy related conditions	Unknown
Awada et al, 1995 [15]	9	3 (33%)			1 (11%)	1 (11%) a		4 (45%)
Sharshar et al, 1995 [12]	15		1 (6,6%) b		7 (47%)	1 (6,6%) c	2 (13,2%) d	4 (26,6%)
Kittner et al, 1996 [16]	17	1 (5,9%) e			4 (23,5%)	6 (35,3%) f		6 (35,3%)
Witlin et al, 1997 [17]	5 g				2 (40%)			
Jiagobin and Silver, 2000 [18]	13	4 (30,7%)	2 (15,3%)	1(8%)	3 h			6 (46%)
Skidmore et al, 2001 [19]	21	5 (23,7%)	2 (9,6%)		3 (14,4%)	5 (23,7%) g		6 (28,6%)
Jeng et al, 2004 [20]	16	9 (56%)	3 (19%)		1 (6%)	1 (6%)		2 (13%)
Liang et al, 2006 [3]	11	4 (36%) h		1(9%)	2 (18%)	3 (27%) i	1 (9%)	

Number of cases (%); a: nephrotic syndrome; b: protein S deficiency; c: cerebral artery dissection; d: 1 postpartum cerebral angiopathy, 1 amniotic fluid embolism; e: mitral valve prolapse; f: 2 primary CNS vasculopathy, 1 cerebral artery dissection, 1 cerebral venous thrombosis, 1 postherpetic vasculitis, 1 thrombotic thrombocytopenic purpura; g: 1 cerebral vasculitis, 1 migrainous infarct, 1 mucormycosis, 1 hypotension, 1 thrombotic thrombocytopenic purpura; h: 2 congenital heart disease, 1 rheumatic heart disease, 1 atrial mixoma; i: cerebral venous thrombosis; l: amniotic fluid embolism; m: 3 patients of 13, since preeclampsia-eclampsia was considered as a risk factor; n: other causes not specified.

Pregnancy-specific Causes of Ischemic Stroke

Preeclampsia and Eclampsia

Preeclampsia-eclampsia, also known as toxemia, is a pregnancy-specific multisystem disorder of unknown cause that occurs in the later stages of pregnancy and in the first 6 to 8 weeks after delivery [28]. It represents a major obstetric problem accounting for a substantial maternal and perinatal morbidity and mortality, especially in developing countries [29].

Preeclampsia affects approximately 6% to 8% of all pregnancies, whereas eclampsia has an incidence of 1/1000 to 1/2000 deliveries in the United States [30]. The proportion of patients with stroke related to preeclampsia-eclampsia during pregnancies varies from 18% to 47% [3, 12, 16]. Moreover, in the Stroke Prevention in Young Women (SPYW) Study women with a history of preeclampsia were 60% more likely to have a non-pregnancy-related ischemic stroke than those without a history of preeclampsia (OR, 1.63; 95% CI, 1.02 to 2.62), suggesting that these patients should be closely monitored and controlled for stroke risk factors beyond the postpartum period [31].

The underlying pathophysiology is complex and not completely understood. This pathological condition is characterized by abnormal vascular response to placentation that is associated with an increased vascular tone and sensitivity to mediators of vasoconstrictions resulting in hypertension, vasospasm and organ hypoperfusion [32-36]. Endothelial cell dysfunction represents another common response including instability of vascular tone, enhanced platelet aggregation and activation of the coagulation system leading to local thrombosis [33, 34, 37]. Therefore, as a consequence of these manifestations, pathological changes (often ischemic changes) may occur in the placenta, liver, brain and kidney.

Pre-eclampsia is usually diagnosed in the presence of elevated gestational blood pressure accompanied by proteinuria. In the absence of proteinuria, pre-eclampsia should be considered when hypertension is associated with persistent cerebral symptoms, epigastric or right upper-quadrant pain with nausea or vomiting, or with thrombocytopenia and abnormal liver enzymes [29]. Although pre-eclampsia is usually asymptomatic, patients may complain of headaches, visual abnormalities, confusion and impairment of consciousness. Eclampsia is defined as the onset of convulsions or coma in women who have either gestational hypertension or pre-eclampsia [29]. About 2 to 12% of patients with eclampsia develop a HELLP syndrome [38], a life-threatening condition characterized by hemolytic anemia (H), elevated liver enzymes (EL), and low platelet count (LP).

In addition, in some patients a manifestation of sudden onset focal neurological deficits may be consistent with a clinical diagnosis of stroke. In these cases, CT is normal or show multiple bilateral and almost symmetrical hypodensities involving the cerebral white matter and the adjacent cerebral cortex, often with posterior predominance, and the basal ganglia [38, 39]. Notwithstanding MR imaging is superior to CT in demonstrating the effects of pre-eclampsia and eclampsia on the brain [39, 40]. The MRI findings include cortical and/or subcortical hyperintensities and even less commonly in the brainstem and cerebellum on T2-weighted sequences. There may or may not be associated enhancement [38, 39].

The pathogenesis of the focal deficits is not clearly understood. Except for women with a persistent neurological deficit consistent with a brain infarction on neuroimaging, the reversibility of the neurological clinical signs and neuroradiological lesions within a few days or weeks in most cases argues against the existence of true cerebral ischemic necrosis. The clinical and neuroimaging findings are more consistent with the presence of reversible vasogenic edema, as reported in most studies using diffusion-weighted MRI in eclampsia [41, 42]. Despite this, loss of endothelial integrity may lead to hemorrhage and severe vasospasm, and thrombosis may lead to infarction. In this regard, it has been showed that vasogenic edema is associated with concurrent foci of infarction in a fourth of eclamptic women [41], documenting a transition between reversible vasogenic edema to irreversible cerebral ischemia and infarction.

The management of pre-eclampsia is aimed at delivery of the fetus and placenta and drug therapy of hypertension. Magnesium sulphate is the first line therapy for seizures, as it prevents vascular spasm, and this could also be used in prophylaxis in pre-eclamptic patients.

Choriocarcinoma

Choriocarcinoma is a malignant neoplasm that arises from placental trophoblastic tissue.

Most choriocarcinomas follow molar pregnancy but the cancer may also follow term delivery, abortion and ectopic pregnancy. It has a tendency to early metastases, especially to the lungs, brain, liver and vagina [43]. Brain metastasis complicates about 20% of choriocarcinomas.

The clinical presentation of cerebral involvement include raised intracranial pressure, intracerebral hemorrhage and cerebral ischemic infarction [44, 45]. Patients may present with headache, focal neurological deficits, seizures, encephalopathy, signs of elevated intracranial pressure, and excessively elevated serum β human choriogonadotrophic hormone level.

Choriocarcinoma is a highly vascular tumor and is extremely prone to hemorrhage. In the brain, trophoblasts may invade blood vessels, just as they would in the uterus. Thrombosis may occur in the damaged vessels with a single or multiple cerebral infarctions as a consequence, or an embolus may fail to lodge and pass distally, leading to transient ischemic attacks. Other vessels may develop neoplastic aneurysms or varicosities resulting in intraparenchymal or subarachnoid space bleeding [27].

Amniotic Fluid Embolism

Amniotic fluid embolism is a rare life-threatening complication of pregnancy that predominates in multiparous women over 30 years of age. The mortality rate varies from 61 to 86% and accounts for approximately 10% of all maternal deaths in the United States [46]. Amniotic fluid embolism has a variable presentation, ranging from mild degrees of organ dysfunction to cardiovascular collapse, coagulopathy and death [46]. Most cases usually present at term during labour and should be suspected in any pregnant patient, specifically those with ruptured membranes, who develop sudden onset dyspnea with hypoxia, acute hypotension and/or cardiac arrest followed by a profound coagulopathy. Seizures occur in 10-20% of cases. The clinical picture is rarely suggestive of a stroke, but focal deficits are possible. The pathophysiology of amniotic fluid embolism remains enigmatic. Paradoxical cerebral amniotic fluid emboli do occur, but their true incidence is unknown [27].

Postpartum Cerebral Angiopathy

Postpartum cerebral angiopathy is part of a group of disorders unified under the term of reversible cerebral vasoconstriction syndrome (RCVS) [47] characterized by prolonged but reversible vasoconstriction of the cerebral arteries, usually associated with acute onset, severe, recurrent headaches, with or without additional neurologic signs and symptoms. Although the pathophysiology is scarcely understood, a disturbance in the control of cerebral vascular tone seems to be a critical element. In the obstetric neurologic literature RCVS in the postpartum period has been described using various labels, including postpartum angiopathy [48-52], postpartum angiitis [53] and puerperal vasospasm [54]. Although a similar syndrome can be seen with preeclampsia or eclampsia [55], most patients with RCVS have a history of uncomplicated pregnancy and normal labor and delivery, followed within days to a few weeks by acute onset of headache with or without various neurologic signs and symptoms. The brain MRI in patients with postpartum angiopathy may show areas of T2/FLAIR hypertensity in any location, but especially in watershed areas between vascular territories and often with corresponding restricted diffusion on apparent diffusion coefficient maps. On both magnetic resonance angiography (MRA) and CT angiography one may see multifocal segmental narrowing of large and medium-size cerebral arteries. Arterial abnormalities are better visualized with CT angiography and conventional invasive catheter angiography, both of which require the use of iodinated contrast material. In postpartum angiopathy, the MRI and MRA features may normalize with time, although extensive infarction may develop [39].

Peripartum Cardiomyopathy

Peripartum cardiomyopathy is a rare dilating cardiomyopathy, that develops in the last gestational month of pregnancy or in the first 5 months after delivery, with no identifiable cause for heart failure and in the absence of heart disease [56]. However, an early development of cardiomyopathy during pregnancy has also been described [57-59]. In the largest database of patients with pregnancy-associated cardiomyopathy diagnosed in United States authors showed that clinical presentation and outcome of patients with a pregnancy-associated cardiomyopathy diagnosed early in pregnancy are similar to those of patients with traditional peripartum cardiomiopathy suggesting that these two conditions may represent a continuum of a spectrum of the same disease [60].

The reported incidence of peripartum cardiomyopathy is widely variable ranging from 1 in 1300 to 1 in 15,000 pregnancies in western countries with a currently accepted incidence in the United States of 1 in 3000 to 1 in 4000 live births [61, 62]. This condition is more common in western Africa with a reported incidence in Nigeria of 1 in 100 pregnancies [63].

Risk factors include advanced age (>30 years), obesity, black race, multiparity, twin pregnancies, preeclampsia and severe hypertension during pregnancy [64, 65]. However, a recent study showed that in United States peripartum cardiomyopathy is not limited to black women and moreover did not support the association with multiparity since almost 40% of cardiomiopathy developed in first pregnancy women and >50% with the first two pregnancies [60].

The etiology of peripartum cardiomyopathy remains uncertain. Many hypotheses have been suggested, including myocarditis, abnormal immune response to pregnancy, maladaptive response to the hemodynamic stresses of pregnancy, stress activated cytokines, viral infection, and prolonged tocolysis [66-72].

Clinical features consist of heart failure with dilated cardiac cavities [73]. However, the diagnosis remains a challenge because many normal women in the last month of a normal pregnancy experience dyspnea, fatigue and pedal edema, symptoms identical to early congestive cardiac failure. A suspicion of heart failure should raise in the presence of symptoms and signs such as paroxysmal nocturnal dyspnea, chest pain, nocturnal cough, new regurgitant murmurs, pulmonary crackles, elevated jugular venous pressure and hepatomegaly. Other late complications of pregnancy such as massive pulmonary embolism, amniotic fluid embolism (most often during labor and delivery), and severe toxemia may also simulate heart failure. Peripartum cardiomyopathy is a diagnosis of exclusion, distinguished by rapid onset, occurrence in the peripartum period, and significant improvement in up to 50% of affected women.

Systemic and pulmonary embolization is frequently associated with this condition with an estimated incidence ranging from 25 to 40% [27]. Neurologic deficits caused by thromboembolism can rarely be the presenting symptoms [74-76]. The incidence of ischemic stroke is about 5% [27]. Additionally, cerebral infarction may result more rarely from cerebral hypoperfusion secondary to cardiac failure [27; 77].

Mortality due to peripatum cardiomyopathy is high. Approximately 20% of women with the disorder either die or survive only because they receive cardiac transplants, the majority recover partially or completely. Recurrences during subsequent pregnancies is common.

Diagnostic Work-up of Ischemic Stroke during Pregnancy

In a pregnant women as in other patients, it is important to differentiate timely hemorrhagic from ischemic stroke, considering the different management implications and to determine as soon as possible the specific etiology, since some of these conditions may need specific management (i.e, eclampsia). In a pregnant woman, besides the few specific causes, stroke has the same etiologies commonly observed in a young non-pregnant woman. As a consequence, the diagnostic work-up should be managed as in non-pregnant state [38] and, as in any young patient, should include a systematic evaluation [78]. Imaging studies should be based on neurological indications despite pregnancy. However, several concerns arise for the clinician when relying on neuroimaging as part of the work-up, but maternal well-being and management should not be compromised because of concerns about fetal exposure to radiation.

Fetal exposure to ionizing radiation from CT of the maternal head is extremely low, corresponding to ~ 0.05 cGy that is even to ~ 1% of the generally accepted maximal threshold dose for safe fetal cumulative exposure [79], and the risk to the fetus is likely to be considerably less than the risk to both the fetus and mother from an acute neurological condition. The harmful effects of radiation depend on the stage of gestation at which the fetus is exposed, the total dose of radiation absorbed, and the rate at which the dose is absorbed [80]. Potential risk of birth defects due to radiation occurs in the first trimester of pregnancy, especially in the first few weeks, the embryogenesis period, when the patient may not be aware of the pregnancy. Radiation-protection precautions for the developing fetus should be used whenever the question of pregnancy arises; during CT the lower abdomen can be surrounded by lead aprons, reducing fetal radiation exposure to approximately 2 mrad, a very low amount [81]. Cerebral angiography requires approximately the same amount of fetal exposure plus whatever results from fluoroscopy during catheter insertion before abdominal shielding begins, which can be limited by skilled hands [81]. Fluoroscopy of the lower abdomen should be specifically avoided during angiography. Digital angiography procedures decrease the X-ray exposure and the amount of administered iodine.

A CT perfusion study increases significantly the X-ray exposure and this procedure should be avoided during pregnancy unless the information is critical to guide therapy.

There are no evidence of adverse fetal effects to the magnetic field exposure for magnetic resonance imaging (MRI) [82]. Theoretical concerns have been raised on the risk due to exposure to very powerful magnetic fields, minimal increases in body temperature and loud tapping noises of the coils [39,83]. However, a possible teratogenic effect has been found in some studies on animal models [84-86]. Thus, the American College of Obstetricians and Gynecologists and the National Radiological Protection Board have stated that there have been no adverse fetal effects reported, but advise against the use of MRI in the first trimester [83]. According to the American College guidelines a MRI study during pregnancy is recommended when it provides information that can not be achieved via safer means, when the data are needed to determine the care of the patient and/or fetus *during* the pregnancy, and when the referring physician does not feel that it is prudent to wait to obtain this data until after the pregnancy [87].

Since the study of the exposure of iodinated and gadolinium-based contrast agents on the human embryo and fetus has been limited, their effects are not completely clear. During pregnancy the exposure to the iodinated contrast agent used in CT studies may pose some risk including maternal allergic reaction, renal toxicity and fetal dehydration due to the high osmolality of the agent for which a good maternal hydration is needed [83,88]. However, low osmolality agents are now available and preferred to reduce the risk. Furthermore, iodinated agents can produce neonatal hypothyroidism but such effects have not been reported from intravenous use [89]. Available data on animal model have not shown teratogenic effects of iodinated contrast agent [90,91] but there are no adequate and well-controlled studies in pregnant women. Nevertheless, the use of iodinated contrast material should be avoided if possible. When contrast must be used, informed written consent is obtained and screening of the neonate for hypothyroidism is indicated.

Regarding the use of gadolinium during MRI study, toxic effects are not known but depositions of the gadolinium ions in fetal tissue raises concern. Moreover, animal reproduction studies showed that gadolinium at high dose have teratogenic effects [83,88]. Therefore, the use of gadolinium should be avoided in a pregnant woman unless specifically indicated in particular situation where the decision must be made after a well-documented and thoughtful risk-benefit analysis [87,92].

Pregnancy does not contraindicate to performance of transoesophageal echocardiography [93].

Differential Diagnosis of Ischemic Stroke in Pregnancy

The major differential diagnosis in pregnant women presenting with focal symptoms besides arterial ischemic stroke are cerebral venous thrombosis and migraine-induced phenomena. Furthermore, a rather common clinical problem for physicians is represented by transient focal neurologic symptoms. Their frequency is 58 of 100,000 pregnancies [94]. They can be attributed to a transient ischemic attack (TIA), raising concern to herald a stroke. The most frequently entertained differential diagnosis is migraine with aura, occurring in the 76% of the patients with transient focal neurological symptoms [95]. However, it may be difficult to distinguish TIA from aura, in particular in cases where headache is absent and in consideration that TIA could be sometimes associated with headache [96]. These two conditions present an overlapping of clinical manifestations but however features like the time course and march of symptoms, the presence of positive and negative symptoms may be helpful.

Although in several studies migraine was resulted to improve during pregnancy [97,98], it worsens in some women [99], and about 2% of patients experience their first migraine attack in this period [100].

Ertresvåg and coworkers in a hospital series of pregnant women with transient focal neurological symptoms reported typical aura without headache in 15% of the patients while 35 % of patients resulted to have typical aura with non migrainous headache, making the migraine diagnosis less obvious and accentuating the diagnostic dilemma in these patients [95].

Other possible diagnosis include multiple sclerosis, partial epilepsy, presincope and carpal tunnel syndrome [95]. Focal transient neurological symptoms in previously healthy pregnant women have a generally benign course.

Treatment of Ischemic Stroke during Pregnancy

Since direct randomized data on stroke prevention during pregnancy are lacking, the choice of agents for prophylactic strategies are largely based upon extrapolations from data reported in other studies, regarding primarily prevention of deep vein thrombosis and the use of anticoagulants in women with high-risk cardiac conditions. However, even in these situations there are no specific randomized controlled trial. Therefore, according to the American Heart Association (AHA) guidelines for pregnant women with ischemic stroke or TIA and high-risk thromboembolic conditions such as coagulopathy and mechanical heart valves, three possible therapeutic options can be used: a) adjusted-dose unfractionated heparin (UFH) throughout pregnancy; b) adjusted-dose low molecular weight heparins (LMWHs) throughout pregnancy; c) either UFH or adjusted-dose LMWHs until week 13, then restarted from the middle of the third trimester until delivery and warfarin at other times [101]. For lower risk conditions, either UFH or LMWH therapy is recommended in the first trimester, followed by low-dose of aspirin for the remainder of the pregnancy [101].

Anticoagulant Therapy

Fetal Complications of Anticoagulants during Pregnancy

Potential complications of maternal anticoagulant therapy include teratogenicity and bleeding. UFH and LMWH do not cross the placenta [102]; thus these agents do not have adverse fetal effects, although bleeding at the utero-placental junction is possible. Several studies strongly suggest that UFH/LMWH therapy is safe for the fetus [103-106]. By contrast, warfarin cross the placenta and can cause bleeding and malformation in the fetus [105,107]. This agent is probable safe if administered during the first 6 weeks of gestation, but confers a risk of embryopathy if given between 6 weeks and 12 weeks of gestation [107]. Besides, warfarin cause an anticoagulant effect in the fetus, which is a concern, particularly at the time of delivery, when the combination with the trauma of delivery can lead to bleeding in the neonate.

Maternal Complications of Anticoagulants during Pregnancy

A major bleeding was reported in about 2% of the pregnant women treated with UFH [106], which is consistent with the observed rate in non pregnant women receiving UFH and warfarin therapy [102]. Since the possibility of a persistent anticoagulant effect (for up to 28 hours after the last injection of heparin), the use of heparin therapy prior to labor may complicate the delivery increasing the risk of bleeding and controindicates epidural analgesia [102].

LMWH therapy is rarely related with bleeding complications and in particular it is not associated with an increased risk of severe peripartum bleeding [108]. In about 3% of non pregnant patients, the UFH therapy can cause the development of the heparin-induced thrombocytopenia (HIT), an acquired immune condition IgG-mediated, which is frequently complicated by extension of the preexisting thrombotic phenomena or new arterial thrombosis [104]. In pregnant women who develop HIT and require ongoing anticoagulant therapy, use of the heparinoid danaparoid sodium is recommended because it is an effective antithrombotic agent, does not cross the placenta and has much less cross-reactivity with UFH and therefore, less potential to produce recurrent HIT than LMWH [102].

Long-term heparin therapy has been associated with the development of osteoporosis and with an increased risk of osteoporotic fracture. In pregnancy the risk of fracture (2.2%) does not seem to be different from that observed in non pregnant women [102]; nevertheless a small randomized trial of pregnant women treated with UFH reported a higher incidence of osteoporotic fracture (15%) which may be due to the older age of the patients than that of the patients of the other studies [109]. Moreover LMWHs are associated with a lower risk of osteoporosis than heparin [108].

Anticoagulants Effects in Nursing Mother

Heparin and LMWHs do not reach the maternal milk and can be safely given to nursing mothers [110]. Reported evidence showed that warfarin therapy administered to a nursing mother does not induce an anticoagulant effect in the breast-fed infant [111,112]. Therefore, the use of warfarin in women who require postpartum anticoagulant therapy is also safe, and women taking this drug should be encouraged to breast feed.

Antiplatelet Therapy

A safe use of aspirin during the first trimester of pregnancy remains unclear. Although in retrospective studies a teratogenic effect has been reported in pregnant women using aspirin, such fetal complication has not been confirmed in prospective studies [27]. Potential complications of aspirin therapy in late pregnancy include fetal and maternal bleeding, premature closure of the ductus arteriosus, prolongation of labour and delay in the onset of labor [27]. According to data reported in a meta-analysis and in a large randomized trial (CLASP study) that enrolled more than 9000 patients, there are no evidence of fetal and maternal adverse effects of low-dose aspirin therapy (60 to 150 mg/d) administered during the second and the third trimester of pregnancy in women at risk for pregnancy-induced hypertension and intrauterine growth retardation [113,114]. Therefore, low-dose aspirin (< 150 mg/die) can be used safely during the second and third trimester; in contrast, the safety of higher dose of aspirin and/or aspirin ingestion during the first trimester is controversial.

Thrombolytic Treatment

In case of an acute ischemic stroke early thrombolysis with intravenous tissue plasminogen activator or intra-arterial thrombolytic therapy with thrombolytic agents or mechanical clot removal is the only approved therapy to establish cerebral reperfusion.

Regarding the use of thrombolytic treatment in pregnancy, no data are available since this conditions was an exclusion criteria from clinical trials that validated these therapies.

Therefore, to date the experience with the use of thrombolytic agents in pregnancy and puerperium is limited only to case reports and case series, including different thromboembolic conditions. In the majority of cases thrombolysis has been carried out in patients with pulmonary embolism, thrombosis of cardiac valve prosthesis, myocardial infarcts, deep venous thrombosis, but also with stroke and in a few pregnant women with cerebral venous sinus thrombosis [115].

Due to its large molecular size rt-PA does not cross the placental barrier and studies on animal model have not shown teratogenic effects [116, 117]. However, fetal adverse effects remain largely unknown. The major concerns regarding the use of thrombolytics during pregnancy include their possible effects on the placenta, possibly resulting in premature labor, placental abruption or fetal demise; other concerns regard the possibility of hemorrhage during parturition or cesarean delivery, if the patient goes into labor within the context sensitive half-time (the time of the drug's effective physiologic and pharmacologic effects in the setting of the disease process being studied) after the administration of the thrombolytic.

In the last years, five single case reports have described the use of rt-PA for acute ischemic stroke in pregnancy (3 intra-venous, 2 intra-arterial) [115, 118-121]. Maternal complications included minor hemorrhagic imbition of infarct area (1 case) [118] and hematoma in basal ganglia (1 case) [119]. Good fetal outcomes were reported overall.

Recently, Murugappan reviewed a series of eight patients who underwent thrombolysis for acute ischemic stroke during pregnancy [122]. Four patients were treated with rt-PA (3 intra-venous, 1 intra-arterial) and 4 received urokinase (3 intra-venous, 1 intra-arterial), two of whom had a cerebral sinus thrombosis. The patients recovered well with one exception due to a fatal malignant infarction as a consequence of a dissection during angioplasty. Maternal complications included one intrauterine hematoma, one buttock hematoma and two asymptomatic small intracranial hemorrhages. Regarding the fetal outcome, three of the seven surviving mothers had therapeutic abortions, two fetuses were miscarried and two babies were delivered healthy.

Moreover, Mendez et al, reported the use of intrarterial urokinase in the post partum period, since fifteen hours after a cesarean delivery, with a good outcome of the patient [123] (Table 4).

However, because of the differences in etiologies, as well as in thrombolytic agents used and way of administration, it is difficult to draw any major efficacy or safety conclusions. The suggestion from these data is that pregnant women generally can be safely treated with thrombolytics for acute ischemic stroke and can have reasonably good outcome in most cases, whereas fetal effects remain unclear. Therefore, thrombolytic therapy should not be withheld for potentially disabling stroke during pregnancy, but in each clinical situation, since experience is limited, the ultimate choice of therapies must be based on careful assessment of the maternal and fetal risks and benefits [115,122,124].

Prognosis and Recurrence

Mortality from pregnancy-related stroke typically results from intracranial hemorrhage or malignant hypertension [12, 17]. Maternal mortality following cerebral infarction has been reported in 0% to 25% of patients [27]. In a previous study of 1968, the maternal mortality immediately after stroke was 26% [13]. More recently, Sharshar et al did not find cases of death among 15 patients with arterial ischemic stroke and 5 of these were discharged with a mild to moderate residual neurological deficit, with a modified Rankin score raging from 1 (3 patients) to 2 (2 patients), and in another patient residual epilepsy was reported [12]. In the study of Jaigobin and Silver all patients with arterial infarct survived [18].

Table 4. Case reports describing the use of thrombolytic treatments in ischemic stroke during pregnancy and puerperium

Author, year		Thrombolysis	Dosage	Maternal age	Gestational age	Maternal complications	Fetal outcome
Dapprich, 2002 [118]		IV rt-PA	0,9 mg/kg	31 y	12 week	hemorrhagic trasformation of infarct area	good
Elford, 2002 [119]		IA rt-PA	15.5 mg	28 y	1 week	hematoma in basal ganglia	good
Johnson, 2005 [126]		IA rt-PA	15 mg	39 y	37 week	none	good
Leonhardt, 2006 [115]		IV rt-PA	0,9 mg/kg	26 y	23 week	basal ganglia infarction	good
Murugappan, 2006 [122]	a	IV rt-PA	0,9 mg/kg	37 y	12 week	none	MTP
	b	IV rt-PA	0,9 mg/kg	31 y	4 week	none	MTP
	c	IV rt-PA	0,9 mg/kg	29 y	6 week	death from dissection during angioplasty	died
	d	IA rt-PA	21 mg	43 y	37 week	none	good
	e	IA UK	600 000 U	28 y	6 week	buttock hematoma	good
	f	local UK	700 000 U	25 y	first trimester	asymptomatic ICH	SA
Wiese, 2006 [121]		IV rt-PA	0,9 mg/kg	33 y	13 week	basal ganglia infarction	good
Mendez, 2008 [123]		IA UK	100 000 U	37 y	fifteen hours after cesarean delivery	none	

IV: intravenous; IA: intraarterial; rt-PA: recombinant tissue plasminogen activator; UK: urokinase; ICH: intracerebral hemorrhage; MTP: medical termination of pregnancy; SA: spontaneous abortion.

Few data are available regarding the influence of pregnancy on the risk of recurrent stroke, thereby making it difficult to counsel women with a history of ischemic stroke regarding future pregnancies. The overall risk of recurrence of stroke associated with subsequent pregnancies is relatively small as showed in a French multi-center study on a group of 489 consecutive women aged 15 to 40 years with a first-ever arterial ischemic stroke or cerebral venous thrombosis [125]. Twenty-eight patients (of 373 with arterial ischemic stroke) had the initial ischemic event during pregnancy or the puerperium. During a mean follow-up period of 5 years, 13 of the whole cohort had a recurrent stroke but only two of these occurred in a subsequent pregnancy, related to rare definite causes of stroke such as essential thrombocytemia and primary antiphospholipid syndrome. The overall risk of recurrence in these patients was 1% within 1 year and 2.3% within 5 years. In line with these results, a descriptive study of a series of 23 patients with a history of a previous ischemic stroke showed no recurrence of ischemic stroke during subsequent pregnancy or after delivery [126].

Assisted Reproductive Technology (ART) and Arterial Cerebral Thromboembolic Complications

ART is related to all treatments or procedures that include the *in-vitro* handling of human oocytes and sperm or embryos for the purpose of establishing a pregnancy [127]. The most common procedure performed to assist reproduction includes *in-vitro* fertilization-embryo transfer (IVF-ET). The process of IVF comprises the administration of exogeneous hormones to achieve cycle control, stimulate the ovaries and support implantation. In the first step of process exogenenous medications as oral contraceptives or a gonadotrophin releasing hormone (GnRH) analog are administered in the cycle preceding the ART cycle. Exogeneous medications are then given to stimulate the formation of follicles in the ovary; these medications include gonadotrophins (LH and FSH), human menopausal gonadotrophins (hMG, which contains both FSH and LH), human chorionic gonadotrophin (hCG) or clomiphene citrate. After oocyte retrieval and *in-vitro* fertilization is achieved, embryo transfer procedure (which occurs three to five days after oocyte retrieval) is carried out. Because the use of GnRH agonist may result in a iatrogenic luteal phase defect by suppressing endogeneous pituitary LH secretion, subsequent secretion of estrogen and progesterone for proper endometrial development may be compromised. Therefore, hormonal supplementation in the form of estrogen, progesterone or hCG has been used in the luteal phase and beyond, in IVF cycles (until the end of the first trimester).

In the last years, it has been assisted an ever increasing ART use in many developed countries (International Committee for Monitoring Assisted Reproductive Technology, 2006). During 2002 over 110,000 ART procedures were performed in the US, resulting in 45,751 infants or 1% of all US infants born that year. This number is only expected to increase with time [128]. Thromboembolic complications associated with the use of ART have been described in several reports [129-131] (Table 5).

The risk of thrombosis, both arterial and venous, has been usually related to the presence of ovarian hyperstimulation syndrome (OHSS), a well-recognized complication of ART [132]; however, in a few cases, the development of thromboembolic complications were seen even in the absence of clinical OHSS [133]. OHSS occurs most often when the ovaries are stimulated with exogeneous gonadotrophins and clomiphene for the purpose of acquiring oocytes for fertilization; notwithstanding, spontaneous form of OHSS has been described but represents a rare event [134]. OHSS usually develops after the administration of hCG during stimulation and oocyte retrieval to enhance luteal function, and it lasts for 10-14 days [132]. The frequency of this syndrome ranges from 1-2% to 30% [132]. In the majority of cases the form is mild, self-limiting and needs no or few therapeutic measures. In OHSS, there are anenlargement of the ovaries, associated with leaky capillaries and a “third-spacing” of fluid, resulting in symptoms from pleural, pericardial or abdominal fluid accumulation. As a consequence of this extravasation of fluid, leukocytosis, hemoconcentration, electrolyte imbalance occurs [132]. This syndrome is also associated with a state of hypercoagulable but its pathogenesis remain unclear [130]. In about 1% of cases the syndrome is severe and can result in thromboembolism, adult respiratory distress syndrome, pleural effusions, significant ascites, renal insufficiency, liver dysfunction and even death [135].

At present, no guidelines regarding the need for thromboprophylaxis in patients who develop OHSS are reported; generally, thromboprophylaxis is initiated in view of the severity and the hospitalization of the patient [132]. Recently, published reports analyzing the association between ART or OHSS and thromboembolic, both arterial and venous, complications were reviewed [136]. Seventy-one episodes of thromboembolic complications in seventy women were gathered. In all but one case, thrombosis occurred after hCG was administered to induce ovulation; in all cases, clomiphene, exogeneous FSH, GnRH or GnRH agonists were administered to cause follicular formation. Pregnancy was attained in 69% (n = 49) of these cases. Twenty-six out 71 events concerned arterial thrombosis and about 60% involved cerebrovascular events. By contrast, myocardial infarcts were less common (2 out of 26). There were two fatalities in patients with arterial ischemic stroke. On average, the timing for arterial thrombosis was 10.5 days after embryo transfer in IVF pregnancies and 8.2 days after post hGC administration for ovulation induction cycles respectively; these arterial events were almost always concurrent with the development of symptoms of OHSS, that was reported in 95% of all cases of arterial thrombotic event for which information was available.

Although data are limited, inherited thrombophilic conditions may also play a role [137].

Another condition that seem to be involved in thrombotic complications in women undergoing ovarian stimulation is a preexisting polycystic ovaries conditions [137], but this may be expected since patients with this condition have often fertility problems.

The mechanism of thrombosis in ART is not completely understood. Ovarian stimulation is likely a trigger factor for arterial and venous thrombotic phenomena since evidences from studies performed on women undergoing controlled ovarian stimulation showed changes in haemostatic system with an increasing in coagulation factors and a decreasing in many markers promoting fibrinolysis; overall these changes suggest that a prothrombotic state could be present over the course of ovarian stimulation. This activation in both coagulation and fibrinolytic systems appears to be exaggerated with the development of OHSS [138], especially if arterial thrombotic complications arise [139].

Table 5. Case reports of cerebral arterial ischemic stroke associated with assisted reproductive techniques

Authors, year	Age	Timing of arterial ischemic stroke (days)	Development of OHSS	Risk factors	Pregnancy outcome and comments
Mozes et al, 1965 [140]	37	5 after last hCG	Yes	None	Not pregnant; death of patient
Rizk et al, 1990 [141]	30	12 after GIFT	Yes	None	Pregnancy completed
Kermode et al, 1993 [142]	34	9 after ET	Yes	Polycistic ovary	Not pregnant
Inbar et al, 1994 [143]	22	11 after hCG	No	Polycistic ovary	Not pregnant
Cluroe et al, 1995 [144]	40	6 after ET	Yes	None	Not pregnant?; death of patient
Aurousseau et al, 1995 [133]	34	7 after ET	ns	None	Therapeutic abortion; previous IVT attempt
Kodama et al, 1996 [145]	30	11 after ET	Yes	None	Successful pregnancy
El Sadek et al, 1998 [146]	24	4 after ET	Yes	None	Not pregnant
Hwang et al, 1998 [147]	22	11 after ET	Yes	None	Therapeutic abortion
Aboulghar et al, 1998 [148]	33	9 after ET	Yes	None	ns
	27	7 after ET	Yes	None	ns
Yoshii et al, 1999 [149]	26	6 after hCG	Yes	Decreased protein S	Therapeutic abortion
Morris et al, 1999 [150]	35	Clomiphene for ovulation induction	Yes	None	
Davies et al, 1999 [151]	33	ns	Yes	None	Not pregnant
Turkistani et al, 2001 [152]	34	12 after hCG	Yes	None	Cesarean twin delivery
Koo et al, 2002 [153]	33	14 after ET	Yes	High IgM anticardiolipin antibody; decreased protein S level	Successful delivery
Elford et al, 2002 [119]	28	7 after ET	Yes	None	Successful delivery; rt-PA treatment
Di Micco et al, 2003 [154]	32	ns	Yes	Heterozygous MTHFR C677T mutation	Not pregnat

ns: not specified; OHSS: ovarian hyperstimulation syndrome; hCG: human chorionic gonadotrophin; ET: embryo transfer; GIFT: gamete intrafallopion transfer; IVT: in vitro fertilization.

Therapeutic approach has been general supportive measures, adequate fluid compensation, cortisone, UH, LMWH, ASA or coumarin drugs. Dosage have been dose commonly used. The appropriate length of therapy, based on the future risk of recurrence in patients who develop these complications, is currently unknown. Data could be extrapolated from studies in pregnant women, and patients counseling accordingly. Moreover, the recognition of OHSS may be the key in preventing the possible devastating development of arterial thromboses and timely intervention critical in maternal and fetal prognosis. In line with this, a case of a successful use of rt-PA to lyse a cerebral arterial thrombus resulting from severe OHSS in a young women undergoing ART procedure was reported [119]. Therapeutic abortion was also a frequent measure utilized in the overall management of these patients.

Although the true incidence of arterial thrombotic complications resulting from ART cannot be determinate, the increasing reporting of these cases in the literature suggests that these complications of ART are not rare. Moreover, it should be noted that with the increasing diffusion of ART in clinical practice, the frequency of these complications will likely also increase and much efforts are needed to reduce the potential devastating consequence of thromboembolic complications related to this elective procedure.

References

[1] Bogousslavsky J, Pierre P. Ischemic stroke in patients under age 45. *Neurol. Clin.* 1992; 10: 113-124

[2] Di Carlo A, Lamassa M, Baldereschi M, Pracucci G, Basile AM, Wolfe CD, Giroud M, Rudd A, Ghetti A, Inzitari D; European BIOMED Study of Stroke Care Group. Sex differences in the clinical presentation, resource use, and 3-month outcome of acute stroke in Europe. Data from a Muticenter Multinational Hospital-Based Registry. *Stroke* 2003;34:1114–1119.

[3] Liang CC, Chang SD, Lai SL, Hsieh CC, Chueh HY, Lee TH. Stroke complicating pregnancy and the puerperium. *Eur. J. Neurol.* 2006;13:1256-1260

[4] James A, Bushnell CD, Jaminson MG, Myers ER. Incidence and risk factors for stroke in pregnancy and puerperium. *Obstet. Gynecol.* 2005;106:509-516

[5] McLaughlin MK, Keve TM. Pregnancy-induced changes in resistance vessels. *Am. J. Obstet. Gynecol.* 1986;155:1296–1299

[6] Cockell A, Poston L. Isolated mesenteric arteries from pregnant rats show enhanced flow-mediated relaxation but normal myogenic tone. *J. Physiol.* 1996;495:545–551

[7] Mackey K, Meyer MC, Stirewalt WS, Starcher BC, McLaughlin MK. Composition and mechanics of mesenteric resistance arteries from pregnant rats. *Am. J. Physiol.* 1992; 263(1 Pt 2):R2-8

[8] Hull AD, Long DM, Longo LD, Pearce WJ. Pregnancy-induced changes in ovine cerebral arteries. *Am. J. Physiol.* 1992;262(1 Pt 2):R137-143

[9] O'Riordan MN, Higgins JR. Haemostasis in normal and abnormal pregnancy. *Best Pract. Res. Clin. Obstet. Gynaecol.* 2003;17:385-396

[10] Bremme KA. Haemostatic changes in pregnancy. *Best Pract. Res. Clin. Haematol.* 2003; 16:153–168
[11] Franchini M. Haemostasis in pregnancy. *Thromb Haemost*. 2006;95: 401–413
[12] Sharshar T, Lamy C, Mas JL, for the Stroke in Pregnancy Group. Incidence and causes of stroke associated with pregnancy and puerperium: a study in public hospitals of Ile de France. *Stroke* 1995;26:930-936
[13] Cross JN, Castro PO, Jennett WB. Cerebral stroke associated with pregnancy and the puerperium. *BMJ* 1968;3:214-218
[14] Wiebers DO, Whisnant JP. The incidence of stroke among pregnant women in Rochester, Minn, 1955 through 1979. JAMA. 1985;254:3055-3057
[15] Awada A, al Rajeh S, Duarte R, Russell N. Stroke and pregnancy. *Int. J. Gynaecol.* Obstet. 1995;48:157-161
[16] Kittner SJ, Stern BJ, Feeser BR, Hebel R, Nagey DA, Buchholz DW, Earley CJ, Johnson CJ, Macko RF, Sloan MA, Wityk RJ, Wozniak MA. Pregnancy and the risk of stroke. *N. Engl. J. Med.* 1996;335:768-774
[17] Witlin AG, Friedman SA, Egerman RS, Frangieh AY, Sibai BM. Cerebrovascular disorders complicating pregnancy-beyond eclampsia. *Am. J. Obstet. Gynecol.* 1997;176: 1139-1145
[18] Jaigobin C, Silver FL. Stroke and pregnancy. *Stroke* 2000;31:2948–2951.
[19] Skidmore FM, Williams LS, Fradkin KD, Alonso RJ, Biller J. Presentation, etiology and outcome of stroke in pregnancy and puerperium. *J. Stroke Cerebrovasc. Dis.* 2001;10:1-10
[20] Jeng JS, Tang SC, Yip PK. Incidence and etiologies of stroke during pregnancy and puerperium as evidenced in Taiwanese women. *Cerebrovasc. Dis*. 2004;18:290–295.
[21] Ros HS, Lichtestein P, Bellocco R, Petersson R, Cnattingius S. Increased risks of circulatory diseases in late pregnancy and puerperium. *Epidemiology* 2001;12:456-460
[22] Lanska DJ, Kryscio RJ. Stroke and intracranial venous thrombosis during pregnancy and puerperium. *Neurology* 1998;51:1622-1628
[23] Kupfermic MJ, Yair D, Bornstein NM, Lessing JB, Eldor A Transient focal neurological deficits during pregnancy in carriers of inherited thrombophilia. Stroke. 2000;31:892-895
[24] Lanska DJ, Kryscio RJ. Risk factors for peripartum and postpartum stroke and intracranial venous thrombosis. *Stroke* 2000;31:1274-1282
[25] Davie CA, O'Brien P. Stroke and pregnancy. *J. Neurol. Neurosurg. Psychiatry* 2008;79: 240-245
[26] Ros HS, Lichtenstein P, Bellocco R, Petersson G, Cnattingius S. Pulmonary embolism and stroke in relation to pregnancy: how can high-risk women be identified? *Am. J. Obstet Gynecol.* 2002;186:198-203
[27] Mas JL, Lamy C. Stroke in pregnancy and the puerperium. J Neurol. 1998;245:305-313
[28] Moodley J, Kalane G. A review of the management of eclampsia: practical issues. *Hypertens Pregnancy* 2006;25:47-62
[29] Sibai B, Dekker G, Kupferminc M. Pre-eclampsia. *Lancet* 2005;365:785-799
[30] Sharma SK. Pre-eclampsia and eclampsia. Sem anesthesia perioperative medicine pain. 2000;19:171-180

[31] Brown DW, Dueker N, Jamieson DJ, Cole JW, Wozniak MA, Stern BJ, Giles WH, Kittner SJ. Preeclampsia and the risk of ischemic stroke among young women. Result from the Stroke Prevention in Young Women Study. *Stroke* 2006;37:1055-1059

[32] Qureshi AI, Frankel MR, Ottenlips JR, Stern BJ. Cerebral hemodynamics in preeclampsia and eclampsia. *Arch Neurol.* 1996;53:1226-1231

[33] Zunker P, Hohenstein C, Deuschl G. Pathophysiology of pre-eclampsia/eclampsia syndrome. *J. Neurol.* 2001;248:437-438

[34] Roberts JM, Cooper DW. Pathogenesis and genetics of pre-eclampsia. *Lancet* 2001;357: 53-56.

[35] Trommer BL, Homer D, Mikhael MA. Cerebral vasospasm and eclampsia. *Stroke* 1988;19:326-329.

[36] Will AD, Lewis KL, Hinshaw DB Jr, Jordan K, Cousins LM, Hasso AN, Thompson JR. Cerebral vasoconstriction in toxemia. *Neurology* 1987;37:1555-1557

[37] McCrae KR, Samuels P, Schreiber AD. Pregnancy-associated thrombocytopenia: pathogenesis and management. *Blood* 1992;80:2697-2714.

[38] Leys D, Lamy C, Lucas C, Henon H, Pruvo JP, Codaccioni X, Mas JL. Arterial ischemic strokes associated with pregnancy and puerperium. *Acta Neurol. Belg.* 1997;97: 5-16

[39] Brass SD, Copen WA.. Neurological disorders in pregnancy from a neuroimaging perspective. *Semin. Neurol.* 2007;27:411-424

[40] Zak IT, Dulai HS, Kish KK. Imaging of neurologic disorders associated with pregnancy and the postpartum period. *Radiographics*. 2007;27:95-108.

[41] Zeeman GG, Fleckenstein JL, Twickler DM, Cunningham FG.) Cerebral infarction in eclampsia. *Am. J. Obstet. Gynecol.* 2004;190:714-20

[42] Cipolla MJ. Cerebrovascular function in pregnancy and eclampsia. *Hypertension* 2007; 50:14-24.

[43] Ilancheran A, Ratnam SS, Baratham G. Metastatic cerebral choriocarcinoma with primary neurological presentation. *Gynecol. Oncol.* 1988;29:361-364

[44] Saad N, Tang YM, Sclavos E, Stuckey SL. Metastatic choriocarcinoma: a rare cause of stroke in the young adult. *Australas Radiol.* 2006;50:481-483

[45] Huang CY, Chen CA, Hsieh CY, Cheng WF. Intracerebral hemorrhage as initial presentation of gestational choriocarcinoma: a case report and literature review. *Int. J .Gynecol. Cancer.* 2007;17:1166-1171

[46] Clark SL, Hankins GD, Dudley DA, Dildy GA, Porter TF. Amniotic fluid embolism: analysis of the national registry. *Am. J. Obstet Gynecol.* 1995;172:1158–1169

[47] Calabrese LH, Dodick DW, Schwedt TJ, Singhal AB. Narrative review: reversible cerebral vasoconstriction syndromes. *Ann. Intern. Med.* 2007;146:34-44

[48] Bogousslavsky J, Despland PA, Regli F, Dubuis PY. Postpartum cerebral angiopathy: reversible vasoconstriction assessed by transcranial Doppler ultrasounds. *Eur. Neurol.* 1989;29:102-105.

[49] Raroque HG Jr, Tesfa G, Purdy P. Postpartum cerebral angiopathy. Is there a role for sympathomimetic drugs? *Stroke* 1993;24:2108-2110

[50] Singhal AB. Cerebral vasoconstriction syndromes. *Top Stroke Rehabil.* 2004;11:1-6.

[51] Konstantinopoulos PA, Mousa S, Khairallah R, Mtanos G. Postpartum cerebral angiopathy: an important diagnostic consideration in the postpartum period. *Am. J. Obstet. Gynecol.* 2004;191:375-377

[52] Williams TL, Lukovits TG, Harris BT, Harker Rhodes C. A fatal case of postpartum cerebral angiopathy with literature review. *Arch Gynecol. Obstet.* 2007;275:67-77

[53] Farine D, Andreyko J, Lysikiewicz A, Simha S, Addison A. Isolated angiitis of brain in pregnancy and puerperium. *Obstet. Gynecol.* 1984;63:586-588

[54] Geraghty JJ, Hoch DB, Robert ME, Vinters HV. Fatal puerperal cerebral vasospasm and stroke in a young woman. *Neurology* 1991;41:1145-1147

[55] Singhal AB. Postpartum angiopathy with reversible posterior leukoencephalopathy. *Arch Neurol.* 2004;61:411-416

[56] Demakis JG, Rahimtoola SH, Sutton GC, Meadows WR, Szanto PB, Tobin JR, Gunnar RM. Natural course of peripartum cardiomyopathy. *Circulation* 1971;44:1053–1061

[57] Brown G, O'Leary M, Douglas I, Herkes R. Perioperative management of a case of severe peripartum cardiomyopathy. *Anaesth. Intensive Care* 1992;20:80–83

[58] Forssell G, Laska J, Olofsson C, Olsson M, Mogensen L. Peripartum cardiomyopathy: three cases. *J. Intern. Med.* 1994;235:493–496

[59] Rizeq MN, Rickenbacher PR, FowlerMB, BillinghamME. Incidence of myocarditis in peripartumcardiomyopathy.*Am. J. Cardiol.* 1994;74:474–477

[60] Elkayam U, Akhter MW, Singh H, Khan S, Bitar F, Hameed A, Shotan A. Pregnancy-associated cardiomyopathy: clinical characteristics and a comparison between early and late presentation. *Circulation* 2005;111:2050-2055

[61] Abboud J, Murad Y, Chen-Scarabelli C, Saravolatz L, M. Scarabelli T. Peripartum cariomyopathy: a comprehensive review. *Int. J. Cardiol.* 2007;118:295–303

[62] Pearson GD, Veille JC, Rahimtoola S, Hsia J, Oakley CM, Hosenpud JD, Ansari A, Baughman KL. Peripartum cardiomyopathy: National Heart, Lung, and Blood Institute and Office of Rare Diseases (National Institutes of Health) workshop recommendations and review. *JAMA* 2000;283:1183—1188.

[63] Cénac A, Djibo A. Postpartum cardiac failure in Sudanese–Sahelian Africa: clinical prevalence in western Niger. *Am. J. Trop. Med. Hyg.* 1998;58:319–323

[64] van Mook WN, Peeters L. Severe cardiac disease in pregnancy, part II: impact of congenital and acquired cardiac diseases during pregnancy. *Curr. Opin. Crit. Care* 2005; 11:435—448

[65] Lang RM, Lampert MB, Poppas A, et al: Peripartal cardiomyopathy. In: Cardiac Problems in Pregnancy. 3rd ed. Elkayam U, Gleicher N (Eds). New York, NY, Wiley-Liss, 1998,

[66] O'Connell JB, Costanzo-Nordin MR, Subramanian R, Robinson JA, Wallis DE, Scanlon PJ, Gunnar RM. Peripartum cardiomyopathy: clinical hemodynamic, histologic and prognostic characteristics. *J. Am. Coll. Cardiol.* 1986;8:52–56

[67] Ansari AA, Neckelmann N, Wang YC, Gravanis MB, Sell KW, Herskowitz A. Immunologic dialogue between cardiac myocytes, endothelial cells, and mononuclear cells. *Clin. Immunol. Immunopathol.* 1993;68:208–214

[68] Ansari AA, Fett JD, Carraway RE, Mayne AE, Onlamoon N, Sundstrom JB. Autoimmune mechanisms as the basis for human peripartum cardiomyopathy. *Clin. Rev. Allergy Immunol.* 2002;23:310–324

[69] Fett JD, Ansari AA, Sundstrom JB, Combs GF. Peripartum cardiomyopathy: A selenium disconnection and an autoimmune connection. *Int. J. Cardiol.* 2002;86:311–316

[70] Sliwa K, Skudicky D, Bergemann A, Candy G, Puren A, Sareli P. Peripartum cardiomyopathy: analysis. *J. Am. Coll. Cardiol.* 2000;35:701-705

[71] Cenac A, Simonoff M, Moretto P, Djibo A. A low plasma selenium is a risk factor for peripartum cardiomyopathy. A comparative study in Sahelian Africa. *Int. J. Cardiol.* 1992 ;36:57—59.

[72] Lampert MB, Hibbard J, Weinert L, Briller J, Lindheimer M, Lang RM. Peripartum heart failure associated with prolonged tocolytic therapy. *Am. J. Obstet. Gynecol.* 1993; 168:493–495.

[73] Homans DC. Peripartum cardiomyopathy. *N. Eng. J. Med.* 1985;312:1432-1437

[74] Heider AL, Kuller JA, Strauss RA, Wells SR. Peripartum cardiomyopathy: a review of the literature. *Obstet. Gynecol. Surv.* 1999;54:526–531

[75] Cunningham FG, Pritchard JA, Hankins GD, Anderson PL, Lucas MJ, Armstrong KF. Peripartum heart failure: idiopathic cardiomyopathy or compounding cardiovascular events? *Obstet. Gynecol.* 1986;67:157—168

[76] Hodgman M, Pessin M, Homans D, Panis W, Prager RJ, Lathi ES, Criscitiello MG. Cerebral embolism as the initial manifestation of peripartum cardiomyopathy. *Neurology* 1982;32:668—671

[77] Connor R, Adams JH. Importance of cardiomyopathy and cerebral ischemia in the diagnosis of fatal coma in pregnancy. *J. Clin. Pathol.* 1966;19:244-249

[78] Kittner SJ, Stern BJ, Wozniak M, Buchholz DW, Earley CJ, Feeser BR, Johnson CJ, Macko RF, McCarter RJ, Price TR, Sherwin R, Sloan MA, Wityk RJ. Cerebral infarction in young adults: the Baltimore-Washington Cooperative Young Stroke Study. *Neurology* 1998;50:890-894

[79] Feske SK. Stroke in pregnancy. *Semin. Neurol.* 2007;27:442-452

[80] Hall EJ, Giaccia AJ. Radiobiology for the radiologist. Philadelphia: Lippincott Williams and Wilkins, 2006

[81] Donaldson JP, Lee NS Arterial and venous stroke associated with pregnancy. In: Yerby MS, Devinsky O (eds) Neurologic clinics. Neurologic complications of pregnancy, vol 12. Saunders, Philadelphia, pp 583-599, 1994.

[82] American College of Radiology Committee on Drugs and Contrast Media. Manual on Contrast Media. 5th ed. Reston VA: American College of Radiology, 2004

[83] ACOG Committee on Obstetric Practice. ACOG Committee Opinion Number 299, September 2004. Guidelines for diagnostic imaging during pregnancy. *Obstet. Gynecol.* 2004;104: 647-651

[84] Heinrichs WL, Fong P, Flannery M, Heinrichs SC, Crooks LE, Spindle A, Pedersen RA. Midgestational exposure of pregnant BALB/c mice to magnetic resonance imaging conditions. *Magn. Reson Imaging.* 1988;6:305-313

[85] Tyndall DA, Sulik KK. Effects of magnetic resonance imaging on eye development in the C57BL/6J mouse. *Teratology* 1991;43:263-275

[86] Yip YP, Capriotti C, Talagala SL, Yip JW. Effects of MR exposure at 1.5 T on early embryonic development of the chick. *J. Magn. Reson. Imaging*. 1994;4:742-748

[87] Kanal E, Borgstede JP, Barkovich AJ, Bell C, Bradley WG, Felmlee JP, Froelich JW, Kaminski EM, Keeler EK, Lester JW, Scoumis EA, Zaremba LA, Zinninger MD; American College of Radiology. American College of Radiology White Paper on MR Safety. *AJR Am. J. Roentgenol.* 2002;178:1335-1347

[88] Webb JA, Thomsen HS, Morcos SK; Members of Contrast Media Safety Committee of European Society of Urogenital Radiology (ESUR). The use of iodinated and gadolinium contrast media during pregnancy and lactation. *Eur. Radiol.* 2005;15:1234-1240.

[89] Bona G, Zaffaroni M, Defilippi C, Gallina MR, Mostert M. Effects of iopamidol on neonatal thyroid function. *Eur. J. Radiol.* 1992;14:22-25

[90] Morisetti A, Tirone P, Luzzani F, de Haën C. Toxicological safety assessment of iomeprol, a new X-ray contrast agent. *Eur. J. Radiol.* 1994;18 Suppl 1:S21-31

[91] Ralston WH, Robbins MS, James P. Reproductive, developmental, and genetic toxicology of ioversol. *Invest. Radiol.* 1989;24 Suppl 1:S16-22

[92] Kanal E, Borgstede JP, Barkovich AJ, Bell C, Bradley WG, Etheridge S, Felmlee JP, Froelich JW, Hayden J, Kaminski EM, Lester JW Jr, Scoumis EA, Zaremba LA, Zinninger MD; American College of Radiology. American College of Radiology White Paper on MR Safety: 2004 update and revisions. *AJR Am. J. Roentgenol.* 2004;182: 1111-1114.

[93] Stoddard MF, Longaker RA, Vuocolo LM, Dawkins PR. Trans-esophageal echocardiography in the pregnant patient. *Am. Heart J.* 1992;124:785-787

[94] Liberman A, Karussis D, Ben-Hur T, Abramsky O, Leker RR. Natural course and pathogenesis of transient focal neurological symptoms during pregnancy. *Arch Neurol.* 2008;65: 218-220

[95] Ertresvåg JM, Zwart JA, Helde G, Johnsen HJ, Bovim G. Migraine aura or transient ischemic attacks? A five-year follow-up case-control study of women with transient central nervous system disorders in pregnancy. *BMC Med.* 2005;5:19.

[96] Loeb C, Gandolfo C, Dall'Agata D. Headache in transient ischemic attacks (TIA). *Cephalalgia* 1985;5 Suppl 2:17-9

[97] Maggioni F, Alessi C, Maggino T, Zanchin G. Headache during pregnancy. *Cephalalgia* 1997;17:765-769

[98] Scharff L, Marcus DA, Turk DC. Headache during pregnancy and in the postpartum: a prospective study. *Headache* 1997;37:203-210

[99] Sances G, Granella F, Nappi RE, Fignon A, Ghiotto N, Polatti F, Nappi G. Course of migraine during pregnancy and postpartum: a prospective study. *Cephalalgia* 2003; 23:197-205.

[100] Ertresvåg JM, Zwart J-A, Helde G, Johnsen H-J, Bovim G. Headache and transient focal neurological symptoms during pregnancy, a prospective cohort. *Acta Neurol. Scand.* 2005:111:233–237

[101]Sacco RL, Adams R, Albers G, Alberts MJ, Benavente O, Furie K, Goldstein LB, Gorelick P, Halperin J, Harbaugh R, Johnston SC, Katzan I, Kelly-Hayes M, Kenton EJ, Marks M, Schwamm LH, Tomsick T; American Heart Association; American Stroke Association Council on Stroke; Council on Cardiovascular Radiology and Intervention; American Academy of Neurology. Guidelines for prevention of stroke in patients with ischemic stroke or transient ischemic attack: a statement for healthcare professionals from the American Heart Association/American Stroke Association Council on Stroke: co-sponsored by the Council on Cardiovascular Radiology and Intervention: the American Academy of Neurology affirms the value of this guideline. *Stroke* 2006; 37:577-617

[102]Bates SM, Greer IA, Hirsh J, Ginsberg JS. Use of antithrombotic agents during pregnancy: the Seventh ACCP Conferenceon antithrombotic and thrombolityc therapy. *Chest* 2004;126:627-644

[103]Lepercq J, Conard J, Borel-Derlon A, Darmon JY, Boudignat O, Francoual C, Priollet P, Cohen C, Yvelin N, Schved JF, Tournaire M, Borg JY. Venous thromboembolism during pregnancy: a retrospective study of enoxaparin safety in 624 pregnancies. *BJOG* 2001; 108:1134–1140

[104]Warkentin TE, Levine MN, Hirsh J, Horsewood P, Roberts RS, Gent M, Kelton JG. Heparin-induced thrombocytopenia in patients treated with low-molecularweight heparin or unfractionated heparin. *N. Engl. J. Med.* 1995;332:1330–1335

[105]Ginsberg JS, Hirsh J, Turner CD, Levine MN, Burrows R. Risks to the fetus of anticoagulant therapy during pregnancy. *Thromb Haemost.* 1989;61:197–203

[106]Ginsberg JS, Kowalchuk G, Hirsh J, Brill-Edwards P, Burrows R. Heparin therapy during pregnancy: Risks to the fetus and mother. Arch Intern Med. 1989;149:2233–2236

[107]Hall JAG, Paul RM, Wilson KM. Maternal and fetal sequelae of anticoagulation during pregnancy *Am. J. Med.* 1980;68:122–140

[108]Greer IA, Nelson-Piercy C. Low-molecular-weight heparins for thromboprophylaxis and treatment of venous thromboembolism in pregnancy: a systematic review of safety and efficacy. *Blood* 2005;106:401-407

[109]Monreal M, Lafoz E, Olive A, del Rio L, Vedia C. Comparison of subcutaneous unfractionated heparin with a low molecular weight heparin (Fragmin) in patients with venous thromboembolism and contraindications for coumarin. *Thromb Haemost.* 1994; 71:7–11

[110]O'Reilly R. Anticoagulant, antithrombotic and thrombolytic drugs. In: Gillman AG, Goodman LS, Gilman A, eds. The pharmacologic basis of therapeutics, 6th ed. New York, NY: Macmillan, 1347, 1980

[111]Orme L'E, Lewis M, de Swiet M, Serlin MJ, Sibeon R, Baty JD, Breckenridge AM. May mothers given warfarin breast-feed their infants? *BMJ* 1977;1:1564–1565

[112]McKenna R, Cole ER, Vasan V. Is warfarin sodium contraindicated in the lactating mother? *J. Pediatr.* 1983;103:325–327

[113]Imperiale TF, Petrulis AS. A meta-analysis of low-dose aspirin for prevention of pregnancy-induced hypertensive disease. *JAMA* 1991;266:260–264

[114]CLASP Collaborative Group. CLASP: a randomised trial of low dose aspirin for the prevention and treatment of preeclampsia among 9,364 pregnant women. *Lancet* 1994; 343:619–629

[115]Leonhardt G, Gaul C, Nietsch HH, Buerke M, Schleussner E. Thrombolytic therapy in pregnancy. *J. Thromb Thrombolysis* 2006;21:271-6

[116]Kojima N, Naya M, Imoto H, Hara T, Deguchi T, Takahira H. Reproduction study of GMK-527 (rt-PA) - (III) Teratogenic Study in rabbits treated intravenously with GMK-527. *Jpn. Pharmacol. Ther.* 1988;16:107–123

[117]Tanaka M, Mizuno F, Ohtsuka T, Komatsu K, Umeshita C, Mizusawa R. Study in rats treated intravenously with GMK-527 (II) Teratogenicity study in rats treated intravenously with GMK-527. *Jpn. Pharmacol. Ther.* 1988;16:93–106

[118]Dapprich M, Boessenecker W. Fibrinolysis with alteplase in a pregnant woman with stroke. *Cerebrovasc. Dis.* 2002;13:290

[119]Elford K, Leader A, Wee R, Stys PK. Stroke in ovarian hyperstimulation syndrome in early pregnancy treated with intra-arterial rt-PA. *Neurology* 2002;59:1270-1272

[120]Johnson DM, Kramer DC, Cohen E, Rochon M, Rosner M, Weinberger J. Thrombolytic therapy for acute stroke in late pregnancy with intra-arterial recombinant tissue plasminogen activator. *Stroke* 2005;36:e53-5

[121]Wiese KM, Talkad A, Mathews M, Wang D. Intravenous recombinant tissue plasminogen activator in a pregnant woman with cardioembolic stroke. *Stroke* 2006; 37: 2168-2169

[122]Murugappan A, Coplin WM, Al-Sadat AN, McAllen KJ, Schwamm LH, Wechsler LR, Kidwell CS, Saver JL, Starkman S, Gobin YP, Duckwiler G, Krueger M, Rordorf G, Broderick JP, Tietjen GE, Levine SR. Thrombolytic therapy of acute ischemic stroke during pregnancy. *Neurology* 2006;66:768-770.

[123]Méndez JC, Masjuán J, García N, de Leciñana M. Successful intra-arterial thrombolysis for acute ischemic stroke in the immediate postpartum period: case report. *Cardiovasc. Intervent. Radiol.* 2008;31:193-195

[124]De Keyser J, Gdovinová Z, Uyttenboogaart M, Vroomen PC, Luijckx GJ. Intravenous alteplase for stroke: beyond the guidelines and in particular clinical situations. *Stroke* 2007; 38:2612-2618.

[125]Lamy C, Hamon JB, Coste J, Mas JL. Ischemic stroke in young women. Risk of recurrence during subsequent pregnancies. *Neurology* 2000;55:269-274

[126]Coppage KH, Hinton AC, Moldenhauer J, Kovilam O, Barton JR, Sibai BM. Maternal and perinatal outcome in women with a history of stroke. *Am. J. Obstet. Gynecol.* 2004; 190:1331-1334

[127]Yen and Jaffe's reproductive endocrinology: physiology, pathophysiology, and clinical management. 5th Edition. W B Saunders Co, 2004

[128]Wright VC, Schieve LA, Reynolds MA, Jeng G. Assisted reproductive technology surveillance in United States, 2002. *MMWR* 2005;54:1-24

[129]Stewart JA, Hamilton PJ, Murdoch AP. Thromboembolic disease associated with ovarian stimulation and assisted conception techniques. *Hum. Reprod.* 1997;12:2167-2173

[130]Baumann P, Diedrich K. Thromboembolic complications associated with reproductive endocrinologic procedures. *Hematol/Oncol. Clin. North Am. April.* 2000;14:431-443.

[131]Mancuso A, De Vivo A, Fanara G, Di Leo R, Toscano A. Upper body venous thrombosis associated with ovarian stimulation: case report and review of the literature. *Clin. Exp. Obstet. Gynecol.* 2005;32:149-154

[132]Whelan JG, Vlahos NF. The ovarian hyperstimulation syndrome. *Fertil. Steril.* 2000;73: 893-896.

[133]Aurousseau MH, Samama MM, Belhassen A, Herve F, Hugues JN Risk of thromboembolism in relation to an in-vitro fertilization programme: three case reports. *Hum. Reprod.* 1995;10:94–97

[134]Todros T, Carmazzi CM, Bontempo S, Gaglioti P, Donvito V, Massobrio M. Spontaneous ovarian hyperstimulation syndrome and deep vein thrombosis in pregnancy: case report. *Hum. Reprod.* 1999;14:2245-2248

[135]Smitz J, Camus M, Devroey P, Erard P, Wisanto A, Van Steirteghem AC. Incidence of severe ovarian hyperstimulation syndrome after GnRH/HMG superovulation for IVF. *Hum. Reprod.* 1990; 5:933–937

[136]Chan WS, Dixon ME. The "ART" of thromboembolism: a review of assisted reproductive technology and thromboembolic complications. *Thromb. Res.* 2008;121: 713-726.

[137]Girolami A, Scandellari R, Tezza F, Paternoster D, Girolami B. Arterial thrombosis in young women after ovarian stimulation: case report and review of the literature. *J. Thromb. Thrombolysis* 2007; 24:169-174.

[138]Kodama H, Fukuda J, Karube H, Matsui T, Shimizu Y, Tanaka T. Status of the coagulation and fibrinolytic systems in ovarian hyperstimulation syndrome. *Fertil. Steril.* 1996; 66:417-424

[139]Phillips LL, Gladstone W, vande Wiele R. Studies of the coagulation and fibrinolytic systems in hyperstimulation syndrome after administration of human gonadotropins. *J. Reprod. Med.* 1975;14:138-143

[140]Mozes M, Bogokowsky H, Antebi E, Lunenfeld B, Rabau E, Serr DM, David A, Salomy M. Thromboembolic phenomena after ovarian stimulation with human gonadotrophins. *Lancet* 1965;2:1213-1215

[141]Rizk B, Meagher S, Fisher AM. Severe ovarian hyperstimulation syndrome and cerebrovascular accidents. *Hum. Reprod.* 1990;5:697-698

[142]Kermode AG, Churchyard A, Carroll WM. Stroke complicating severe ovarian hyperstimulation syndrome. *Aust. N. Z. J. Med.* 1993;23:219-220

[143]Inbar OJ, Levran D, Mashiach S, Dor J. Ischemic stroke due to induction of ovulation with clomiphene *citrate and menotropins without evidence of ovarian hyperstimulation syndrome. Fertil.* Steril. 1994;62:1075-1076

[144]Cluroe AD, Synek BJ. A fatal case of ovarian hyperstimulation syndrome with cerebral infarction. *Pathology* 1995;27:344-346

[145]Kodama H, Fukuda J, Karube H, Matsui T, Shimizu Y, Tanaka T. In vitro fertilization of in vitro matured oocytes obtained from the follicles without hCG exposure for prevention of severe ovarian hyperstimulation syndrome: a case report. *J. Obstet. Gynaecol. Res.* 1996; 22:61-65

[146]El Sadek MM, Amer MK, Fahmy M. Acute cerebrovascular accidents with severe ovarian hyperstimulation syndrome. *Hum. Reprod.* 1998;13:1793-1795

[147]Hwang WJ, Lai ML, Hsu CC, Hou NT. Ischemic stroke in a young woman with ovarian hyperstimulation syndrome. *J. Formos. Med. Assoc.* 1998;97:503-506

[148]Aboulghar MA, Mansour RT, Serour GI, Amin YM. Moderate ovarian hyperstimulation syndrome complicated by deep cerebrovascular thrombosis. *Hum. Reprod.* 1998; 13: 2088-2091

[149]Yoshii F, Ooki N, Shinohara Y, Uehara K, Mochimaru F. Multiple cerebral infarctions associated with ovarian hyperstimulation syndrome. *Neurology* 1999;53:225-227

[150]Morris RS, Paulson RJ. Increased angiotensin-converting enzyme activity in a patient with severe ovarian hyperstimulation syndrome. *Fertil. Steril.* 1999;71:562-563

[151]Davies AJ, Patel B. Hyperstimulation--brain attack. *Br. J. Radiol.* 1999;72:923-924

[152]Turkistani IM, Ghourab SA, Al-Sheikh OH, Abuel-Asrar AM. Central retinal artery occlusion associated with severe ovarian hyperstimulation syndrome. *Eur. J. Ophthalmol.* 2001; 11:313-315

[153]Koo EJ, Rha JH, Lee BI, Kim MO, Ha CK. A case of cerebral infarct in combined antiphospholipid antibody and ovarian hyperstimulation syndrome. *J. Korean Med. Sci.* 2002; 17:574-576

[154]Di Micco P, D'Uva M, Romano M, Di Marco B, Niglio A. Stroke due to left carotid thrombosis in moderate ovarian hyperstimulation syndrome. *Thromb. Haemost.* 2003;90: 957-960

In: Cerebral Ischemia in Young Adults
Editors: A. Pezzini and A. Padovani
ISBN 978-1-60741-627-2

Chapter 10

Cervical Artery Dissection

Caspar Grond-Ginsbach[1*], Christoph Lichy[1] and Tobias Brandt[2]
1. Department of Neurology,
University of Heidelberg, Heidelberg, Germany
2. Kliniken Schmieder,
Teaching Hospital of the University of Heidelberg, Germany

Abstract

Cervical artery dissection (CAD) is an important cause of cerebral ischemia in young adults. The distal internal carotid artery is most commonly affected, followed by the distal extracranial vertebral artery. Dissections of the common carotid artery and of the intracranial parts of the carotid and vertebral arteries are rarer. CAD pathogenesis is largely unknown, but trauma, hypertension, migraine, recent infection, and connective tissue alterations appear to be risk factors. The clinical spectrum of CAD varies considerably (from pain with or without local signs like a Horner's syndrome to severe brain infarction). Clinical diagnosis of CAD is usually confirmed by non-invasive techniques, including Doppler studies and magnetic resonance (MRI) angiography. Delayed MRI with fat suppressed sequences enables to prove CAD by identification of a hematoma in the arterial wall. Treatment of CAD is empiric, as controlled clinical trials have not yet been performed. After initial anticoagulation with intravenous heparin, oral warfarin with a target INR of 2-3 is given in most centers, usually limited to 3-6 months if follow up studies reveal(s) recanalization or stable occlusion of the affected vessel.

[*] Correspondence: Caspar Grond-Ginsbach, Im Neuenheimer Feld 400, D-69120 Heidelberg, Germany. Tel: +49-6221-568213, Email: Caspar.Grond-Ginsbach@med.uni-heidelberg.de.

Introduction

A cervical arterial dissection (CAD) is thought to occur by a rupture within the arterial wall leading to an intramural haematoma. Possible consequence is an acute obstruction of the vessel inducing a high risk for local thrombus formation and cerebral embolism, or, alternatively, hemodynamic insufficiency. The clinical spectrum of CAD is very broad. Some patients merely present with local pain, isolated Horner's syndrome or caudal cranial nerve palsy, but most patients suffer cerebral ischemia. Due to increased clinical awareness and diagnostic sensitivity, CAD is nowadays probably the most common cause of ischemic stroke in young adults (<45 years) in Western countries. In this chapter we discuss the epidemiology and pathogenesis of CAD and present an overview of the clinical manifestation, diagnosis, treatment and prognosis of this common cause of stroke in the young.

Definitions

- Dissecting aneurysm = arterial dissection: a disease of the arterial wall, defined by a flap-like tear in the intimal layer or by an hematoma in the medial layer. Arterial dissections have been described for many types of arteries, in particular for the aorta and the cervical arteries
- Fibromuscular dysplasia (FMD): a rare segmental non-inflammatory non-atherosclerotic vascular disease that most often affects the renal and carotid arteries, although almost any artery can be involved. Affected blood vessels characteristically resemble a string of beads on angiography. In patients with CAD the prevalence of fibromuscular dysplasia is increased.
- Intimal flap: a layer of intimal tissue, that separates the true lumen from the false lumen or that is partially torn of from the vessel wall with one free end flapping in the blood stream. The demonstration of an intimal flap is considered as the single best criterion for the diagnosis of aortic dissection. In CAD, however, an intimal flap is visualized only in a minority of cases. The detection of an intramural hematoma is therefore considered as the single best criterion for the diagnosis of a dissection of the vertebral or carotid artery.
- Intramural hematoma: a collection of blood resulting from an internal bleeding within or into the arterial wall.
- Pseudoaneurysm (= false aneurysm): an outpouching of a blood vessel involving a defect in the two innermost tissue layers (tunica media and tunica intima). A true aneurysm, in contrast, is a localized abnormal dilatation of an artery due to a weakness in the arterial wall containing all three tissue layers (intima, media and adventitia).

Unfortunately there is some discordance in the terminology and definitions used in literature. For instance, well defined notions with slightly different meaning were proposed by Lee et al [1].

Epidemiology

The annual incidence of CAD was estimated at about 3 per 100.000 [1, 2]. The true incidence might be somewhat higher since patients with isolated cervical pain or headaches but without neurological deficits are not always suspected to have a CAD and, therefore, are not screened for flow abnormalities by Doppler sonography [3]. Moreover, the accidental finding of additional asymptomatic dissections in other cervical arteries of the patients during the acute phase or during follow-up studies [4] demonstrated that dissections can occur without any signs or symptoms.

CAD affects all age groups, including children, but there is a peak in the fifth decade of life. There are more male CAD patients (ratio men/women is about 1.5/1) but as a rule affected women are somewhat younger than male patients [5]. Familial occurrence of CAD is rare [6]. Some studies revealed that the incidence of CAD shows seasonal variation with an slight excess of cases in autumn or winter [7,8].

The incidence of vertebral artery (VA) dissection is in most studies reported to be roughly one third of ICA (internal carotid artery) dissection [5, 2], but some larger consecutive series contain particularly high numbers of VA dissections [1, 9, 10]. This might perhaps partially reflect the usually more specific signs and symptoms found in ICA dissection and the technically more challenging evaluations of the vertebral arteries by means of Doppler sonography.

Extracranial artery dissection is far more frequent than intracranial dissection in Western populations (however, see [11]). Simultaneous dissection of more than one vessel or multiple dissections within a few weeks may occur in about 15-25% of the patients [4], whereas recurrent CAD at a later stage is much less frequent [3]. Usually recurrent CAD affects a vessel different from the first site of CAD manifestation. Dissections of the common carotid artery [12] are very rare.

In the ICA, sites of predilection are the 2-3 centimeters distal to the carotid artery bifurcation and before entrance into the cranium. This might be due to increased shear forces and stretching in this part of the carotid artery, which is located in the highly mobile neck region but is fixed at its distal part by the surrounding bone of the skull. The site of predilection for dissection is different from the site with strongest atherosclerotic lesions, which is usually found at the carotid bifurcation. This typical, but not pathognomonic difference can be helpful for the clinical interpretation of both Doppler and angiographic studies of ICA dissections.

Of a total of 195 VA dissections, 174 were located in the extracranial part of the artery [13], mostly in the V2 or V3 segments. Dissections of the proximal V1 segment or of the intracranial V4 segment are much less frequent.

The most common intracranial locations for dissections are the intracranial ICA, the middle cerebral arteries and the intracranial vertebral arteries (often with spread to the basilar artery) [14].

Pathogenesis

Two different mechanisms might explain the development of the intramural haematoma in a cervical artery: (1) blood might have penetrated from the arterial lumen into the vessel wall (after a rupture of the intimal layer of the arterial wall); or (2) the hematoma might have developed from a bleeding caused by a ruptured vas vasorum. During later stages of CAD pathogenesis, the initial damage within the medial layer of the arterial wall might further develop in such a way that the original damage cannot be recognized anymore: The intramural hematoma may subsequently enlarge into other layers of the vessel wall and reconnect with the true lumen of the artery. Moreover, the initial damage of the intima might heal and the origin of the intramural blood becomes untraceable. In fact both pathomechanisms may have occurred in different patients. We like to emphasize at this occasion that dissections of the aorta or of other arteries might have at least partially different pathologies, as some signs (for instance an intimal flap or a second lumen) are often seen in a dissected aorta, but only rarely in a dissected carotid or vertebral artery. Whereas neurologists consider an intramural hematoma in a cervical artery as a pathognomonic sign for a dissection, some vascular surgeons and cardiologists tend to consider aortic intramural hematomas and aortic dissections as two distinct etiologic entities [15, 16]. An aortic intramural hematoma might develop (if an intimal tear occurs) into an aortic dissection, but it might also completely regress before a dissection occurs or develop into a pseudo-aneurysm, into a saccular or into a fusiform aneurysm. The aortic intramural hematoma itself is thought to be either the result of a bleeding from the vasa vasorum or the consequence a penetrating atherosclerotic ulcer. According to this model of the pathogenesis of aortic dissections the intimal tear is considered to develop after the formation of the intramural hematoma [15]. However, according to the definition of an arterial dissection as it was proposed in the introduction of this current chapter, the intramural hematoma was regarded as a result of an arterial dissection.

CAD is probably a multifactorial disease with environmental and congenital risk factors. Its pathogenesis remains unknown in most individual cases [17]. CAD may develop spontaneously in otherwise healthy individuals with no risk factors for stroke at all. Hypertension [18], migraine [19,20] or recent previous infections [21-23] are found more frequently in CAD patients than in healthy control subjects and were therefore considered as associated risk factors. However, no association was found between CAD and hypertension, smoking and hypercholesterolemia in a recent case control study [24] Moreover, many patients report a mild mechanical stress such as sudden head movement, coughing, or sport activities prior to the dissection [14,25]. In many circumstances, very mild trauma preceding CAD is felt inadequate to cause such injury in an otherwise healthy vessel. Mechanical injury like blunt trauma to the neck, acceleration/deceleration trauma, prolonged child delivery and (suicidal) strangulation can lead to “traumatic” CAD [26]. Chiropractic maneuvers also have been associated with CAD, in particular with dissections of the vertebral arteries. However, it cannot be excluded that some of the patients presenting with ischemic stroke after a chiropractic treatment suffered from neck pain because of (unrecognized, but already pre-existing) CAD [27]. The chiropractic maneuver might not have caused CAD itself, but might have induced its ischemic complication.

Iatrogenic dissections or pseudo-aneurysms might occur as rare (1-2%) periprocedural complications during diagnostic catheter angiography or endovascular recanalization procedures [28, 29]. Stretching of the neck of anesthetized patients [30] or during medical treatment [31,32] was followed by CAD in some published cases.

In most CAD patients no physical challenge can be found at all. Hence, an underlying arteriopathy has often been postulated in these patients with "spontaneous" CAD [2,17]. Structural aberrations of the arterial walls and defective extracellular matrix components in the surrounding connective tissue leading to a so called "weakness of the vessel wall" have been assumed. Some experimental findings indeed confirm the presence of chronic pathologic changes in ICA wall from CAD patients. Carotid arteries from CAD patients were shown to be stiffer than arteries from healthy control persons [33-35]. Angiographic signs of fibromuscular dysplasia are found in up to 15% in patients with CAD [2,36]. Post-mortem examinations of affected and non-affected arteries from CAD patients were not often performed. In the few published studies pronounced histopathological abnormalities are typical for carotid arteries of CAD patients [37,38], predominantly in the medial layer of the arterial wall. The localization of the major aberrations in the medial layer of the arterial wall suggests that CAD is not directly related to atherosclerotic alterations. Morphologic abnormalities were also found in other (non-cervical) arteries from CAD patients [37,39] which suggests the presence of a generalized arterial disease. The observed pathology resembles the findings which were described as segmental mediolytic arteriopathy (SMA) in arteries of patients with inherited connective tissue syndromes, a condition with similarities to the cystic medial degeneration or mucoid media necrosis originally described by Erdheim and Gsell in aorta preparations from patients with Marfan-like pathology. Carotid dissection, often accompanied by dissection of the innominate artery, can also occur as a sequela of aortic dissection [40].

Investigation of the connective tissue components of skin biopsies by electron microscopy revealed ultrastructural abnormalities in the collagen and elastic fibres morphology in the majority (50-60%) of the patients with spontaneous CAD [41-44] (Figure 1).

None of the patients in these studies [40,41] had clinical signs of known hereditary connective tissue disorders, which are anyway rare amongst CAD patients [44]. The finding of connective tissue alterations in skin biopsies from CAD patients but not in biopsies from healthy controls was recently confirmed by independent biochemical methods [45], but alterations of skin elasticity, as they were diagnosed in patients with Ehlers Danlos syndrome, could not be measured in CAD patients [46]. Since the morphologic alterations in the dermal connective tissue of CAD patients are generally very mild, their detection depends on a sophisticated technology (electron microscopy and light microscopy) and its evaluation is a matter of specialists. The association of CAD with morphologic connective tissue alterations in skin biopsies was also confirmed by morphometric studies [47].The authors of this latter study rightly emphasize that the presence or absence of electron microscopic alterations alone is not pathognomonic for CAD.

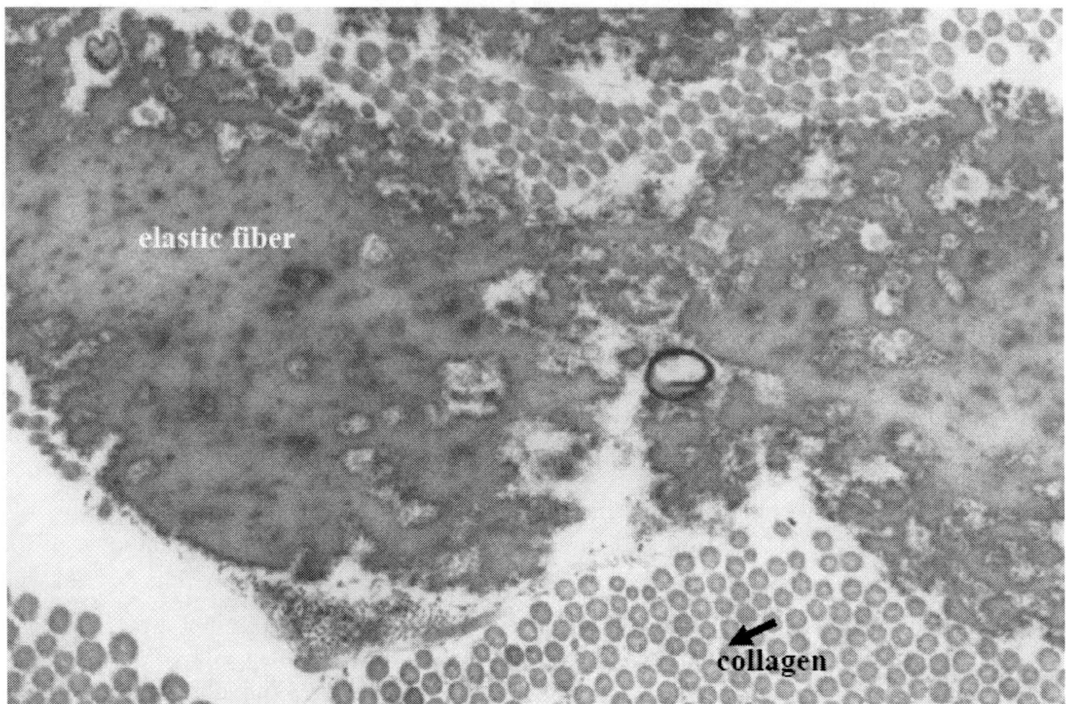

Figure 1. Electron microscopy of connective tissue elements from a skin biopsy of a CAD patient. Note the irregular morphology of the elastic fiber (moth eaten appearance) with the minicalcification (arrow) (figure courtesy of Ingrid Hausser).

In their initial work Brandt, Hausser and colleagues [41,48] emphasized the morphologic alterations of the collagen fibers (flower like appearance of the composite fibers in cross section). Similar morphologic alterations were observed in additional independent studies of CAD patients [43,49,50] During the study of larger series of CAD patients and of patients with intracranial aneurysms [51] two additional but less frequent patterns of connective tissue aberrations in CAD patients were observed [42]. In skin biopsies from these latter patients, the electron microscopic alterations affect predominantly the elastic material, as is illustrated in the above micrograph.

Electron microscopic study of the connective tissue in CAD patients and their healthy relatives revealed an autosomal dominant segregation of the connective tissue phenotype in some analyzed families [42,52]. These observations support the hypothesis of a primary arteriopathy in CAD patients with a genetic background. According to this hypothesis inherited weakness of the arterial wall and the surrounding extracellular matrix may predispose to arterial dissections. However, analysis of several candidate genes involved in connective tissue disorders or involved in the biosynthesis of connective tissue structures did not yet lead to the identification of disease causing mutations (see below).

The pathologic morphology of the arterial wall in patients with a hereditary connective tissue disorder must not necessarily be the consequence of a defective bio-synthesis of a particular connective tissue element, as it can also be caused by degenerative processes. In a mouse model of Marfan syndrome, for instance, the defective morphology of the aorta developed within the first days after birth and was accompanied by inflammatory infiltration.

The recombinant fibrillin-1 molecules of this mouse strain were shown to acts as chemotactic stimuli for macrophages [53]. These experiments might perhaps throw light on the observation that both connective tissue alterations (which is a rare condition) and previous infections (that are unspecific and common) were found to be associated with CAD [21-23]. Acute CAD patients without previous apparent infectious diseases nevertheless revealed mild but significant elevation of several acute phase markers [54,55]. This finding underlines the possible importance of inflammation in the etiology of CAD.

Genetics of CAD

If there are genetic variants that predispose to a disease, a positive family history of that disease should be a risk factor for the disease itself. Stated another way, the disease should cluster within pedigrees if genetic risk factors exist. Unfortunately, the number of reported familial CAD cases is very low. Due to the low prevalence of CAD, systematic studies of the prevalence of CAD were not performed. Hence it is unclear whether there is any clustering within pedigrees or whether the few familial cases occurred by accident in one and the same family. A single family with three first degree relatives affected with CAD [52], however, suggested that common familial factors predisposing to CAD might seem to exist. The low prevalence of familial cases indicates that CAD is no Mendelian disorder with highly penetrant disease-causing mutations. We rather expect that CAD is a complex disease with several predisposing genetic variants that each contribute in a modest way to its pathogenesis.

Three main research strategies were developed to identify disease-associated or disease causing genetic factors.

Genetic Linkage Analysis

The clear definition of a biologically homogeneous disease phenotype or the identification of a subclinical phenotype is the first step of each successful genetic analysis. In fact the connective tissue phenotype described by Brandt and Hausser can be considered as such an intermediate phenotype. Familial CAD is very rare [6] and therefore classical linkage studies to identify unknown candidate genes cannot be performed, due to lack of family material. However, the CAD-associated connective tissue phenotype shows a classical Mendelian segregation with a regular autosomal dominant pattern, which finding opened the way to classical genome wide linkage studies [52,56,57]. Unfortunately the invasive diagnosis of a connective tissue requires a skin biopsy and is inappropriate for a broad screen of patients and their families. The search for additional intermediate phenotypes or associated traits might be interesting as potential phenotypic markers for genetic linkage studies.

Genetic Association of Candidate Genes

Association analyses are generally designed as case control studies, comparing the prevalence of a genetic variant (an allele) between disease group and control group. The value of such studies depends on the choice of the candidate alleles to be studied as well as on the sizes of the study groups (number of analyzed individuals), which determines the statistical power of the study. The choice of the candidate alleles generally depends on some assumptions concerning the pathophysiology of CAD. Since the effect of a single genetic polymorphism on the disease risk is expected to be modest, large study populations will be required to demonstrate these modest effects with high probability. The study of sufficient large series of patients and healthy controls will probably result in the future to the identification of genetic risk factors for CAD. Candidates for such genetic association studies might be selected from genetic pathways involved in connective tissue biosynthesis, inflammation, or endothelial function. Positive findings in related diseases (stroke, aneurysms etc) or interesting candidate regions from positional studies (for instance chromosome 15q [52,58] might also suggest further candidate variants to be tested in CAD patients.

Genome Wide Association Studies

Detailed information about the tremendous genetic variation in the whole human genome and the technology to genotype hundred thousands of such variants on a single glass slide (Gene Chip) opened the way for genome wide association studies (GWAS). An advantage of this kind of genetic case control studies (compared to candidate studies) is that the GWAS approach is not hypothesis-bound and thus permits the identification of new and unexpected genetic variants. However, as control group and disease group must be compared pair wise for each of the genetic variants, the number of performed statistical tests in a GWAS will be very large (usually > hundred thousand) and as a consequence the number of false positive test results will increase correspondently. Indeed, many genetic association studies have yielded irreproducible results [59,60] and questions regarding the methodology of these studies (patient's selection, phenotype, sample size, statistical evaluation) must be carefully considered [61,62]. No GWAS with CAD patients has been performed yet, but large series of patients are currently recruited by the CADISP consortium (see below) with the aim to perform for such kinds of studies.

Until now, most candidate gene association studies were performed with small series of (< 100) CAD patients. Moreover, most genetic variants were tested only in a single study. For a recent overview of the analyzed genes see [63,64]. Positive associations were reported for variants in COL3A1 [50], MTHFR [65-67] in ICAM-1 [68] and in LOXL1 [58]. However, the positive association of the 2bp deletion in the COL3A1 transcript was not confirmed in a subsequent larger study with >200 CAD patients and > 200 healthy control subjects (Christiane Wagner, doctoral thesis in preparation). The finding of a significant association of the ICAM-1 469E allele with CAD observed in the German population was not reproduced in an independent sample of CAD patients from Italy (Pezzini and Grond-Ginsbach, unpublished). The reported association between LOXL1 and CAD was based on a nominal significance level of 5% found for a single SNP (rs3825942) in the LOXL1 gene, whereas 11 further variants in the same gene were not significantly associated with CAD. Amazingly, this very SNP rs3825942 (that was informative in the large pedigree studied by genome wide linkage before) did not co-segregate with the disease phenotype in that study [52]. Moreover, no mutations were found in the LOXL1 gene [52,58]. The author's tentative conclusion that genetic variation in LOXL1 might play a role as a risk factor for sCAD [58] seems therefore not too firmly established. The reported association between the MTHFR 677T genotype and CAD [67], albeit not reproduced in one study [69], appeared to be the only genetic association with CAD that has been confirmed in several independent investigations [65,66,70,71].

Several genes involved in connective tissue biosynthesis or in the etiology of inherited connective tissue disorders have been studied or are currently being studied by SSCP (single strand conformation polymorphism) analysis and/or sequencing analysis to look for disease mutations (COL1A1 [72], COL3A1 [56, 73], COL5A1 [74], COL5A2 [75], COL8A1 [76], COL8A2 [76], ELN [77], CSPG4 [52], ABCC6 [78], MYH11, TGFBR2, ACTA2 [Wiest et al, unpublished data]). Apart from observed mutations in some rare patients [6,72,79], these mutation search studies remained without positive results. Moreover, these few patients with a detected mutation presented several clinical aspects that are not typical for CAD patients. A COL1A1 glycine substitution was found in one patient who presented with dissections of all cervical arteries and with minor signs of Osteogenesis imperfecta [72]. A comparable missense mutation in COL3A1 was found in a young patient with familial dissection [6]. The effect of the glycine substitution in the helical region of the alpha2 chain of type V procollagene found in a patient with bilateral dissection remains unclear and we cannot firmly substantiate, that this variant does play any role in the etiology of CAD. A presumed COL5A1 mutation found in one CAD patient [74] turned out to be rare variant probably without phenotypic effect as we analysis a larger series of control subjects for another study [6].

Clinical Manifestations

CAD can occur as mono- or oligosymptomatic form with isolated new onset of pain or a cranial nerve deficit but also as full hemispheric or brainstem syndrome with diagnosis of CAD only on further diagnostic work-up including MRI. Characteristic and possibly differentiating features from other etiologies of stroke are the younger age of patient (< 60 years, with a maximum of 35-45 years) in association with a painful Horner´s syndrome (Table 1).

The pain is commonly described as unusual, unilateral, severe or sharp in all localizations of CAD and might occur as isolated symptom [80]. With dissection of the ICA the pain is localized in the antero-lateral area of the neck, often including the mastoid area and lateral mandible. In dissection of the VA, frequency of neck pain with a dorsolateral localization is higher with up to 50%. Concomitant headaches are severe and mostly described as unusual by the patients, sometimes throbbing but mostly sharp and continuous, and in 80% ipsilateral to the CAD. In up to 70% of the patients headaches are the initial symptoms of CAD. A pulsatile ipsilateral tinnitus might occur with CAD of the ICA and VA [81].

A local sign of CAD is a Horner´s syndrome by compression of the periadvential sympatic nerve plexus occuring in up to 50% with ICA dissection [81,1]. Thus, for ICA dissection, the most characteristic and potentially differentiating features from other stroke etiologies are young age and presence of a painful Horner´s syndrome. Another local symptom is an ipsilateral cranial nerve deficit. Involvement of all single cranial nerves is described with dissection of the ICA, but lower cranial nerve deficits are far more frequent. Also isolated cranial nerve deficits are described, e.g. for the hyopglossus nerve. The combination of ipsilateral cranial nerve findings and contralateral hemispheric deficits in dissection of the ICA imitating brain stem ischemia is described as "false localising sign" [82]. Local symptoms often precede ischemic events for several days up to 4 weeks [81].

In summary, unusual local neck pain or headaches in combination with a new onset of an ipsilateral Horner syndrom or cranial nerve deficit could be called the specific warning syndrome of acute CAD and is present *initially* in approximately 20% of all patients with CAD.

Table 1. Characteristic clinical signs and symptoms of ICA and VA Dissection

Symptoms
Unusual and unilateral sharp neck pain
ICA: antero-lateral neck radiating to mandible, mastoid and ear (20-40%)
VA: dorsal neck (about 50%)
Headaches (80%)
ICA: unilateral, mostly dull and severe, sometimes throbbing; frontal, retroorbital VA: neck and occiput
Pulsatile tinnitus (10-15%, more common in ICA dissection)
Transient monocular blindness (10-15% in ICA dissection)
TIA (10-20%, in 40% preceding to cerebral infarction)
Signs
Horner´s syndrome (ICA dissection: 40-50%, presenting symptom in 20%; VA dissection: central Horner´s syndrome in 20-30%)
Cranial nerve deficits (ICA dissection: 5-12% III-XII, contralateral to hemispheric deficits as “false localizing sign”, lower cranial nerves more frequent. VA dissection: >50%)
Cerebral infarction (40-90% in selected patient populations)

TIAs associated with CAD are present in about 10%: amaurosis fugax, and hemispheric symptoms for CAD of the ICA whereas dizziness, nausea, double vision, or gait abnormalities for CAD of the VA with brain stem ischemia [13,83,84].

Ischemic infarcts of the distal territories are frequent with CAD and found in 50 to 90% in selected patients. Outcome is mostly benign [1,10]. Due to distal ICA occlusion, however, also life threatening large hemispheric infarction might result. Bogousslavsky and coworkers found in 12% out of 208 large MCA infarcts CAD of the ICA [85]. In a series of 51 patients with basilar artery occlusion in 5 (10%) CAD of the VA was the cause [81]. Asymptomatic forms of CAD detected by Doppler sonography or MRI, however, are described and their incidence might be underestimated in cases with isolated neck or head pain. Patients with intracranial arterial dissections present with either subarachnoid hemorrhage (rare) or brain infarction [14]. Intracerebral vasculitis is a major and difficult differential diagnosis with normaly no mural hematoma to vizualize in these cases prompting cerebral angiography and other studies as spinal fluid analysis and in some cases even menigeal biopsy.

Diagnosis

Ultrasound and Neuroradiological Tools

Clinical diagnosis of CAD is usually confirmed by non-invasive techniques. Doppler sonography is a highly sensitive first diagnostic screening method to confirm a clinically suspected CAD. Typical finding is a high resistance flow pattern in the distal ICA. The use of a transcranial 2 MHz probe for insonation of the distal vessel might be helpful. This flow pattern in combination with characteristic clinical findings and in absence of arteriosclerosis in the carotid bifurcation is highly suggestive for CAD. Pathognonomic signs like a double lumen, a mural hematoma (Figure 2), or an intimal flap of the dissected vessel are rarely observed by color-coded duplex sonography. In the vertebral arteries, presence of a hypoplastic artery (defined as less than 2 mm of diameter, found in about 10% of the healthy population) or a vessel ending in the posterior inferior cerebellar artery might be mistaken as "disturbed flow" in Doppler sonography. Color-coded duplex sonography and / or MR angiography can help to avoid such misinterpretations.

MRI enables to prove dissection by identification of a circular or semilunar-shaped hematoma in the arterial wall (Figure 3) on axial slices 3 days after the event and up to approximately 6 months later. Therefore, if an acute dissection is suspected but not proven by means of sonography, it is advisable to delay MRI studies for the search of specific findings for 2-3 days.

MRI fat-supression sequences are the most sensitive sequences to visualize an intramural hematoma. Spiral CT angiography proved also to be diagnostic by demonstrating an intramural hematoma as well as a string sign and might be positive already in the very first days of CAD. However, the high burden of radiation exposure should be considered. Conventional angiography nowadays rarely is indicated for the diagnosis of CAD, even if historically it had widely been used for this purpose. Typical findings like a "string sign", an intimal flap, or a double lumen have been described (Table 2).

Skin Biopsy and other Advanced Diagnostic Tools

Unfortunately, the extent of the ultrastructural changes in the connective tissue of CAD patients could not be associated with any clinical aspect of the disease. In particular, there is no relationship with the risk of multiple or recurrent dissections or with the occurrence of familiar dissections. Therefore, routine evaluation of skin biopsy cannot be recommended for diagnostic purposes.

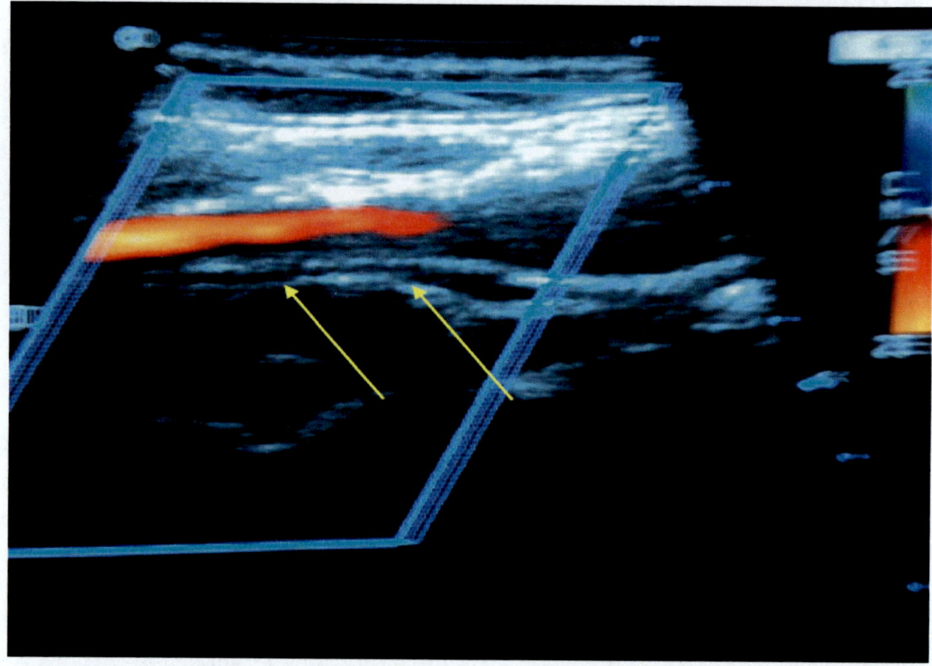

Figure 2. Color-coded duplex sonography. Mural hematoma as a hypoechogenic semilunar perivascular structure.

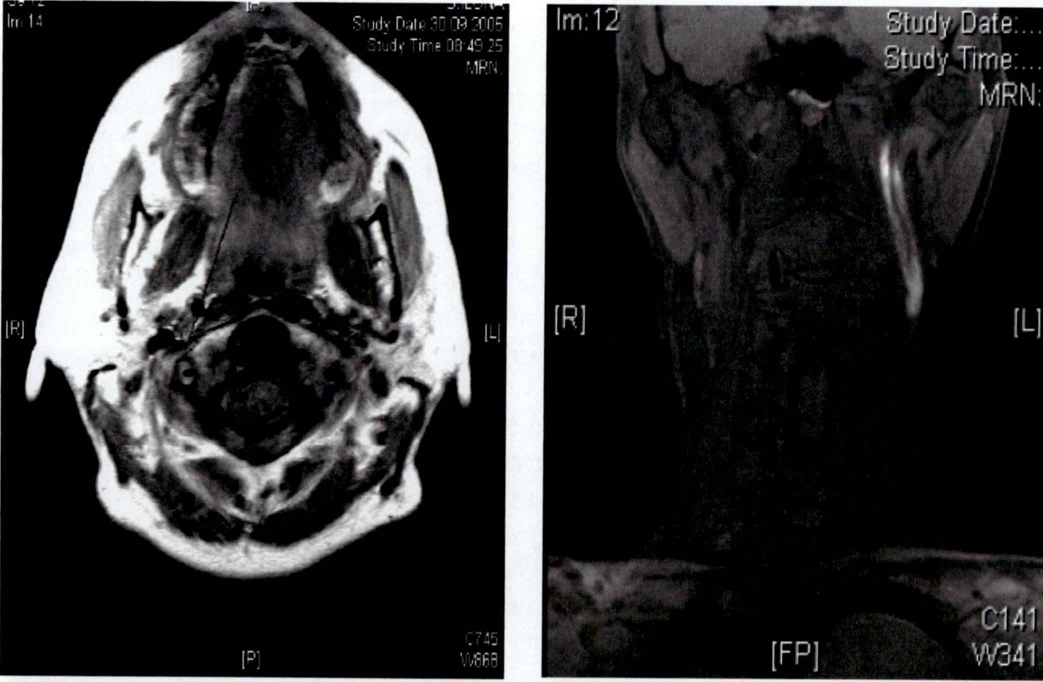

Figure 3. Axial fat suppressed MR imaging of right VA dissection (left picture: arrow) and coronar imaging of left ICA dissection (courtesy Prof. Klaus Sartor).

The investigation of a skin biopsy is indicated to exclude known connective tissue diseases. There is an increased, albeit low (about 2%), incidence of CAD and other neurovascular complications in patients with vascular Ehlers-Danlos syndrome, a known heritable connective tissue disorder [86]. The association of CAD with other connective tissue disorders (Marfan syndrome, osteogenesis imperfecta, or alpha-1-antitrypsin deficiency) was suggested by some case reports but could not be confirmed in a systematic review of the association between CAD and rare connective tissue disorders [87].

Table 2. Diagnosis: characteristic Doppler and imaging findings

Duplex sonography

distal high resistance flow pattern (cw-Doppler, frequent finding, high sensitivity, characteristic follow-up with recanalization >60%)

distal stenosis (TCD 2 MHz-probe)

intimal flap

mural hematoma as a hypoechogenic semilunar perivascular structure (very rare, color-coded duplex)

none or insignificant arteriosclerosis on duplex

Angiography

flame-shaped or tappered occlusion or long segmental stenosis (string sign) distal to carotid bifurcation, in V3-segment of VA (less frequent on origin of the VA in V1-segment)

pseudoaneurysm (5-30%)

signs of FMD (10-15%)

ICA redundancies (coiling/ kinking in about 30% of cases)

CTA/ MRI

semilunar mural hematoma (hyperintensity signal on T1-weighted MRI) as confirmation of diagnosis, MRI with axial and coronal sections including sensitive fat-suppression sequences; MRI sensitive only about 3 days up to 6-9 months after dissection

CTA early detection possible; no differentiation of complete vessel occlusion of intraluminal thrombus vs intramural hematoma (course on follow-up)

The finding of profound connective tissue alterations in a patient with CAD after severe trauma (for instance after a car accident with whiplash injury or due to chiropractic treatment) has sometimes been used as an argument in a legal expert opinion against the exclusive role of trauma in the etiology of CAD. In an investigation of an 29-year-old woman who died from a right hemispheric infarction caused by dissection and subsequent thrombosis of the internal carotid artery after chiropractic manipulations of the neck, Peters and coworkers found in several arteries of muscular and elastic type a mediolytic arteriopathy with widespread mucoid degeneration and cystic transformation of the vessel wall caused by segmental degeneration of smooth muscle cells of the tunica media [38]. The authors hypothesized that mediolytic arteriopathy was a predisposing factor for the dissection of the internal carotid artery after chiropractic manipulations in this patient. This study underlines that CAD has a complex etiology: therefore the finding of one single positive risk factor (albeit a MTHFR 677TT genotype, an infection during the week before onset, a trauma or an aberrant morphology of the dermal connective tissue) is as a rule not sufficient to explain the appearance of the disease (for discussion see [88,89]).

Treatment

Medical Treatment

Use of intravenous rt-PA for acute stroke attributable to CAD has been reported in more than 50 patients. It appears to be safe and effective. Systemic thrombolysis does apparently not increase the risk of wall hematoma extension in CAD. Importantly, no new or worsening focal deficits, subarachnoid hemorrhage, or rupture of the internal carotid artery were observed [90].

There is no controlled study for the best treatment or managment of CAD [91,92]. The rates of recurrent stroke and of recurrent CAD are low. Therefore, huge numbers of patients would be required to perform a randomized controlled trial with sufficient power to compare CAD secondary prevention strategies [91]. Initial empiric treatment which is generally accepted in acute CAD to prevent secondary embolism is PTT-guided anticoagulation with intravenous heparin followed by oral warfarin (or other cumarins like e.g. phenprocoumon). Target INR is 2.5 with a range of 2-3 similarly to the use in atrial fibrillation. Stop of anticoagulation is indicated when complete recanalization by Doppler sonography is diagnosed or no further change of hemodynamics and risk of embolism are to be expected in occluded vessels (as a rule after 3-6 months). However, lack of evidence-based treatment guidelines prompted several national advisory boards to consider anticoagulation and other antithrombotic therypies as equivalent [91]. The finding of a pseudo-aneurysm following CAD is apparently not associated with an increased risk and, therefore, not necessarily an indication for long-term anticoagulation. Aspirin as secondary prophylaxis is prescribed in some cases for several further years.

Interventional Procedures

The use of carotid angioplasty by ballon dilatation and stenting in selected cases of persisting vessel narrowing mostly after traumatic CAD is described in case reports but studies in larger series of patients are lacking. Carotid angioplasty might be useful in selected patients who have persistent brain ischemia due to unilateral severe ICA stenosis or bilateral lumen obstruction. Prior diffusion/ perfusion weighted MRI and transcranial Doppler assessment with CO2-reactivitiy for assessment of intracerebral hemodynamic impairment are recommended to further quantify the probable risk for hemodynamic infarction and the necessity of the intervention.

Surgery

Carotid surgery for treatment of CAD is not anymore recommended with the possible exception of presisting severe stenosis of the proximal ICA. Only one large series with 48 surgically treated patients with CAD and persistent high-grade ICA stenosis is published [93]. Rationale for indication for surgical treatment can be a presistent high-grade ICA stenosis (>70%, corresponding to the symptomatic carotid artery stenosis trials) for at least 6 months or embolization with sufficient anticoagulation. For exposure of the ICA at the base of the skull, the digastric muscle has to be divided. If further exposure is necessary fracture of the styloid at its base is required mostly without removal. Before resection of the dissected segment the artery is clamped proximally to avoid thrombosis and mechanical embolization. Saphneous vein graft replacement is performed in most cases. In 20% early occlusion occured with an 80% overall patency rate after surgery. Infrequently, thrombendarterectomy with patch angioplasty or ligation of the artery is performed. After operation, low-dose heparinization is administered for one week without further anticoagulation thereafter.

Perioperative death was 2% rate in 48 patients caused by intracranial hemorrhage [93]. Risk of perioperative stroke is 10%, early cranial nerve damage occured in 58% of the patients: mostly cranial nerve IX followed by cranial nerves X and XII; infrequently cranial nerve impairment: VII and XI, and Horner´s syndrome. Long-term damage was present in 35% of the patients mostly with hoarseness and minor dysphagia. There is no evidence that pseudoaneurysms increase the risk for embolic complication and there is no evidence for surgery in patients with pseudoaneurysms [94]. Before surgical treatment is considered regression of the stenosis by spontaneous recanalization has to be excluded by doppler sonography for some months.

Prognosis

The prognosis of CAD patients mainly depends on the severity of the initial stroke and on the risk of subsequent stroke. Multivessel CAD or recurrent CAD within the first few weeks is observed in 10-25% of the patients [4]. Clinical outcome after CAD can vary considerably but is most often benign [1]. In a subgroup of patients, however, CAD might also cause occlusion of the distal ICA resulting in large hemispheric infarction or artery-to artery occlusion of the basilar artery with brain stem infarction [85,95]. In a survey of the literature on outcome after CAD of the ICA in 466 patients Saver found for 76% of the patients mild or no deficits, in 18% moderate, and in 5% of the patients major deficits or death [96].

Recently, the Swiss group around Georgiadis reported a very benign outcome in 298 patients with spontaneous CAD at 3 months. Only 1 patient had an ischemic stroke(0.3%); TIA (3.4%)and retinal ischemia (1%) were also very rare. Importantly, 96 of these patients were treated with ASA and had even less recurrencies as compared to those on anticoagulation (2.1% vs. 5.9%). Also, early ischemic events were extremly rare in patients without inital ischemia (1.1% vs. 6.2%). Thus, the authors conclude within the limitations of a nonrandomized study that oral anticoagulation may be not necessary in patients with spontaneous CAD [97].

Recurrence rate for CAD is low with < 10% (8 years) varying from 4 to 8%. Recurrent dissection of the formerly affected artery is very rare and most often occurs in other cervicocerebral arteries. No risk factors for recurrency besides familial dissection and presence of a hereditary connective tissue disorder could be identified yet. Intense sport activities, however, such as e.g. trampoline exercises should probably be avoided. The same is true for oral contraceptives known to possibly cause abnormalities in the intima in the arterial wall. The late recurrency of dissections up to 14 years after the initial event with potential ischemic sequela underlines the necessity of close follow-up.

Outlook

During the last two decades CAD has increasingly been recognized as a major cause of brain ischemia in young adults. Its clinical diagnosis is definitely confirmed by the demonstration of an intramural hematoma in magnetic resonance imaging. CAD is now one of the best defined stroke etiologies and therefore the subject of a growing number of scientific studies. Moreover, there is considerably progress in the research of some other diseases that might be related to CAD, like intracranial aneurysm, aorta dissection or vascular Ehlers-Danlos syndrome. Progress might be expected in various research areas:

1. Further developments in high resolution imaging [98] combined with functional studies of the arterial elasticity and of the endothelial function [33,34] will perhaps open the way to study the pathologic transformations in the medial layer of the carotid and vertebral arteries before the dissection event occurs. This is particularly important during the acute phase, since in a considerable number of patients (15-25%) a subsequent dissection occurs within a few weeks [4].
2. The search for common genetic variants with a modest impact on the risk for CAD and for rare mutations with a strong effect on the risk for CAD will be intensified during the next few years. Mutations were recently found in patients with aorta dissections (in ACTA2, TGFBR1, TGFBR2, MYH11) and these genes will be also promising candidates for mutation search analysis in CAD patients. Larger series of CAD patients are being enrolled in the CADISP (Cervical Artery Dissection and Ischemic Stroke Patients – www.chazard.org/cadisp) study, which will enable to perform genetic association studies with sufficient power. The CADISP was established in 2004 to coordinate and intensify research on CAD. Centers from eight European countries (Belgium, Finland, France, Germany, Great-Britain, Italy, Switzerland and Turkey) are currently participating. The CADISP consortium harbors neurologists as well as specialists from a variety of other disciplines (genetics, dermatology, neuro-immunology, epidemiology, electron microscopy, neuro-radiology, neuro-rehabilitation). CADISP is a steadily growing network, open to integrate additional centers that are interested in collaborative research and that are willing to contribute to the central documentation and DNA-databases.

3. The analysis of large cohorts of patients (for instance [5,24]) yielded already extremely valuable data on epidemiology, prognosis and natural history of CAD. Additional large series will be analyzed in the near future, amongst other from the CADISP consortium. These data will perhaps enable the distinction of various subgroups of CAD patients with different risk profiles. Moreover, they might help to rationalize the treatment strategies currently used for secondary prevention of CAD.

Acknowledgments

We are indebted to Dr. Ingrid Hausser and Prof. Marius Hartmann for the illustrations and to Prof. Werner Hacke for excellent working conditions. We are grateful to Drs. Marie-Luise Arnold, Tina Wiest, Manja Kloss and Alessandro Pezzini for critical reading of the manuscript and for valuable suggestions.

References

[1] Lee VH, Brown RD, Mandrekar JN, Mokri B. Incidence and outcome of cervical artery dissection: A population-based study. *Neurology* 2006;67:1809-1812.

[2] Schievink WI. Spontaneous dissection of the carotid and vertebral arteries. *N. Engl. J. Med.* 2001;344:898-906.

[3] Touzé E, Gauvit JY, Moulin T, Meder JF, Bracrad S, Mas JL. Multicenter survey on Natural History of Cervical Artery Dissection. *Neurology* 2003;61:1347-1351.

[4] Dittrich R, Nassenstein I, Bachmann R, Maintz D, Nabavi DG, Heindel W, Kuhlenbaumer G, Ringelstein EB. Polyarterial clustered recurrence of cervical artery dissection seems to be the rule. *Neurology* 2007;69:180-6.

[5] Arnold M, Kappeler L, Georgiadis D, Berthet K, Keserue B, Bousser MG, Baumgartner RW. Gender differences in spontaneous cervical artery dissection. *Neurology* 2006;67:1050-2.

[6] Martin JJ, Hausser I, Lyrer P, Busse O, Schwarz R, Schneider R, Brandt T, Kloss M, Schwaninger M, Engelter S, Grond- Ginsbach C. Familial cervical artery dissections – clinical, morphologic and genetic studies. *Stroke* 2006;37:2924-9.

[7] Paciaroni M, Georgiadis D, Arnold M, Gandjour J, Keseru B, Fahrni G, Caso V, Baumgartner RW. Seasonal variability in spontaneous cervical artery dissection. *J. Neurol. Neurosurg. Psychiatry* 2006;77:677–9.

[8] Schievink WI, Wijdicks EF, Kuiper JD. Seasonal pattern of spontaneous cervical artery dissection. *J. Neurosurg.* 1998;89:101-3.

[9] Arauz A, Hoyos, L, Espinoza C, Cantú C, Barinagarrementeria F, Román G. Dissection of cervical arteries: Long-term follow-up study of 130 consecutive cases. *Cerebrovasc. Dis.* 2006;22:150-4.

[10] Leys D, Bandu L, Henon H, Lucas C, Mounier-Vehier F, Rondepierre P, Godefroy O. Clinical outcome in 287 consecutive young adults (15 to 45 years) with ischemic stroke. *Neurology* 2002;59:26-33.

[11] Metso TM, Metso AJ, Helenius J, Haapaniemi E, Salonen O, Porras M, Hernesniemi J, Kaste M, Tatlisumak T. Prognosis and safety of anticoagulation in intracranial artery dissections in adults. *Stroke* 2007;38:1837-42.

[12] Hirth K, Sander S, Hörmann K. Common carotid artery dissection: a rare cause for cervical pain. *J. Laryngol. Otol.* 2002;116:309-11.

[13] Arnold M, Bousser MG, Fahrni G, Fischer U, Georgiades D, Gandjour J, Benninger D, Sturzenegger M, Mattle HP, Baumgartner RW. Vertebral Artery Dissection. Presenting Findings and Predictors of Outcome. *Stroke* 2006;37:2499-2503.

[14] Caplan LR. Dissections of brain-supplying arteries. *Nat. Clin. Pract. Neurol.* 2008;4:34-42.

[15] Evangelista A, Dominguez R, Sebastiá C, Salas A, Permayer-Miralda G, Avegliano G, Elorz C, González-Alujas T, García del Castillo H, Soler-Soler J. Long-Term Follow-Up of Aortic Intramural Hematoma. Predictors of Ourcome. *Circulation* 2003;108:583-9.

[16] Vilacosta I, San Roman JA, Ferreiros J,. Aragoncillo P, Mendez R, Castillo JA,. Rollan MJ, Batlle E, Peral V, Sanchez-. Harguindey L. Natural history and serial morphology of aortic intramural hematoma: a novel variant of aortic dissection. *Am. Heart J.* 1997; 134:495-507.

[17] Brandt T, Grond-Ginsbach C. Spontaneous Cervical Artery Dissection – from risk factors towards pathogenesis. *Stroke* 2002;33:657-8.

[18] Pezzini A, Caso V, Zanferrari C, Del Zotto E, Paciaroni M, Bertolino C, Grassi M, Agnelli G, Padovani A. Arterial hypertension as risk factor for spontaneous cervical artery dissection. A case–control study. *J. Neurol. Neurosurg. Psychiatry* 2006;77:95-7.

[19] Pezzini A, Granella F, Grassi M, Bertolino C, Del Zotto E, Immovilli P, Bazzoli E, Padovani A, Zanferrari C. History of migraine and risk of spontaneous cervical artery dissection. *Cephalalgia* 2005;25:575-80.

[20] Tzourio C, Benslamia L, Guillon B, Aidi S, Bertrand M, Berthet K, Bousser MG. Migraine and the risk of cervical artery dissection: a case-control study. *Neurolog.* 2002;59:435-7.

[21] Grau AJ, Brandt T, Forsting M, Winter R, Hacke W. Infection-associated cervical artery dissection. Three cases. *Stroke* 1997;28:453-5.

[22] Grau AJ, Brandt T, Buggle F, Orberk E, Mytilineos J, Werle E, Conradt, Krause M, Winter R, Hacke W. Association of cervical artery dissection with recent infection. *Arch Neurol.* 1999;56:851-6.

[23] Guillon B, Berthet K, Benslamia L, Bertrand M, Bousser MG, Tzourio C. Infection and the risk of spontaneous cervical artery dissection: a case-control study. *Stroke* 2003; 34:79-81.

[24] Arnold M, Pannier B, Chabriat H, Nedeltchev K, Stapf C, Buffon F, Crassard I, Thomas F, Guize L, Baumgartner RW, Bousser MG. Vascular risk factors and morphometric data in cervical artery dissection: a case-control study. J Neurol Neurosurg Psychiatry. 2009;80:232-4.

[25] Dittrich R, Rohsbach D, Heidbreder A, Heuschmann P, Nassenstein I, Bachmann R, Ringelstein EB, Kuhlenbäumer G, Nabavi DG. Mild mechanical traumas are possible risk factors for cervical artery dissection. *Cerebrovasc. Dis.* 2006;23:275- 81.
[26] Rubinstein SM, Peerdeman SM, van Tulder MW, Riphagen I, Haldeman S. A systematic review of the risk factors for cervical artery dissection. *Stroke* 2005;36:1575-80.
[27] Rothwell DM, Bondy SJ, Williams JI. Chiropractic manipulation and stroke: a population-based case-control study. *Stroke* 2001;32:1054-60.
[28] Gupta R, Schumacher HC, Mangla S, Meyers PM, Duong H, Khandji AG, Marshall RS, Mohr JP, Pile-Spellman J. Urgent endovascular revascularization for symptomatic intracranial atherosclerotic stenosis. *Neurology* 2003;61:1729 -35.
[29] Le Roux PD, Elliott JP, Eskridge JM, Cohen W, Winn HR. Risks and benefits of diagnostic angiography after aneurysm surgery: a retrospective analysis of 597 studies. *Neurosurgery* 1998;42:1248-54.
[30] Gould DB, Cunningham K. Internal carotid artery dissection after remote surgery. Iatrogenic complications of anesthesia. *Stroke* 1994;25:1276-8.
[31] Cerrato P, Giraudo M, Bergui M, Baima C, Grasso M, Rizzuto A, Lentini A, Gallo G, Bergamasco B. Internal carotid artery dissection after mandibular third molar extraction. *J. Neurol.* 2004;251:348-9.
[32] Siwiec RM, Solomon GD. Bilateral carotid artery dissection after dental work. *Headache* 2007;47:1449-50.
[33] Baumgartner RW, Lienhardt B, Mosso M, Gandjou J, Michael N, Georgiadis D. Spontaneous and Endothelial-Independent Vasodilation Are Impaired in Patients With Spontaneous Carotid Dissection. A Case-control Study. *Stroke* 2007;38:405-6.
[34] Calvet D, Boutouyrie P, Touze E, Laloux B, Mas JL, Laurent S. Increased stiffness of the carotid wall material in patients with spontaneous cervical artery dissection. *Stroke* 2004;35:2078-2082.
[35] Lucas C, Lecroart JD, Gautier C, Leclerc X, Dauzat M, Leys D, Deklunder G. Impairment of endothelial function in patients with spontaneous cervical artery dissection: evidence for a general arterial wall disease. *Cerebrovasc. Dis.* 2004;17:170-4.
[36] Dziewas R, Konrad C, Drager B, Evers S, Besselmann M, Ludemann P, Kuhlenbaumer G, Stogbauer F, Ringelstein EB. Cervical artery dissection–clinical features, risk factors, therapy and outcome in 126 patients. *J. Neurol.* 2003;250:1179-84.
[37] Brandt T, Morcher M, Hausser I. Association of cervical artery dissection with connective tissue abnormalities in skin and arteries. *Front Neurol. Neurosci.* 2005; 20:16-29.
[38] Peters M, Bohl J, Thömke F, Kallen KJ, Mahlzahn K, Wandel E, Meyer zum Büschenfelde KH. Dissection of the internal carotid artery after chiropractic manipulation of the neck. *Neurology* 1995;45:2284-6.
[39] Völker W, Besselmann M, Dittrich R, Navabi D, Konrad C, Dziewas R, Evers S, Grewe S, Krämer C, Bachmann R, Stögbauer F, Ringelstein EB, Kuhlenbäumer G. Generalized arteriopathy in patients with cervical artery dissection. *Neurology* 2005; 64:1508-13.

[40] Zirkle PK, Wheeler JR, Gregory RT, Snyder SO Jr, Gayle RG, Sorrell K. Carotid involvement in aortic dissection diagnosed by duplex scanning. *J. Vasc. Surg*. 1984;1: 700-3.

[41] Brandt T, Orberk E, Weber R, Werner I, Busse O, Muller B, Wigger F, Grau A, Grond-Ginsbach C, Hausser I: Pathogenesis of cervical artery dissections: Association with connective tissue abnormalities. *Neurology* 2001;57:24-30.

[42] Hausser I, Muller U, Engelter S, Lyrer P, Pezzini A, Padovani A, Moormann B, Busse O, Weber R, Brandt T, Grond-Ginsbach C. Different types of connective tissue alterations associated with cervical artery dissections. *Acta Neuropathol.* (Berl) 2004;107:509-14.

[43] Ulbricht D, Diederich NJ, Hermanns-Le T, Metz RJ, Macian F, Pierard GE. Cervical artery dissection: An atypical presentation with Ehlers-Danlos-like collagen pathology? *Neurology* 2004;63:1708-10.

[44] Dittrich R, Heidbreder A, Rohsbach D, Schmalhorst J, Nassenstein I, Maintz D, Ringelstein EB, Nabavi DG, Kuhlenbäumer G. Connective tissue and vascular phenotype in patients with cervical artery dissection. *Neurology* 2007;68:2220-4.

[45] Uhlig P, Bruckner P, Dittrich R, Ringelstein EB, Kuhlenbäumer G, Hansen U. Aberrations of dermal connective tissue in patients with cervical artery dissection (sCAD). *J. Neurol.* 2008;255:340-6.

[46] Heidbreder AE, Ringelstein EB, Dittrich R, Navabi D, Metze D, Kuhlenbäumer G. Assessment of skin extensibility and joint hypermobility in patients with spontaneous cervical artery dissection and Ehlers-Danlos syndrome. *J. Clin. Neurosci.* 2008;15:650-3

[47] Völker W, Ringelstein EB, Dittrich R, Maintz D, Nassenstein Il, Heindel W, Grewe S Kuhlenbaumer G. Morphometric Analysis of Collagen Fibrils in Skin of Spontaneous Cervical Artery Dissection Patients. *J. Neurol. Neurosurg. Psychiatry* 2008 Sep;79: 1007-12.

[48] Brandt T, Hausser I, Orberk E, Grau A, Hartschuh W, Anton-Lamprecht I, Hacke W. Ultrastructural connective tissue abnormalities in patients with spontaneous cervicocerebral artery dissections. *Ann. Neurol.* 1998;44:281-5.

[49] Ogura K, Maegaki Y, Morino S, Ogawa T, Ohno K, Oka A. Vertebral artery dissection in an infant: ultrastructural aberrations in connective tissue components. *Neuropediatrics* 2003;34:307-10.

[50] Sengoku R, Sato H, Honda H, Inoue K, Ono S. Skin collagen abnormalities in a Japanese patient with extracranial internal carotid artery dissection followed by extracranial vertebral artery dissection. *Rinsho Shingeigaku*. 2006;46:140-3.

[51] Grond-Ginsbach C, Schnippering H, Hausser I, Weber R, Werner I, Steiner H, Lüttgen N, Busse O, Grau A, Brandt T. Ultrastructural connective tissue aberrations in patients with intracranial aneurysms. *Stroke* 2002; 33:2192-6.

[52] Wiest T, Hyrenbach S, Bambul P, Erker B, Pezzini A, Hausser I, Arnold M-L, Martin JJ, Engelter S, Lyrer P, Busse O, Brandt T, Grond-Ginsbach C. Genetic analysis of familial connective tissue alterations associated with cervical artery dissections suggests locus heterogeneity. *Stroke* 2006;37:1697-702.

[53] Guo G, Booms P, Halushka M, Dietz H, Ney A, Stricker S, Hecht J, Mundlos S, Robinson RN. Induction of macrophage chemotaxis by aortic extracts of the mgR Marfan mouse model and a GxxPG-containing fibrillin-1 fragment. *Circulation* 2006;114:1855-62.

[54] Forster K, Poppert H, Conrad B, Sander D. Elevated inflammatory laboratory parameters in spontaneous cervical artery dissection as compared to traumatic dissection: a retrospective case-control study. *J. Neurol.* 2006;253:741-5.

[55] Genius J, Dong-Si T, Grau AP, Lichy C. Postacute C-reactive protein levels are elevated in cervical artery dissection. *Stroke* 2005;36:42-4.

[56] von Pein F, Välkkilä M, Schwarz R, Morcher M, Klima B, Grau A, Ala-Kokko L, Hausser I, Brandt T, Grond-Ginsbach C. Analysis of the COL3A1 gene in patients with spontaneous cervical artery dissections. *J. Neurol.* 2002;249:862-6.

[57] Grond-Ginsbach C, Klima B, Weber R, Striegel J, Fischer Chr, Hacke W, Brandt T, Hauser I. Exclusion mapping of the genetic predisposition for cerebral artery dissections by linkage analysis. *Ann. Neurol.* 2002;52:359-64.

[58] Kuhlenbäumer G, Friedrichs F, Kis B, Berlit P, Maintz D, Nassenstein I, Nabavi D, Dittrich R, Stoll M, Ringelstein EB. Association between Single Nucleotide Polymorphisms in the Lysyl Oxidase-Like 1 (LOXL1) gene and Spontaneous Cervical Artery Dissection (sCAD). *Cerebrovascular. Disease* 2007;24:343-8.

[59] Ioannidis JP, Ntzani EE, Trikalinos TA, Contopoulos-Ioannidis DG: Replication validity of genetic association studies. *Nat. Genet.* 2001;29:306-9.

[60] Ioannidis JP. Why most published research findings are false. *PLoS Med.* 2005;2:124.

[61] McCarthy MI, Abecasis GR, Cardon LR, Goldstein DB, Little J, Ioannidis JP, Hirschhorn JN. Genome-wide association studies for complex traits: consensus, uncertainty and challenges. *Nat. Rev. Genet.* 2008;9:356-69.

[62] Zondervan KT, Cardon LR. Designing candidate gene and genome-wide case control association studies. *Nat. Protoc.* 2007;2:2492-501.

[63] Grond-Ginsbach C, Debette S, Pezzini A. Genetic approaches in the study of risk factors for cervical artery dissection. *Front Neurol. Neurosci.* 2005;20:30-43.

[64] Debette S, Markus H. The genetics of cervical artery dissection: a systematic review. Stroke. 2009;40:e459-66

[65] Arauz A, Hoyos L, Cantúd C, Jara A, Martínez L, García I, de los Ángeles Fernández M, Alonso E. Mild Hyperhomocysteinemia and Low Folate Concentrations as Risk Factors for Cervical Arterial Dissection. *Cerebrovasc. Dis.* 2007;24:210-4.

[66] Kloss M, Wiest T, Hyrenbach S, Werner I, Arnold M-L, Lichy C, Grond Ginsbach C. MTHFR 677TT genotype increases the risk for cervical artery dissections. *J. Neurol. Neurosurg. Psychiatry.* 2006;77:951-952.

[67] Pezzini A, Del Zotto E, Archetti S, Negrini R, Bani P, Alberini A, Grassi M, Assanelli D, Gasparotti R, Vignolo LA, Magoni M, Padovani A. Plasma homocysteine concentration, C677T MTHFR genotype and 844ins68bp CBS genotype in young adults with spontaneous cervical artery dissection and atherothrombotic stroke. *Stroke* 2002;33:664-9.

[68] Longoni M, Grond-Ginsbach C, Grau AJ, Genius J, Debette S, Schwaninger M, Ferrarese C, Lichy C. The ICAM-1 E469K gene polymorphism is a risk factor for spontaneous cervical artery dissection. *Neurology* 2006;66:1273-5.

[69] Konrad C, Müller GA, Langer C, Kuhlenbäumer G, Berger K, Nabavi DG, Dziewas R, Stögbauer F, Ringelstein EB, Junker R. Plasma homocysteine, MTHFR C677T, CBS 844ins68bp, and MTHFD1 G1958A polymorphisms in spontaneous cervical artery dissections. *J. Neurol.* 2004;251:1242-8.

[70] Pezzini A, Grassi M, Del Zotto E, Giossi A, Monastero R, Della Volta G, Archetti S, Zavarise P, Camarda C, Gasparotti R, Magoni M, Cararda R, Padovani A. Migraine mediates the influence of C677T MTHFR genotype on ischemic stroke risk with a stroke subtype effect. *Stroke* 2007;38:3145-51.

[71] McGolgan, Sharma P. The genetics of carotid dissection: meta-analysis of a MTHFR/C677T common molecular variant. Cerebrovasc Dis. 2008;25:561-5

[72] Mayer SA, Rubin BS, Starman BJ, Byers PH. Spontaneous multivessel cervical artery dissection in a patient with a substitution of alanine for glycine (G13A) in the alpha 1(I) chain of type I collagen. *Neurology* 1996;47:552-6.

[73] Kuivaniemi H, Prockop DJ, Wu Y, Madhatheri SL, Kleinert C, Earley JJ, Jokinen A, Stolle C, Majamaa K, Myllyla VV, Norrgard O, Schievink WI, Mokri B, Fukawa O, ter Berg JWM, De Paepe A, Lozano AM, Leblanc R, Ryynanen M, Baxter BT, Shikata H, Ferell RE, Tromp G. Exclusion of mutations in the gene for type III collagen (COL3A1) as a common cause of intracranial aneurysms or cervical artery dissections: results from sequence analysis of the coding sequences of type III collagen from 55 unrelated patients. *Neurology* 1993;43:2652–8.

[74] Grond-Ginsbach C, Weber R, Haas J, Orberk E, Kunz S, Busse O, Hausser I, Brandt T, Wildemann B. Mutations in the COL5A1 coding sequence are not common in patients with spontaneous cervical artery dissections (sCAD). *Stroke* 1999; 30:1887-90.

[75] Grond-Ginsbach C, Wigger F, Morcher M, von Pein F, Grau A, Hausser I, Brandt T. Sequence analysis of the COL5A2 gene in patients with spontaneous cervical artery dissections. *Neurology* 2002;58:1103-5.

[76] Kuhlenbaumer G, Muller US, Besselmann M, Rauterberg J, Robenek H, Hunermund G, Brandt T, Ringelstein EB, Stogbauer F, Hausser I. Neither collagen 8A1 nor 8A2 mutations play a major role in cervical artery dissection. A mutation analysis and linkage study. *J. Neurol.*. 2004;251:357-9.

[77] Grond-Ginsbach C, Thomas-Feles C, Werner I, Hausser I, Weber R, Wigger F, Brandt T. Mutations in the tropoelastin gene (ELN) were not found in patients with spontaneous cervical artery dissections. *Stroke* 2000;31:1935-8.

[78] Morcher M, Hausser I, Brandt T, Grond-Ginsbach C. Heterozygous carriers of Pseudoxanthoma elasticum were not found among patients with cervical artery dissections. *J. Neurol.* 2003;250:983-6.

[79] Wagner C, Kloss M, Lichy C, Grond-Ginsbach C. A glycine-valine substitution in alpha2 type V procollagen associated with recurrent cervical artery dissection. *J. Neurol.* 2008;255:1421-2.

[80] Arnold M, Cumurciuc R, Stapf C, Favrole P, Berthet K, Bousser MG. Pain as the only symptome of cervical artery dissection. *J. Neurol. Neurosurg. Psychiatry* 2006;77: 1021-4.

[81] Biousse V, D'Anglejan-Chatillon J, Touboul PJ, Amarenco P, Bousser MG. Time course of symptoms in extracranial carotid artery dissections. A series of 80 patients. *Stroke* 1995;26:235-9.

[82] Hess DC,Sehti KD,Nichols FT (1990) Carotid dissection:a new false localising sign. *J Neurol. Neurosurg. Psychiatry* 1990;53:804-5.

[83] Baumgartner RW; Arnold M, Baumgartner I, Mosso M, Gönner F, Studer A, Schroth G, Schuknecht B, Sturzenegger M. Carotid dissection with and without ischemic events: local symptoms and cerebral artery findings. *Neurology* 2001;57:827-32.

[84] Baumgartner RW, Bogousslavsky J. Clinical manifestations of carotid dissection. *Front Neurol. Neurosci.* 2005;20:70-6.

[85] Heinsius T, Bogousslavsky J, van Melle G. Large infarcts in the middle cerebral artery territory. Etiology and outcome patterns. *Neurology* 1998;50:341-350.

[86] Pepin M, Schwarze U, Superti-Furg, A, Byers PH. Clinical and Genetic Features of Ehlers-Danlos Syndrome Type IV, the Vascular Type. *N. Engl. J. Med.* 2000;342:673-80.

[87] Grond-Ginsbach C, Debette S. The association of connective tissue disorders with cervical artery dissections. *Curr. Mol. Med.* 2009;9:210-4.

[88] Bacigaluppi S, Rusconi R, Rampini P, Annoni F, Zavanone ML, Carnelli V, Gaini SM.Vertebral artery dissection in a child. Is "spontaneous" still an appropriate definition? *Neurol. Sci.* 2006;27:364-8.

[89] Pezzini A, Hausser I, Brandt T, Padovani A, Grond-Ginsbach C. Internal carotid artery dissection after French horn playing. Spontaneous or traumatic event? *J. Neurol.* 2003; 250:1004-1005.

[90] De Keyser J, Gdovinová Z, Uyttenboogaart M, Vroomen PC, Luijckx GJ. Intravenous Alteplase for Stroke. Beyond the Guidelines and in Particular Clinical Situations. *Stroke* 2007;38:2612-8.

[91] Engelter ST, Brandt T, Debette S, Caso V, Lichy C, Pezzini A, Abboud S, Bersano A, Dittrich R, Grond-Ginsbach C, Hausser I, Kloss M, Grau A, Tatlisumak T, Leys D, Lyrer PA. Antiplatelets versus anticoagulation in cervical artery dissection - pathophysiological considerations, observational data, systematic review findings and conclusions by analogy. *Stroke* 2007;38:2605-11.

[92] Georgiadis D, Caso V, Baumgartner RW. Acute therapy and prevention of stroke in spontaneous carotid dissection. *Clin. Exp. Hypertens.* 2006;28:365-70.

[93] Müller BT, Luther B, Hort S, Neumann-Haefelin T, Aulich A, Sandmann W. Surgical treatment of 50 carotid dissections: indications and results. *J. Vasc. Surg.* 2000;31:980-8.

[94] Guillon B, Brunereau L, Biousse V, Djouhri H, Levy C, Bousser MG. Long-term follow-up of aneurysms developed during extracranial internal carotid artery dissection. *Neurology* 1999;53:117-22.

[95] Brandt T, von Kummer R, Müller-Küppers M, Hacke W. Thrombolytic therapy of acute basilar artery occlusion. Variables affecting recanalization and outcome. *Stroke* 1996;27:875-81.

[96] Saver JL, Easton JD, Hart RG. Dissections and trauma of cervicocerebral arteries. In Barnett HJM, Mohr JP, Stein BM, Yatsu FM (eds). Stroke: Pathophysiology, Diagnosis and Management. New York, Churchill Livingstone, 1998, 3rd edition, pp 769-90.

[97] Georgiadis D, Arnold M, von Buedingen HC, Valko P, Sarikaya H, Rousson V, Mattle HP, Bousser MG, Baumgartner RW. Aspirin vs anticoagulation in carotid artery dissection: a study of 298 patients. Neurology. 2009;72:1810-5.

[98] Bachmann R, Nassenstein I, Kooijman H, Dittrich R, Stehling C, Kugel H, Niederstadt T, Kuhlenbaumer G, Ringelstein EB, Kramer S, Heindel W. High resolution magnetic resonance imaging (MRI) at 3.0 Tesla in the short-term follow-up of patients with proven cervical artery dissection. *Invest. Radiol.* 2007;42:460-6.

In: Cerebral Ischemia in Young Adults
Editors: A. Pezzini and A. Padovani
ISBN 978-1-60741-627-2

Chapter 11

Vasculitis

Marta Altieri[1]*, Roberta Priori[2], Alessio Mercurio[1], Guido Valesini[2] and Vittorio Di Piero[1]
1. Department Neurological Sciences, "La Sapienza" University, Rome, Italy
2. Rheumatology Unit, "La Sapienza" University, Rome, Italy

Abstract

Vasculitis of the central nervous system (CNS) is a potentially devastating condition representing a diagnostic and therapeutic challenge. Any age, including children, can be affected by the inflammatory process. The overall annual incidence is estimated to be 31–47 cases/million, but is as low as 1–5 cases/million for rare types such as Churg-Strauss.

Almost all forms of vasculitis can involve the vessels feeding the brain parenchyma and cause stroke-like episodes, but the frequency of CNS involvement is highly variable. Indeed, vasculitis is a rare cause of stroke, even in the young age groups.

CNS vasculitis can occur as isolated event of unknown cause (primary CNS vasculitis-PCNSV), or be associated with a known systemic condition (secondary CNS vasculitis) such as an infectious disease, systemic vasculitis, connective tissue autoimune disease, or malignancy.

In these chapter we will discuss the pathogenesis, clinical features and general principles of treatments of PCNSV and other forms of cerebral vasculitis associated with systemic vasculitis and connective tissue diseases.

* Correspondence: Marta Altieri, Clinica Neurologica A, Viale dell'Università 30, 00185 Rome, Italy. Tel +390649914989, Fax +39064457376, marta.altieri@uniroma1.it.

Introduction

The vasculitides are a heterogeneous group of disorders characterized by inflammation and necrosis of the blood vessels. Such angiocentric inflammation may either result to tissue ischemic injury or cause vessel rupture with resultant hemorrhage [1,2].

The vasculitides that affect the central nervous system (CNS) are one of the most intriguing diagnostic and therapeutic challenge for physicians, because their clinical manifestations are highly variable, and correct diagnosis requires a high degree of suspicion coupled with knowledge of other diseases that may mimic vasculitis.

CNS vasculitides are usually classified in two main cathegories: 1) primary (isolated) vasculitis of the CNS (PACNS) - when vasculitis is confined to the CNS-, and 2) secondary vasculitis of the CNS [2,3].

They may affect blood vessels of varying calibre, from the aorta to capillaries and veins, and the classic core histopathological change consists of an inflammatory infiltrate within the vessel wall, in association with fibrinoid necrosis, precipitating vascular occlusion and then infarction which, in turn, accounts for the clinical manifestation (Table 1).

Primary (Isolated) Vasculitis of the CNS

Definitive diagnosis of PACNS is one of the most difficult tasks facing the neurologist. The difficulty has many causes: 1) no pathognomonic clinical presentation of PACNS; 2) neuroimaging, including MRI and MRA, may disclose a pattern consistent with "vasculitis" in a diverse range of non-vasculitic conditions; 3) the results of routine laboratory testing are non-specific or even normal in many patients with PACNS; 4) cerebral angiography is neither sensitive nor specific for vasculitis.

In 1988 Calabrese proposed the following criteria for the diagnosis of PACNS wich are still actual [3]:

The presence of an acquired and otherwise unexplained neurologic deficit

with

Either classic angiographic or histopathologic features of angiitis within the CNS

with

No evidence of systemic vasculitis or any condition that could elicit the angiographic features

PACNS was initially described in the 1950s as a progressive, fatal disorder characterized histologically by granulomatous necrotizing vasculitis [4]. Over time, it was recognized that different clinical subtests of PACNS exist, define by clinical, laboratory, angiographic, and pathologic findings.

Granulomatous Angiitis of the CNS (GACNS)

Granulomatous angiitis of the CNS (GACNS) is the most severe form of PACNS, and accounts for approximately 22% of all patients with PACNS. It is primarily a leptomeningeal and cortical vasculitis, involving the small and medium arteries. Pathologic findings include the classic granulomatous angiitis with Langhans' or foreign body giant cells, necrotizing vasculitis, or lymphocytic vasculitis. The pathological involvement is confined to the brain and spinal cord, though autopsy studies have revealed subclinical extracranial involvement, which may explain the occasional features of fever, rigors, weight loss, raised plasma viscosity [1,5,6].

The range of symptoms, signs, and ancillary test results that have been described in proven GACNS is various. About 70% of patients are male, and the mean age is 46 years. The most common clinical features are decreased cognition (80%), diffuse neurological dysfunction such as encephalopathy (68%), and headache (55%). Isolated stroke occurs in a minority of cases of GACNS; about 15% have ischemic stroke and 11% have intracerebral hemorrhage in the absence of more diffuse symptoms and signs. More often, sudden onset focal deficits due to stroke occur in the setting of progressive, global neurological dysfunction. Seizures occur in about one third of patients. Isolated cases of TIA-like episodes, and cranial neuropathies, have been sporadically described. The true incidence of these symptoms is unknown. Importantly, an acute presentation of GANCS is distinctly unusual and majority of patients have subacute or chronic symptoms. The median time from first symptom onset to definitive diagnosis is 5 months [7].

Salvarani and collegues retrospectively studied the incidence, clinical findings and outcome of 101 patients with PACNS during a 21-year period. They found that mortality rate and disability at last follow-up was greater in those who presented with a focal neurological deficit, cognitive impairment, cerebral infarctions, and angiographic large-vessel involvement and lower in those with prominent gadolinium-enhanced lesions at MRI. The annual incidence rate was 2.4/1000000 person-year [8].

Diagnosting Testing in GACNS

Despite CSF analysis and MRI are usually abnormal, no diagnostic test for GACNS has 100% sensitivity. Routine laboratory testing is unremarkable, and serologic testing for systemic vaculitides is rarely useful unless historical or physical examination findings are suggestive of systemic involvement. The erythrocyte sedimentation rate (ESR) is normal in 35% of biopsy-proven cases of PACNS or less [9].

In pathologically verified GACNS, CSF is abnormal in 80-90% of cases. The median protein is 177 mg/dl, with a median cell count of 55/cc [1]. While the spinal fluid is usually abnormal there are no specific tests to confirm angiitis. Nonetheless, serial CSF analysis can be a useful indicator of disease activity during immunosuppressive treatment [10].

MRI is abnormal in >95% of biopsy-confirmed cases of GACNS, although the findings are non-specific. The most common findings are multiple, bilateral, small cerebral infarctions in the cortex or white matter [11]. Depending on disease activity some, but not all, may be positive on DWI sequences. Some lesions may enhance, suggesting subacute brain infarction.

MRA is generally not useful for diagnosing GACNS. It may reveal multiple areas of stenosis in distal arterial branches, but these findings may be seen in atherosclerosis. Many patients with abnormal catheter angiograms have normal MR angiograms because the vascular pathology is distal to the arteries that are well-visualized by the latter modality.

Angiograms are normal in 40% of cases of GACNS [12]. Of the 60% of cases with abnormal angiograms, one third do not show the “classic” findings of alternating areas of stenosis and ectasia in leptomeningeal vessels [7]. The specificity of an abnormal angiogram is about 25% [13]. Many angiographic mimics of “vasculitis” exist, including vasospasm, reversible cerebral vasoconstriction and atypical atherosclerosis. In biopsy confirmed cases with abnormal angiography, serial angiograms may sometimes be used to objectively verify disease progression or regression [14].

Though CSF and MRI are not specific for GACNS, the combination of normal spinal fluid and normal MRI essentially rules out the diagnosis of GACNS [7].

Biopsy remains the gold standard for diagnosis, and in “biopsy proven” GACNS, the sensitivity is by definition 100%. Biopsy may show granulomatous angiitis, necrotizing vasculitis, or both coexisting in a single specimen [9]. In their cohort Salvarani and Collegues found that 90% of bioptised patients had a granulomatous pattern, 27.6% had a lymphocytic pattern and 17% had an acute necrotizing pattern [8]. Biopsy specimens with a granulomatous pattern were identified more frequently in older-onset patients and for those presenting initially with altered cognition. Because vasculitis is a patchy disease, false negative biopsies occur. One series of autopsy-confirmed cases of GACNS revealed a false negative biopsy rate of 25% [15].

In this box are summarized the main clinical/instrumental features of GACNS:

1. Male-predominant
2. Mean age 45 (wide range)
3. MRI abnormal in 95% biopsy-confirmed cases
4. MRA normal/not useful
5. Angiography 40% normal
6. CSF abnormal 80% (not specific)
7. Biopsy 100% sensitivity
8. False-negative rate 25%
9. Bad prognosis

Treatment of GACNS

There have been no controlled trials of therapy in GACNS. The standard recommendation for treatments involves the combination of glucocorticoids and cyclophosphamide. The most common treatment is high dose intravenous methylprednisolone 1 g/day for 3 to 7 days followed by oral prednisolone 60 mg, together with oral cyclophosphamide (2-2.5 mg/kg/day), or i.v. cyclophosphamide. Azatioprine and methotrexate are recommended as glucocotricoid sparing drugs [16].

Benign Angiopathy of the CNS (BACNS)

BACNS accounts for about 20% of all PACNS and has been considered for a long time as a subset of PACNS on the basis of a characteristic set of clinical findings and a classic or high-probability angiogram [17].

In the box below are summerized the main clinical and instrumental characteristics of BACNS

1. Female-predominant
2. Mean age 35
3. Previous histories of headaches
4. Heavy nicotine or caffeine use
5. Over–the–counter cold remedy use
6. Oral contraceptive
7. MRI normal/abnormal
8. MRA characteristic
9. Angiography
10. CSF normal or slightly abnormal
11. Biopsy negative
12. Good prognosis

Clinically, headache is present in about 90% of cases, stroke or TIA in 40% of patients, seizures in 20%, visual disturbances (diplopia) in 14%, ataxia in 14% and speech abnormality in 7%. Changes in cognition/consciousness may be present in up to 40% of cases [2].

Angiography is characteristic and should present areas of ectasia and narrowings in multiple vascular beds. To satisfy the diagnostic criteria these finding must be reversible within 3 to 4 months of symptom onset [18]. Parenchimal MRI is frequently abnormal: lacunar infarcts may be present in 30% of cases, white matter signal changes in 20%, intracranial hemorrhage in 15%, subaracnoid hemorrhage in 8% [19,20].

Since clinical and instrumental characteristics of GACNS and BACNS are completely different (as summarized in Table 1) and being BACNS more similar to the so called "reversible vasoconstriction syndrome" than to PACNS, there is now strong belief that GACNS and BACNS might be two different clinical entities.

Table 1. comparison between clinical and instrumental characteristics of GACNS and BACNS

GACNS	BACNS
Angiitis	Angiopathy
Male-predominant	Female-predominant
Subacute symptoms' onset	Acute symptoms' onset
MRA not specific	MRA specific
Bad prognosis	Good prognosis

Treatment of BACNS

To date there are no clinical trials on treatment of BACNS. Calcium channel blockers have been used: Verapamil 240 mg/day once daily increasing if symptoms (headaches) are not controlled, or oral Nimodipine 60 mg every 4 hours. The addition of glucocorticoids should be reserved to non-responders patients [1].

Secondary Vasculitis of the CNS Related to Primary Systemic Vasculitis

Among the systemic vasculitides interesting secondarily the CNS, we should distinguish between *primary* and *secondary* variants, being the first idiopathic, and the latter associated with connective tissue disorders.

Along the last few years, some reports have been published proposing new classification systems and criteria for secondary vasculitis of the CNS, based on serology rather than clinical syndromes and involving the abandonment of a longstanding eponymic diagnostic terminology [21].

Recently, primary systemic vasculitides have been categorized into: 1) large vessel vasculitis, causing chronic granulomatous inflammation predominantly of the aorta and its major branches, 2) medium sized vessel vasculitis causing necrotizing inflammation predominantly of mid-sized arteries, and 3) small vessel vasculitis provoking necrotizing inflammation of predominantly capillaries, venules, arterioles, and small arteries [16,22,23].

Large Vessel Vasculitides (Chronic Granulomatous Arteritides)

The two major categories of large vessel vascultis are the Giant Cell Arteritis (GCA) and the Takayasu Arteritis (TA).

Giant Cell Arteritis

Both the American College of Rheumatology (ACR) [24] and the Chapel Hill nomenclature [25] system advocate using the term of GCA (or Horton's disease) rather than temporal arteritis because vasculitides other than giant cell can cause temporal arteritis, and not all patients with giant cell arteritis have temporal artery involvement. Indeed, in same cases vessels other than the temporal arteries, especially the aorta and its primary branches, may be involved [26].

According to the ACR the diagnosis of GCA requires the presence of at least 3 of the following factors [24]:

1. Age at disease onset >50 years
2. New headache
3. Claudication of the jaw and tongue and difficulties with deglutition
4. Temporal artery tenderness to palpation or decreased pulsation
5. Erythrocyte sedimentation rate (ESR) >50 mm/h
6. Temporal artery biopsy showing vasculitis characterized by a predominance of mononuclear cell or granulomatous inflammation, usually with multinucleated giant cells.

Vasculitis can be found along the ophthalmic, posterior ciliary, superficial temporal, occipital, facial, and internal maxillary arteries, primarily in old individuals of either sex.

Temporal artery biopsy is still the better approach for confirming or supporting the diagnosis and a segment approximately 3 cm long should be obtained for reasonable sensitivity. The degree of pathologic injury seems to have a prognostic relevance. As a matter of fact, patients with intense chronic inflammation and numerous multinucleated giant cells seem to have more frequently major complications, such as blindness and cerebrovascular accidents, than those with only chronic inflammation and no giant cells [26,27].

The ESR may be used to monitor treatment response, though cases of low ESR inactive phase are not uncommon.

Classically it manifests as temporal headache with tender, pulseless, nodular temporal arteries and, more rarely, systemic symptoms such as general malaise, jaw claudication and features of polymyalgia reumatica. Blindness occurs in about 1/6 of patients and is the consequence of anterior ischemic optic neuropathy after vasculitic involvement of the posterior ciliary arteries and/or the ophthalmic artery. The typical picture comprises loss of acuity, often with an altitudinal field defect and the fundal appearance varies from normal to mild swelling. In about 30% of cases other neurological manifestation such as neuropsychiatric syndromes, peripheral neuropathies, spinal cord lesions, medullary infarction are observed. Moreover, patients can experience concomitant symptoms of polymyalgia rheumatica [26-29].

Cerebrovascular ischemic events have been reported in 3–7% of patients with GCA, commonly occurring in elderly patients. The vertebrobasilar territory is most frequently involved (carotid/vertebrobasilar rate 3:2 instead of 5:1 of the general population) [27-29]. In the Lausanne Stroke Registry among 4086 patients only 6 (0.15%) had a stroke due to GCA

[30]. All patients were > 50 years and 5/6 were man. The ESR was increased to >50 mm/h only in 3 patients, thus confirming previous results indicating that a normal ESR can also be seen even during the active period of GCA [30].

Clinical and pathologic findings suggest that the ischemic events are due to the involvement of extradural vertebral and carotid arteries with high-grade stenosis or occlusion rather than intracranial vasculitis. The underlying pathologic process in GCA may be an autoimmune reaction involving arterial elastic tissue, which could account for the sparing of the intracranial arteries that have little or no elastic tissue in their two outer coats [31-33]. Only 9 patients are described in literature of GCA involving the intracranial arteries. The presence of intracranial vasculitis in GCA seems to characterize a group of patients whose disease tend to follow a catastrophic course with no response to corticosteroids [33].

Corticosteroids represent the mainstay of treatment for GCA, and prolonged therapy is often necessary. The therapeutic scheme is the following: Prednisolone (60-80 mg daily) for 4-7 days than gradually reduced by 5 mg weekly to reach a maintenance dose of 10 mg daily with the clinical response and the ESR as a guide [34]. However, disease relapses and steroid-related adverse effects are common [35]. Recent retrospective studies as well as experimental models indicate that prevention of platelet aggregation with low-dose aspirin is potentially effective in preventing ischemic complications of GCA. The risk of visual loss and cerebrovascular accidents seems to be decreased in patients receiving aspirin without increasing the risk of bleeding [36,37]. There is still no evidence concerning the use of anticoagulants. Steroid sparing or disease-modifying agents such as methotrexate, azathiprine, cycolsporine A, and anti-TNF-α antagonists, have been used in GCA with conflicting results [34].

Takayasu Arteritis (TA)

TA is an uncommon disease of young women, characterized by granulomatous vasculitis of medium and large arteries with predilection for the aorta and its primary branches. The inflammatory disease primarily involves the media and adventitia of vessel walls and thus results in luminal abnormalities (stenosis, occlusion, aneurysm formation) [38].

In addition to constitutional symptoms, TA presents with several clinical manifestations, such as arm claudication, decreased arterial pulses, carotidynia and hypertension.

Neurological involvement is sporadically reported, and the occurrence of neurological syndromes at onset is even more sporadic. Approximately 10–20% of patients with TA have ischaemic stroke or TIAs [39,40] due to a steno-occlusive vasculitic lesion, thromboembolism, or malignant hypertension [41,42]. Some patients present subaracnoid hemorrhage due to ruptured intracranial aneurysms [43-46].

Accurate diagnosis depends on imaging studies: the use of both MRA and 18-fluorodeoxyglucose PET scan can respectively detect luminal diameter changes, and disparities in vessel metabolic activity. These are indicative of early inflammation, and will probably supersede standard angiography for the diagnosis of TA [47-49].

Traditional treatment is performed with steroid and immunosoppressants but evidence has accumulated that new therapeutic agents, such as anti-TNF α, may provide alternative treatments in refractory patients [50].

Medium Sized Vessel Vasculitides (Necrotizing Arteritides)

The two major forms of medium sized vessel vasculitis are Polyarteritis Nodosa (PAN) and Kawasaki disease (KD). According to the Chapel Hill nomenclature they are necrotizing arteritis confined predominantly to the arteries [25].

Polyarteritis Nodosa

PAN is a rare necrotizing vasculitis affecting small and medium arteries but never arterioles, capillaries and venules, which can present with a wide spectrum of symptoms, mostly aspecific. For this reason, it represents a true diagnostic challenge for the clinicians. This entity has been definitely separated from microscopic polyangiitis which seems to be more frequent.

It is believed that damage is initiated by immune complex deposition; fibrinoid necrosis is typical but not diagnostic. About 30% of patients have hepatitis B antigen or antibody in serum. ANCA antibodies are characteristically negative [51].

According to the ACR 1990 classification criteria, patients with systemic vasculitis can be classified as PAN if they present at least 3 of the following 10 criteria [24]:

1. weight loss above 4 kg
2. livedo reticularis, testicular pain/tenderness
3. myalgias
4. weakness or leg tenderness
5. mononeuropathy or polyneuropathy
6. diastolic blood pressure above 99 mm Hg
7. elevated urea and creatinine
8. HBV
9. arteriographic abnormality
10. biopsy of a small or medium sized artery containing polymorphonuclear neutrophils

The peripheral nervous system is involved in around 70% of cases (mono-polineuropaties), followed by muscle and cutaneous engagement, which is found in about 50% of patients [51].

The most frequent manifestations of CNS involvement are focal lesions localized in the cortex, brain stem and cerebellum due to hyperplasia and occlusion of the small-medium vessel, especially great vessel fork. Vision loss, headache in various form, and encephalopathy with seizures are also common [52].

There are also organ-limited varieties of PAN, such as the cutaneous form or the CNS form, in which are mainly involved the medium-sized arteries. In contrast to what happens for small PACNS, this medium vessel variety can be diagnosed by angiography [53].

The prognosis is heavily dependent on the severity and organ distribution at time of diagnosis. A five-factor prognostic factor has been developed which, besides renal and gastrointestinal involvement, also includes CNS and cardiac engagement [54]. Patients having ≥2 organs involved have the worse prognosis [54].

Strokes occur in 13 to 17% of PAN patients but no specific stroke syndrome has been delineated [55]. They are mainly lacunar, followed by pure lobar hematoma and large ischemic infarcts. Recent reports indicate that stroke can be the inaugural or chief manifestation of PAN and should no longer be considered a late complication. Stroke can be due by atherosclerosis-like mechanism or, more rarely, by segmental inflammation. Corticosteroids may have a detrimental effect in the acute phase, causing an enequal reduction in the production of TXA2 and prostacyclin PG12 [55].

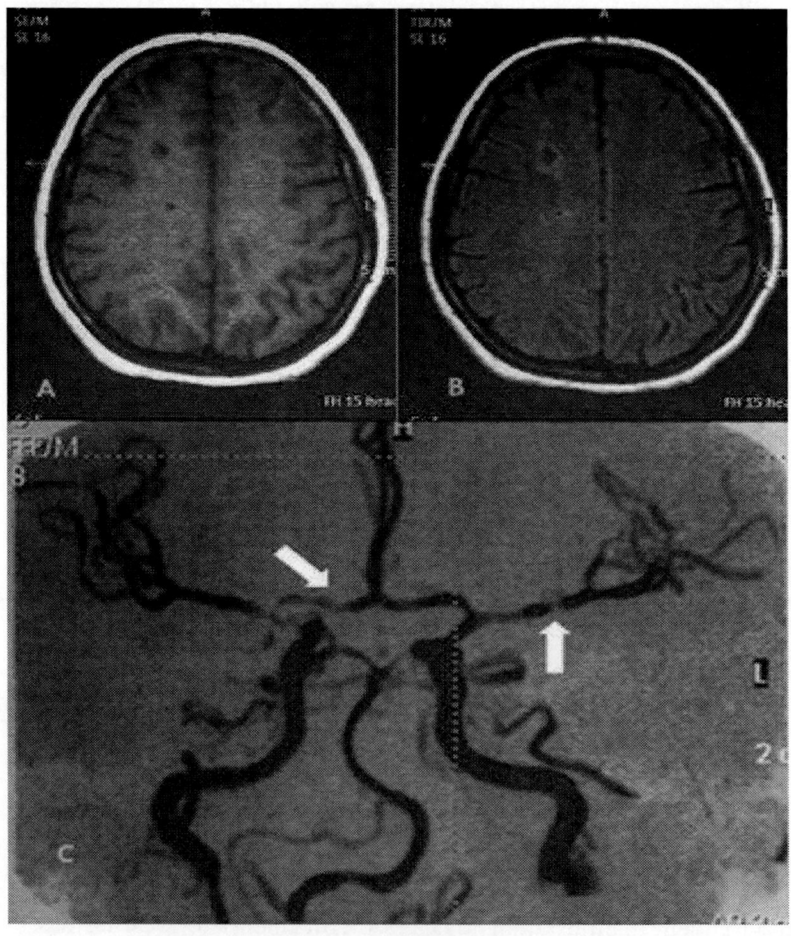

Figure 1.

Cyclophosphamide is indicated when there are negative prognostic factors present, such as renal and gastrointestinal engagement, or when corticosteroids fail to control the disease. Anti tumor necrosis factor-α agents, intravenous γ-globulin infusions and plasmapheresis have been used for refractory cases [56].

Figure 1 shows two lacunar lesions in the right centrum ovale (1A: T1-SE; 1B: T2 Flair) and multiple bilateral narrowings of the middle cerebral arteries (1C: MRA TOF) in a 45 years old Pakistanian woman with PAN admitted to our hospital because of the sudden onset of thunderclap headache followed by multiple episodes of transient left hand paresis and dysarthria.

Kawasaki Disease

KD is a necrotizing medium sized vessel vasculitis affecting mainly chidren under the age of 12 years; however, it has been occasionally reported in adults [57]. KD is quite unusual in the Western countries being far more frequent in Japan.

The etiology and pathophysiology are still unknown though a number of epidemiologic and clinical observations suggest it might be triggered by one or more infectious agents [58].

A complex network of cytokines, endothelin, and other vasoactive mediators resulting in the development of vascular endothelial changes are implicated in leaving a permanent damage on vascular integrity [59].

To date no specific laboratory tool is available for the diagnosis of KD but recently the 2006 EULAR/PreS classification system for childhood vasculitis has proposed the following classification criteria: fever persisting for at least 5 days (mandatory criterion) in addition to four of the five features (unless coronary artery involvement is documented which requires fewer criteria) desquamation in peripheral extremities or perianal region, polymorphous exanthema, conjunctival injection, changes in the oral or pharyngeal mucosa, and cervical lymphadenopathy [60].

Coronary artery involvement is a life threatening complication and should be treated promptly. Indeed, KD is the most common cause of acquired cardiovascular disease in children in the United States [61,62].

CNS complications are unfrequent: patients can have irritability or lethargy while meningitis, facial palsy, subdural effusion, and cerebral infarction have been rarely reported [63-68].

Appropriate therapy with intravenous immunoglobulins and aspirin reduces the incidence of coronary abnormalities to less than 5% dramatically improving the prognosis. Immunoglobulins have been shown to be highly effective in reducing disease symptoms or their severity and chiefly in reducing the rate of coronary artery aneurysm development. Aspirin is firstly used in high dose for its anti-inflammatory properties and then in low dose for its anti-thrombotic effects [69].

Small Vessel Vasculitides (Necrotizing Polyangiitides)

The major forms of small vessel vasculitis are the Wegener's Granulomatosis (WG), Churg-Strauss syndrome (CS), Henoch-Schönlein purpura (HSP), Microscopic Polyangiitis (MPA), Mixed Essential Cryoglobulinemia (MEC) and the Inflammatory Bowel Disease (IBD)-associated vasculitis. This group of vasculitides was found to be closely related to circulating ANCA antibodies. Nevertheless, cases of ANCA-negative small vessels vasculitis have been described.

Wegener's Granulomatosis

WG is a necrotizing granulomatous vasculitis primarily involving the upper and lower respiratory tract and the kidney; however, WG can affect almost any organ, including the nervous system with a prevalence ranging from 30 to 50% according to the different studies. Most frequently it presents with peripheral neuropathies, cranial nerves palsy and optic neuritis as the result from vasculitis of the anterior and posterior ciliary and retinal vessels [51].

CNS impairment is less frequent and occurs in 2–8% of patients. Three major pathogenetic mechanisms can be considered: CNS vasculitis, spreading of granulomas from the adjacent anatomical areas (paranasal cavities, orbit), and new formation of granulomas in brain tissue [70-71]. Contiguous extension from nasal and paranasal sinus cavity granulomas can occur through the orbit leading to pseudotumor with exophthalmos, or may involve extraocular muscles, optic and oculomotor nerves, whereas extension through the temporal bone can destroy the middle ear [51].

The incidence of cerebrovascular accidents in WG is rather low. In one of the oldest studies available so far, 9% of patients with WG experienced cerebrovascular events [70]. These included intracerebral hemorrage (ICH) (3%), subarachnoid hemorrhage (SAH) (2%), cerebral arterial thrombosis (3%), and venous thrombosis (1%). More recent studies confirm the low prevalence of cerebrovascular accidents in WG [72]. All these complications might be linked to a weakening of cell wall by the inflammatory process that eventually leads to the rupture of the involved vessels [73]. Unfortunately, since the small size of the vessels (50–300 MCM) typically involved in WG is below the sensitivity of routine angiography, cerebral angiogram, fails to reveal vasculitic features. [74]. Infarcts may also result from renal failure induced hypertension, emboli from endocarditis or vessel occlusion by a skull base granuloma [75]. Cerebrovascular accidents are reported to occurr also while the patient is under treatment with immunosuppressive agents; Rituximab has proved to be effective in one case of WG with massive intracerebral hemorrage [76].

The lesions of WG begin as minute foci of granular necrosis and fibrinoid degeneration with polymorphonuclear leukocytes followed by histiocytes and giant cells along the margin of granulomas of the upper airway and in the renal glomeruli [51].

The detection of antineutrophil cytoplasmic antibodies directed against proteinase 3 (PR3-ANCA) is highly specific for WG. ANCA positivity is found only in about 50% of the patients with localized WG (which is restricted to the respiratory tract and affects ≤5% of the patients), whereas PR3-ANCA positivity is seen in 95% of the patients with generalized WG [51,70].

MRI is a fundamental tool to the possible presence of central nervous system vasculitis, or the direct spread to the meninges from the orbital, nasal and paranasal localizations of the disease and, exceptionally, the new formation of granulomas; MRI technique is also useful in evaluating the local efficacy of treatment [75-77].

The most widely used immunosuppressive treatment for WG is either the daily administration of low-dose oral cyclophophamide (CY) or high-dose pulse CY, both combined with corticosteroids [78] but other drugs have been successfully used to treat WG such as cyclosporine A, azathioprine, methotrexate, mycophenolate, and the new biologic agents directed against TNF-alpha and CD20+ B-lymphocytes [79-83].

Churg-Strauss Syndrome

CS is characterized by pulmonary and systemic small-vessel necrotizing vasculitis, vascular and/or extravascular eosinophil-rich granulomas, blood eosinophilia occurring in individuals with asthma and often allergic rhinitis or sinusal polyposis. The most frequent clinical findings are transient and patchy pulmonary infiltrates, peripheral neuropathy (50-78%), generally mononeuritis multiplex, and skin lesions such as palpable purpura.

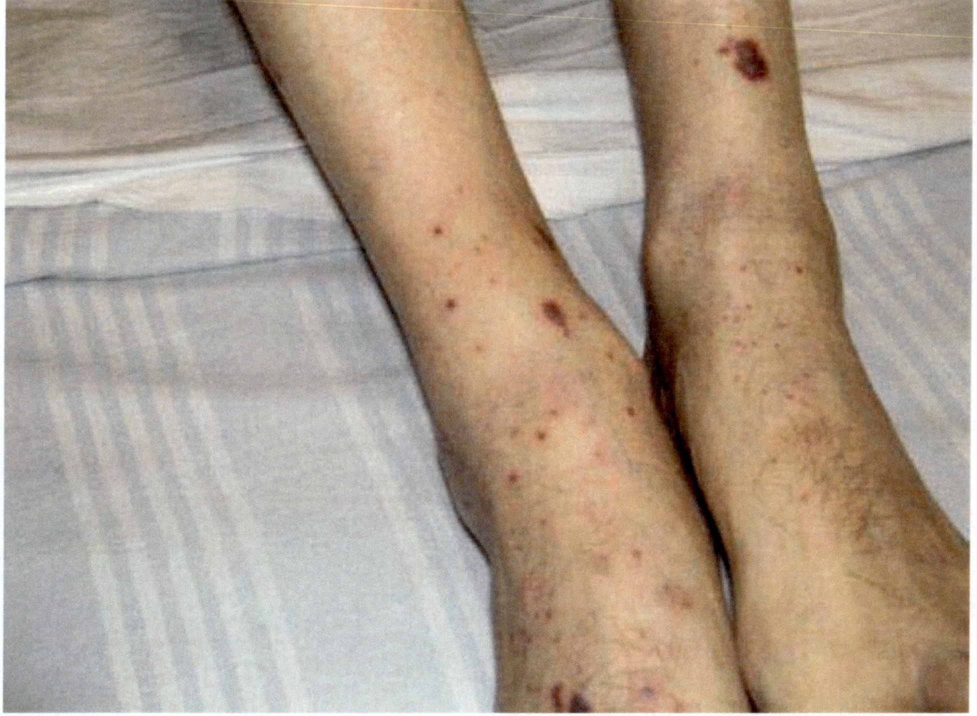

Figure 2.

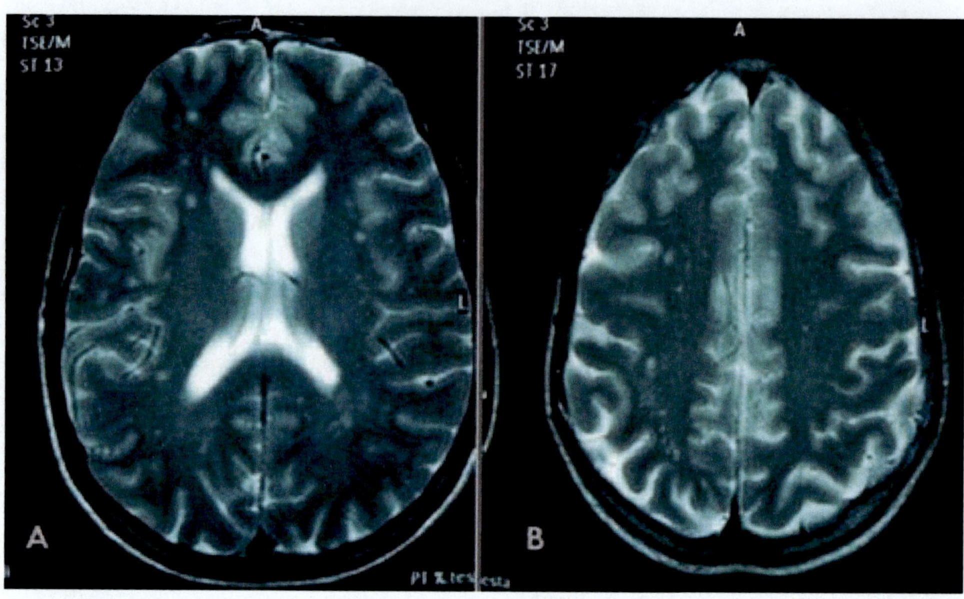

Figure 3.

CNS involvement is rather rare, usually presenting as cerebral infarctions, cerebral haemorrhages, cranial neuropathies, cognitive disturbances, epilepsies and coma. A few cases of intracerebral and subarachnoid hemorrage probably due to vasculitis have been described [84-87] as well as some other few cases of stroke [88-91].

ANCA can be detected in 38–50% of patients, generally with a perinuclear immunofluorescent- labeling pattern, most frequently (92–100%) directed to myeloperoxidase (MPO) on enzyme-linked immunofluorescence assay [92].

The pathogenesis of CS syndrome also has different potential mechanisms: asthma, involving Th2 lymphocytes, the contribution of ANCA in the development of vasculitis lesions, and, finally, the role of eosinophils which appear to be activeted during the active phase of the disease. The mainstay of treatment include corticosteroids and immunosuppressors according to the severity of the disease [51,92].

Figure 2 shows a purpuric rash at the inferior limbs, in a patient with CS syndrome, which had onset with asthma and peripheral polyneuropathy.

Henoch-Schönlein Purpura

HSP is a multisystem immunoglobulin A-mediated vasculitis with a self-limited course affecting the skin, joints, gastrointestinal tract, and kidneys. HSP occurs most often in children between the ages of 3 and 10 years, and presents classically with a unique distribution of the rash to the lower extremities and the buttocks area. However, also adults can have HSP with a worse long term prognosis [93]. Severe renal and CNS disease may lead to life-threatening conditions, and in these cases immunosuppressive agents and plasmapheresis may be needed. Up to now, treatment of brain involvement in HSP is mainly based on anecdotal reports.

Actually, nervous system manifestations are usually mild and transient while permanent sequelae are rare. The most frequent finding in adult-onset Schönlein Disease patients are headache and behavioral changes followed by seizures, focal neurologic deficits, mononeuropathies, and polyradiculoneuropathies. However, severe neurologic manifestations such as seizures, intracerebral hemorrhage, hemiplegia, and encephalopathy are rare, but potentially fatal complications [94-103]. Some of such manifestations could result from cerebral vasculitis but, so far, no ultrastructural or immunofluorescence studies of the central nervous system in HSP are available even though it may be assumed that IgA immune complex deposition initiates arteriolar inflammation in the cerebral vasculature as well as in the systemic vessels.

MRI is the diagnostic tool of choice for cerebral vasculitis complicating HSP [104,105].

Microscopic Polyangiitis (MPA)

MPA is a systemic small vessel p-ANCA positive vasculitis, although 10-20% patients with the clinical and pathological features of MPA results pANCA negative [106-111]. Middle sized vessels may be rarely involved [108].

p-ANCA titer increases before an activity phase of the disease and decreases during the remission phases [109,111-113]. Several studies in literature have showed that p-ANCA play a pathogenic role in MPA by means of neutrophil activation, degranulation and ROS production [109; 113-118].

MPA is uncommon but possible in the youth, being the peak of incidence between 65 and 70 years. Genetic and environmental factors are important in the etiology: infections and drugs, such as propiltiouracil, may provoke p-ANCA positivity, sometimes associated with a frank MPA, remitting after the drug withdrawal [119-121].

The most common clinical feature is extracapillary necrotizing glomerulonephritis or crescentic glomerulonephritis, with epithelial crescents and glomerulosclerosis, reported in 90-100% patients, rapidly evolving in renal failure, without a treatment [122,123]. Isolated renal involvement may be detected in a high rate of patients (necrotizing crescentic glomerulonephritis) [111,122]. The presence of clinical and hystopathological features of isolated rapidly-progressive renal MPA, in the absence of p-ANCA positivity is defined paucimmune glomerulonephritis [123-125].

Even a skin vasculitis is very common (40-70% patients) [108]. The cutaneous involvement is present at an early stage of microscopic polyangiitis [126]. It consists of erythematous macules or papules, purpura and ulcers, more commonly localized at the limbs. Skin biopsy specimens reveal a neutrophil infiltrate, interesting the small sized vessels with the aspect of leukocytoclastic vasculitis. The isolated dermatological involvement is, therefore, termed: cutaneous leukocytoclastic vasculitis [108,121,126]. The otolaryngological involvement, with oral or nasal ulcers and epistaxis, and the pulmonary involvement with alveolar hemorrhages and hemoptysis, are possible, although less commonly than in other ANCA positive vasculitides. [127-129]. Other clinical features reported are: scleritis, uveitis, pericarditis and arthritis [108]. The neurological involvement is more commonly peripheral, with sensori-motor axonal neuropathy, symmetric or asymmetric, reported in 15-60% patients, while only 10% patients develop CNS disorders [107,108,121].

The most common CNS clinical pictures are acute brain ischemia and vascular cognitive impairment [108,130]. Hypertrophic pachymeningitis, cranial polyneuritis and temporal artery involvement, similar to Horton's arteritis, are also reported [131,132]. Rare, but possible, is the encephalitic-like presentation [133].

The treatment is performed firstly with glucocorticoids, eventually associated with methotrexate or ciclophosphamide pulse-therapy [106,134,135]. Plasma exchange and immunoglobulins are, usually, reserved to the resistant cases and to those patients with more rapid renal functional impairment [106,134,136]. New promising treatment options effective for the induction therapy are represented by mycophenolate mofetil [137], rituximab [138] and TNF-receptor antagonist infliximab [106,139]. The mantainance is obtained with azatioprin or methotrexate associated with low-dose steroid [106,134].

Inflammatory Bowel Disease (IBD)-related Vasculitis

p-ANCA, immunological markers of small vessels necrotizing vasculitides, have been also detected inflammatory bowel disease (IBD), associated with both ulcerative colitis (UC) and Crohn's disease (CD) [140-143]. These autoantibodies are implied in the immunologic aggression of the bowel by neutrophil activation, including: the engagement of Fc gamma receptors, neutrophil degranulation and ROS release and neutrophil-endothelial interactions [109,113-118,140]. ANCA levels are useful to monitor disease: significant increase in ANCA titres should alert the clinicians [111].

The pANCA associated with IBD have different antigens if compared with those commonly isolated from patients with small vessels necrotizing vasculitides. Atypical p-ANCA recognize a nuclear, and not perinuclear, target antigen [144]. Another possible target is represented by bactericidal/permeability-increasing protein (BPI), an endotoxin-binding protein contained in leukocyte granules and characterized by antibacterial properties [145].

The presence of anti-endohelial cells antibodies (AECA) supports a vasculitic mechanism in the pathogenesis of IBD [146]. The serologic responses seen in IBD disease include antibodies directed to the intestinal flora due to the higher mucosal permeability observed in these patients. Saccharomyces cerevisiae, mycobacteria, bacteroides and E. coli are common targets of the immune response. Besides p-ANCA may react with epitopes of H1 histone, Bacteroides caccae (Ton-B linked outer membrane protein), Pseudomonas fluorescens-associated bacterial protein I-2, mycobacterial histone 1 homologue called Hup B [147].

IBD may be complicated by neurological manifestations, due to vasculitic mechanisms [148,149]. The cerebrovascular complications of IBD are well recognized, in particular venous thrombosis, but also: retinal branch artery occlusions, transient brainstem ischemia and brainstem or cerebral infarction [150-155]. Patients with IBD disease usually have one or more features of a hypercoagulable state, which may increase the risk of ischemic damage. It has been suggested that a hypercoagulable state is associated with clinical activity of the disease, with elevation of factors V, VIII, fibrinogen and platelets and a lowering of anti-thrombin III [156]. Hyperhomocysteinemia is significantly more common in patients with IBD compared with healthy controls, and is associated with lower (but not necessarily deficient) vitamin B12 levels [157,158]. Higher rates of pS deficiency and antiphospholipids syndrome have been reported [159,160]. Besides the cytokine environment in IBD can favor the activation of the clot cascade [156]. Cerebral hemorrhage due to IBD vascultic involvement is rare but possible [161].

Another possible neurological feature observed in patients with IBD is represented by: multiple focal white matter lesions, due to small vessels vasculitis, sometimes necessitating a differential diagnosis with multiple sclerosis. Epilepsy, chronic inflammatory polyneuropathies, and muscle involvement are also reported [148,149].

The treatment is based on: 5-aminosalicylic acid derivatives, corticosteroids and immunomodulators). Emerging therapies include: biological agents directed to cytokines (infliximab, adalimumab, certolizumab) or receptors (eg, visilizumab, abatacept) involved in T-cell activation; selective adhesion molecule blockers (eg, natalizumab, alicaforsen); anti-inflammatory cytokines (interleukin 10), modulation of the intestinal flora (antibiotics, prebiotics, probiotics) and leucocyte apheresis and many more monoclonal antibodies [162]. Peripheral arthritis, erythema nodosum, and episcleritis respond to the treatment of the underlying IBD. Spondilitis, pyoderma gangrenosum, and uveitis do not. Anti-TNF agents may be useful in these cases [163,164].

The treatment in neurological involvement is that of the underlying disorder, although cerebrovascular accidents necessitate of antithrombotic and symptomatic therapy.

Mixed Essential Cryoglobulinemia (MEC)

Cryoglobulins are serum proteins, which precipitate at temperatures below 37° C (often around 4° C) and redissolve at 37° C [165]. The presence of cryoglobulins in the serum is called cryoglobulinemia [166]. The most common clinical features of cryoglobulinemias are dependent by systemic vasculitis, secondary to the deposition of immunocomplexes and increased plasma viscosity: purpura, ulcers of the extremities, arthralgia, proteinuria, oligo-anuria, hemorrhagic diathesis, abdominal pain, congestive heart failure, confusion and coma [165-169].

According to the nature of the autoantibodies cryoglobulinemias have been classified by Brouet as:

1. *Type 1* (25%): Monoclonal; >50% IgM against monoclonal IgG; generally related to neoplastic diseases of the lymphoid tissue.
2. *Type 2* (25%): Monoclonal; 90%; IgM against polyclonal IgG; generally associated with neoplasms of the lymphoid tissue and connective tissue disorders.
3. *Type 3* (50%): Polyclonal against polyclonal; generally related to infections, such as: CMV, EBV, HBV, HIV, adenoviruses, subacute batterial endocarditis, sifilis, LGV, malaria, toxoplasmosis, kala-azar, schistosomiasis) [170-172].

The most common form of cryoglobulinemia is MEC (type 2 variant), which is usually associated with HCV infection (80-90% patients) [167,172-174]. The autoantibodies are IgM directed against a neo-antigen, resulting by the interaction HCV/VLDL which permits the access of the virus into the hepatocytes [168,175].

Although cryoglobulins are detected in 40-60% of HCV patients, the clinical features of cryoglobulinaemic vasculitis are reported in only 5-10% of the cases [167,176].

The peripheral nervous system is more often involved, producing either axonal or demyelinating, sensory or sensorimotor, polyneuritis or mononeuritis multiplex [177-182].

The main pathophysiologic mechanism of CNS involvement is ischemia (or rarely hemorrhage) due to diffuse or segmental vasculitis of the small cerebral vessels [178,179,183-186]. Testing for hepatitis C virus and cryoglobulins should be considered in selected patients with cerebral ischemia of undetermined cause [185]. Several reports of myelitis, encephalitis and CNS lymphoma associated with MEC are reported.

HCV may be the etiologic virus of progressive encephalomyelitis with rigidity, a rare disorder similar to stiff-man syndrome [179].

Antiviral therapy with interferon alpha and ribavirin may be active, but sustained responses are rare. In case of rapidly progressive disease a short course of steroids and cytotoxic drugs, with or without plasmapheresis, may be needed. Once the acute phase has been controlled, antiviral therapy may be administered to eradicate HCV. If antiviral therapy is ineffective, contraindicated or not tolerated, rituximab, a monoclonal anti-CD20 antibody, may represent an alternative to standard immunosuppression [166,167].

Secondary Vasculitides of the Nervous System Related to other Diseases

Necrotizing and non-necrotizing vasculitis may occur during the clinical course of connective tissue disorders, such as: systemic lupus erythematosus (SLE), scleroderma (SS), rheumatoid arthritis (RA), Sjögren syndrome (SjS), mixed connective tissue disease (MCD), and dermatomyositis (DM).

Secondary Vasculitides of the CNS Associated with Connective Tissue Disorders

A vasculitis process in the course of connective tissue disorder is frequently observed, due to the precipitation of immunocomplexes in the vascular wall, the direct action of cross-reacting autoantibodies with endothelial antigens and to cell-mediated immunopathogenetic mechanisms.

Rheumatoid Arthritis (RA)

RA is a common form of chronic inflammatory arthritis, actually in the context of a multisystemic disorder, potentially involving every organ [187]. The risk of cardiovascular disease (CVD) is increased in patients with RA [188-191].

A recent study demonstrated that RA patients experienced an approximate doubled risk for myocardial infarction and stroke and a 30% increase in CVD death in comparison to subjects without RA [192].

A frank inflammatory vasculitis of the CNS is exceedingly rare in RA and the symptoms may be misleading. Most of the reported cases occurr in males with long-standing, nodular, destructive, rheumatoid factor-positive disease where severe constitutional symptoms and other extraarticular manifestations of vasculitis are usually present [193-195]. However, sporadic cases in pediatric age have been described [196]. Some cases of cerebral vasculitis occurring after the use of anti-TNF alpha agents have been recently described [197]. Methotrexate have been successfully used to treat cerebral vasculitis in RA [198].

Systemic Lupus Erythematosus (SLE)

SLE is a multisystem autoimmune disorder characterized by an explosion of autoantibodies in the serum [199] and commonly involving skin, joints, kidney, heart, blood, CNS and PNS [200]. The ARC classification criteria for SLE require for diagnosis the presence of at least 4 of the following: malar rash, discoid rash, photosensitivity, oral ulcers, arthritis, serositis, renal disease, neurological disorder, hematological disease, immunological changes, and antinuclear antibodies [24].

Neurological manifestation of SLE are varies, and the same patient may have more than one syndrome. While a frank vasculitis involving the brain vessels is not common, cerebrovascular diseases, headaches, and seizures are frequently observed and seem to be caused by circulating IgG and IgM antiphospholipid antibodies, which are present in 30 up to 50% of SLE patients [201]. The ACR has proposed case definitions and classification criteria for 19 CNS and PNS syndromes which are defined as neuropsychiatric SLE (NPSLE) [202]. These guidelines have eliminated the old term lupus cerebritis because actually a diffuse involvement of the brain is quite rare. The prevalence of cerebrovascular disease in SLE based on these criteria range from 2% to 17%.

The pathogenesis of NPSLE is still unclear and probably multifactorial involving autoantibodies [203], intrathecal production of inflammatory cytokines, and microangiopathy. Anti-phospholipid (aPL) antibodies are implicated in microvascular, thromboembolic damage and clinically in most cases of seizures, stroke and chorea [204].

aPL antibodies, which include anti-cardiolipin antibodies and lupus anticoagulant (LA), are the laboratory hallmark of the aPL syndrome, also called Hughes syndrome, which is defined as a constellation of at least one clinical criterion among thrombosis, livedo reticularis and recurrent pregnancy loss [205,206]. aPL abs are detectable in 25-40% of SLE patients while at least 30% of SLE patients have an associated aPL syndrome [207]. Thromboses were the leading cause of death in the latter 5 years of a prospective national lupus cohort study. Strokes accounted for 11.8% of these events and were associated with aPL antibodies in a young predominantly female cohort (age 37 at study entry) [208].

Another recent study assessing the importance of various factors influencing the development of clinical thrombotic events in SLE demonstrated that LAC, constant and cumulative presence of aPL and previous thrombosis are positive predictors for the development of thrombotic complication in lupus patients [209]. According to one recent study, CVD, headache and seizures are independently associated with aPL antibodies [210], while in a further Italian study, even if patients with CVD have higher levels of antiphospholipid antibodies the difference does not reach the significativity [211].

Other antibodies have been claimed to play a role such as anti-endothelial cell antibodies for the vessel wall damage [212] or anti-ribosomal P protein antibodies, controversially linked to a diffuse CNS involvement in NPSLE [213-216].

Neuropathological studies of SLE are very few, due to improved prognosis and the most frequent histopathologic finding is a mild microvasculopathy with vessel tortuosity, cuffing of the small vessels, vascular hyalinization, endothelial proliferation and perivascular gliosis. However, a wide spectrum of abnormalities can be found in the brain, first of all gross or multifocal small infarcts, but also cortical atrophy, hemorrage, ischemic demyelinization and patchy multiple sclerosis-like lesions [217-226].

There is no a single test specific and sensitive enough for the diagnosis of NPSLE and the assessment of a patient with the suspect of NPSLE is based on clinical evaluation, detection of autoantibodies, psychiatric and neuropsychiatric evaluation and brain imaging. These tools are useful also to rule out other alternative explanations and to monitor disease progression; they also have the potential of providing guidance for therapeutic decisions [227].

Different neuroimaging techniques, both morphological and functional, have been used to evaluate NPSLE: MRI, which is usually normal in patients with diffuse psychiatric manifestations, SPECT and ^{18}FDG-PET. The most frequent MRI abnormality in NPSLE is the presence of small focal lesions localized in periventricular and subcortical white matter. More recently, magnetic resonance spectroscopy (MRS) has revealed neurometabolic abnormalities in white and grey matter also in patients with a normal conventional MRI [228,229]. MRS as well as SPECT and PET have been reported to have sensitivities as high as 100% for active NPSLE, but are much less specific in diagnosing NPSLE when compared to MRI [230-232].

The most common classes of drugs used to treat SLE include non-steroidal anti-inflammatory drugs, antimalarials, corticosteroids, and immunosuppressive agents (cyclosporine A, azathioprine, cyclophosphamide, mycophenolate mophetil) [233-237].

In some cases of NPSLE resistant to conventional treatment the adjunction of plasmapheresis has proved to be effective in remission induction [238]. Autologous hematopoietic stem cell transplantation, with its potential to eliminate autoreactive lymphocytes, may be a good therapeutic option for patients with refractory disease [239]. More recently some biologic agents have been used with the advantage of targeting specific pathways that contribute to the inflammatory response, such as Rituximab, a chimeric mouse–human monoclonal antibody directed against the B lymphocyte surface antigen CD20, Epratuzumab, a fully humanized antibody against CD22, a B lymphocyte restricted type I transmembrane sialoglycoprotein of the immunoglobulin (Ig) superfamily, CTLA4Ig (abatacept), a recombinant fusion protein developed to take advantage of the co-inhibitory nature of CTLA4 [240,241].

Sjögren's Syndrome (SjS)

SjS is a chronic inflammatory process that primarily involves the exocrine glands. Its clinical manifestations range from autoimmune exocrinopathy to extraglandular (systemic) involvement affecting the lungs, kidneys, blood vessels, and muscles; it can occur alone (primary SjS) or in association with other autoimmune diseases, more frequently RA, SLE, and autoimmune thyroid diseases [242-244].

PNS involvement is a well-documented complication in SjS [245] while the relevance of CNS disease is still a controversial issue, with a reported prevalence ranging from 1.5% to 62% [246,247].

The most frequently observed CNS disorders are 'non-focal' manifestations such as migraine, cognitive defects, psychiatric abnormalities [248] supporting the pathogenetic hypothesis of diffuse vascular-mediated damage. Also focal defects such as meningoencephalitis, transverse myelitis, and subarachnoid hemorrhage have been described [249-253].

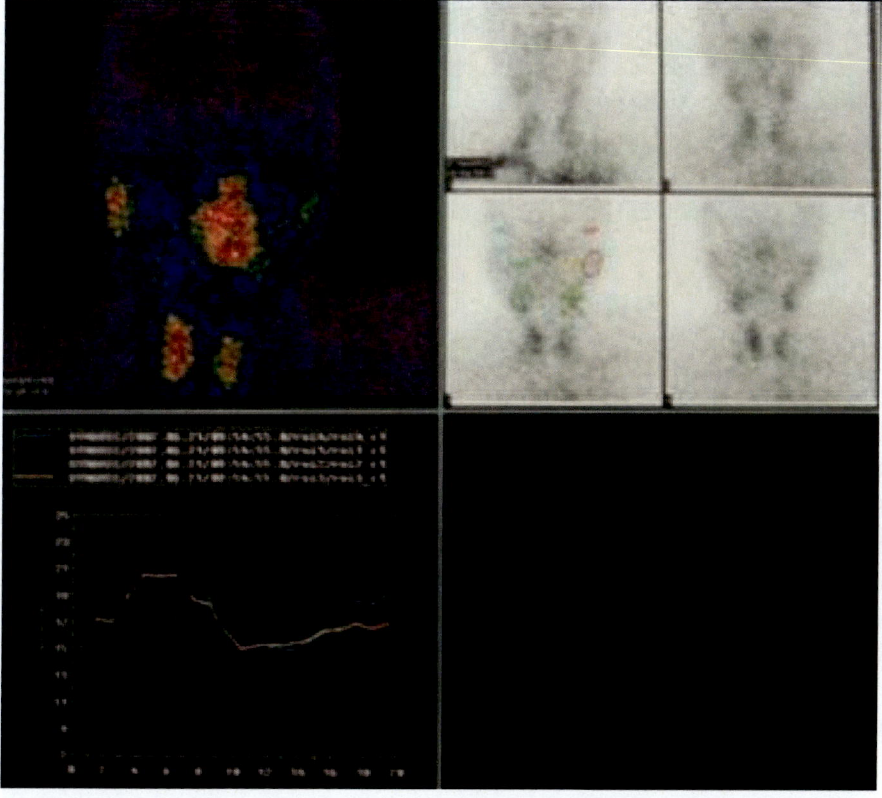

Figure 4.

Cerebral lesions can be focal or multifocal and may be acute (stroke-like), progressive or remittent (multiple sclerosis-like) [251-255]. CNS manifestations can be the presenting symptoms of the disease, representing a true challenge for the neurologist.

No correlation have been found between the clinical findings and the results of the radiological investigations or CSF study, which are normal or show only unspecific abnormalities, (such as high signals on T2 images within periventricular or subcortical white matter and increased protein level and/or mild lymphocytosis) [256].

Anti-Ro/SSA antibodies have been related to more severe and progressive cases and to the presence of MRI, CT and angiographic abnormalities, while other autoantibodies such as aPL and anti-P ribosomal protein appear to have a secondary role in SjS [257].

In Figure 3 and 4 are represented the MRI pattern and salivary-gland scintigraphy of a 60 years old woman presenting since 2004 recurrent sensation of sand in the eyes, dry mouth, headache and hearing loss. The MRI showed multiple lesions hyperintense in T2 in the white matter and centrum ovale (Figure 3A-B), while the salivary-gland scintigraphy showed decreased accumulation in the submandibulary gland and decreased secretion by the parotid gland (Figure 4).

Other Vasculitides with Nervous System Involvement

Behçet disease (BD), Buerger disease (Tromboangiitis obliterans, TAO), Cogan's syndrome, Sneddon's syndrome (a variant of the antiphospholipid antibodies syndrome with endothelial proliferation and microvascular occlusion [258], Amyloid angiopathy (AA), Susac's syndrome and familial Mediterranean fever (FMF) are uncommon disorders with a vascular involvement similar to vasculitides and are usually included in "other vasculitides with nervous system involvement" [16]. This heterogeneous group of vascular disorders present features similar to vasculitides, although the different ethiopathogenesis and immunopathologic findings.

Behçet Disease

BD is a multi-system inflammatory disease of unknown etiology, more diffused in the Middle-East, involving also great and small arteries and veins and the microcirculation. The clinical course consists of recurrent acute inflammatory attacks, resulting in oral and genital ulcers and ophthalmologic involvement. According to the International Study Group, diagnosis requires recurrent oral ulcerations (97-100%), plus two of four additional features: recurrent genital ulcerations (85%), eye lesions (50%) (uveitis, vitreous cells, retinal vasculitis), skin lesions (85%) (e.nodosum, pseudofolliculitis, acneiform nodules), or positive pathology test (60%) (interpreted by a physician at 24-48 hours). Other clinical features include arthritis (50%), thrombophlebitis (25%), epididymitis (5%), and GI lesions (1-30%) [259].

There is a slight male predominance (1.4 to 1), and onset most commonly is in the third decade.

Neurologic involvement occurs in 5 to 13% of cases, and is more common in men (4 to 1). It generally follows recurrent oral aphthous ulcers. CNS involvement has been described in 10-49% of the cases and its clinical expression varies widely. Two forms are commonly described: parenchymal involvement, *neuro-BD*, and non-parenchymal involvement, also called *angio-BD* [259,261].

Neuro-BD: Parenchymal involvement includes brainstem, hemispheric, spinal inflammatory lesions, and meningoencephalitis; *angio-BD* includes dural sinus thrombosis, arterial occlusion, and/or aneurysms [260,261*]*.

Clinically, *angio-BD* is more often relapsing-remitting, resembling multiple sclerosis, but it can also become progressive in later years, or, rarely, be progressive from onset. Neurologic problems may be primary (headache, dural venous sinus thrombosis, parenchymal involvement, PNS involvement, psychiatric disease, subclinical CNS involvement) or secondary (reflecting complications of treatment or of the systemic disease). Intra-axial CNS involvement results from small vessel inflammatory disease, more commonly presenting as a subacute brainstem syndrome. MRI often reveals iso-/hypointense lesions in T1-weighted images and hyperintense lesions in T2-weighted images, mostly in the mesodiencephalic junction, cerebellar peduncles, and other parts of the brainstem. MR allows also to evaluate the effects of treatment in BD [261,262].

Angio-BD: During the course of BD, arterial involvement is rare (1±5%) and more commonly peripheral, with aneurysm and pseudo-aneurysm formation or thrombosis referable to a vasculitis of vasa vasorum, with mononuclear and/or neutrophilic infltration, endothelial cell proliferation, destruction of internal elastic lamina, fibrinoid necrosis and thrombus formation [262]. However venous involvement, consisting in thromboembolic events, is more common than the arterial one [51, 262].

Cerebral arteries and veins are a potential target of the wide-spreading inflammatory process: both the extracranial and the intracranial circulation may be involved. Thus arterial and venous stroke, aneurisms rupture resulting in intraparenchimal or subarachnoidal hemorrhage are possible [261-264].

In conclusion, BD should be considered in the differential diagnosis of stroke in young adults, multiple sclerosis, movement disorders, intracranial hypertension and other neurologic syndromes. Corticosteroids and immunosuppressive agents are used for parenchymal manifestations, and corticosteroids and anticoagulants are used for treatment of dural sinus thrombosis [265-268].

Prognostic features have been identified. Male sex, young age at onset, onset with cerebellar syndrome, progressive course, repeated attacks, incomplete recovery, and high CSF cell count and protein level have all been associated with worse prognosis. In contrast, headache at the onset, venous sinus thrombosis and a single neurologic episode are associated with more favorable course [261].

Buerger Disease (Tromboangiitis Obliterans, TAO)

Buerger's disease or TAO is a peculiar vasculitis characterized by a granoulomatous necrotizing inflammation, starting at the avventitial surface and progressively involving not only the arterial wall, but also the satellite lymphatic, vein and nerve. [269]. Patients are generally young male (M/F=7.5:1; median age at the onset < 50 years) affected by recurrent attacks of acute arterial thrombosis of the legs, commonly interesting the most distal vessels and evolving in chronic ischemia with gangrene, necessitating the limb amputation [270-273].

TAO present a peculiar geographical distribution: very rare in North America and North Europe, it is common in the Mediterranean region and very common in the Orient [270,271].

The etiopathogenesis still remains unknown: higher antibody titre directed against periodontal pathogens has been reported in patients with Buerger's disease, if compared with normal subjects [274]. Even p-ANCA, antiphospholipid anti-endothelial antibodies have been reported, with a higher titre during the active phases [275-277]. Tobacco smoke has a role in onset and clinical progression, being this disease more diffused among cigarettes smokers and the risk directly proportional to the daily number of cigarettes consumed and to the duration of the habitude [278-280]. A vasculitis with features very similar to TAO has been reported among cannabis and cocaine abusers [281,282]. Actually the most trustable explanation is the contamination with chemical poisons or heavy metals, such as arsenic [283-285].

The most common clinical features of TAO are: ischemia involving the lower (100%; 50% isolated) and/or the upper limbs (30-40%; 10% isolated); migrating superficial thrombophlebitis (40-60%), which often represents a warning sign; Raynaud's phenomenon; mesenteric ischemia; TIA/Stroke; myocardial ischemia (uncommon); venous thromboembolisms; arthritis; nephritis with mesangial IgA deposition; systemic features such as: malaise, fever, dizziness, headache, arthromyalgias, etc. [270-272,286].

Even an isolated CNS involvement is possible, although rare, and is termed Spatz-Linderberg syndrome, characterized by recurrent strokes producing a vascular dementia [287,288].

Diagnosis requires clinical and instrumental investigations: absence of the peripheral pulses or a positive Allen test (i.e.: hand ischemia evoked by the compression of either radial or ulnar arteries) in a young person are highly suggestive of Buerger's disease [272,273].

The most common angiographic finding is represented by multiple stenoses with preferential involvement of the distal arteries at the leg or the wrist, with an attenuation of the palmar and the pedal arch [289].

Cerebral angiography may evidence multiple segments of arterial narrowing, in the distal portions of intracranial arteries, with massive collateral circulation ("tree root" or "corkscrew" vessels) [290]. Even cases of cerebral venous thrombosis are reported in patients with TAO [291].

Shionoya proposed the following diagnostic criteria: (1) smoking history; (2) onset before the age of 50 years; (3) infra-popliteal arterial occlusion; (4) superficial thrombophlebitis and/or arterial upper limb involvement and/or Raynaud's phenomenon, together with the exclusion of atherosclerotic risk facxtors other than smoke (i.e.: diabetes mellitus, atheromatous lesions, potential source of embolism, entrapment syndrome, auto-immune diseases, myeloproliferative disorders, hypercoagulability states [292]. Mills and Porter have successively introduced more accurate and strict diagnostic criteria: the Oregon criteria [270] while Papa and colleagues have developed a more flexible numerical score [293].

The therapy is still controversial and tobacco abstinence remains the cornerstone of treatment, also at the present moment, inducing a sustained remission of the disease [270-273]. In refractory cases the treatments of choice are antithrombotics (aspirin or anticoagulant) [294] and/or vasodilators, particularly prostaglandin analogues such as iloprost [294-297] and limaprost [298], with both vasodilating and anti-platelet action [294,295]. Also immunosuppressant drugs, corticosteroids and thrombolytics has been proposed, but the results of these studies are controversial [294].

Cogan's Syndrome

Cogan's syndrome is a rare clinical disease, primarily affecting white young adults, characterized by the association between nonsyphilitic interstitial keratitis and acute vestibuloauditory dysfunction resembling Meniere's syndrome and naturally evolving in deafness in a 60% patients [299-302].

Also an atypical form is possible, presenting as scleritis, episcleritis, retinal artery occlusion, choroiditis, retinal hemorrhages, papilloedema, exophthalmos, or tenonitis with or without interstitial keratitis [301-303].

Systemic vasculitis is present in 12-15% patients, involving vessels of all sizes, more commonly the large vessels but also the coronary arteries and the small kidney vasculature [304]. The differential diagnosis is with the TA since it may affect the aortic thoracic tract and valve [302,305,306].

All organs and systems may be interested, even the CNS with vasculitic infarctions [178, 307]. The variety of systemic manifestations is large and includes fever, eosinophilia, hypertension, gastrointestinal and respiratory features, skin lesions, splenomegaly, lymphadenopathy, and musculoskeletal symptoms [301,302,305].

An autoimmune pathogenesis has been postulated due to the presence of autoantibodies [308-310] and the common referred history of upper respiratory tract infections [302].

MR and CT represent the instrumental investigations of choice, revealing the narrowing or the obliteration of the vestibular labyrinth and/or cochlea, with contrast enhancement of the same structures [311]. The cerebral angiographic investigations reveal multiple stenoses or tortuosity of the interested vessels [312].

The mainstay of treatment in Cogan's syndrome is corticosteroids, topically for interstitial keratitis and systemically for inner ear dysfunction, neurologic or systemic feature. Early treatment is critical to preserve hearing. In patients resistant to steroids a possibility is the association with orally or IV (pulse therapy = 0.9-1 g/monthly) cyclophosphamide [299-302] or IV metothrexate (7.5-25 mg/weekly) [313]. TNFα-receptor blockers as infliximab or etanercept have been showed highly effective in patients resistant to the treatments [314].

Cochlear implants can partially restore auditory function and have been a salvation for patients who suffer from deafness as a result of permanent cochlear damage [300].

Susac's Syndrome

Susac's syndrome consists of the clinical triad of encephalopathy, branch retinal artery occlusions and hearing loss, due to an autoimmune microangiopathy affecting the precapillary arterioles of the brain, retina, and inner ear (cochlea and vestibulus). More common among young women (F/M= 3:1) the presenting feature is often represented by migraine-like headache, with or without aura [315-321]. Multifocal neurological signs and symptoms, psychiatric disturbances, cognitive disorders, memory loss and confusion, represents the most common features associated with CNS involvement, sometimes rapidly progressing to dementia [318-320].

Diagnosis is based on the following investigations: the audiogram may reveal a bilateral sensorineural hearing loss [317], funduscopy and fluorangiography stenoses or interruptions in the distal branches of the retinal artery [315,316,322] and brain MRI may evidence multiple lacunar lesion, often clinically silent and always affecting the corpus callosum. The lacunae may appear as linear defects (spokes) and large round lesions (snowballs). Frequently, the lesions enhance and if recent are evident on diffusion weighted imaging (DWI) [323]. Elevated levels of Factor VIII and von Willebrand Factor Antigen reflect the endothelial perturbation. Despite extensive evaluations, a procoagulant state has never been demonstrated [315].

High-dose corticosteroid therapy is the mainstay of treatment, but additional therapies such as intravenous immunoglobulin, mycophenolate mofetil, and cyclophosphamide are often necessary [324,325]. Rituximab is the newest therapy to consider. Aspirin at high dosages can be added to immunomodulatory therapy [325].

Treatment should be prompt, aggressive, and sustained to avoid the dreaded residuals of dementia, deafness, and blindness. Course is self-limiting after an active fluctuating phase and 50% patients return to normal life using an aggressive therapeutical approach [326].

References

[1] Molloy ES, Hajj-Ali RA. Primary angiitis of the central nervous system. *Curr. Treat Options Neurol.* 2007 May;9(3):169-75.

[2] Calabrese LH, Molloy ES, Singhal AB. Primary central nervous system vasculitis: progress and questions. *Ann. Neurol.* 2007 Nov;62(5):430-2.

[3] Calabrese LH, Mallek JA. Primary angiitis of the central nervous system. Report of 8 new cases, review of the literature, and proposal for diagnostic criteria. *Medicine* (Baltimore). 1988 Jan;67(1):20-39.

[4] Cravioto H, Feigin I. Noninfectious granulomatous angiitis with a predilection for the nervous system. *Neurology* 1959 Sep;9:599-609.

[5] Calabrese LH. Vasculitis of the central nervous system. *Rheum. Dis. Clin. North Am.* 1995 Nov;21(4):1059-76.

[6] Lie JT. Primary (granulomatous) angiitis of the central nervous system: a clinicopathologic analysis of 15 new cases and a review of the literature. *Hum. Pathol.* 1992 Feb;23(2):164-71.

[7] Calabrese LH, Duna GF, Lie JT. Vasculitis in the central nervous system. *Arthritis and Rheumatism* 1997;40:1189-1201.

[8] Salvarani C, Brown RD Jr, Calamia KT, Christianson TJ, Weigand SD, Miller DV, Giannini C, Meschia JF, Huston J 3rd, Hunder GG.Primary central nervous system vasculitis: analysis of 101 patients. *Ann. Neurol.* 2007 Nov;62(5):442-51.

[9] Lie JT. Classification and histopathologic spectrum of central nervous system vasculitis. *Neurologic Clinics* 1997;15:805-819.

[10] Oliveira V, Povoa P, Costa A, Ducla-Soares J. Cerebrospinal fluid and therapy of isolated angiitis of the central nervous system. *Stroke* 1994;25:1693-1695.

[11] Wynne PJ, Younger DS, Khandji A, Silver AJ. Radiographic features of central nervous system vasculitis. *Neurologic Clinics* 1997;15:779-804.

[12] Vollmer TL, Guarnaccia J, Harrington W, Pacia SV, Petroff OA. Idiopathic granulomatous angiitis of the central nervous system. Diagnostic challenges. *Archives of Neurology* 1993;50:925-930.

[13] Duna GF, Calabrese LH. Limitations of invasive modalities in the diagnosis of primary angiitis of the central nervous system. *Journal of Rheumatology* 1995;22:662-667.

[14] Alhalabi M, Moore PM. Serial angiography in isolated angiitis of the central nervous system. *Neurology* 1994;44:1221-1226.

[15] Calabrese LH, Furlan AJ, Gragg LA, Ropos TJ. Primary angiitis of the central nervous system: diagnostic criteria and clinical approach. *Cleveland Clinic Journal of Medicine* 1992;59:293-306.

[16] Siva A. Vasculitis of the nervous system. *J. Neurol.* 2001;248:451-468.

[17] Calabrese LH, Gragg LA, Furlan AJ. Benign angiopathy: a distinct subset of angiographically defined primary angiitis of the central nervous system. *J. Rheumatol.* 1993 Dec;20(12):2046-50.

[18] Jolly M, Curran JJ, Ellman M. Benign Angiopathy of the Central Nervous System. *J. Clin. Rheumatol.* 2004 Apr;10(2):80-82.

[19] Cloft HJ, Phillips CD, Dix JE, McNulty BC, Zagardo MT, Kallmes DF. Correlation of angiography and MR imaging in cerebral vasculitis. Acta Radiol. 1999 Jan;40(1):83-7.

[20] Koopman K, Uyttenboogaart M, Luijckx GJ, De Keyser J, Vroomen PC. Pitfalls in the diagnosis of reversible cerebral vasoconstriction syndrome and primary angiitis of the central nervous system. *Eur. J. Neurol.* 2007 Oct;14(10):1085-7.

[21] Ozen S, Ruperto N, Dillon MJ, et al. EULAR/PReS endorsed consensus criteria for the classification of childhood vasculitides. *Ann. Rheum. Dis.* 2006; 65:936–941.

[22] Younger DS. Vasculitis of the nervous system. *Curr. Opin. Neurol.* 2004;17:317-336.

[23] Jennette JC, Falk RJ. Nosology of primary vasculitis. *Curr. Opin. Rheumatol.* 2007;19: 10-16.

[24] Hunder GG, Arend WP, Bloch DA, Calabrese LH, Fauci AS, Fries JF, Leavitt RY, Lie JT, Lightfoot RW Jr, Masi AT, et al. The American College of Rheumatology 1990

criteria for the classification of vasculitis. Introduction. *Arthritis Rheum*. 1990;33:1065-1067.

[25] Jennette JC, Falk RJ, Andrassy K, Bacon PA, Churg J, Gross WL, Hagen EC, Hoffman GS, Hunder GG, Kallenberg CG, et al. Nomenclature of systemic vasculitides. Proposal of an international consensus conference. *Arthritis Rheum*. 1994;37:187-92.

[26] Bongartz T, Matteson EL. Large-vessel involvement in giant cell arteritis. *Curr. Opin. Rheumatol*. 2006 Jan;18(1):10-7.

[27] Caselli RJ, Hunder GG, Whisnant JP. Neurologic disease in biopsy-proven giant cell (temporal) arteritis. *Neurology* 1988;38:352–9.

[28] Gonzalez-Gay MA, Blanco R, Rodriguez-Valverde V, Martinez- Taboada V, Delgado-Rodriguez M, Figueroa M, et al. Permanent visual loss and cerebrovascular accidents in giant cell arteritis: predictors and response to treatment. *Arthritis Rheum*. 1998;41: 1497–504.

[29] Wilkinson IM, Russell RW. Arteries of the head and neck in giant cell arteritis: a pathological study to show the pattern of arterial involvement. *Arch Neurol*. 1972;27: 378–91.

[30] Wiszniewska M, Devuyst G, Bogousslavsky J.Giant cell arteritis as a cause of first-ever stroke. *Cerebrovasc. Dis*. 2007;24(2-3):226-30.

[31] Hu Z, Yang Q, Yang L, Li J, Tang J, Zhang H. Cerebral infarction due to giant cell arteritis-three case reports. *Angiology* 2004;55:227-31

[32] Thielen KR, Wijdicks EF, Nichols DA. Giant cell (temporal) arteritis: involvement of the vertebral and internal carotid arteries. *Mayo Clin. Proc*. 1998;73:444–6.

[33] Salvarani C, Giannini C, Miller DV, Hunder G. Giant cell arteritis: Involvement of intracranial arteries. *Arthritis Rheum*. 2006 Dec 15;55(6):985-9.

[34] Warrington KJ, Matteson EL. Management guidelines and outcome measures in giant cell arteritis (GCA). *Clin. Exp. Rheumatol*. 2007;25:6 Suppl 47:137-41.

[35] Warrington KJ,; Staunton H, Stafford F, Leader M, O'Riordain D. Deterioration of giant cell arteritis with corticosteroid therapy. *Arch Neurol*. 2000 Apr; 57(4):581-4.

[36] Lee MS, Smith SD, Galor A, Hoffman GS: Anti-platelet and anti-coagulant therapy in patients with giant cell arteritis. *ArthritisRheum*. 2006;54:3306-9.

[37] Nesher G, Berkun Y, Mates M, Baras M, Rubinow A, Sonnenblick M: Low-dose aspirin and prevention of cranial ischemic complications in giant cell arteritis. *Arthritis Rheum*. 2004;50:1332-7.

[38] Seko Y. Giant cell and Takayasu arteritis. *Curr. Opin. Rheumatol*. 2007;19:39-43.

[39] Sikaroodi H, Motamedi M, Kahnooji H, Gholamrezanezhad A, Yousefi N Stroke as the first manifestation of Takayasu arteritis *Acta Neurol. Belg*. 2007;107:18-2.

[40] Kerr GS, Hallahan CW, Giordano J, et al. Takayasu arteritis. *Ann. Intern. Med*. 1994; 120:919-29.

[41] Kim HJ, Suh DC, Kim JK, Kim SJ, Lee JH, Choi CG, Yoo B, Kwon SU, Kim JS. Correlation of neurological manifestations of Takayasu's arteritis with cerebral angiographic findings. *Clin. Imaging* 2005;29:79-85.

[42] Ringleb PA, Strittmatter EI, Loewer M, Hartmann M, Fiebach JB, Lichy C, Weber R, Jacobi C, Amendt K, Schwaninger M. Cerebrovascular manifestations of Takayasu arteritis in Europe Rheumatology 2005;44:1012-5.

[43] Molnar P, Hegedus K: Direct involvement of intracerebral arteries in Takayasu's arteritis. *Acta Neuropathol.* (Berl) 1984;63:83-86.

[44] Ringleb PA, Strittmatter EI, Loewer M, Hartmann M, Fiebach JB, Lichy C, Weber R, Jacobi C, Amendt K, Schwaninger M: Cerebrovascular manifestations of Takayasu arteritis in Europe. *Rheumatology* (Oxford) 2005;44:1012-1015.

[45] Klos K, Flemming KD, Petty GW, Luthra HS: Takayasu's arteritis with arteriographic evidence of intracranial vessel involvement. *Neurology* 2003;60:1550-1551.

[46] Kanda M, Shinoda S, Masuzawa T: Ruptured vertebral artery-posterior inferior cerebellar artery aneurysm associated with pulseless disease--case report. *Neurol. Med. Chir.* 2004;44:363-367.

[47] Webb M, Chambers A, A AL-N, Mason JC, Maudlin L, Rahman L, Frank J: The role of 18F-FDG PET in characterising disease activity in Takayasu arteritis. *Eur. J. Nucl. Med. Mol. Imaging* 2004;31:627-634.

[48] Kissin EY, Merkel PA: Diagnostic imaging in Takayasu arteritis. *Curr. Opin. Rheumatol.* 2004;16:31-37.

[49] Andrews J, Mason JC. Takayasu's arteritis--recent advances in imaging offer promise. *Rheumatology* 2007;46:6-15.

[50] Tanaka F, Kawakami A, Iwanaga N, Tamai M, Izumi Y, Aratake K, Arima K, Kamachi M, Nakamura H, Huang M, Ida H, Origuchi T, Eguchi K. Infliximab is effective for Takayasu arteritis refractory to glucocorticoid and methotrexate. *Intern. Med.* 2006;45: 313-6.

[51] Scolding N: The neurological vasculitides. In: Schapira AHV Neurology and clinical neuroscience, publisher Mosby (Elsevier), 2007.

[52] Bouvard B, Lavigne C, Marc G, Menei P, Debray JM, Dubas F. Two consecutive episodes of intracerebral hemorrhage as the presenting feature of polyarteritis nodosa. *Rev. Med. Interne.* 2007;28:651-4.

[53] MacLaren K, Gillespie J, Shrestha S, et al. Primary angiitis of the central nervous system: emerging variants. *QJM* 2005;98:643–654.

[54] Gayraud M, Guillevin L, le Toumelin P, Cohen P, Lhote F, Casassus P, Jarrousse B; French Vasculitis Study Group. Long-term follow-up of polyarteritis nodosa, microscopic polyangiitis, and Churg-Strauss syndrome: analysis of four prospective trials including 278 patients. *Arthritis Rheum.* 2001;44:666-675.

[55] Reichart MD, Bogousslavsky J, Janzer RC. Early lacunar strokes complicating polyarteritis nodosa: thrombotic microangiopathy.: *Neurology* 2000 Feb 22;54(4):883-9.

[56] M Segelmark, D Selga The challenge of managing patients with polyarteritis nodosa *Curr. Opin. Rheumatol.* 2007; 19:33–38.

[57] Wolff AE, Hansen KE, Zakowski L Acute Kawasaki disease: not just for kids. *J. Gen. Intern. Med.* 2007;22:681-4.

[58] Rowley AH, Shulman ST New developments in the search for the etiologic agent of Kawasaki disease. *Curr. Opin. Pediatr.* 2007;19:71-4.

[59] Gedalia A. Kawasaki disease: 40 years after the original report. *Curr. Rheumatol. Rep.* 2007;9:336-4.

[60] Ozen S, Ruperto N, Dillon MJ, et al. EULAR/PReS endorsed consensus criteria for the classification of childhood vasculitides. *Ann. Rheum. Dis*. 2006;65:936–941.

[61] Satou GM, Giamelli J, Gewitz MH. Kawasaki disease: diagnosis, management, and long-term implications. *Cardiol. Rev*. 2007;15:163-9.

[62] Wood L, Tulloh R. Kawasaki disease: diagnosis, management and cardiac sequelae. *Expert Rev. Cardiovasc. Ther*. 2007;5:553-6.

[63] Suda K, Matsumura M, Ohta S. Kawasaki disease complicated by cerebral infarction. *Cardiol. Young* 2003;13:103-5.

[64] Fujiwara S, Yamano T, Hattori M, Fujiseki Y, Shimada M. Asymptomatic cerebral infarction in Kawasaki disease. *Pediatr. Neurol*. 1992;8:235-6.

[65] Laxer RM, Dunn HG, Flodmark O. Acute hemiplegia in Kawasaki disease and infantile polyarteritis nodosa. *Dev. Med. Child Neurol*. 1984;26:814-8.

[66] Husain E, Hoque E. Meningoencephalitis as a presentation of Kawasaki disease. *J. Child Neurol*. 2006;21:1080-1.

[67] Bailie NM, Hensey OJ, Ryan S, Allcut D, King MD. Bilateral subdural collections--an unusual feature of possible Kawasaki disease. *Eur. J. Paediatr Neurol*. 2001;5:79-81.

[68] Tabarki B, Mahdhaoui A, Selmi H, Yacoub M, Essoussi AS. Kawasaki disease with predominant central nervous system involvement. *Pediatr Neurol*. 2001;25:239-41.

[69] De Rosa G, Pardeo M, Rigante D. Current recommendations for the pharmacologic therapy in Kawasaki syndrome and management of its cardiovascular complications. *Eur. Rev. Med. Pharmacol. Sci*. 2007;11:301-8.

[70] Drachman DA. Neurologic involvement in Wegener's granulomatosis. *Arch Neurol*. 1963;8:145–155.

[71] Murphy JM, Gomez-Anson B, Gillard JH, Antoun NM, Cross J, Elliott JD et al. Wegener granulomatosis: MR imaging findings in brain and meninges. *Radiology* 1999;213:794–799.

[72] Nishimo H, Rubino FA, DeRemee RA, et al. Neurological involvement in Wegener's granulomatosis: an analysis of 324 consecutive patients at the Mayo Clinic. *Ann. Neurol*. 1993;33:4–9.

[73] Granziera C, Michel P, A, Rossetti O, Lurati F, Reymond S, Bogousslavsky J. Wegener Granulomatosis presenting with haemorragic stroke in a young adult. *J. Neurol*. 2005; 252:615–616.

[74] Memet B, Rudinskaya A, Krebs T, Oelberg D, Wegener Granulomatosis With Massive Intracerebral Hemorrhage. *J. Clin. Rheumatol*. 2005;11:314–318.

[75] Provenzale JM, Allen NB. Wegener's granulomatosis: CT and MR findings. *AJNR Am. J. Neuroradiol*. 1996;17:785–92.

[76] Memet B ; Rudinskaya A; Krebs T; Oelberg D. Wegener Granulomatosis With Massive Intracerebral Hemorrhage: Remission of Disease in Response to Rituximab. *J. Clin. Rheumatol*. 2005;11:314-8.

[77] Murphy JM, Gomez-Anson B, Gillard JH, Antoun NM, Cross J, Elliott JD, Lockwood M. Wegener granulomatosis: MR imaging findings in brain and meninges. *Radiology* 1999;213:794-9.

[78] Guillevin l, Cordier jf, Lhote f, et al .: A prospective multicenter, randomized trial comparing steroids and pulse cyclophosphamide versus steroids and oral

cyclophosphamide in the treatment of generalized Wegener's granulomatosis. *Arthritis Rheum.* 1997;40:2187-98.

[79] Riccieri V, Spadaro A, Parisi G, Benfari G, Trasimeni G, Taccari MD, Valesini G. Imaging evidence of successful multiple immunosuppressive treatment of cerebral involvement in Wegener's granulomatosis. *Clin. Exp. Rheumatol.* 2002;20:578-9.

[80] Antoniu SA Treatment options for refractory Wegener's granulomatosis: a role for rituximab? *Curr. Opin. Investig Drugs* 2007;8:927-32.

[81] Hellmich B, Lamprecht P, Gross WL. Advances in the therapy of Wegener's granulomatosis. *Curr. Opin. Rheumatol.* 2006;18:25-32.

[82] Benenson E, Fries JW, Heilig B, Pollok M, Rubbert A. High-dose azathioprine pulse therapy as a new treatment option in patients with active Wegener's granulomatosis and lupus nephritis refractory or intolerant to cyclophosphamide. *Clin. Rheumatol.* 2005;24: 251-7.

[83] Langford CA, Talar-Williams C, Sneller MC. Mycophenolate mofetil for remission maintenance in the treatment of Wegener's granulomatosis. *Arthritis Rheum.* 2004; 15; 51:278-83.

[84] Tyvaert L, Devos P, Deloizy M, Belhadia A, Stekelorom T. Peripheral and central neurological manifestations in a case of Churg Strauss Syndrome. *Rev. Neurol.* 2004; 160:89-92.

[85] Liou HH, Liu HM, Chiang IP, Yeh TS, Chen R Churg-Strauss syndrome presented as multiple intracerebral hemorrhage. *Lupus* 1997;6(3):279-82.

[86] Calvo-Romero JM, del Carmen Bonilla-Gracia M, Bureo-Dacal P. Churg-Strauss syndrome presenting as spontaneous subarachnoid haemorrhage. *Clin. Rheumatol.* 2002;21:261-3.

[87] Sakamoto S, Ohba S, Eguchi K, Shibukawa M, Kiura Y, Okazaki T, Kajihara Y, Arita K, Kurisu K Churg-Strauss syndrome presenting with subarachnoid hemorrhage from ruptured dissecting aneurysm of the intracranial vertebral artery. *Clin. Neurol. Neurosurg.* 2005;107:428-31.

[88] Dinç A, Soy M, Pay S, Simsek I, Erdem H, Sobaci G. A case of Churg-Strauss syndrome presenting with cortical blindness. *Clin. Rheumatol.* 2000;19(4):318-20.

[89] Kang DW, Kim DE, Yoon BW, Seo JW, Roh JK. Delayed diagnosis: recurrent cerebral infarction associated with Churg-Strauss syndrome. *Cerebrovasc. Dis.* 2001;12:280-1.

[90] Winek J, Zych J, Wiatr E, Oniszh K, Roszkowski-Sliz K. Stroke as a predominant symptom at Churg-Strauss syndrome Pneumonol Alergol. Pol. 2007;75(2):191-6.

[91] Sonneville R, Lagrange M, Guidoux C, Michel M, Khellaf M, Russel S, Hosseini H. The association of cardiac involvement and ischemic stroke in Churg Strauss Syndrome. *Rev. Neurol.* 2006;162:229-32.

[92] Pagnoux C, Guilpain P, Guillevin L. Churg–Strauss syndrome. *Curr. Opin. Rheumatol.* 2007;19:25–32.

[93] Saulsbury F T. Clinical update: Henoch-Schönlein purpura. *Lancet* 2007;369:976-9.

[94] Elinson P, Foster KW, Kaufman DB. Case report: magnetic resonance imaging of central system vasculitis. *Acta Paediatr. Scand.* 1990;70:710–713.

[95] Ha TS, Cha SH Cerebral vasculitis in Henoch-Schönlein purpura: a case report with sequential magnetic resonance imaging. *Pediatr. Nephrol.* 1996;10:634–636.

[96] Woolfen AR, Hukin J, Poskitt KJ, Connolly MB Encephalopathy complicating Henoch-Schönlein purpura: reversible MRI changes. *Pediatr. Neurol.* 1998;19:74–78.

[97] Bakkaloglu SA, Ekim M, Tumer N, Deda G, Erden I, Erdem T Cerebral vasculitis in Henoch-Schönlein purpura. *Nephrol. Dial Transplant.* 2000;15:246–248.

[98] Bulun A, Topaloglu R, Duzova A, Saatci I, Besbas N, Bakkaloglu A Ataxia and peripheral neuropathy: rare manifestations in Henoch-Schönlein purpura. *Pediatr. Nephrol.* 2001;16:1139–1141.

[99] Perez C, Maravi E, Olier J MRI imaging of encephalopathy in adult Henoch-Schönlein purpura. *Am. J. Rheumatol.* 2000;175:922–923.

[100] Chen CL, Chiou YH, Wu CY, Lai PH, Chung HM Cerebral vasculitis in Henoch-Schönlein purpura: a case report with sequential magnetic resonance imaging changes and treated with plasmapheresis alone. *Pediatr. Nephrol.* 2000;15:276–278.

[101] Gianviti A, Trompeter RS, Barratt TM, Lythgoe MF, Dillon MJ Retrospective study of plasma exchange in patients with idiopathic rapidly progressive glomerulonephritis and vasculitis. *Arch Dis. Child* 1996;75:186–190.

[102] Ng CC, Huang SC, Huang LT Henoch-Schönlein purpura with intracerebral hemorrhage: case report. *Pediatr Radiol.* 1996;26:276–277.

[103] Wen YK, Yang Y, Chang CC. Cerebral vasculitis and intracerebral hemorrhage in Henoch-Schönlein purpura treated with plasmapheresis. *Pediatr Nephrol.* 2005;20:223–225.

[104] Chen CL, Chiou YH, Wu CY, Lai PH, Chung HM.. Cerebral vasculitis in Henoch-Schonlein purpura: a case report with sequential magnetic resonance imaging changes and treated with plasmapheresis alone. *Pediatr Nephrol.* 2000;15:276-8.

[105] Eun SH, Kim SJ, Cho DS, Chung GH, Lee DY, Hwang PH. Cerebral vasculitis in Henoch-Schonlein purpura: MRI and MRA findings, treated with plasmapheresis alone. *Pediatr Int.* 2003;45:484-7.

[106] Jayne D. Challenges in the management of microscopic polyangiitis: past, present and future. *Curr. Opin. Rheumatol.* 2008 Jan;20(1):3-9.

[107] Haubitz M. ANCA-associated vasculitis: diagnosis, clinical characteristics and treatment. *Vasa.* 2007 May;36(2):81-9.

[108] Puéchal X. Antineutrophil cytoplasmic antibody-associated vasculitides. *Joint Bone Spine.* 2007 Oct;74(5):427-35.

[109] Bosch X, Guilabert A, Font J. Antineutrophil cytoplasmic antibodies. *Lancet* 2006 Jul 29;368(9533):404-18.

[110] Seo P, Stone JH. The antineutrophil cytoplasmic antibody-associated vasculitides. *Am. J. Med.* 2004 Jul 1;117(1):39-50.

[111] Radice A, Sinico RA. Antineutrophil cytoplasmic antibodies (ANCA). *Autoimmunity* 2005 Feb;38(1):93-103.

[112] Gaskin G, Savage COS, Ryan JJ, et al. Anti-neutrophil cytoplasmic antibodies and disease activity during long-term follow-up of 70 patients with systemic vasculitis. *Nephrol. Dial Transplant.* 1991;6:689–94.

[113] Han WK, Choi HK, Roth RM, McCluskey RT, Niles JL. Serial ANCA titers: useful tool for prevention of relapses in ANCA-associated vasculitis. *Kidney Int.* 2003;63: 1079–85.

[114]Falk RJ, Terrell RS, Charles LA, Jennette JC. Anti-neutrophil cytoplasmic autoantibodies induce neutrophils to degranulate and produce oxygen radicals in vitro. *Proc. Natl. Acad. Sc.i USA* 1990;87:4115–9.

[115]Charles LA, Caldas ML, Falk RJ, Terrell RS, Jennette JC. Antibodies against granule proteins activate neutrophils in vitro. *J. Leukoc. Biol.* 1991;50:539–46.

[116]Mulder AH, Heeringa P, Brouwer E, Limburg PC, Kallenberg CGM. Activation of granulocytes by anti-neutrophil cytoplasmic antibodies (ANCA): a Fc gamma RII-dependent process. *Clin. Exp. Immunol.* 1994;98:270–8.

[117]Savage COS, Pottinger BE, Gaskin G, Pusey CD, Pearson JD. Autoantibodies developing to myeloperoxidase and proteinase 3 in systemic vasculitis stimulate neutrophil cytotoxicity toward cultured endothelial cells. *Am. J. Pathol.* 1992;141:335–42.

[118]Ewert BH, Jennette JC, Falk RJ. Anti-myeloperoxidase antibodies stimulate neutrophils to damage human endothelial cells. *Kidney Int.* 1992 Feb;41(2):375-83.

[119]Lane SE, Watts R, Scott DG. Epidemiology of systemic vasculitis. *Curr. Rheumatol. Rep.* 2005 Aug;7(4):270-5.

[120]Chen YX, Yu HJ, Ni LY, Zhang W, Xu YW, Ren H, Chen XN, Wang XL, Li X, Pan XX, Wang WM, Chen N. Propylthiouracil-associated antineutrophil cytoplasmic autoantibody-positive vasculitis: retrospective study of 19 cases. *J. Rheumatol.* 2007 Dec;34(12):2451-6.

[121]Guillevin L, Durand-Gasselin B, Cevallos R, Gayraud M, Lhote F, Callard P, Amouroux J, Casassus P, Jarrousse B. Microscopic polyangiitis: clinical and laboratory findings in eighty-five patients. *Arthritis Rheum.* 1999 Mar;42(3):421-30.

[122]Morgan MD, Harper L, Williams J, Savage C. Anti-neutrophil cytoplasm-associated glomerulonephritis. *J. Am. Soc. Nephrol*. 2006 May;17(5):1224-34.

[123]Lionaki S, Jennette JC, Falk RJ. Anti-neutrophil cytoplasmic (ANCA) and anti-glomerular basement membrane (GBM) autoantibodies in necrotizing and crescentic glomerulonephritis. *Semin. Immunopathol*. 2007 Nov;29(4):459-74.

[124]Eisenberger U, Fakhouri F, Vanhille P, Beaufils H, Mahr A, Guillevin L, Lesavre P, Noël LH. ANCA-negative pauci-immune renal vasculitis: histology and outcome. *Nephrol. Dial Transplant.* 2005 Jul;20(7):1392-9.

[125]Chen M, Yu F, Wang SX, Zou WZ, Zhao MH, Wang HY. Antineutrophil cytoplasmic autoantibody-negative Pauci-immune crescentic glomerulonephritis. *J. Am. Soc. Nephrol.* 2007 Feb;18(2):599-605.

[126]Kawakami T, Soma Y, Saito C, Ogawa H, Nagahuchi Y, Okazaki T, Ozaki S, Mizoguchi M. Cutaneous manifestations in patients with microscopic polyangiitis: two case reports and a minireview. *Acta Derm. Venereol.* 2006;86(2):144-7.

[127]Brown KK. Pulmonary vasculitis. *Proc. Am. Thorac. Soc*. 2006;3(1):48-57.

[128]Pesci A, Manganelli P. Respiratory system involvement in antineutrophil cytoplasmic-associated systemic vasculitides: clinical, pathological, radiological and therapeutic considerations. *Drugs* R D. 2007;8(1):25-42.

[129]Manganelli P, Fietta P, Carotti M, Pesci A, Salaffi F. Respiratory system involvement in systemic vasculitides. *Clin. Exp. Rheumatol.* 2006 Mar-Apr;24(2 Suppl 41):S48-59.

[130]Mattioli F, Capra R, Rovaris M, Chiari S, Codella M, Miozzo A, Gregorini G, Filippi M. Frequency and patterns of subclinical cognitive impairment in patients with ANCA-associated small vessel vasculitides. *J. Neurol. Sci.* 2002 Mar 30;195(2):161-6.

[131]Morinaga A, Ono K, Komai K, Yamada M. Microscopic polyangitis presenting with temporal arteritis and multiple cranial neuropathies. *J. Neurol. Sci.* 2007 May 15;256(1-2):81-3.

[132]Takuma H, Shimada H, Inoue Y, Ishimura E, Himuro K, Miki T, Nishizawa Y. Hypertrophic pachymeningitis with anti-neutrophil cytoplasmic antibody (p-ANCA), and diabetes insipidus. *Acta Neurol. Scand.* 2001 Dec;104(6):397-401.

[133]Nagata H, Teramoto K, Suwa A, Abe T, Kimura T, Shibata R. A 73-year-old man with confusion, fever, and positive MPO-ANCA. Keio J Med. 2004 Jun;53(2):103-14.

[134]Belmont HM. Treatment of ANCA-associated systemic vasculitis. *Bull. NYU Hosp. Jt Dis.* 2006;64(1-2):60-6.

[135]Ozaki S. ANCA-associated vasculitis: diagnostic and therapeutic strategy. *Allergol. Int.* 2007 Jun;56(2):87-96.

[136]Aries PM, Hellmich B, Gross WL. Intravenous immunoglobulin therapy in vasculitis: speculation or evidence? *Clin. Rev. Allergy Immunol.* 2005 Dec;29(3):237-45.

[137]Hu W, Liu C, Xie H, Chen H, Liu Z, Li L. Mycophenolate mofetil versus cyclophosphamide for inducing remission of ANCA vasculitis with moderate renal involvement. *Nephrol. Dial Transplant.* 2008 Apr;23(4):1307-12.

[138]Walsh M, Jayne D. Rituximab in the treatment of anti-neutrophil cytoplasm antibody associated vasculitis and systemic lupus erythematosus: past, present and future. *Kidney Int.* 2007 Sep;72(6):676-82.

[139]Huugen D, Cohen Tervaert JW, Heeringa P. TNF-alpha bioactivity-inhibiting therapy in ANCA-associated vasculitis: clinical and experimental considerations. *Clin. J. Am. Soc. Nephrol.* 2006 Sep;1(5):1100-7.

[140]Reumaux D, Duthilleul P, Roos D. Pathogenesis of diseases associated with antineutrophil cytoplasm autoantibodies. *Hum. Immunol.* 2004 Jan;65(1):1-12.

[141]Ozaki S. ANCA in inflammatory bowel disease. *J. Gastroenterol.* 2000;35(9):721-3.

[142]Abad E, Tural C, Mirapeix E, Cuxart A. Relationship between ANCA and clinical activity in inflammatory bowel disease: variation in prevalence of ANCA and evidence of heterogeneity. *J. Autoimmun.* 1997 Apr;10(2):175-80.

[143]Wiik A. Neutrophil-specific autoantibodies in chronic inflammatory bowel diseases. *Autoimmun. Rev.* 2002 Feb;1(1-2):67-72.

[144]Terjung B, Worman HJ, Herzog V, Sauerbruch T, Spengler U. Differentiation of antineutrophil nuclear antibodies in inflammatory bowel and autoimmune liver diseases from antineutrophil cytoplasmic antibodies (p-ANCA) using immunofluorescence microscopy. *Clin. Exp. Immunol.* 2001 Oct;126(1):37-46.

[145]Schultz H, Weiss J, Carroll SF, Gross WL. The endotoxin-binding bactericidal/permeability-increasing protein (BPI): a target antigen of autoantibodies. *J. Leukoc. Biol.* 2001 Apr;69(4):505-12.

[146]Aldebert D, Notteghem B, Reumaux D, Lassalle P, Lion G, Desreumaux P, Duthilleul P, Colombel JF. Anti-endothelial cell antibodies in sera from patients with inflammatory bowel disease. *Gastroenterol. Clin Biol.* 1995 Nov;19(11):867-70.

[147]Nakamura RM, Matsutani M, Barry M. Advances in clinical laboratory tests for inflammatory bowel disease. *Clin. Chim. Acta* 2003 Sep;335(1-2):9-20.

[148]Levine JB, Lukawski-Trubish D. Extraintestinal considerations in inflammatory bowel disease. *Gastroenterol. Clin. North Am.* 1995 Sep;24(3):633-46.

[149]Ghezzi A, Zaffaroni M. Neurological manifestations of gastrointestinal disorders, with particular reference to the differential diagnosis of multiple sclerosis. *Neurol. Sci.* 2001 Nov;22 Suppl 2:S117-22.

[150]Schneiderman JH, Sharpe JA, Sutton DM. Cerebral and retinal vascular complications of inflammatory bowel disease. *Ann. Neurol.* 1979 Apr;5(4):331-7.

[151]Joshi D, Dickel T, Aga R, Smith-Laing G. Stroke in inflammatory bowel disease: a report of two cases and review of the literature. *Thromb J.* 2008 Mar 21;6(1):2.

[152]Haas S. Venous thromboembolism in medical patients--the scope of the problem. *Semin. Thromb Hemost.* 2003 Dec;29 Suppl 1:17-21.

[153]Hasegawa H, Yokomori H, Tsuji T, Hirose R. Hemorrhagic cerebral sinus thrombosis in a case of controlled ulcerative colitis. *Intern. Med.* 2005 Feb;44(2):155.

[154]Fukuhara T, Tsuchida S, Kinugasa K, Ohmoto T. A case of pontine lacunar infarction with ulcerative colitis. *Clin. Neurol. Neurosurg.* 1993 Jun;95(2):159-62.

[155]Freilinger T, Riedel E, Holtmannspötter M, Dichgans M, Peters N. Ischemic stroke and peripheral arterial thromboembolism in a patient with Crohn's disease: a case presentation. *J. Neurol. Sci.* 2008 Mar 15;266(1-2):177-9.

[156]Pounder RE. The pathogenesis of Crohn's disease. *J. Gastroenterol.* 1994 Jul;29 Suppl 7:11-5.

[157]Romagnuolo J, Fedorak RN, Dias VC, Bamforth F, Teltscher M. Hyperhomo cysteinemia and inflammatory bowel disease: prevalence and predictors in a cross-sectional study. *Am. J. Gastroenterol.* 2001 Jul;96(7):2143-9.

[158]Younes-Mhenni S, Derex L, Berruyer M, Nighoghossian N, Philippeau F, Salzmann M, Trouillas P. Large-artery stroke in a young patient with Crohn's disease. Role of vitamin B6 deficiency-induced hyperhomocysteinemia. *J. Neurol. Sci.* 2004 Jun 15;221(1-2):113-5.

[159]Mevorach D, Goldberg Y, Gomori JM, Rachmilewitz D. Antiphospholipid syndrome manifested by ischemic stroke in a patient with Crohn's disease. *J. Clin. Gastroenterol.* 1996 Mar;22(2):141-3.

[160]Vaezi MF, Rustagi PK, Elson CO. Transient protein S deficiency associated with cerebral venous thrombosis in active ulcerative colitis. *Am. J. Gastroenterol.* 1995 Feb;90(2):313-5.

[161]Karacostas D, Mavromatis J, Artemis K, Milonas I. Hemorrhagic cerebral infarct and ulcerative colitis. A case report. *Funct. Neurol.* 1991 Apr-Jun;6(2):181-4.

[162]Baumgart DC, Sandborn WJ. Inflammatory bowel disease: clinical aspects and established and evolving therapies. *Lancet* 2007 May 12;369(9573):1641-57.

[163]Kethu SR. Extraintestinal manifestations of inflammatory bowel diseases. *J. Clin. Gastroenterol.* 2006 Jul;40(6):467-75.

[164]Watson B. TNF inhibitors: a review of the recent patent literature. *IDrugs* 2002 Dec;5(12):1151-61.

[165] Dammacco F, Miglietta A, Lobreglio G, Bonomo L. Cryoglobulins and pyroglobulins: an overview. *Ric. Clin. Lab.* 1986 Apr-Jun;16(2):247-67.

[166] Tedeschi A, Baratè C, Minola E, Morra E. Cryoglobulinemia. *Blood Rev.* 2007 Jul;21 (4):183-200.

[167] Schott P, Hartmann H, Ramadori G. Hepatitis C virus-associated mixed cryoglobulinemia. Clinical manifestations, histopathological changes, mechanisms of cryoprecipitation and options of treatment. *Histol. Histopathol.* 2001 Oct;16(4):1275-85.

[168] Ferri C, Mascia MT. Cryoglobulinemic vasculitis. *Curr. Opin. Rheumatol.* 2006 Jan; 18(1):54-63.

[169] Arena MG, Ferlazzo E, Bonanno D, Quattrocchi P, Ferlazzo B. Cerebral vasculitis in a patient with HCV-related type II mixed cryoglobulinemia. *J. Investig. Allergol. Clin. Immunol.* 2003;13(2):135-6.

[170] Brouet JC. Cryoglobulinemias. *Presse Med.* 1983 Dec 24;12(47):2991-6.

[171] Brouet JC, Clauvel JP, Seligmann M. Cryoglobulinemias. Clinical and biological correlations. *Ann. Med. Interne* (Paris). 1975 Aug-Sep; 126 (8-9):563-7.

[172] Invernizzi F, Pietrogrande M, Sagramoso B. Classification of the cryoglobulinemic syndrome. *Clin. Exp. Rheumatol.* 1995 Nov-Dec;13 Suppl 13:S123-8.

[173] Cacoub P, Maisonobe T, Thibault V, Gatel A, Servan J, Musset L, Piette JC. Systemic vasculitis in patients with hepatitis C. *J. Rheumatol.* 2001 Jan;28(1):109-18.

[174] Cacoub P, Saadoun D. Hepatitis C Virus Infection Induced Vasculitis. *Clin. Rev. Allergy Immunol.* 2008 Jan 11.

[175] Sasso EH. The rheumatoid factor response in the etiology of mixed cryoglobulins associated with hepatitis C virus infection. *Ann. Med. Interne* (Paris). 2000 Feb;151 (1):30-40.

[176] Saadoun D, Landau DA, Calabrese LH, Cacoub PP. Hepatitis C-associated mixed cryoglobulinaemia: a crossroad between autoimmunity and lymphoproliferation. *Rheumatology* (Oxford). 2007 Aug;46(8):1234-42.

[177] Abramsky O, Slavin S. Neurologic manifestations in patients with mixed cryoglobulinemia. *Neurology* 1974 Mar;24(3):245-9.

[178] Nadeau SE. Neurologic manifestations of systemic vasculitis. *Neurol. Clin.* 2002 Feb; 20(1):123-50,vi.

[179] Khella SL, Souayah N. Hepatitis C: a review of its neurologic complications. *Neurologist* 2002 Mar;8(2):101-6

[180] Heckmann JG, Kayser C, Heuss D, Manger B, Blum HE, Neundörfer B. Neurological manifestations of chronic hepatitis C. *J. Neurol.* 1999 Jun;246(6):486-91.

[181] Gemignani F, Brindani F, Alfieri S, Giuberti T, Allegri I, Ferrari C, Marbini A. Clinical spectrum of cryoglobulinaemic neuropathy. *J. Neurol. Neurosurg. Psychiatry* 2005 Oct;76(10):1410-4.

[182] Boukhris S, Magy L, Senga-mokono U, Loustaud-ratti V, Vallat JM. Polyneuropathy with demyelinating features in mixed cryoglobulinemia with hepatitis C virus infection. *Eur. J. Neurol.* 2006 Sep;13(9):937-41.

[183]Filippini D, Colombo F, Jann S, Cornero R, Canesi B. Central nervous system involvement in patients with HCV-related cryoglobulinemia: literature review and a case report. *Reumatismo* 2002 Apr-Jun;54(2):150-5.

[184]Pines A, Kaplinsky N, Goldhammer E, Frankl O. Cerebral involvement in primary mixed cryoglobulinaemia. *Postgrad. Med. J.* 1982 Jun;58(680):359-61.

[185]Petty GW, Duffy J, Houston J 3rd. Cerebral ischemia in patients with hepatitis C virus infection and mixed cryoglobulinemia. Mayo Clin Proc. 1996 Jul;71(7):671-8. Erratum in: *Mayo Clin. Proc.* 1996 Aug;71(8):824.

[186]Marshall Rj, Malone Rg. Cryoglobulinaemia with cerebral purpura. *Br. Med. J.* 1954 Jul 31;2(4882):279-80.

[187]Scrivo R, Di Franco M, Spadaro A, Valesini G. The immunology of rheumatoid arthritis. *Ann. N. Y. Acad. Sci.* 2007;1108:312-22.

[188]Solomon DH, Karlson EW, Rimm EB, Cannuscio CC, Mandl LA, Manson JE, et al. Cardiovascular morbidity and mortality in patients with rheumatoid arthritis. *Circulation* 2003;107:1303–7;.

[189]Del Rincon I, Williams K, Stern MP, Freeman GL, O'Leary DH, Escalante A. Association between carotid atherosclerosis and markers of inflammation in rheumatoid arthritis patients and healthy subjects. *Arthritis Rheum.* 2002;48:1833–40.

[190]Krishnan E, Lingala VB, Singh G. Declines in mortality from acute myocardial infarction in successive incidence and birth cohorts of patients with rheumatoid arthritis. *Circulation* 2004;110:1774–9.

[191]Goodson NJ, Marks J, Lunt M, Symmons DPM. Cardiovascular admissions and mortality in an inception cohort of patients with rheumatoid arthritis with an onset in the 1980's and 1990's. *Ann. Rheum. Dis.* 2005;64:1595–601.

[192]Solomon DH, Goodson NJ, Katz JN, Weinblatt ME, Avorn J, Setoguchi S, Canning C, Schneeweiss S. Patterns of cardiovascular risk in rheumatoid arthritis. *Ann. Rheum. Dis.* 2006;65:1608–1612.

[193]Mrabet D, Meddeb N, Ajlani H, Sahli H, Sellami S. Cerebral vasculitis in a patient with rheumatoid arthritis. *Joint Bone Spine* 2007;74:201-4.

[194]Singleton JD, West SG, Reddy VV, Rak KM. Cerebral vasculitis complicating rheumatoid arthritis. *South Med. J.* 1995;88:470-4.

[195]Ando Y, Kai S, Uyama E, Iyonaga K, Hashimoto Y, Uchino M, Ando M Involvement of the central nervous system in rheumatoid arthritis: its clinical manifestations and analysis by magnetic resonance imaging *Intern. Med.* 1995;34:188-91.

[196]Pedersen RC, Person DA. Cerebral vasculitis in an adolescent with juvenile rheumatoid arthritis. *Pediatr Neurol.* 1998;19:69-73.

[197]Saint Marcoux B, De Bandt M. Vasculitides induced by TNFalpha antagonists: a study in 39 patients in France. *Joint Bone Spine* 2006;73:710-3.

[198]Ohno T, Matsuda I, Furukawa H, Kanoh T. Recovery from rheumatoid cerebral vasculitis by low-dose methotrexate. *Intern. Med.* 1994t;33:615-20.

[199]Sherer Y, Gorstein A, Fritzler MJ, Shoenfeld Y. Autoantibody explosion in systemic lupus erythematosus: more than 100 different antibodies found in SLE patients. *Semin. Arthritis Rheum.* 2004;34:501-37.

[200]T Borchers, C A. Aoki, S M. Naguwa, C L. Keen, Y Shoenfeld, M.E Gershwin Neuropsychiatric features of systemic lupus erythematosus. *Autoimmunity Reviews* 2005 Jul;4(6):329–344.

[201]D'Cruz DP, Khamashta MA, Hughes GR. Systemic lupus erythematosus. *Lancet* 2007;369:587-596.

[202]ACR Ad Hoc Committee on Neuropsychiatric Lupus Nomenclature. The American College of Rheumatology nomenclature and case definitions for neuropsychiatric lupus syndromes. *Arthritis Rheum.* 1999;42:599–608.

[203]Greenwood DL, Gitlits VM, Alderuccio F, Sentry JW, Toh BH. Autoantibodies in neuropsychiatric lupus. *Autoimmunity* 2002;35:79-86.

[204]Sanna G, Bertolaccini ML, Cuadrado MJ, Khamashta MA, Hughes GR. Central nervous system involvement in the antiphospholipid (Hughes) syndrome. *Rheumatology* 2003;42:200-213.

[205]Miyakis S , Atsumi T, Branch DW, Brey RL, Cervera R, Derksen RHWM, De Groot PG, Koike T, Meroni PL, Reber G, Shoenfeld Y, Tincani A, Vlachoyiannopoulos PG, Krilis SA. International consensus statement on an update of the classification criteria for definite antiphospholipid syndrome (APS) *Journal of Thrombosis and Haemostasis*;4:295–306.

[206]Drijkoningen J, Damoiseaux J, van Paassen P, Tervaert JWC. Clinical manifestations of the anti-phospholipid syndrome as defined by the updated Sapporo classification criteria Ann Rheum Dis 2007; 66: 1407–1408. Petri M. Epidemiology of the antiphospholipid antibody syndrome. *J. Autoimmun.* 2000;15:145–51.

[207]Petri M. Epidemiology of the antiphospholipid antibody syndrome. *J. Autoimmun.* 2000 Sep;15(2):145-51.

[208]Cervera R, Khamashta MA, Font J et al. Morbidity and mortality in systemic lupus erythematosus during a 10-year period: a comparison of early and late manifestations in a cohort of 1,000 patients. *Medicine* 2003;82:299–308.

[209]T Tarr, G Lakos, H P Bhattoa, Y Shoenfeld, G Szegedi and E Kiss. Analysis of risk factors for the development of thrombotic complications in antiphospholipid antibody positive lupus patients. *Lupus* 2007;16:39–45.

[210]Sanna G, Bertolaccini ML, Cuadrado MJ et al. Neuropsychiatric manifestations in systemic lupus erythematosus: prevalence and association with antiphospholipid antibodies. *J. Rheumatol.* 2003;30:985–992.

[211]Afeltra A, Garzia P, Mitterhofer AP et al. Neuropsychiatric lupus syndromes: relationship with antiphospholipid antibodies. *Neurology* 2003;61:108–110.

[212]Margutti P, Sorice M, Conti F, Delunardo F, Racaniello M, Alessandri C, Siracusano A, Riganò R, Profumo E, Valesini G, Ortona E. Screening of an endothelial cDNA library identifies the C-terminal region of Nedd5 as a novel autoantigen in systemic lupus erythematosus with psychiatric manifestations. *Arthritis Res. Ther.* 2005;7:R896-903.

[213]Karassa FB, Afeltra A, Ambrozic A, Chang DM, De Keyser F, Doria A, Galeazzi M, Hirohata S, Hoffman IE, Inanc M, Massardo L, Mathieu A, Mok CC, Morozzi G, Sanna G, Spindler AJ, Tzioufas AG, Yoshio T, Ioannidis JP. Accuracy of anti-

ribosomal P protein antibody testing for the diagnosis of neuropsychiatric systemic lupus erythematosus: an international meta-analysis. *Arthritis Rheum.* 2006;54:312-24.

[214] Yoshio T, Hirata D, Onda K, Nara H, Minota S.Antiribosomal P protein antibodies in cerebrospinal fluid are associated with neuropsychiatric systemic lupus erythematosus; *J. Rheumatol.* 2005;32:34-9.

[215] Isshi K, Hirohata S. Association of anti-ribosomal P protein antibodies with neuropsychiatric systemic lupus erythematosus. *Arthritis Rheum.* 1996;39:1483-90.

[216] Mahler M, Kessenbrock K, Szmyrka M, Takasaki Y, Garcia-De La Torre I, Shoenfeld Y, Hiepe F, Shun-le C, von Mühlen CA, Locht H, Höpfl P, Wiik A, Reeves W, Fritzler MJ. International multicenter evaluation of autoantibodies to ribosomal P proteins. *Clin. Vaccine Immunol.* 2006;13:77-83.

[217] Hanly JG, Walsh NMG, Sanglang V Brain pathology in SLE. *J. Rheumatol.* 1992; 19:732-41.

[218] Belmont HM, Abramson SB, Lie JT Pathology and pathogenesis of vascular injury in SLE: interactions of inflammatory cells and activated endothelium. *Arthr. Rheum.* 1996;39:9-22.

[219] Devinsky O, Petito CK, Alonso DR. Clinical and neuropathological findings in systemic lupus erythematosus: the role of vasculitis, heart emboli, and thrombotic thrombocytopenic purpura. *Ann. Neurol.* 1988;23:380–384.

[220] Ellis SG, Verity MA. Central nervous system involvement in systemic lupus erythematosus: review of neuropathological findings in 57 cases 1955–1957. *Semin. Arthritis Rheum.* 1979;8:212–221.

[221] Suzuki Y, Kitagawa Y, Matsuoka Y, Fukuda J, Mizushima Y. Severe cerebral and systemic necrotizing vasculitis developing during pregnancy in a case of systemic lupus erythematosus. *J. Rheumatol.* 1990;17:1408–1411.

[222] Suwabe H, Moriuchi J, Hoshina Y, Iwata Y, Ichikawa Y, Arimori S. Renal and cerebral infarctions in a patient with systemic lupus erythematosus without antiphospholipid antibodies. *Ryumachi.* 1993;33:335–340.

[223] Wolf J, Neidermaier N, Bergner R, Lowitzsch K. Cerebral vasculitis as the initial manifestation of systemic lupus erythematosus. *Dtsch Med. Wochenschr* 2001;126: 947–950.

[224] Mimenza-Alvarado AJ, Tellez-Zenteno JF, Cantu Brito C, Garcia-Ramos G. Systemic lupus erythematosus with affection to brainstem: report of three cases. *Rev. Neurol.* 2002;35:128–131.

[225] Sipek-Dolnicar A, Hojnik M, Bozic B, Vizjak A, Rozman B, Ferluga D. Clinical presentations and vascular histopathology in autopsied patients with systemiclupus erythematosus and anticardiolipin antibodies. *Clin. Exp. Rheumatol.* 2002;20:335–342.

[226] Goel D, Rajashekhar Reddy S, Sundaram C, K Prayaga A, Rajasekhar L, Narsimulu G. Active necrotizing cerebral vasculitis in systemic lupus erythematosus. *Neuropathology* 2007;27:561–565.

[227] Otte A, Weiner SM, Hoegerle S, Wolf R, Juengling FD, Peter HH, Nitzsche EU. Neuropsychiatric systemic lupus erythematosus before and after immunosuppressive treatment: a FDG PET study. *Lupus* 1998;7:57-9.

[228]Sibbitt Jr WL, Sibbitt RR, Brooks WM. Neuroimaging in neuropsychiatric systemic lupus erythematosus. *Arthritis Rheum*. 1999;42:2026– 38.

[229]Govoni M, Castellino G, Padovan M, Borrelli M, Trotta F. Recent advances and future perspective in neuroimaging in neuropsychiatric systemic lupus erythematosus. *Lupus* 2004;13:149– 58.

[230]Kao CH, Ho YJ, Lan JL, Changlai SP, Liao KK, Chieng PU. Discrepancy between regional cerebral blood flow and glucose metabolism of the brain in systemic lupus erythematosus patients with normal brain magnetic resonance imaging findings. *Arthritis Rheum*. 1999;42:61–8.

[231]Chen JJ, Yen RF, Kao A, Lin CC, Lee CC. Abnormal regional cerebral blood flow found by technetium-99m ethyl cysteinate dimer brain single photon emission computed tomography in systemic lupus erythematosus patients with normal brain MRI findings. *Clin. Rheumatol*. 2002;21:516–9.

[232]Handa R, Sahota P, Kumar M, Jagannathan NR, Bal CS, Gulati M, et al. In vivo proton magnetic resonance spectroscopy (MRS) and single photon emission computerized tomography (SPECT) in systemic lupus erythematosus (SLE). *Magn. Reson Imaging* 2003; 21:1033–1037.

[233]Steens SC, Steup-Beekman GM, Bosma GP, Admiraal-Behloul F, Olofsen H, Doornbos J, Huizinga TW, van Buchem MA. The effect of corticosteroid medication on quantitative MR parameters of the brain. *AJNR Am. J. Neuroradiol*. 2005;26:2475-80.

[234]Jose J, Paulose BK, Vasuki Z, Danda D; Mycophenolate mofetil in neuropsychiatric systemic lupus erythematosus. *Indian J. Med. Sci*. 2005;59:353-6.

[235]Barile-Fabris L, Ariza-Andraca R, Olguín-Ortega L, Jara LJ, Fraga-Mouret A,Miranda-Limón JM, Fuentes de la Mata J, Clark P, Vargas F, Alocer-Varela J.Controlled clinical trial of IV cyclophosphamide versus IV methylprednisolone in severe neurological manifestations in systemic lupus erythematosus. *Ann. Rheum. Dis*. 2005;64:620-5.

[236]Baca V, Lavalle C, García R, Catalán T, Sauceda JM, Sánchez G, Martínez I, Ramírez ML, Márquez LM, Rojas JC.Favorable response to intravenous methylprednisolone and cyclophosphamide in children with severe neuropsychiatric lupus. *J. Rheumatol*. 1999; 26:432-9.

[237]Neuwelt CM, Lacks S, Kaye BR, Ellman JB, Borenstein DG. Role of intravenous cyclophosphamide in the treatment of severe neuropsychiatric systemic lupus erythematosus. *Am. J. Med*. 1995;98:32-41.

[238]Bartolucci P, Bréchignac S, Cohen P, Le Guern V, Guillevin L. Adjunctive plasma exchanges to treat neuropsychiatric lupus: a retrospective study on 10 patients. *Lupus* 2007;16:817-22.

[239]Lehnhardt FG, Scheid C, Holtik U, Burghaus L, Neveling M, Impekoven P, Rüger A, Hallek M, Jacobs AH, Rubbert A. Autologous blood stem cell transplantation in refractory systemic lupus erythematodes with recurrent longitudinal myelitis and cerebral infarction. *Lupus* 2006;15:240-3.

[240]Mount GR, Gilliland WR. Emerging Biological Therapies in Systemic Lupus Erythematosus. *Clin. Pharmacol. Ther*. 2008;83:167-171.

[241]Tokunaga M, Saito K, Kawabata D, Imura Y, Fujii T, Nakayamada S, Tsujimura S, Nawata M, Iwata S, Azuma T, Mimori T, Tanaka Y. Efficacy of rituximab (anti-CD20) for refractory systemic lupus erythematosus involving the central nervous system. *Ann. Rheum. Dis*. 2007; 66: 470-5.

[242]Tzioufas AG, Voulgarelis M. Update on Sjögren's syndrome autoimmune epithelitis: from classification to increased neoplasias. *Best Pract. Res. Clin. Rheumatol.* 2007;21: 989-1010.

[243]Fox PC. Autoimmune diseases and Sjogren's syndrome: an autoimmune exocrinopathy. *Ann. N. Y. Acad. Sci*. 2007;1098:15-21.

[244]Ramos-Casals M, Brito-Zerón P, Font J. The overlap of Sjögren's syndrome with other systemic autoimmune diseases. *Semin. Arthritis Rheum.* 2007 Feb;36:246-55.

[245]Mellgren SI, Göransson LG, Omdal R. Primary Sjögren's syndrome associated neuropathy. *Can. J. Neurol. Sci.* 2007;34:280-7.

[246]Govoni M, Bajocchi G, Rizzo N, Tola M. R, Caniatti L, Tugnoli V, Colamussi P, Trotta F. Neurological Involvement in Primary Sjögren’s Syndrome: Clinical and Instrumental Evaluation in a Cohort of Italian Patients. *Clin. Rheumatol.* 1999;18:299–303.

[247]Delalande S, de Seze J, Fauchais A, Hachulla E, Stojkovic T, Ferriby D, Dubucquoi S, Pruvo JP, Vermersch P, Hatron PY. Neurologic Manifestations in Primary Sjögren Syndrome: A Study of 82 Patients. *Medicine* 2004;83:280–291.

[248]Malinow KL, Molina R, Gordon B, et al. Neuropsychiatric dysfunction in primary Sjogren’s syndrome. *Ann. Intern. Med.* 1985;103:344–9.

[249]Escudero D, Latorre P, Codina M, Coll-Canti J, Coll J. Central nervous system disease in Sjogren’s syndrome. *Ann. Med. Interne*. (Paris) 1995;146:239-42.

[250]Belin C, Moroni C, Caillat-Vigneron N, Debray M, Baudin M, Dumas JL, et al. Central nervous system involvement in Sjogren’s syndrome: evidence from neuropsychological testing and HMPAO-SPECT. *Ann. Med. Interne*. (Paris) 1999;150: 598-604.

[251]Alexander EL, Craft C, Dorsch C, Moser RL, Provost TT, Alexander GE. Necrotizing arteritis and spinal subarachnoid hemorrhage in Sjogren syndrome. *Ann. Neurol.* 1982; 11:632-5.

[252]Alexander EL, Alexander GE. Aseptic meningoencephalitis in primary Sjogren’s syndrome. *Neurology* 1983;33:593-8.

[253]Konttinen YT, Kinnunen E, von Bonsdorff M, Lillqvist P, Immonen I,Bergroth V, et al. Acute transverse myelopathy successfully treated with and prednisone in a patient with primary Sjogren’ssyndrome. *Arthritis Rheum*. 1987;30:339-44.

[254]Alexander EL, Malinow K, Lejewski JE, Jerdan MS, Provost TT, Alexander GE. Primary Sjögren’s syndrome with central nervous system disease mimicking multiple sclerosis. *Ann. Intern. Med*. 1986;104:323–330.

[255]Bragoni M, Di Piero V, Priori P, Valesini G, Lenzi GL (1994). Sjögren’s syndrome presenting as ischemic stroke. *Stroke* 25:2276–2279.

[256]Alexander EL. Central nervous system disease in Sjögren’s syndrome. New insights into immunopathogenesis. *Rheum. Dis. Clin. North Am*. 1992;18:637–672.

[257] Ranzenbach MR, Kumar A, Rosembaum AE, et al. Anti-Ro(SS-A) autoantibodies (A-RoAb) in the immunopathogenesis of serious focal CNS disease in Sjogren's syndrome (CNS-SS). *Arthritis Rheum.* 1992;35:S168.

[258] Lewandowska E, Wierzba-Bobrowicz T, Wagner T, Boguslawska R, Rudnicka A, Leszczyńska A, Pasennik E, Lechowicz W, Stepień T, Kuran W. Sneddon's syndrome as a disorder of the small arteries with endothelial cells proliferation: ultrastructural and neuroimaing study. *Folia Neuropathol.* 2005;43(4):345-354.

[259] International Study Group for Behcet's Disease. Criteria for diagnosis of Behcet's disease. *Lancet* 1990;335:1078-1080.

[260] Borhani Haghighi A, Pourmand R, Nikseresht AR. Neuro-Behçet disease. A review. *Neurologist.* 2005;11:80-9.

[261] Akman-Demir G, SerdarogÆ lu P, Tas i B and the Neuro-Behcet Study Group. Clinical patterns of neurological involvement in Behcet's disease: evaluation of 200 patients. *Brain* 1999;122:2171-2181.

[262] Matsumoto T, Uekusa T, Fukuda Y. Vasculo-Behcet's disease: a pathologic study of eight cases. *Human Pathol.* 1991;22:45-51.

[263] Nishimura M, Satoh K, Suga M, Oda M. Cerebral angio- and neuro- Behcet's syndrome: neuroradiological and pathological study of one case. *J. Neurol. Sci.* 1991; 106:19-24.

[264] Krespi Y, Akman-Demir G, Poyraz M, Tugcu B, Coban O, Tuncay R, Serdaroglu P, Bahar S. Cerebral vasculitis and ischaemic stroke in Behcet's disease: report of one case and review of the literature. *European Journal of Neurology* 2001;8:719-722.

[265] Diri E, Espinoza LR. Neuro-Behçet's syndrome: differential diagnosis and management. *Curr. Rheumatol. Rep.* 2006;8:317-22.

[266] Mizukami K, Shiraishi H, Tanaka Y, Terashima Y, Kawai N, Baba A, Arai T, Koizumi CNS changes in neuro-Behçet's disease: CT, MR, and SPECT findings. *J. Comput. Med. Imaging Graph.* 1992;16:401-6.

[267] Akman-Demir G, Bahar S, Coban O, Tasci B, Serdaroglu P. Cranial MRI in Behçet's disease: 134 examinations of 98 patients. *Neuroradiology* 2003;45:851-9.

[268] Patel DV, Neuman MJ, Hier DB. Reversibility of CT and MR findings in neuro-Behçet disease. *J. Comput. Assist. Tomogr.* 1989;13:669-73.

[269] Kurata A, Franke FE, Machinami R, Schulz A. Thromboangiitis obliterans: classic and new morphological features. *Virchows Arch* 2000 Jan;436(1):59-67.

[270] Mills JL Sr. Buerger's disease in the 21st century: diagnosis, clinical features, and therapy. *Semin. Vasc. Surg.* 2003 Sep;16 (3):179-89.

[271] Puéchal X, Fiessinger JN. Thromboangiitis obliterans or Buerger's disease: challenges for the rheumatologist. *Rheumatology* (Oxford). 2007 Feb;46(2):192-9.

[272] Olin JW, Shih A. Thromboangiitis obliterans (Buerger's disease). *Curr. Opin. Rheumatol.* 2006 Jan;18(1):18-24.

[273] Olin JW. Thromboangiitis obliterans (Buerger's disease). *N. Engl. J. Med.* 2000 Sep 21;343(12):864-9.

[274] Chen YW, Iwai T, Umeda M, Nagasawa T, Huang Y, Takeuchi Y, Ishikawa I. Elevated IgG titers to periodontal pathogens related to Buerger disease. *Int. J. Cardiol.* 2007 Oct 31;122(1):79-81.

[275]Maslowski L, McBane R, Alexewicz P, Wysokinski WE. Antiphospholipid antibodies in thromboangiitis obliterans. *Vasc. Med.* 2002;7(4):259-64.

[276]Eichhorn J, Sima D, Lindschau C, Turowski A, Schmidt H, Schneider W, Haller H, Luft FC. Antiendothelial cell antibodies in thromboangiitis obliterans. *Am. J. Med. Sci.* 1998 Jan;315(1):17-23.

[277]Halacheva KS, Manolova IM, Petkov DP, Andreev AP. Study of anti-neutrophil cytoplasmic antibodies in patients with thromboangiitis obliterans (Buerger's disease). *Scand. J. Immunol.* 1998 Nov;48(5):544-50.

[278]Cooper LT, Henderson SS, Ballman KV, Offord KP, Tse TS, Holmes DR, Hurt RD. A prospective, case-control study of tobacco dependence in thromboangiitis obliterans (Buerger's Disease). *Angiology* 2006 Jan-Feb;57(1):73-8.

[279]Börner C, Heidrich H. Long-term follow-up of thromboangiitis obliterans. *Vasa* 1998 May;27(2):80-6.

[280]Puchmayer V. Smoking as a risk factor for the development of arterial occlusive disease. *Acta Univ. Carol. Med. Monogr.* 1984;105:1-134.

[281]Schneider HJ, Jha S, Burnand KG. Progressive arteritis associated with cannabis use. *Eur. J .Vasc. Endovasc. Surg.* 1999 Oct;18(4):366-7.

[282]Marder VJ, Mellinghoff IK. Cocaine and Buerger disease: is there a pathogenetic association? *Arch Intern. Med.* 2000 Jul 10;160(13):2057-60.

[283]Adar R, Papa MZ, Schneiderman J. Thromboangiitis obliterans: an old disease in need of a new look. *Int. J. Cardiol.* 2000 Aug 31;75 Suppl 1:S167-70;discussion:S171-3.

[284]Tseng CH, Chong CK, Chen CJ, Tai TY. Dose-response relationship between peripheral vascular disease and ingested inorganic arsenic among residents in blackfoot disease endemic villages in Taiwan. *Atherosclerosis* 1996 Feb;120(1-2):125-33.

[285]Narang AP, Greval RS, Goyal SC. Arsenic adulteration in Indian tobacco. *Indian J. Med. Sci.* 1995 Mar;49(3):55-7.

[286]Puéchal X, Fiessinger JN, Kahan A, Menkès CJ. Rheumatic manifestations in patients with thromboangiitis obliterans (Buerger's disease). *J. Rheumatol.* 1999 Aug;26(8): 1764-8.

[287]Zhan SS, Beyreuther K, Schmitt HP. Vascular dementia in Spatz-Lindenberg's disease (SLD): cortical synaptophysin immunoreactivity as compared with dementia of Alzheimer type and non-demented controls. *Acta Neuropathol.* 1993;86(3):259-64.

[288]Larner AJ, Kidd D, Elkington P, Rudge P, Scaravilli F. Spatz-Lindenberg disease: a rare cause of vascular dementia. Stroke. 1999 Mar;30(3):687-9.

[289]Suzuki S, Yamada I, Himeno Y. Angiographic findings in Buerger disease. *Int. J. Cardiol.* 1996 Aug;54 Suppl:S189-95.

[290]No YJ, Lee EM, Lee DH, Kim JS. Cerebral angiographic findings in thromboangiitis obliterans. *Neuroradiology* 2005 Dec;47(12):912-5.

[291]Bischof F, Kuntz R, Melms A, Fetter M. Cerebral vein thrombosis in a case with thromboangiitis obliterans. *Cerebrovasc. Dis.* 1999 Sep-Oct;9(5):295-7.

[292]Shionoya S. Diagnostic criteria of Buerger's disease. *Int. J. Cardiol.* 1998 Oct 1;66 Suppl 1:S243-5;discussion S247.

[293]Papa MZ, Rabi I, Adar R. A point scoring system for the clinical diagnosis of Buerger's disease. *Eur. J. Vasc. Endovasc. Surg.* 1996 Apr;11(3):335-9.

[294] Paraskevas KI, Liapis CD, Briana DD, Mikhailidis DP. Thromboangiitis obliterans (Buerger's disease): searching for a therapeutic strategy. *Angiology* 2007 Feb-Mar; 58(1):75-84.

[295] Paraskevas KI. Treatment-of-choice for Buerger's disease (thromboangiitis obliterans): still an unresolved issue. *Clin. Rheumatol.* 2008 Apr;27(4):547.

[296] Fiessinger JN, Schäfer M. Trial of iloprost versus aspirin treatment for critical limb ischaemia of thromboangiitis obliterans. The TAO Study. *Lancet* 1990 Mar 10; 335(8689):555-7.

[297] Bozkurt AK, Köksal C, Demirbas MY, Erdoğan A, Rahman A, Demirkiliç U, Ustünsoy H, Metin G, Yillik L, Onol H, Cinar B, Karaçelik M, Erdinç I, Bolcal C, Sayin AG; Turkish Buerger's Disease Research Group. A randomized trial of intravenous iloprost (a stable prostacyclin analogue) versus lumbar sympathectomy in the management of Buerger's disease. *Int. Angiol.* 2006 Jun;25(2):162-8.

[298] Swainston Harrison T, Plosker GL. Limaprost. *Drugs* 2007;67(1):109-18;discussion: 119-20.

[299] Cundiff J, Kansal S, Kumar A, Goldstein DA, Tessler HH. Cogan's syndrome: a cause of progressive hearing deafness. *Am. J. Otolaryngol.* 2006 Jan-Feb;27(1):68-70.

[300] St Clair EW, McCallum RM. Cogan's syndrome. *Curr. Opin. Rheumatol.* 1999 Jan; 11(1):47-52.

[301] García Berrocal JR, Vargas JA, Vaquero M, Ramón y Cajal S, Ramírez-Camacho RA. Cogan's syndrome: an oculo-audiovestibular disease. *Postgrad. Med. J.* 1999 May; 75(883):262-4.

[302] Grasland A, Pouchot J, Hachulla E, Blétry O, Papo T, Vinceneux P; Study Group for Cogan's Syndrome. Typical and atypical Cogan's syndrome: 32 cases and review of the literature. *Rheumatology* (Oxford). 2004 Aug;43(8):1007-15.

[303] Shah P, Luqmani RA, Murray PI, Honan WP, Corridan PG, Emery P. Posterior scleritis--an unusual manifestation of Cogan's syndrome. *Br. J. Rheumatol.* 1994 Aug;33(8):774-5.

[304] Cheson BD, Bluming AZ, Alroy J. Cogan's syndrome: a systemic vasculitis. Am. J Med 1976;60:549-555.

[305] Gaubitz M, Lübben B, Seidel M, Schotte H, Gramley F, Domschke W. Cogan's syndrome: organ-specific autoimmune disease or systemic vasculitis? A report of two cases and review of the literature. *Clin. Exp. Rheumatol.* 2001 Jul-Aug;19(4):463-9.

[306] Gelfand ML, Kantor T, Gorstein F. Cogan's syndrome with cardiovascular involvement: aortic insufficiency. Bull N Y Acad Med. 1972 May;48(4):647-60.

[307] Bicknell JM, Holland JV. Neurological manifestation of Cogan's syndrome. *Neurology* 1978;28:278-281.

[308] Benvenga S, Trimarchi F, Facchiano A. Cogan's syndrome as an autoimmune disease. *Lancet* 2003 Feb 8;361(9356):530-1.

[309] Ikeda M, Okazaki H, Minota S. Cogan's syndrome with antineutrophil cytoplasmic autoantibody. *Ann. Rheum. Dis.* 2002 Aug;61(8):761-2.

[310] Helmchen C, Arbusow V, Jäger L, Strupp M, Stöcker W, Schulz P. Cogan's syndrome: clinical significance of antibodies against the inner ear and cornea. *Acta Otolaryngol.* 1999; 119(5):528-36.

[311]Majoor MH, Albers FW, Casselman JW. Clinical relevance of magnetic resonance imaging and computed tomography in Cogan's syndrome. *Acta Otolaryngol.* 1993 Sep; 113(5):625-31.

[312]Albayram MS, Wityk R, Yousem DM, Zinreich SJ. The cerebral angiographic findings in Cogan syndrome. *AJNR Am. J. Neuroradiol.* 2001 Apr;22(4):751-4.

[313]Matteson EL, Fabry DA, Facer GW, Beatty CW, Driscoll CL, Strome SE, McDonald TJ. Open trial of methotrexate as treatment for autoimmune hearing loss. *Arthritis Rheum.* 2001 Apr;45(2):146-50.

[314]Aeberli D, Oertle S, Mauron H, Reichenbach S, Jordi B, Villiger PM. Inhibition of the TNF-pathway: use of infliximab and etanercept as remission-inducing agents in cases of therapy-resistant chronic inflammatory disorders. *Swiss Med. Wkly* 2002 Jul 27;132(29-30):414-22.

[315]Susac JO, Egan RA, Rennebohm RM, Lubow M. Susac's syndrome: 1975-2005 microangiopathy/autoimmune endotheliopathy. *J. Neurol. Sci.* 2007 Jun 15;257(1-2):270-2.

[316]Susac JO. Susac's syndrome. *AJNR Am. J. Neuroradiol.* 2004 Mar;25(3):351-2.

[317]Susac JO, Calabrese LH, Baylin E, Prayson RA, Medeiros NE, Hull RP, Tucker JP. Branch retinal artery occlusions as the presenting feature of primary central nervous system vasculitis. *Clin. Exp. Rheumatol.* 2004;22,6 Suppl 36:S70-4.

[318]Gross M, Banin E, Eliashar R, Ben-Hur T. Susac syndrome. *Otol. Neurotol.* 2004 Jul; 25(4):470-3.

[319]Do TH, Fisch C, Evoy F. Susac syndrome: report of four cases and review of the literature. *AJNR Am. J. Neuroradiol.* 2004 Mar;25(3):382-8.

[320]Saw VP, Canty PA, Green CM, Briggs RJ, Cremer PD, Harrisberg B, McCluskey P, O'Day J, Paine M, Wakefield D, Watson JD.Susac syndrome: microangiopathy of the retina, cochlea and brain. *Clin. Experiment Ophthalmol.* 2000 Oct;28(5):373-81.

[321]Flammer J, Kaiser H, Haufschild T. Susac syndrome: a vasospastic disorder? *Eur. J. Ophthalmol.* 2001 Apr-Jun;11(2):175-9.

[322]Egan RA, Ha Nguyen T, Gass JD, Rizzo JF 3rd, Tivnan J, Susac JO. Retinal arterial wall plaques in Susac syndrome. *Am. J. Ophthalmol.* 2003 Apr;135(4):483-6.

[323]Susac JO, Murtagh FR, Egan RA, Berger JR, Bakshi R, Lincoff N, Gean AD, Galetta SL, Fox RJ, Costello FE, Lee AG, Clark J, Layzer RB, Daroff RB. MRI findings in Susac's syndrome. *Neurology* 2003 Dec 23;61(12):1783-7.

[324]Rennebohm RM, Egan RA, Susac JO. Treatment of Susac's Syndrome. *Curr. Treat Options Neurol.* 2008 Jan;10(1):67-74.

[325]Fox RJ, Costello F, Judkins AR, Galetta SL, Maguire AM, Leonard B, Markowitz CE. Treatment of Susac syndrome with gamma globulin and corticosteroids. *J. Neurol. Sci.* 2006 Dec 21;251(1-2):17-22.

[326]Aubart-Cohen F, Klein I, Alexandra JF, Bodaghi B, Doan S, Fardeau C, Lavallée P, Piette JC, Hoang PL, Papo T. Long-term outcome in Susac syndrome. *Medicine* (Baltimore). 2007 Mar;86(2):93-102.

In: Cerebral Ischemia in Young Adults
Editors: A. Pezzini and A. Padovani

ISBN 978-1-60741-627-2

Chapter 12

Moyamoya Disease in Young Adults

***Satoshi Kuroda*[*1] *and Kiyohiro Houkin*[2]**

1. Department of Neurosurgery,
Hokkaido University Graduate School of Medicine (SK), Japan
2. Department of Neurosurgery, Sapporo Medical University (KH), Japan

Abstract

In this chapter, the authors describe various aspects of moyamoya disease in young adults, including its definition, epidemiology, pathophysiology, clinical symptoms, radiological findings, surgical treatment and prognosis. Moyamoya disease is characterized by progressive occlusion of the bilateral carotid forks associated with a fine vascular network at the base of brain, called as the "moyamoya" vessels. Its etiology is still unclear, although recent studies have suggested the involvement of some genetic factor in disease onset. Although the incidence of moyamoya disease is not so high in Western countries, neurologists and neurosurgeons should always take into consideration as one of probable etiology when they take care of young adult patients who develop ischemic or hemorrhagic stroke. Precise analysis of their neurological and radiological findings is essential to determine therapeutic strategies and improve their long-term outcome. Surgical revascularization improves cerebral hemodynamics and metabolism and reduces the risk for subsequent ischemic stroke. In near future, an ongoing randomized clinical trial in Japan would clarify whether surgical revascularization also reduce the risk for recurrence of hemorrhagic stroke.

* Correspondence: Satoshi Kuroda, North 15 West 7, Kita-ku, Sapporo 060-8638, Japan. Tel: +81-11-706-5987, Fax: +81-11-708-7737. E-mail: skuroda@med.hokudai.ac.jp.

Introduction

Moyamoya disease is characterized by progressive occlusion of the bilateral carotid forks associated with a fine vascular network at the base of brain, called as the "moyamoya" vessels [1]. In the literature, Takeuchi and Shimizu (1957) reported the first case of moyamoya disease as hypoplasia of the bilateral internal carotid arteries (ICAs) [2]. Subsequently, Suzuki and Takaku (1969) established this disease as a novel entity of occlusive cerebrovascular disease and named it as moyamoya disease, based on its angiographical appearances. "Moyamoya" is a Japanese word that means something puffy, hazy, obscure, or vague, such as a puff of cigarette smoke drifting in the air [1].

Numerous numbers of studies have clarified that the essential pathology of moyamoya disease is progressive stenosis of the terminal portion of ICAs. Nowadays, "moyamoya" vessels are considered as the dilated perforating arteries that function as collateral pathway in response to reduced cerebral perfusion pressure [3]. As described below, moyamoya disease is a very unique disorder because of its own specific clinical features, and often involves young adults. Although its incidence is not so high, appropriate understandings on its diagnosis and treatments are essential to improve their long-term prognosis. Various aspects of moyamoya disease in young adults are discussed in this chapter.

Definition

The Research Committee on Spontaneous Occlusion of the Circle of Willis (Moyamoya Disease) has published the guidelines for diagnosis of moyamoya disease in English in 1997 [4]. Thus, moyamoya disease is defined as having (1) stenosis or occlusion at the terminal portion of the internal carotid artery or the proximal portion of the anterior or the middle cerebral arteries and (2) abnormal vascular networks demonstrated in the arterial phase in the vicinity of the occlusive or stenotic lesions on cerebral angiography.

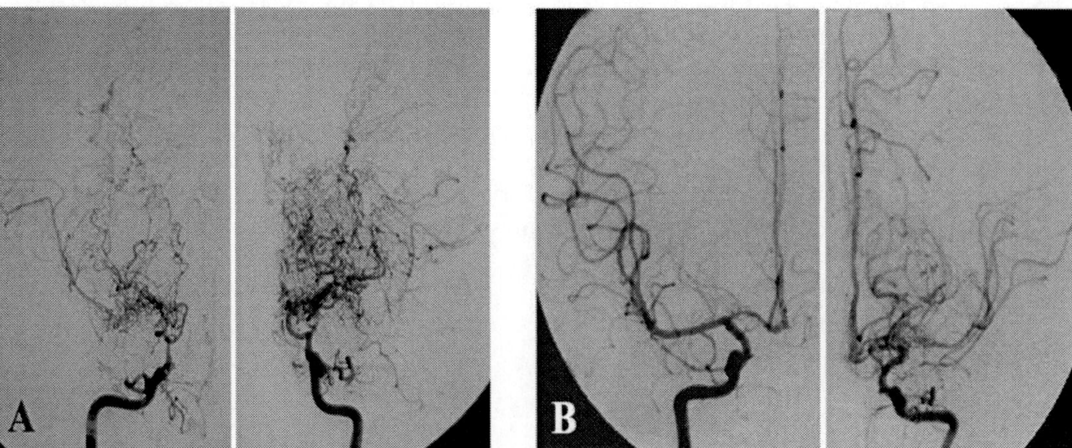

Figure 1. Cerebral angiography in "definite" case with bilateral involvement (A) and "probable" case with unilateral involvement (B). Note that right internal carotid angiogram is intact in "probable" case.

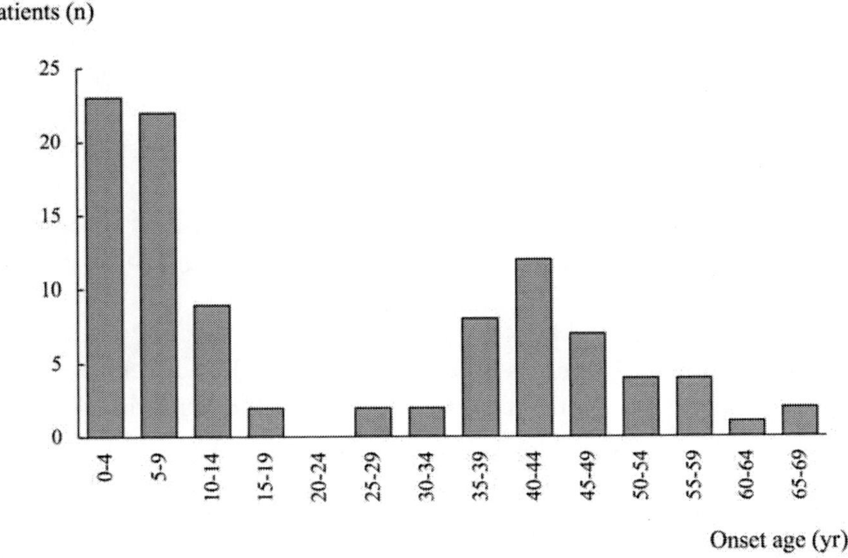

Figure 2. Age distribution of the patients who were admitted to Hokkaido University Hospital due to moyamoya disease between 1979 and 2000.

The patients with bilateral lesions are diagnosed as "definite" cases, while those with unilateral lesions are diagnosed as "probable" cases (Figure 1). Because the etiology of this disease is unknown, cerebrovascular disease with the following basic diseases or conditions should thus by eliminated and is usually categorized as quasi-moyamoya disease: atherosclerosis, autoimmune disease, meningitis, brain neoplasm, Down syndrome, von Recklinghausen's disease, head trauma, irradiation to the head and others. When 1.0- or 1.5-Tesla MR imaging (MRI) and MR angiography (MRA) clearly demonstrate all of angiographical findings, conventional cerebral angiography is not essential.

Epidemiology

Disease Distribution over the World

It is well known that the incidence of moyamoya disease is particularly high among far-east Asia including Japan and Korea. A nationwide, questionnaires-based survey in Japan was conducted in 1995 and revealed that its prevalence and incidence rates were 3.16 and 0.35 per 100,000 populations, respectively. The sex ratio (female to male) was 1.8. The peak of age distribution of the patients was observed in 10-14 years old and a smaller peak in 40-50 years old. Familial occurrence was observed in 15.4% of patients [5]. Figure 2 shows the age distribution of 91 patients who were admitted to Hokkaido University Hospital due to moyamoya disease between 1979 and 2000, supporting two-peak distribution of their age.

However, based on recent data all-inclusive survey of moyamoya disease in Hokkaido, one of main islands in Japan, Baba et al. (2007) reported that both prevalence and incidence rates are higher than those described before and that the highest peak of age distribution is observed in 45-49 years old [6]. There are several explanations for the discrepancy. First, the survey methodology is different among the studies. Thus, most of previous epidemiological studies are based on the data obtained from questionnaires survey in large-volume hospitals, while Baba et al. (2007) collected the data from all-inclusive survey in Hokkaido Island with approximately 5.6 million populations [6]. Second, recent widespread use of non-invasive MR examination may increase the opportunity to detect asymptomatic moyamoya disease in adults, although the incidence of asymptomatic moyamoya disease was considered very low until recently (see below). Finally, epidemiological features in moyamoya disease may gradually change.

Based on the literature review, Goto and Yonekawa (1992) collected 1,063 patients with moyamoya disease from the countries other than Japan, and found 625 patients in Asia, 201 in Europe, 176 in North and South America, 52 in Africa, and 9 in Australia in the literature [7]. Subsequently, precise information on epidemiological features in the world, including South Korea, Taiwan, Hawaii, the United States, and Europe, was reported in 1997 [8-13]. According to these reports, epidemiological features in South Korea, but not in Taiwan, are very similar to those in Japan [10, 11]. Numaguchi et al. (1997) identified ethnic background in 54 patients in the United States, and reported that 35 patients were Caucasians, eight Asians, five African-Americans, three Haitians and three Hispanics [12]. However, Graham and Matoba (1997) analyzed epidemiological features of moyamoya disease in Hawaii with high percentage of Asians and Pacific Islanders (56%), and reported that the incidence and prevalence are higher in Hawaii than in the rest of the United States because of the larger percentage of Asians. They suggested that genetic rather than environment factors explain the increased moyamoya disease in Hawaii [9].

Familial Moyamoya Disease

Another epidemiological feature of moyamoya disease is the high incidence of familial occurrence. As aforementioned, familial occurrence has been recognized in approximately 15% of patients [14]. According to recent literature review, 172 familial cases of 76 pedigrees have been reported. Of these, 38 parent-offspring pairs of 16 pedigrees and 128 sibling pairs of 51 pedigrees have been described [15, 16]. Compared with general population, first- or second-degree relatives are known to have a 30- to 40-fold significantly increased risk of moyamoya disease [17]. Identical twins associated with moyamoya disease have also been reported [18].

We recently reviewed 155 Japanese patients with moyamoya disease, including 24 familial cases (10 family pedigrees) and 131 sporadic cases. As the results, the male-to-female ratios were 1:5.0 and 1:1.6 in familial and sporadic cases, respectively. Therefore, a female preponderance was significantly more prominent in familial group than in sporadic group. Onset age ranged from 1 to 36 years (11.8 ± 11.7 years) in familial group, whereas onset age ranged from 1 to 78 years (30.0 ± 20.9 years) in sporadic group. Kaplan-Meier analysis and Mantel-Cox log-rank statistics also showed that age at onset was significantly lower in familial group than in sporadic group. Furthermore, we investigated analyzed the clinical features of familial moyamoya disease to characterize their genetic properties. Of 10 pedigrees, there were 8 parent-offspring pairs, all of which were mother-offspring pairs. The parents presented with the symptoms related to moyamoya disease when they were 22 to 36 years (30.7 ± 7.5 years). On the other hands, their children presented with the symptom when they were 5 to 11 years (7.2 ± 2.7 years). Thus, mean age at onset age was significantly lower in the second generation than in the first generation. These results strongly suggest that anticipation may be closely associated with familial moyamoya disease [16].

Pathology and Pathophysiology

Pathology

The histopathological findings in the circle of Willis are fibrocellular thickening of the intima, an irregular undulation (waving) of the internal elastic lamina, and the attenuation of the media (Figure 3), suggesting that the disease process occurs mainly in the intima [19]. The "moyamoya" vessels in the basal ganglia and thalamus show either dilated, thin-walled arteries or obstruction from recent thrombi or mural thickening with our without elastosis or fibrosis. Moreover, similar lesions can be found in the vessels of the other organs such as heart and kidney in some cases [20].

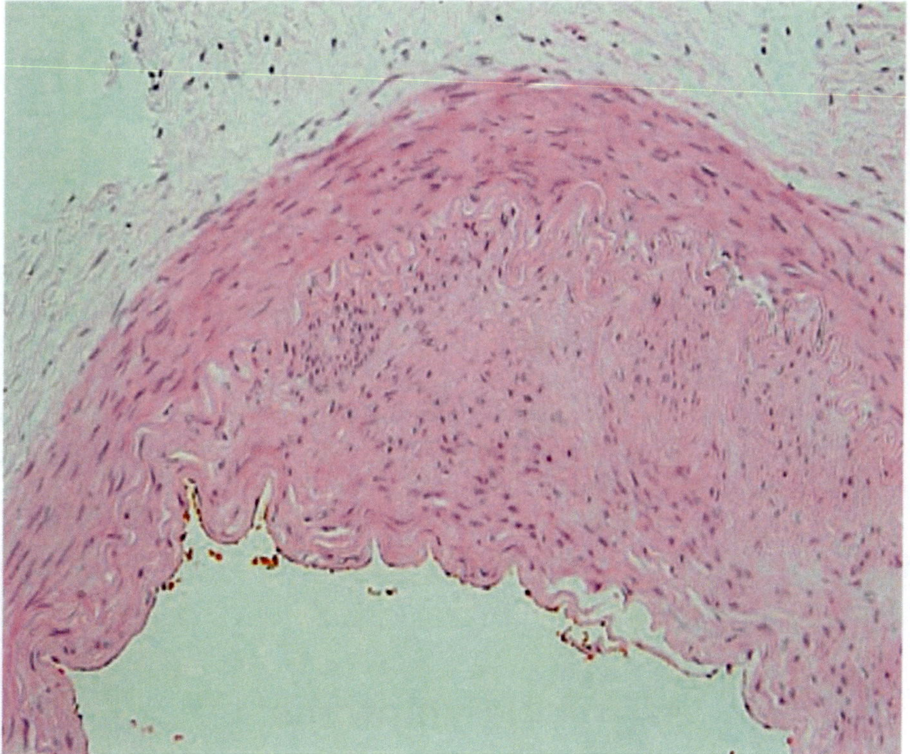

Figure 3. HE staining of the terminal portion of the ICA in a 34-year-old female who developed fetal intracranial hemorrhage due to moyamoya disease. Note intimal thickening, irregular undulation of the internal elastic lamina, and the attenuation of the media (original magnification; x100).

Increased Cytokines in Cerebrospinal Fluid in Moyamoya Disease

Previous studies have shown that certain growth factors or cytokines are elevated in the CSF of patients with moyamoya disease. Expression of basic fibroblast growth factor (bFGF) is reported to increase in the cerebrospinal fluid (CSF) and in the intra- and extracranial arteries [21-25]. Houkin et al. (1998) showed that bFGF was highly expressed in the surface of the thickened intima in the terminal portion of the internal carotid artery [22]. Soriano et al. (2002) reported that CSF levels of soluble vascular cell adhesion molecule Type 1 (VCAM-1), intercellular adhesion molecule Type 1 (ICAM-1), and E-selectin are elevated in moyamoya disease, and suggested ongoing inflammatory processes in the central nervous system [26]. Kim et al (2003) also characterized a specific protein, cellular retinoic acid-binding protein (CRABP)-I, from the CSF of patients moyamoya disease [27]. Very recently, we found that CSF level of hepatocyte growth factor (HGF) was 820±319.0 pg/ml in patients with moyamoya disease, being significantly higher than 443.2±193.5 pg/ml in those with ICA occlusion. Both HGF and its specific receptor, c-Met were widely expressed in the media and thickened intima of the carotid fork in patients with moyamoya disease, but not in control patients [28]. The distribution was quite different from that of bFGF, which was localized only in the single layer of endothelial cells in the carotid forks of moyamoya disease [22]. These findings strongly suggest that enhanced expression of HGF in the vascular smooth muscle cells may promote intimal thickening and their migration into the intima in the carotid fork of moyamoya disease and be closely related to pathogenesis of moyamoya disease [28].

Etiology

Underlying pathogenesis is still obscure [3]. However, several epidemiological studies suggest the infection in head and neck regions may be related to moyamoya disease, although a certain infectious pathogen has not been determined [29]. Some genetic factors may also play an important role in pathogenesis of moyamoya disease. As described above, the hypothesis is based on the facts that familial occurrence is recognized in approximately 15% of patients [30], and that the incidence of moyamoya disease is much higher in Far East than in western countries [7]. Clinical studies of familial cases have suggested that moyamoya disease is most likely inherited in a polygenic mode or an autosomal dominant fashion with a low penetrance. Microsatellite linkage analysis has recently identified the genetic loci on chromosomes 3, 6, and 17 [30-32]. However, the responsible genes have not been identified yet [33].

Clinical Symptoms

It is well known that both children and adults can be involved by moyamoya disease, but their clinical features often differ. Thus, most pediatric patients develop transient ischemic attack (TIA) or cerebral infarction. On the other hands, about half of adult patients develop intracranial bleeding, although the remainders suffer from TIA and/or cerebral infarction. As shown in Figure 2, the age distribution of adult patients with moyamoya disease has a peak between 35 and 45 years, indicating the importance to always remind that moyamoya disease may be involved in the onset of ischemic and hemorrhagic stroke in young adults.

TIA and Ischemic Stroke

The carotid forks are predominantly involved in moyamoya disease, leading to cerebral ischemia in the territory of the internal carotid artery (see below). As the result, young adult patients with moyamoya disease often develop TIA or ischemic stroke and exhibit a variety of neurological deficits, including speech disturbance and motor weakness of the upper and lower extremities. Therefore, once young adults develop focal neurological symptoms, moyamoya disease should be taken into consideration as one of probable causes, even if their symptoms are transient or mild. The posterior cerebral arteries are also involved in about 25% of adult patients with ischemic type of moyamoya disease [34]. Some of them develop homonymous hemianopsia due to cerebral infarction in the occipital lobe.

Although it is well known that cerebral infarction disturbs intellectual development in pediatric patients with moyamoya disease [35,36], a certain subpopulation of adult patients also develop cognitive dysfunction including short memory disturbance, irritability and agitation. They are often misdiagnosed as psychiatric disorders including schizophrenia, depression and personality disorder [37,38]. Furthermore, moyamoya disease may provoke involuntary movement and paroxysmal exercise-induced dyskinesia [39]. It should be reminded that moyamoya disease can potentially cause these rare symptoms in young adults [40].

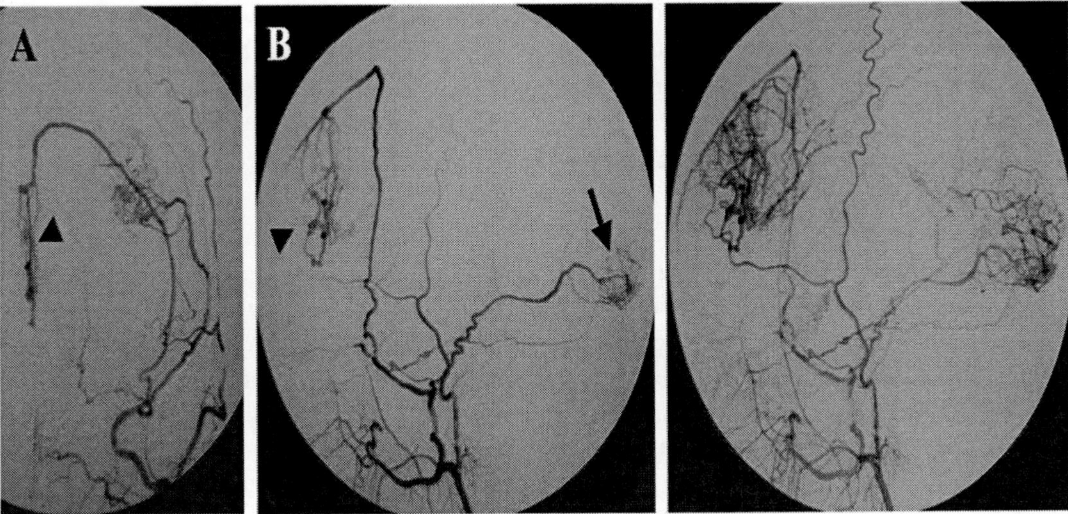

Figure 4. Towne's view (A) and lateral view (B) of left external carotid angiogram in a 34-year-old female who experienced transient right hemiparesis. Note that the branches of the left ACA (arrowheads) and MCA (arrow) are opacified through the dilated middle meningeal artery ("vault" moyamoya).

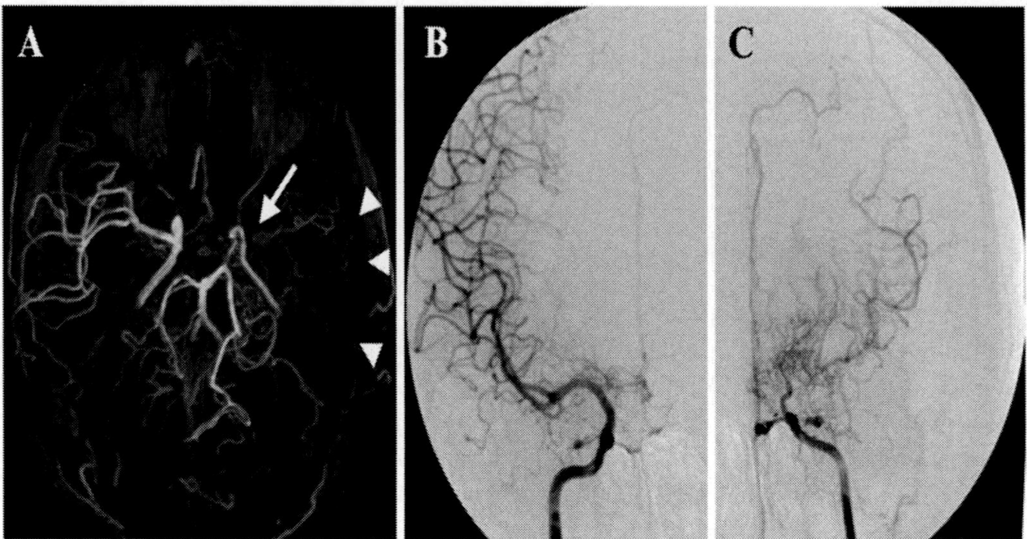

Figure 5. Radiological findings of a 36-year-old male who were diagnosed as asymptomatic moyamoya disease. (A) MR angiography reveals the stenosis of the bilateral ACA and the left MCA and "basal" moyamoya vessels around the left carotid fork (arrow). Note a marked attenuation of flow signals in the branches of the left MCA (arrow heads). (B) Right internal carotid angiogram shows the marked stenosis of the right ACA and faint "basal" moyamoya vessels (stage II). (C) Left internal carotid angiogram shows marked stenosis of the left carotid fork and development of "basal" moyamoya vessels. The branches of the left ACA and MCA are opacified through the moyamoya vessels (stage IV), correlating with the findings on MR angiography.

Intracranial Bleeding

About half of adult patients with moyamoya disease develop intracranial bleeding, while it is quite rare in pediatric patients. There are two main causes of intracranial bleeding in moyamoya disease. First, intracranial bleeding is known to occur from the dilated, fragile moyamoya vessels due to persistent hemodynamic stress and to occur in the basal ganglia, thalamus or periventricular region [41-43]. Intraventricular hemorrhage (IVH) is often complicated (Figure 4).

Yamashita et al. (1983) examined histological findings of the "moyamoya" vessels of 22 patients. As the results, they found that the ruptured vessels were dilated and had fibrin deposits in the wall, fragmented elastic laminae and attenuated media [44]. Of these, a certain subpopulation of patients have the "peripheral" aneurysms located within the collaterals or moyamoya vessels, although its incidence is not so high [45-50]. Pathological examination performed in 8 cases clarified that the "peripheral" aneurysms were true aneurysms in 5 cases and pseudo-aneurysms in 3 [51]. Pseudo-aneurysm is most likely secondary to the rupture of the fragile moyamoya vessels. Intracranial bleeding from the collaterals or moyamoya vessels leads to a variety of neurological symptoms, including headache, consciousness disturbance, hemiparesis and speech disturbance, and the severity depends on the site and degree of bleeding.

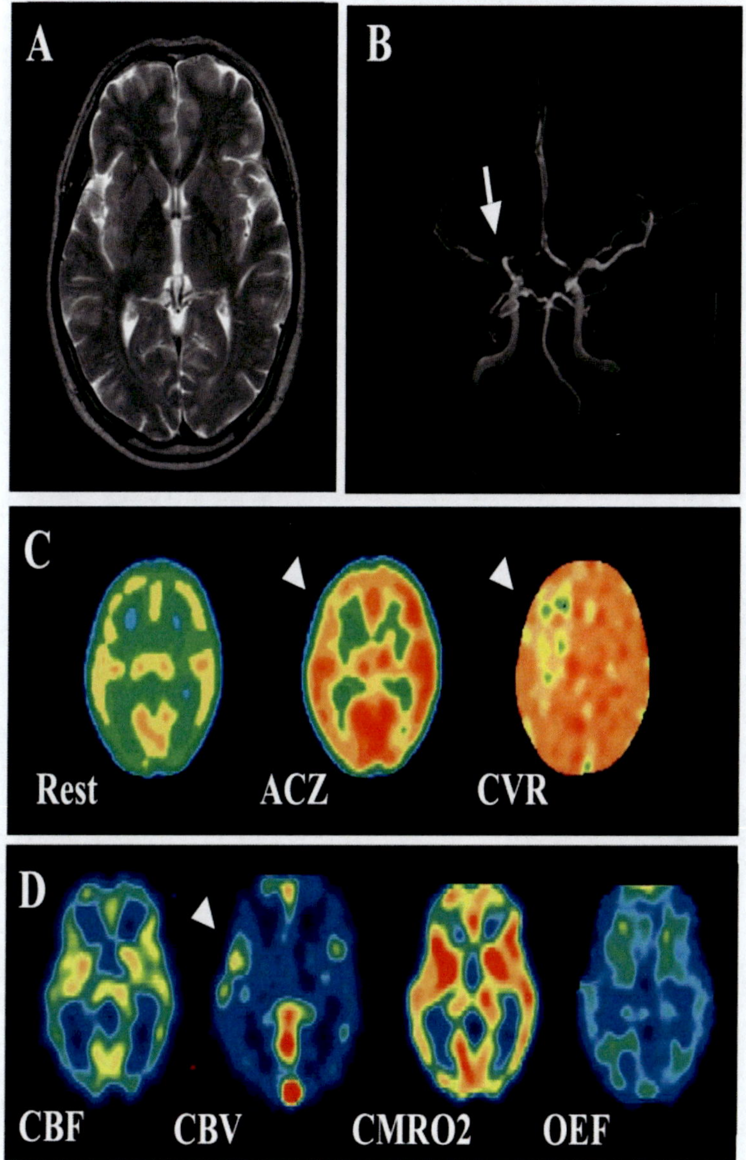

Figure 6. Radiological findings of a 45-year-old male who experienced transient left hemiparesis. (A) T2-weighted MRI reveals no parenchymal lesions. (B) MR angiography shows marked stenosis of the right carotid fork. (C) ^{123}I-IMP SPECT demonstrates normal CBF distribution at resting state, but a decreased cerebrovascular reactivity (CVR) to acetazolamide (ACZ) in the right frontal lobe (arrowheads). (D) ^{15}O-gas PET demonstrates an elevated CBV in the right frontal lobe, representing Powers' stage I.

Another source of bleeding are the aneurysms located around the Willis' circle, especially in the basilar artery bifurcation or basilar artery-superior cerebellar artery junction. Vertebrobasilar system is playing an important role as collateral circulation in moyamoya disease. Thus, hemodynamic stress can induce the saccular, true aneurysm in the vertebrobasilar system (Figure 5). Rupture of such aneurysm causes subarachnoid hemorrhage (SAH), which is same as bleeding from ordinary saccular aneurysm [45, 46, 52].

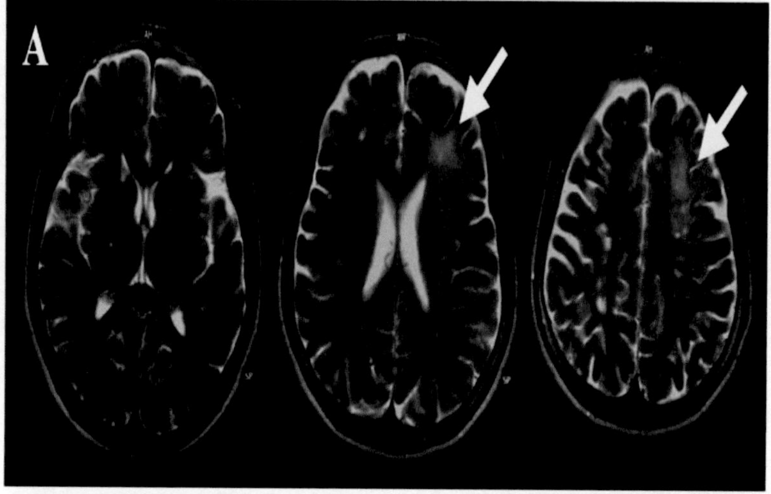

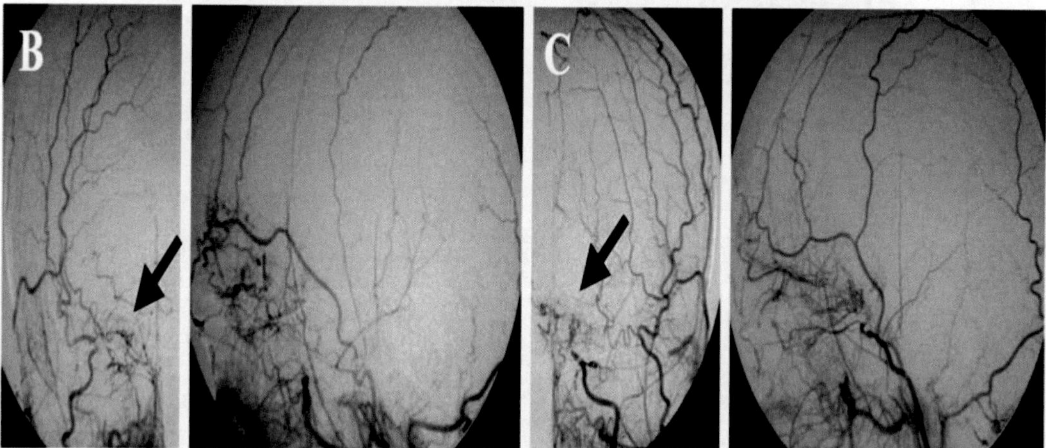

Figure 7. Radiological findings of a 56-year-old female who developed transient motor aphasia lasting for 30 minutes. (A) T2-weighted MRI shows cerebral infarction in the left MCA-ACA watershed zone (arrows). (B) Right common carotid angiogram demonstrates complete occlusion of the right ICA and "ethmoidal" moyamoya vessels (stage VI, arrow). (C) Left common carotid angiogram demonstrates the occlusion of the left ICA at the terminal portion and faint "basal" moyamoya vessels (stage V, arrow).

Recently, there is increasing evidence that adult moyamoya disease may induce SAH localized over the cerebral cortex in spite of the absence of intracranial aneurysm [53-55]. The dilated collateral arteries on the brain surface may rarely rupture, being the third cause of intracranial bleeding in adult patients with moyamoya disease [55].

It is well known that pregnancy provokes dramatic changes in cardiopulmonary functions. For example, both total blood volume and cardiac output increase up to 40-50% during the second and third trimesters of pregnancy [56,57]. Increased serum level of estrogen also causes the vasodilatation of the anomalous vasculature [58]. Based on these considerations, pregnant women are at higher risk for hemorrhagic stroke during pregnancy (Figure 6). In fact, a certain number of female patients have been reported to develop intracranial bleeding during pregnancy and delivery [59,60]. Therefore, once pregnant women develop intracranial bleeding, moyamoya disease should be taken into consideration as one of probable causes, even if they had no history suggesting moyamoya disease.

Asymptomatic Adult Patients

The recent development of non-invasive diagnostic modalities, including MRI and MRA, has led to the realization that the incidence of asymptomatic moyamoya disease may be higher than previously thought [61-64]. Recent nation-wide survey in Japan enrolled 40 asymptomatic adult patients. As the results, cerebral infarction and disturbed cerebral hemodynamics were detected in about 20% and 40% of the involved hemispheres, respectively. Angiographical stage was more advanced in more elderly patients. Of 34 non-surgically treated patients, seven experienced TIA (n = 3), ischemic stroke (n = 1) or intracranial bleeding (n = 3) during follow-up periods (mean, 43.7 months). The annual risk for any stroke was 3.2%. Disease progression was associated with ischemic events or silent infarction in four of five patients (see also the "Prognosis" section). No cerebrovascular event occurred in the six patients who underwent surgical revascularization [65]. These findings revealed that asymptomatic moyamoya disease is not a silent disorder and may potentially cause ischemic or hemorrhagic stroke. Asymptomatic patients with moyamoya disease should be carefully followed up to further clarify their outcome and to establish the management guideline for them.

Radiological Findings

Precise analysis of radiological findings in adult patients with moyamoya disease is essential to diagnose, predict their outcome and determine therapeutic strategies.

CT/MRI

CT and MRI are very useful modalities to localize ischemic and hemorrhagic lesions in the brain. Cerebral infarction develops in the MCA-ACA or MCA-PCA borderzone area in patients with mild ischemia (Figure 7), but extends to the frontal, temporal and parietal cortex in those with severe ischemia [66- 68].

As described above, the posterior cerebral artery is involved in about 25% of adult patients with moyamoya disease. Cerebral infarction can more frequently be found in the temporal and occipital lobes in such patients [34].

As shown in Figure 8, MRI is practical to identify occlusive lesion around the Willis' circle and the dilated moyamoya vessels [68,69]. Leptomeningeal contrast enhancement is frequently observed over the cerebral cortex in moyamoya disease and becomes less prominent after bypass, which may represent the dilated pial arterioles [70]. Diffusion-weighted MRI can also detect the irreversibly damaged tissue in acute stage of cerebral ischemia.

Cerebral Angiography

Even now, cerebral angiography is accepted as a gold standard for diagnosis of moyamoya disease. Typically, cerebral angiography demonstrates stenosis or occlusion of the terminal portion of the ICA (C1-C2 portion) and the proximal portion of the ACA and MCA (A1 and M1 portion) bilaterally (Figure 1). As described above, the proximal portion of the PCA (P1-P2 portion) is also involved in about 25% of patients with moyamoya disease.

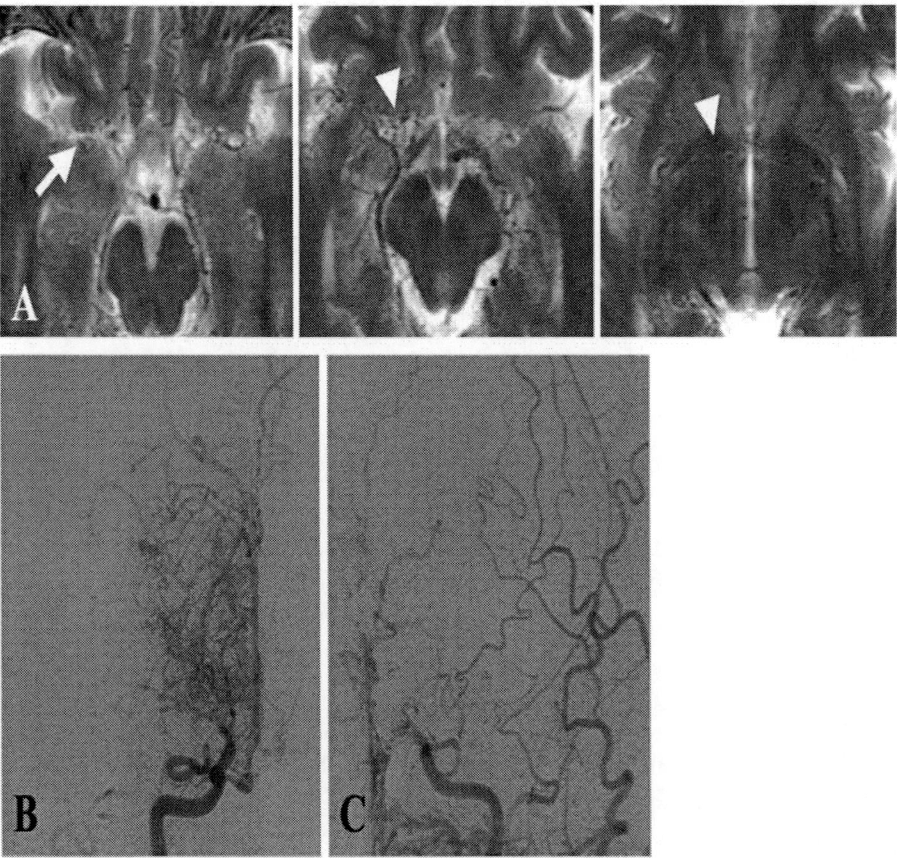

Figure 8. Radiological findings of a 38-year-old female who experienced transient weakness of the left extremities lasting for 5 minutes. (A) T2-weighted MRI reveals the disappearance of flow void signal of the horizontal portion of the MCA (arrow) and numerous numbers of small flow void signals in the basal cistern and basal ganglia suggesting "basal" moyamoya vessels. "Basal" moyamoya vessels are more prominent in the right side (arrowheads). (B) Right internal carotid angiogram shows near occlusion of the right ICA and "basal" moyamoya vessels. The ACA is faintly opacified through "basal" moyamoya vessels (stage IV). (C) Left common carotid angiogram demonstrates occlusion of the left ICA and "ethmoidal" moyamoya vessels (stage V).

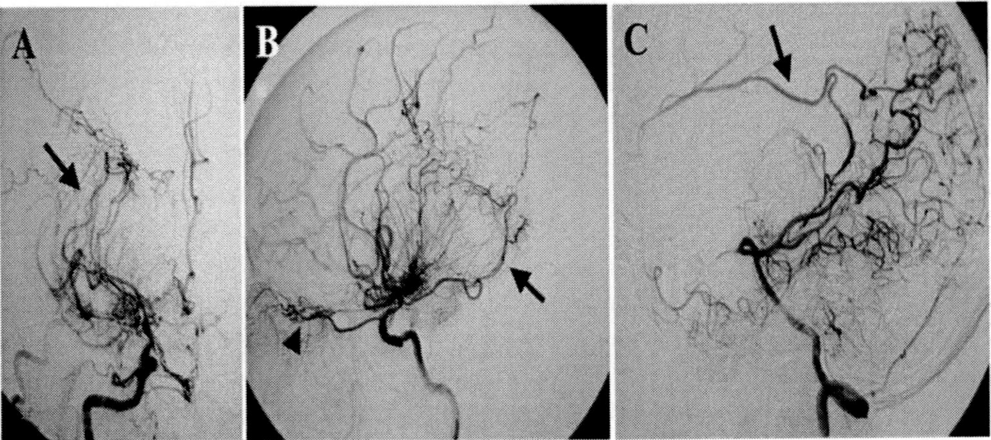

Figure 9. Radiological findings of a 45-year-old male who developed moderate left hemiparesis due to cerebral infarction. (A) Towne's view of right internal carotid angiogram shows marked development of "basal" moyamoya vessels. The branches of MCA and ACA are opacified through moyamoya vessels (stage IV). Note the marked dilated moyamoya vessels that is visible in the subventricular zone (arrow). (B) Lateral view of right internal carotid angiogram shows marked dilatation of the right anterior choroidal artery (arrow) and development of "ethmoidal" moyamoya vessels (arrowhead).

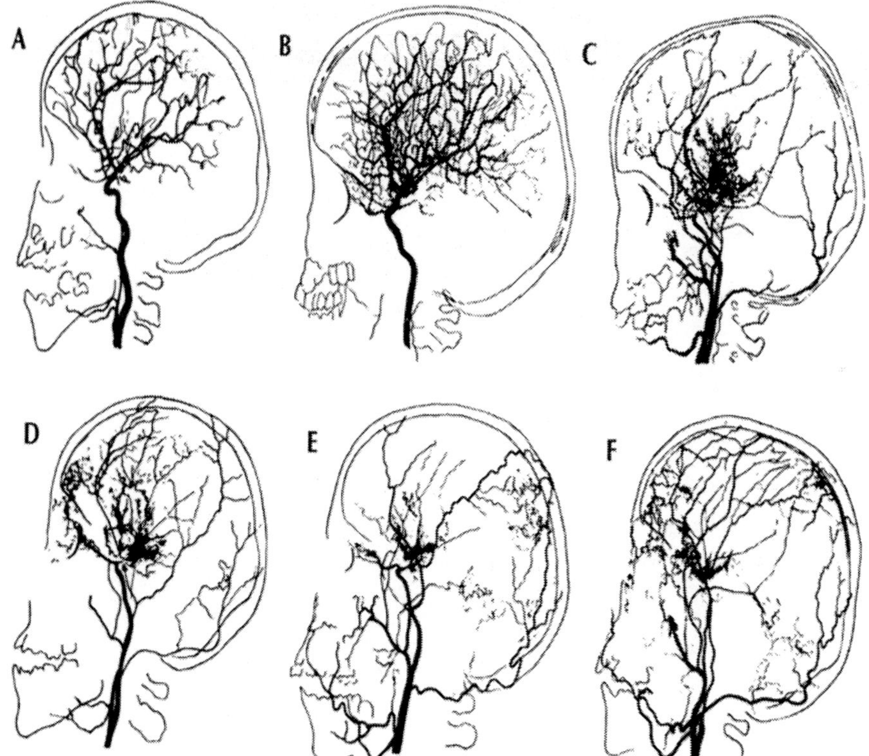

Referred from Suzuki and Takaku (115).

Figure 10. Diagram of Suzuki's six-stage classification on cerebral angiography. Stage I (A), stage II (B), stage III (C), stage IV (D), stage V (E) and stage VI (F).

Moyamoya disease is characterized by extensive developments of "pathognomonic" collateral pathways through various routes in response to these progressive, stenotic changes in the carotid forks [1]. Growth factors such as bFGF and HGF may be involved in such collateral developments in moyamoya disease [21-25]. First, the perforating arteries such as the lenticulo-striate artery and thalamo-perforating artery abnormally dilate in the basal ganglia and thalamus, called as "basal moyamoya" (Figure 1). In some case, markedly dilated perforating arteries can be observed in the subventricular zone (Figure 9).

Second, the anterior choroidal artery and posterior pericallosal artery are markedly dilated and function as collateral circulation in the majority of patients with moyamoya disease. Dilated choroidal artery may be one of risk factors for intracranial bleeding in moyamoya disease (Figure 9) [41]. Third, the anterior and posterior ethmoidal arteries also function as collateral pathways mainly from the ophthalmic arteries to the ACA branches, called as "ethmoidal moyamoya" (Figure 9) [71]. Finally, moyamoya disease often induces an abnormal vascular network at the cranial vault, which enables blood supply from the dural arteries to pial arteries. This collateral pathway is called as "vault moyamoya". Vault moyamoya is often observed in patients with advanced stage of disease (Figure 4).

Table 1.

ICA		
	Normal	0
	Stenosis of C1	1
	Discontinuity of C1 signal	2
	Invisible	3
MCA		
	Normal	0
	Stenosis of M1	1
	Discontinuity of M1 signal	2
	Invisible	3
ACA		
	Normal A2 and its distal	0
	A2 and its distal signal decrease or loss	1
	Invisible	2
PCA		
	Normal A2 and its distal	0
	A2 and its distal signal decrease or loss	1
	Invisible	2
Total		0~10

MRA scores by Houkin et al (2005).

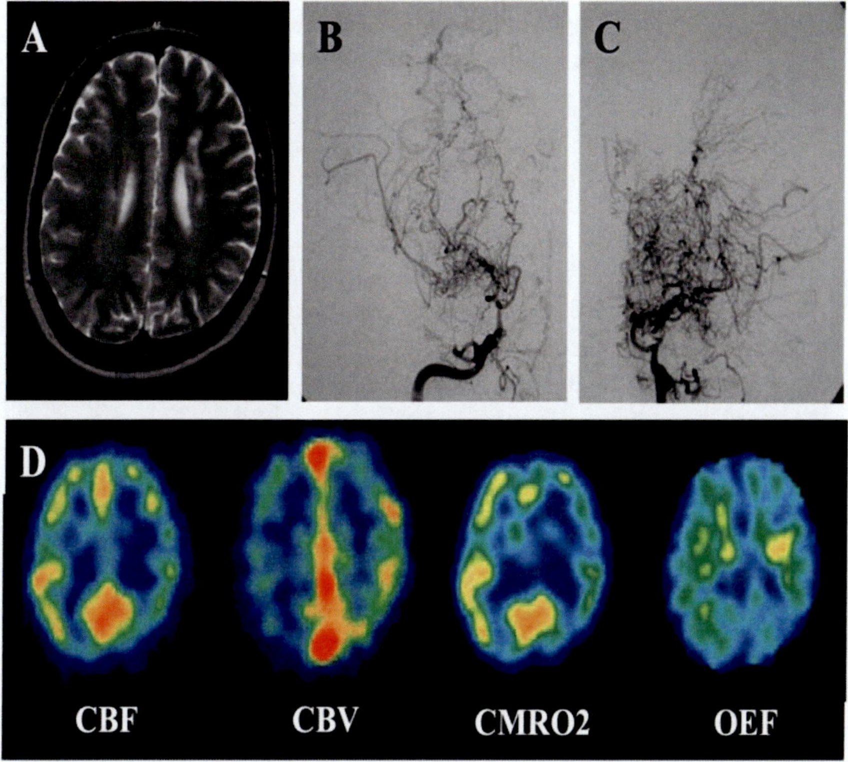

Figure 11. Radiological findings of a 37-year-old female who presented with transient right hemiparesis. (A) T2-weighted MRI reveals cerebral infarction in the left MCA-ACA watershed zone. Right (B) and left (C) carotid angiograms show marked stenosis of the bilateral carotid forks and well-developed "basal" moyamoya vessels (stage III). (D) ^{15}O-gas PET demonstrates a marked CBF decrease in the bilateral ICA territories. The finding is more distinct in the left side. The CBV is elevated and $CMRO_2$ is attenuated in the left cerebral hemisphere. The OEF is increased in the left deep frontal lobe.

Suzuki's six-stage classification on cerebral angiography is well known and is still widely used in clinical situation. Suzuki et al. precisely analyzed serial changes in angiographical findings of moyamoya disease and classified moyamoya disease into six stages [1]. Scheme of Suzuki's six-stage classification is shown in Figure 10. First, mild stenosis occurs in the carotid fork (Stage I). Then, all the main branches of MCA and ACA start to dilate, and very slight moyamoya vessels appear around the carotid fork (Stage II). Occlusive changes in the carotid fork progress and the branches of MCA and ACA start to disappear, and distinct moyamoya vessels can be seen at the base of the brain. Basal moyamoya is most distinct at this stage (Stage III). Occlusive changes in the carotid fork further progress, and the branches of MCA and ACA are faintly opacified through moyamoya vessels. However, the moyamoya vessels become coarse during this stage (Stage IV). Subsequently, the carotid fork is completely occluded and the branches arising form the ICA disappear on cerebral angiography. There is no or, if any, minimal moyamoya vessels around the carotid siphon (Stage V). Finally, the carotid siphon and moyamoya vessels completely disappear on cerebral angiography, and the ICA territory is fed by the posterior circulation and vault moyamoya (Stage VI).

Furthermore, cerebral angiography is quite useful to precisely evaluate the effects of surgical revascularization. Postoperative findings on cerebral angiography are described in the "Surgical Treatment" section.

MR Angiography

MR angiography (MRA) is a newly developed modality and is valuable to diagnose moyamoya disease non-invasively. As aforementioned, the guideline by the Research Committee on Spontaneous Occlusion of the Circle of Willis (Moyamoya Disease) determines that when MRI and MRA clearly demonstrate all the following findings, conventional cerebral angiography is not mandatory:

a) Stenosis or occlusion at the terminal portion of the internal carotid artery or at the proximal portion of the anterior and middle cerebral arteries on MRA and an abnormal vascular network in the basal ganglia on MRA.
b) An abnormal vascular network can also be diagnosed when more than two apparent flow voids are seen by MRI in the basal ganglia on the same side.
c) Findings a) and b) above are seen bilaterally.

However, it should be reminded that the image quality of MRA largely depends on the strength of the static magnetic field. The new diagnostic criteria for moyamoya disease require MRA with a 1.5-tesla machine. MRA with 0.5- and 1.0-tesla machines is not recommended [66,72-75].

MRA is very sensitive to stenotic lesion in the carotid fork, but its specificity is not so high because of its imaging principle. Thus, MRA may overestimate stenotic lesion in the carotid fork. In early stage of moyamoya disease, the branches of MCA and ACA can clearly be seen on MRA in spite of carotid fork stenosis. As the disease stage progresses, however, their flow signals start to become invisible (Figure 5). MRA can clearly identify the moyamoya vessels that are considered as dilated perforating arteries such as lenticulo-striate artery and thalamo-perforating artery (Figure 5) [72]. On behalf of the Research Committee on Spontaneous Occlusion of the Circle of Willis (Moyamoya Disease), Houkin et al. (2005) recently proposed a novel stage grading on MRA in moyamoya disease. MRA scores were assigned based on the severity of occlusive changes of the ICA, the horizontal portion of the MCA, ACA and PCA, and the flow signals of the distal branches of these arteries (Table 1). Total points ranged from 0 (normal) to 10 (most severe). As the results, MRA scores (0-10) correlated with Suzuki's six-stage classification on cerebral angiography, with high sensitivity and specificity [76].

Needless to say, one of great advantages of MRA is its non-invasiveness. Therefore, MRA is quite useful modality to repeat the examinations serially and to detect asymptomatic patients in the pedigree of familial moyamoya disease [73]. As well as cerebral angiography, MRA can identify the development of collateral circulation after surgical revascularization. Postoperative findings on MRA are described in the "Surgical Treatment" section.

Cerebral Hemodynamics and Metabolism

Single photon emission computed tomography (SPECT) and positron emission tomography (PET) are major two modalities to be widely employed to analyze cerebral hemodynamics and metabolism. The basic theory of SPECT and PET is beyond the scope of this chapter. SPECT is widely used in clinical situation, using a radioactive tracer such as ^{133}xenon, ^{99m}Tc-HMPAO and ^{123}I-IMP, and can quantify cerebral blood flow (CBF). Acetazolamide (ACZ) is a specific cerebral vasodilator and increase CBF in a dose-dependent manner by inhibiting the erythrocyte carbonic anhydrase. Intravenous injection of 10 mg/kg or 1,000 mg of ACZ induces more than 20% of CBF at resting state within 15 minutes [77, 78]. Acetazolamide injection does not alter blood pressure and can estimate vasodilatory capacity, although CO_2 inhalation may modify the result because of blood pressure augmentation [79]. Based on these observations, acetazolamide has been widely used to assess cerebral perfusion reserve in patients with occlusive vascular disorder, since Vorstrup et al. reported its usefulness in 1986 [80-84]. On the other hands, PET can quantitatively determine CBF, cerebral blood volume (CBV), cerebral metabolic rate for oxygen ($CMRO_2$), and oxygen extraction fraction (OEF), using ^{15}O gas or $H_2{}^{15}O$ as a positron-emitting tracer. Although PET cannot be widely available, PET provides a lot of information on cerebral hemodynamics and metabolism in occlusive vascular disorders, including moyamoya disease. Especially, OEF is a direct indicator for the balance between blood supply and metabolic demand in the brain. When CPP moderately falls, compensatory cerebral vasodilatation occurs and keeps CBF constant. Under this condition, cerebral vasodilatation is expressed as an increase of CBV, called as Powers' stage I [85]. When CPP further declines, autoregulatory vasodilatation can no longer compensate for CPP reduction, leading to a blood flow decline. Under this condition, blood supply cannot satisfy metabolic demand and cerebral oxygen metabolism is kept constant by increasing OEF. Such metabolic compensation is called as misery perfusion or Powers' stage II [85, 86].

Significant numbers of studies have been reported on cerebral hemodynamics and metabolism in adult patients with moyamoya disease. According to these studies, the disturbances in cerebral hemodynamics and metabolism are usually less prominent in adult patients than in pediatric patients [87, 88]. However, hemodynamic and metabolic status of moyamoya disease is not uniform, and severe hemodynamic compromise is observed in a certain subgroup of patients (Figures 6 and 11) [89]. The CBF is significantly lower than control values in the ICA territories, especially in the frontal lobes, in the majority of adult patients with moyamoya disease. Therefore, their CBF distribution is dominant in posterior circulation [90]. Cerebrovascular reactivity (CVR) to acetazolamide or CO_2 is usually impaired in the ICA territories more widely [88, 91-94].

PET studies have revealed that CBV is diffusely elevated in the ICA territories including the basal ganglia in most of adult patients with moyamoya disease, suggesting that compensatory vasodilatation occurs in response to CPP reduction [88, 95-97]. However, OEF was reported to be within normal limits in the majority of adult patients (Figures 10 and 11) [97]. Cerebral hemodynamics and metabolism are more extensively impaired in patients with Suzuki's stage III and IV than in those in Suzuki's stage V and VI [96].

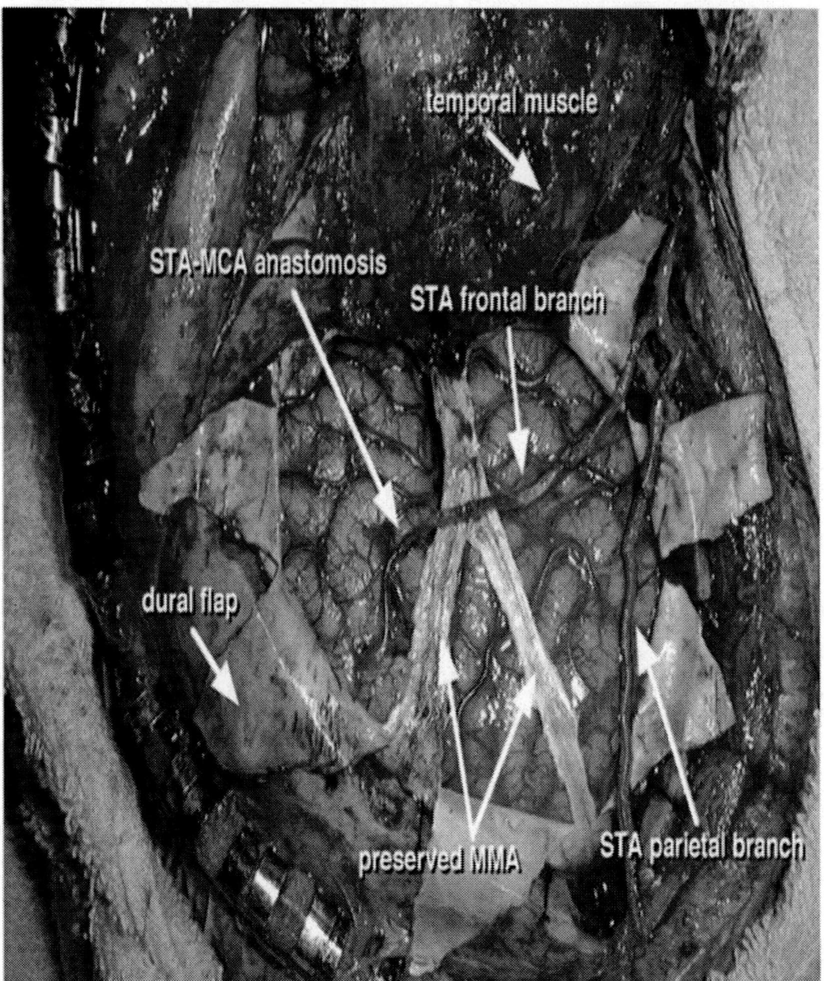

Figure 12. Intraoperative photograph of STA-MCA anastomosis and EDAMS. Note that the main branches of the middle meningeal artery (MMA) are preserved.

Surgical Treatment

Surgical Procedures

Surgical procedures for moyamoya disease can largely be classified into three categories: direct bypass, indirect bypass, and combined bypass. Direct bypass procedures include superficial temporal artery to middle cerebral artery (STA-MCA) anastomosis. The STA can also be anastomosed to the branch of anterior cerebral artery (ACA) in patients who have severe ischemia in the ACA area [98, 99]. The concept and surgical technique are very similar to those for the patients with atherosclerotic, occlusive carotid artery diseases. Direct bypass such as STA-MCA anastomosis can improve cerebral hemodynamics and resolve ischemic attacks immediately after surgery. However, the patients should be carefully managed after surgery, because postoperative dramatic changes in cerebral hemodynamics may induce hyperperfusion syndrome especially in the patients with markedly reduced CPP before surgery. Preoperative SPECT/PET studies would be essential [100-103].

On the other hands, indirect bypass procedures are very specific for moyamoya disease. Previously, significant numbers of procedures have been reported, including encephalo-duro-arterio-synangiosis (EDAS) [104-106], encephalo-myo-synangiosis (EMS) [107], encephalo-duro-arterio-myo-synangiosis (EDAMS) [108], encephalo-galeo-synangiosis (EGS) [109, 110], and multiple burr-hole surgery [111]. Indirect bypass surgery induces the angiogenesis between the brain surface and the vascularized donor tissues and functions as collateral pathways. Indirect bypass is technically simple. However, surgical effect cannot be obtained just after surgery, because the development of surgical collaterals requires three to four months [112, 113]. Surgical design is also quite important, because the extent of surgical collateral pathways depends on the size of craniotomy and indirect bypass [36, 114-116]. Furthermore, it must be reminded that collateral pathways through indirect bypass does not develop in about 40 to 50% of adult patients, although indirect bypass provides extensive surgical collaterals in most all of pediatric patients. Thus, direct bypass is quite important in adult moyamoya disease [117, 118].

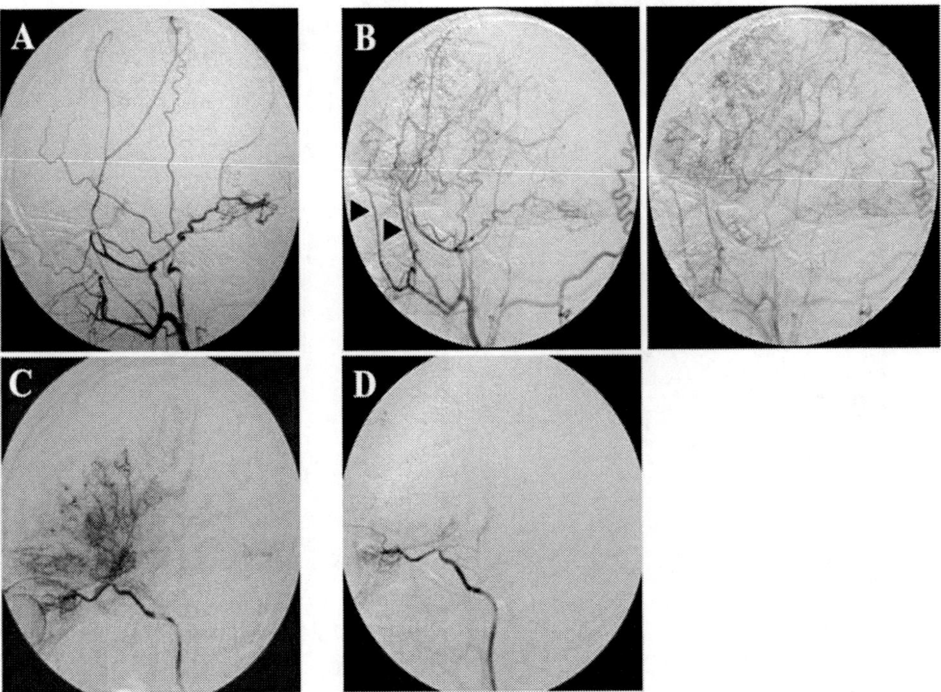

Figure 13. Radiological findings of a 34-year-old female who experienced transient right hemiparesis. (A) Preoperative right external carotid angiogram shows “vault” moyamoya vessels in the occipital region. (B) Postoperative left external carotid angiograms demonstrates well-developed collateral pathways through the STA, MMA and deep temporal artery (DTA). Note the marked increase in the caliber of the DTA after surgery (arrowheads). (C) Preoperative right internal carotid angiogram demonstrates near occlusion of the right ICA and marked development of “basal” and “ethmoidal” moyamoya vessels. (D) Postoperative right external carotid angiogram shows a disappearance of “basal” moyamoya vessels, suggesting that surgical collaterals effectively supply blood flow into the right hemisphere.

Combined bypass procedures include both direct and indirect bypass, and serves the merits of both procedures (Figure 12) [119].

Postoperative Radiological Evaluations

Cerebral angiography is still very useful to evaluate the development of collateral pathways through direct and/or indirect bypass. Effective bypass surgery leads to the disappearance or reduction of moyamoya vessels, because they no longer need to function as collateral pathways (Figure 13).

Postoperative angiography should be planned at least 3 months after surgery, because the development of collateral pathways through indirect bypass requires 3 to 4 months after surgery (see above).

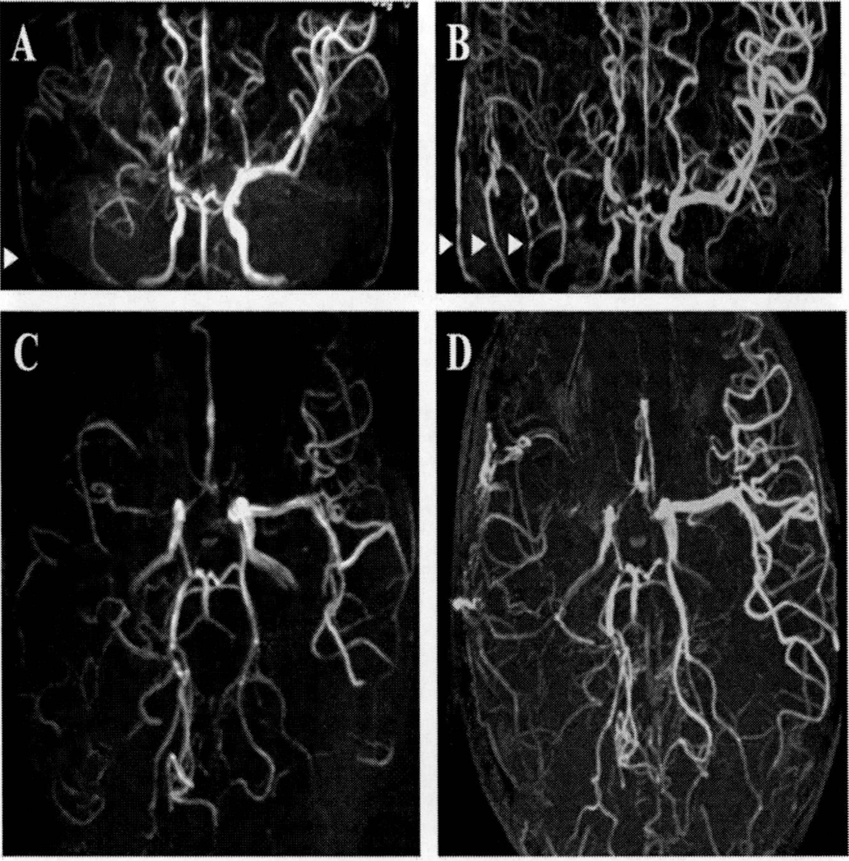

Figure 14. Pre- and postoperative MR angiography of a 40-year-old male who developed left hemiparesis. Coronal (A) and axial views of MR angiography before surgery (C) show a marked stenosis of the right carotid fork and a mild stenosis of the left ACA. Note a marked decrease in flow signals of the branches of the right MCA. The caliber of the right STA is very small (A, arrowhead). Coronal (B) and axial views of MR angiography 4 months after surgery (D) demonstrate the marked increase in the calibers of the right STA, DTA, and MMA (B, arrowheads). Note a significant increase in flow signals of the branches of the right MCA.

Alternatively, MRA is a useful modality to evaluate the development of collateral pathways after surgery. MRA can be repeated after surgery serially and non-invasively. As the results, MRA has clarified how collateral pathways are produced after surgery. Houkin et al. (2004) reported that moyamoya vessels start to decrease one month after combined bypass surgery, and that the deep temporal artery and the middle meningeal artery increase their calibers and can be identified 3 months after surgery. Stenotic change in the carotid forks rapidly progresses after surgery (Figure 14). Thus, a reciprocal relationship between neovascularization surgically induced by bypass surgery and moyamoya vessels can be observed [113].

Cerebral hemodynamics and metabolism have also been known to dramatically change after effective surgical revascularization in adult patients with moyamoya disease. Thus, both CBF and its reactivity to acetazolamide markedly improve or normalize after surgery. After surgery, OEF often normalizes in patients with an elevated OEF prior to surgery [95, 120-124].

Prognosis

According to several studies, the incidence of cerebrovascular events, including both ischemic and hemorrhagic stroke, is quite high in conservatively treated adult patients with moyamoya disease [125-127]. Hallemieier et al. (2006) reviewed 34 adult patients with moyamoya disease and reported that the 5-year risk of recurrent ipsilateral stroke was 65% in medically treated symptomatic hemispheres. Especially, the 5-year risk increased up to 82% in adult patients with bilateral involvement and ischemic symptoms [126].

Adult patients with unilateral moyamoya disease should be carefully followed up to overlook the progression to bilateral lesions. The incidence may be higher than considered previously [128-130]. Furthermore, recent cohort study has clarified that disease progression occurred in 15 of 63 adult patients (23.8% per patient) during follow-up period. Occlusive arterial lesions progressed in both anterior and posterior circulations, in both symptomatic and asymptomatic patients, and in both bilateral and unilateral types. Eight of 15 adult patients developed ischemic or hemorrhagic events in relation to disease progression. Multivariate analysis revealed that odds ratio conferred by male patient was 0.20 (95% confidence interval [CI], 0.04 to 0.97). Careful follow-up would be essential to prevent further stroke occurrence in medically treated adult patients with moyamoya disease, even if they are asymptomatic or are diagnosed as unilateral moyamoya disease [131].

On the other hands, surgical revascularization is believed to improve cerebral hemodynamics and metabolism and lower the incidence of subsequent ischemic stroke, although randomized clinical trials have not been conducted to confirm it. Transient ischemic attacks and ischemic stroke almost disappear in the majority of adult patients, when surgical revascularization is effectively performed [95, 121, 126, 127, 132-134, 135]. Recurrent hemorrhagic stroke (rebleeding) is still one of serious problems in adult patients with moyamoya disease. During follow-up periods, rebleeding occurs in about 30 to 65% of patients during follow-up periods of 2 to 20 years [136-139]. Rebleeding significantly worsens their functional outcome and increases the mortality [137, 139]. Rebleeding can occur at the original bleeding site and at the different site [42, 117]. Some of clinical studies have suggested that surgical revascularization may reduce the incidence of rebleeding to 12.5 to 20%, although their evidence level is not so high [117, 134, 135, 139]. Direct or combined bypass (see above) may have the potential to reduce the risk of rebleeding and to resolve the "peripheral" aneurysms located within the collaterals or moyamoya vessels [47, 140]. At present, Japan Adult Moyamoya (JAM) Trial, a multi-center, randomized clinical trial, has been started to evaluate whether direct or combined bypass surgery can reduce the risk of rebleeding in adult patients with moyamoya disease [141].

References

[1] Suzuki J, Takaku A: Cerebrovascular "moyamoya" disease. Disease showing abnormal net-like vessels in base of brain. *Arch Neurol.* 1969;20:288-299

[2] Takeuchi K, Shimizu K: Hypoplasia of the bilateral internal carotid arteries. *No To Shinkei.* 1957;9:37-43

[3] Fukui M: Current state of study on moyamoya disease in Japan. *Surg. Neurol.* 1997; 47:138-143

[4] Fukui M: Guidelines for the diagnosis and treatment of spontaneous occlusion of the circle of Willis ('moyamoya' disease). Research Committee on Spontaneous Occlusion of the Circle of Willis (Moyamoya Disease) of the Ministry of Health and Welfare, Japan. *Clin. Neurol. Neurosurg.* 1997;99 Suppl 2:S238-240

[5] Wakai K, Tamakoshi A, Ikezaki K, Fukui M, Kawamura T, Aoki R, Kojima M, Lin Y, Ohno Y: Epidemiological features of moyamoya disease in Japan: findings from a nationwide survey. *Clin. Neurol. Neurosurg.* 1997;99 Suppl 2:S1-5

[6] Baba T, Houkin K, Kuroda S: Novel epidemiological features of moyamoya disease. *J. Neurol. Neurosurg. Psychiatry*, 2007.

[7] Goto Y, Yonekawa Y: Worldwide distribution of moyamoya disease. *Neurol. Med. Chir. (Tokyo).* 1992;32:883-886

[8] Edwards-Brown MK, Quets JP: Midwest experience with moyamoya disease. *Clin. Neurol. Neurosurg.* 1997;99 Suppl 2:S36-38

[9] Graham JF, Matoba A: A survey of moyamoya disease in Hawaii. *Clin. Neurol. Neurosurg.* 1997;99 Suppl 2:S31-35

[10] Hung CC, Tu YK, Su CF, Lin LS, Shih CJ: Epidemiological study of moyamoya disease in Taiwan. *Clin. Neurol. Neurosurg.* 1997;99 Suppl 2:S23-25

[11] Ikezaki K, Han DH, Kawano T, Inamura T, Fukui M: Epidemiological survey of moyamoya disease in Korea. *Clin. Neurol. Neurosurg.* 1997;99 Suppl 2:S6-10

[12] Numaguchi Y, Gonzalez CF, Davis PC, Monajati A, Afshani E, Chang J, Sutton CL, Lee RR, Shibata DK: Moyamoya disease in the United States. *Clin. Neurol. Neurosurg.* 1997;99 Suppl 2:S26-30

[13] Yonekawa Y, Ogata N, Kaku Y, Taub E, Imhof HG: Moyamoya disease in Europe, past and present status. *Clin. Neurol. Neurosurg.* 1997;99 Suppl 2:S58-60

[14] Yamauchi T, Houkin K, Tada M, Abe H: Familial occurrence of moyamoya disease. *Clin. Neurol. Neurosurg.* 1997;99 Suppl 2:S162-167

[15] Nanba R, Kuroda S, Ishikawa T, Iwasaki Y, Tada M, Kiyohiro H: [Familial moyamoya disease--clinical features and current study]. *No Shinkei Geka*. 2004;32:7-16
[16] Nanba R, Kuroda S, Tada M, Ishikawa T, Houkin K, Iwasaki Y: Clinical features of familial moyamoya disease. *Childs Nerv. Syst*. 2006;22:258-262
[17] Kanai N: [A genetic study of spontaneous occlusion of the circle of Willis (moyamoya disease)]. *J. Tokyo Women Med. Univ*. 1992;62:1227-1258
[18] Kaneko Y, Imamoto N, Mannoji H, Fukui M: Familial occurrence of moyamoya disease in the mother and four daughters including identical twins. *Neurol. Med. Chir. (Tokyo)*. 1998;38:349-354
[19] Fukui M, Kono S, Sueishi K, Ikezaki K: Moyamoya disease. *Neuropathology* 2000;20 Suppl:S61-64
[20] Ikeda E: Systemic vascular changes in spontaneous occlusion of the circle of Willis. *Stroke* 1991;22:1358-1362
[21] Hoshimaru M, Takahashi JA, Kikuchi H, Nagata I, Hatanaka M: Possible roles of basic fibroblast growth factor in the pathogenesis of moyamoya disease: an immunohistochemical study. *J. Neurosurg*. 1991;75:267-270
[22] Houkin K, Yoshimoto T, Abe H, Nagashima K, Nagashima M, Takeda M, Isu T: Role of basic fibroblast growth factor in the pathogenesis of moyamoya disease. *Neurosurg. Focus*. 1998;5:1-5
[23] Malek AM, Connors S, Robertson RL, Folkman J, Scott RM: Elevation of cerebrospinal fluid levels of basic fibroblast growth factor in moyamoya and central nervous system disorders. *Pediatr. Neurosurg*. 1997;27:182-189
[24] Takahashi A, Sawamura Y, Houkin K, Kamiyama H, Abe H: The cerebrospinal fluid in patients with moyamoya disease (spontaneous occlusion of the circle of Willis) contains high level of basic fibroblast growth factor. *Neurosci. Lett*. 1993;160:214-216
[25] Yoshimoto T, Houkin K, Takahashi A, Abe H: Angiogenic factors in moyamoya disease. *Stroke* 1996;27:2160-2165
[26] Soriano SG, Cowan DB, Proctor MR, Scott RM: Levels of soluble adhesion molecules are elevated in the cerebrospinal fluid of children with moyamoya syndrome. *Neurosurgery* 2002;50:544-549
[27] Kim SK, Yoo JI, Cho BK, Hong SJ, Kim YK, Moon JA, Kim JH, Chung YN, Wang KC: Elevation of CRABP-I in the cerebrospinal fluid of patients with Moyamoya disease. *Stroke* 2003;34:2835-2841
[28] Nanba R, Kuroda S, Ishikawa T, Houkin K, Iwasaki Y: Increased expression of hepatocyte growth factor in cerebrospinal fluid and intracranial artery in moyamoya disease. *Stroke* 2004;35:2837-2842
[29] Yamada H, Deguchi K, Tanigawara T, Takenaka K, Nishimura Y, Shinoda J, Hattori T, Andoh T, Sakai N: The relationship between moyamoya disease and bacterial infection. *Clin. Neurol. Neurosurg*. 1997;99 Suppl 2:S221-224
[30] Yamauchi T, Tada M, Houkin K, Tanaka T, Nakamura Y, Kuroda S, Abe H, Inoue T, Ikezaki K, Matsushima T, Fukui M: Linkage of familial moyamoya disease (spontaneous occlusion of the circle of Willis) to chromosome 17q25. *Stroke* 2000; 31:930-935

[31] Ikeda H, Sasaki T, Yoshimoto T, Fukui M, Arinami T: Mapping of a familial moyamoya disease gene to chromosome 3p24.2-p26. *Am. J. Hum. Genet*. 1999;64:533-537

[32] Inoue TK, Ikezaki K, Sasazuki T, Matsushima T, Fukui M: Linkage analysis of moyamoya disease on chromosome 6. *J. Child Neurol*. 2000;15:179-182

[33] Nanba R, Tada M, Kuroda S, Houkin K, Iwasaki Y: Sequence analysis and bioinformatics analysis of chromosome 17q25 in familial moyamoya disease. *Childs Nerv. Syst*. 2005;21:62-68

[34] Kuroda S, Ishikawa T, Houkin K, Iwasaki Y: [Clinical significance of posterior cerebral artery stenosis/occlusion in moyamoya disease]. *No Shinkei Geka*. 2002;30: 1295-1300

[35] Bowen M, Marks MP, Steinberg GK: Neuropsychological recovery from childhood moyamoya disease. *Brain Dev*. 1998;20:119-123

[36] Kuroda S, Houkin K, Ishikawa T, Nakayama N, Ikeda J, Ishii N, Kamiyama H, Iwasaki Y: Determinants of intellectual outcome after surgical revascularization in pediatric moyamoya disease: a multivariate analysis. *Childs Nerv. Syst*. 2004;20:302-308

[37] Lubman DI, Pantelis C, Desmond P, Proffitt TM, Velakoulis D: Moyamoya disease in a patient with schizophrenia. *J Int Neuropsychol Soc*. 2003;9:806-810

[38] Nagata T, Harada D, Aoki K, Kada H, Miyata H, Kasahara H, Nakayama K: Effectiveness of carbamazepine for benzodiazepine-resistant impulsive aggression in a patient with frontal infarctions. *Psychiatry Clin. Neurosci*. 2007;61:695-697

[39] Lyoo CH, Kim DJ, Chang H, Lee MS: Moyamoya disease presenting with paroxysmal exercise-induced dyskinesia. *Parkinsonism Relat. Disord*. 2007;13:446-448

[40] Bruno A, Adams HP, Jr., Biller J, Rezai K, Cornell S, Aschenbrener CA: Cerebral infarction due to moyamoya disease in young adults. *Stroke* 1988;19:826-833

[41] Irikura K, Miyasaka Y, Kurata A, Tanaka R, Fujii K, Yada K, Kan S: A source of haemorrhage in adult patients with moyamoya disease: the significance of tributaries from the choroidal artery. *Acta Neurochir (Wien)*. 1996;138:1282-1286

[42] Iwama T, Morimoto M, Hashimoto N, Goto Y, Todaka T, Sawada M: Mechanism of intracranial rebleeding in moyamoya disease. *Clin. Neurol. Neurosurg*. 1997;99 Suppl 2:S187-190

[43] Oka K, Yamashita M, Sadoshima S, Tanaka K: Cerebral haemorrhage in Moyamoya disease at autopsy. *Virchows Arch A Pathol. Anat. Histol*. 1981;392:247-261

[44] Yamashita M, Oka K, Tanaka K: Histopathology of the brain vascular network in moyamoya disease. *Stroke* 1983;14:50-58

[45] Kawaguchi S, Sakaki T, Morimoto T, Kakizaki T, Kamada K: Characteristics of intracranial aneurysms associated with moyamoya disease. A review of 111 cases. *Acta Neurochir (Wien)*. 1996;138:1287-1294

[46] Konishi Y, Kadowaki C, Hara M, Takeuchi K: Aneurysms associated with moyamoya disease. *Neurosurgery* 1985;16:484-491

[47] Kuroda S, Houkin K, Kamiyama H, Abe H: Effects of surgical revascularization on peripheral artery aneurysms in moyamoya disease: report of three cases. *Neurosurgery* 2001;49:463-467; discussion 467-468

[48] Kwak R, Emori T, Nakamura T, Kadoya S: [Significance of intracranial aneurysms associated with moyamoya disease. (Part II). Cause and site of hemorrhage--review of the literature]. *Neurol. Med. Chir (Tokyo).* 1984;24:104-109

[49] Kwak R, Ito S, Yamamoto N, Kadoya S: [Significance of intracranial aneurysms associated with moyamoya disease. (Part I). Differences between intracranial aneurysms associated with moyamoya disease and usual saccular aneurysms--review of the literature]. *Neurol. Med. Chir (Tokyo).* 1984;24:97-103

[50] Yuasa H, Tokito S, Izumi K, Hirabayashi K: Cerebrovascular moyamoya disease associated with an intracranial pseudoaneurysm. Case report. *J. Neurosurg.* 1982;56: 131-134

[51] Hamada J, Hashimoto N, Tsukahara T: Moyamoya disease with repeated intraventricular hemorrhage due to aneurysm rupture. Report of two cases. *J. Neurosurg.* 1994;80:328-331

[52] Kawaguchi S, Sakaki T, Kakizaki T, Kamada K, Shimomura T, Iwanaga H: Clinical features of the haemorrhage type moyamoya disease based on 31 cases. *Acta Neurochir (Wien).* 1996;138:1200-1210

[53] Dietrichs E, Dahl A, Nyberg-Hansen R, Russell D, Rootwelt K, Veger T: Cerebral blood flow findings in moyamoya disease in adults. *Acta Neurol. Scand.* 1992;85:318-322

[54] Marushima A, Yanaka K, Matsuki T, Kojima H, Nose T: Subarachnoid hemorrhage not due to ruptured aneurysm in moyamoya disease. *J. Clin. Neurosci.* 2006;13:146-149

[55] Osanai T, Kuroda S, Nakayama N, Yamauchi T, Houkin K, Iwasaki Y: Moyamoya disease presenting with subarachnoid hemorrhage localized over the frontal cortex: case report. *Surg. Neurol.* 2008;69:197-200

[56] Mashini IS, Albazzaz SJ, Fadel HE, Abdulla AM, Hadi HA, Harp R, Devoe LD: Serial noninvasive evaluation of cardiovascular hemodynamics during pregnancy. *Am. J. Obstet Gynecol.* 1987;156:1208-1213

[57] Metcalfe J, McAnulty JH, Ueland K: Cardiovascular physiology. *Clin. Obstet Gynecol.* 1981;24:693-710

[58] Letterman G, Schurter M, Barter RH, Martin SS: Hemangiomas of pregnancy. *South Med. J.* 1957;50:594-599

[59] Komiyama M: Moyamoya disease and pregnancy. *J. Nucl. Med.* 1999;40:214-215

[60] Mehrkens JH, Steiger HJ, Strauss A, Winkler PA: Management of haemorrhagic type moyamoya disease with intraventricular haemorrhage during pregnancy. *Acta Neurochir (Wien).* 2006;148:685-689; discussion 689

[61] Akasaki T, Kagiyama S, Omae T, Ohya Y, Ibayashi S, Abe I, Fujishima M: Asymptomatic moyamoya disease associated with coronary and renal artery stenoses--a case report. *Jpn. Circ. J.* 1998;62:136-138

[62] Aoki T, Saiki M, Ishizaki R, Sato T: [A case report of the adult patient with asymptomatic moyamoya disease]. *Pract. Curren. Neurosurg.* 2004;14:597-602

[63] Nanba R, Kuroda S, Takeda M, Shichinohe H, Nakayama N, Ishikawa T, Houkin K, Iwasaki Y: [Clinical features and outcomes of 10 asymptomatic adult patients with moyamoya disease]. *No Shinkei Geka.* 2003;31:1291-1295

[64] Yamada M, Fujii K, Fukui M: [Clinical features and outcomes in patients with asymptomatic moyamoya disease--from the results of nation-wide questionnaire survey]. *No Shinkei Geka*. 2005;33:337-342

[65] Kuroda S, Hashimoto N, Yoshimoto T, Iwasaki Y: Radiological findings, clinical course, and outcome in asymptomatic moyamoya disease: results of multicenter survey in Japan. *Stroke* 2007;38:1430-1435

[66] Hasuo K, Mihara F, Matsushima T: MRI and MR angiography in moyamoya disease. *J. Magn. Reson. Imaging*. 1998;8:762-766

[67] Suto Y, Caner BE, Nakatsugawa S, Katsube Y, Ishii Y, Torizuka K: Evaluation of MRI in moyamoya disease. *Radiat. Med*. 1990;8:92-95

[68] Yamada I, Suzuki S, Matsushima Y: Moyamoya disease: diagnostic accuracy of MRI. *Neuroradiology* 1995;37:356-361

[69] Harada A, Fujii Y, Yoneoka Y, Takeuchi S, Tanaka R, Nakada T: High-field magnetic resonance imaging in patients with moyamoya disease. *J. Neurosurg*. 2001;94:233-237

[70] Komiyama M, Nakajima H, Nishikawa M, Yasui T, Kitano S, Sakamoto H: Leptomeningeal contrast enhancement in moyamoya: its potential role in postoperative assessment of circulation through the bypass. *Neuroradiology* 2001;43:17-23

[71] Suzuki J, Kodama N: Cerebrovascular "Moyamoya" disease. 2. Collateral routes to forebrain via ethmoid sinus and superior nasal meatus. *Angiology* 1971;22:223-236

[72] Houkin K, Aoki T, Takahashi A, Abe H: Diagnosis of moyamoya disease with magnetic resonance angiography. *Stroke* 1994;25:2159-2164

[73] Houkin K, Tanaka N, Takahashi A, Kamiyama H, Abe H, Kajii N: Familial occurrence of moyamoya disease. Magnetic resonance angiography as a screening test for high-risk subjects. *Childs Nerv. Syst*. 1994;10:421-425

[74] Yamada I, Matsushima Y, Suzuki S: Moyamoya disease: diagnosis with three-dimensional time-of-flight MR angiography. *Radiology* 1992;184:773-778

[75] Yamada I, Suzuki S, Matsushima Y: Moyamoya disease: comparison of assessment with MR angiography and MR imaging versus conventional angiography. *Radiology* 1995;196:211-218

[76] Houkin K, Nakayama N, Kuroda S, Nonaka T, Shonai T, Yoshimoto T: Novel magnetic resonance angiography stage grading for moyamoya disease. *Cerebrovasc. Dis*. 2005;20:347-354

[77] Vorstrup S, Henriksen L, Paulson OB: Effect of acetazolamide on cerebral blood flow and cerebral metabolic rate for oxygen. *J. Clin. Invest*. 1984;74:1634-1639

[78] Vorstrup S, Jensen KE, Thomsen C, Henriksen O, Lassen NA, Paulson OB: Neuronal pH regulation: constant normal intracellular pH is maintained in brain during low extracellular pH induced by acetazolamide--31P NMR study. *J. Cereb. Blood Flow Metab*. 1989;9:417-421

[79] Kazumata K, Tanaka N, Ishikawa T, Kuroda S, Houkin K, Mitsumori K: Dissociation of vasoreactivity to acetazolamide and hypercapnia. Comparative study in patients with chronic occlusive major cerebral artery disease. *Stroke* 1996;27:2052-2058

[80] Kuroda S, Houkin K, Kamiyama H, Mitsumori K, Iwasaki Y, Abe H: Long-term prognosis of medically treated patients with internal carotid or middle cerebral artery occlusion: can acetazolamide test predict it? *Stroke* 2001;32:2110-2116

[81] Kuroda S, Kamiyama H, Abe H, Houkin K, Isobe M, Mitsumori K: Acetazolamide test in detecting reduced cerebral perfusion reserve and predicting long-term prognosis in patients with internal carotid artery occlusion. *Neurosurgery* 1993;32:912-918; discussion 918-919

[82] Kuroda S, Kamiyama H, Abe H, Takigawa S, Mitsumori K, Nomura M, Saitoh H: Drug-induced hypotension SEP test and acetazolamide test using 133Xe SPECT in patients with occlusive carotid disease--selection of candidates for extracranial-intracranial bypass. *Neurol. Med. Chir (Tokyo).* 1991;31:7-12

[83] Vorstrup S, Boysen G, Brun B, Engell HC: Evaluation of the regional cerebral vasodilatory capacity before carotid endarterectomy by the acetazolamide test. *Neurol. Res.* 1987; 9:10-18

[84] Vorstrup S, Brun B, Lassen NA: Evaluation of the cerebral vasodilatory capacity by the acetazolamide test before EC-IC bypass surgery in patients with occlusion of the internal carotid artery. *Stroke* 1986;17:1291-1298

[85] Powers WJ, Grubb RL, Jr., Raichle ME: Physiological responses to focal cerebral ischemia in humans. *Ann. Neurol.* 1984;16:546-552

[86] Baron JC, Bousser MG, Rey A, Guillard A, Comar D, Castaigne P: Reversal of focal "misery-perfusion syndrome" by extra-intracranial arterial bypass in hemodynamic cerebral ischemia. A case study with 15O positron emission tomography. *Stroke* 1981; 12:454-459

[87] Kuwabara Y, Ichiya Y, Otsuka M, Tahara T, Gunasekera R, Hasuo K, Masuda K, Matsushima T, Fukui M: Cerebral hemodynamic change in the child and the adult with moyamoya disease. *Stroke* 1990;21:272-277

[88] Kuwabara Y, Ichiya Y, Sasaki M, Yoshida T, Masuda K, Ikezaki K, Matsushima T, Fukui M: Cerebral hemodynamics and metabolism in moyamoya disease--a positron emission tomography study. *Clin. Neurol. Neurosurg.* 1997;99 Suppl 2:S74-78

[89] Nariai T, Matsushima Y, Imae S, Tanaka Y, Ishii K, Senda M, Ohno K: Severe haemodynamic stress in selected subtypes of patients with moyamoya disease: a positron emission tomography study. *J. Neurol. Neurosurg. Psychiatry* 2005;76:663-669

[90] Ogawa A, Yoshimoto T, Suzuki J, Sakurai Y: Cerebral blood flow in moyamoya disease. Part 1: Correlation with age and regional distribution. *Acta Neurochir (Wien).* 1990;105:30-34

[91] Hoshi H, Ohnishi T, Jinnouchi S, Futami S, Nagamachi S, Kodama T, Watanabe K, Ueda T, Wakisaka S: Cerebral blood flow study in patients with moyamoya disease evaluated by IMP SPECT. *J. Nucl. Med.* 1994;35:44-50

[92] Ogawa A, Nakamura N, Yoshimoto T, Suzuki J: Cerebral blood flow in moyamoya disease. Part 2: Autoregulation and CO2 response. *Acta Neurochir (Wien).* 1990;105: 107-111

[93] Watanabe H, Ohta S, Oka Y, Kumon Y, Sakaki S, Sugawara Y, Tanada S: Changes in cortical CBF and vascular response after vascular reconstruction in patients with adult onset moyamoya disease. *Acta Neurochir (Wien).* 1996;138:1211-1217

[94] Yamashita T, Kashiwagi S, Nakashima K, Ishihara H, Kitahara T, Nakano S, Ito H: Modulation of cerebral hemodynamics by surgical revascularization in patients with moyamoya disease. *Acta Neurol. Scand. Suppl.* 1996;166:82-84

[95] Morimoto M, Iwama T, Hashimoto N, Kojima A, Hayashida K: Efficacy of direct revascularization in adult Moyamoya disease: haemodynamic evaluation by positron emission tomography. *Acta Neurochir (Wien).* 1999;141:377-384

[96] Piao R, Oku N, Kitagawa K, Imaizumi M, Matsushita K, Yoshikawa T, Takasawa M, Osaki Y, Kimura Y, Kajimoto K, Hori M, Hatazawa J: Cerebral hemodynamics and metabolism in adult moyamoya disease: comparison of angiographic collateral circulation. *Ann. Nucl. Med.* 2004;18:115-121

[97] Taki W, Yonekawa Y, Kobayashi A, Ishikawa M, Kikuchi H, Nishizawa S, Senda M, Fukuyama H, Harada K, et al.: Cerebral circulation and oxygen metabolism in moyamoya disease of ischemic type in children. *Childs Nerv. Syst.* 1988;4:259-262

[98] Ishikawa T, Kamiyama H, Kuroda S, Yasuda H, Nakayama N, Takizawa K: Simultaneous superficial temporal artery to middle cerebral or anterior cerebral artery bypass with pan-synangiosis for Moyamoya disease covering both anterior and middle cerebral artery territories. *Neurol. Med. Chir (Tokyo).* 2006;46:462-468

[99] Iwama T, Hashimoto N, Tsukahara T, Miyake H: Superficial temporal artery to anterior cerebral artery direct anastomosis in patients with moyamoya disease. *Clin. Neurol. Neurosurg.* 1997;99 Suppl 2:S134-136

[100] Fujimura M, Kaneta T, Mugikura S, Shimizu H, Tominaga T: Temporary neurologic deterioration due to cerebral hyperperfusion after superficial temporal artery-middle cerebral artery anastomosis in patients with adult-onset moyamoya disease. *Surg. Neurol.* 2007;67:273-282

[101] Fujimura M, Shimizu H, Mugikura S, Tominaga T: Delayed intracerebral hemorrhage after superficial temporal artery-middle cerebral artery anastomosis in a patient with moyamoya disease: possible involvement of cerebral hyperperfusion and increased vascular permeability. *Surg. Neurol,* 2008.

[102] Kuroda S, Kamiyama H, Abe H, Asaoka K, Mitsumori K: Temporary neurological deterioration caused by hyperperfusion after extracranial-intracranial bypass--case report and study of cerebral hemodynamics. *Neurol. Med. Chir (Tokyo).* 1994;34:15-19

[103] Yoshimoto T, Houkin K, Kuroda S, Abe H, Kashiwaba T: Low cerebral blood flow and perfusion reserve induce hyperperfusion after surgical revascularization: case reports and analysis of cerebral hemodynamics. *Surg. Neurol.* 1997;48:132-138; discussion 138-139

[104] Matsushima Y, Aoyagi M, Fukai N, Tanaka K, Tsuruoka S, Inaba Y: Angiographic demonstration of cerebral revascularization after encephalo-duro-arterio-synangiosis (EDAS) performed on pediatric moyamoya patients. *Bull. Tokyo Med. Dent. Univ.* 1982;29:7-17

[105] Matsushima Y, Fukai N, Tanaka K, Tsuruoka S, Inaba Y, Aoyagi M, Ohno K: A new surgical treatment of moyamoya disease in children: a preliminary report. *Surg. Neurol.* 1981;15:313-320

[106]Scott RM, Smith JL, Robertson RL, Madsen JR, Soriano SG, Rockoff MA: Long-term outcome in children with moyamoya syndrome after cranial revascularization by pial synangiosis. *J. Neurosurg.* 2004;100:142-149

[107]Karasawa J, Kikuchi H, Furuse S, Sakaki T, Yoshida Y: A surgical treatment of "moyamoya" disease "encephalo-myo synangiosis". *Neurol. Med. Chir (Tokyo).* 1977; 17:29-37

[108]Kinugasa K, Mandai S, Kamata I, Sugiu K, Ohmoto T: Surgical treatment of moyamoya disease: operative technique for encephalo-duro-arterio-myo-synangiosis, its follow-up, clinical results, and angiograms. *Neurosurgery* 1993;32:527-531

[109]Ishii R: [Surgical treatment of moyamoya disease]. *No Shinkei Geka.* 1986;14:1059-1068

[110]Park JH, Yang SY, Chung YN, Kim JE, Kim SK, Han DH, Cho BK: Modified encephaloduroarteriosynangiosis with bifrontal encephalogaleoperiosteal synangiosis for the treatment of pediatric moyamoya disease. Technical note. *J. Neurosurg.* 2007; 106:237-242

[111]Kawaguchi T, Fujita S, Hosoda K, Shose Y, Hamano S, Iwakura M, Tamaki N: Multiple burr-hole operation for adult moyamoya disease. *J. Neurosurg.* 1996;84:468-476

[112]Houkin K, Kuroda S, Ishikawa T, Abe H: Neovascularization (angiogenesis) after revascularization in moyamoya disease. Which technique is most useful for moyamoya disease? *Acta Neurochir (Wien).* 2000;142:269-276

[113]Houkin K, Nakayama N, Kuroda S, Ishikawa T, Nonaka T: How does angiogenesis develop in pediatric moyamoya disease after surgery? A prospective study with MR angiography. *Childs Nerv. Syst.* 2004;20:734-741

[114]Matsushima T, Inoue T, Katsuta T, Natori Y, Suzuki S, Ikezaki K, Fukui M: An indirect revascularization method in the surgical treatment of moyamoya disease--various kinds of indirect procedures and a multiple combined indirect procedure. *Neurol. Med. Chir (Tokyo).* 1998;38 Suppl:297-302

[115]Matsushima T, Inoue T, Suzuki SO, Fujii K, Fukui M, Hasuo K: Surgical treatment of moyamoya disease in pediatric patients--comparison between the results of indirect and direct revascularization procedures. *Neurosurgery* 1992;31:401-405

[116]Takahashi A, Kamiyama H, Houkin K, Abe H: Surgical treatment of childhood moyamoya disease--comparison of reconstructive surgery centered on the frontal region and the parietal region. *Neurol. Med. Chir (Tokyo).* 1995;35:231-237

[117]Houkin K, Kamiyama H, Abe H, Takahashi A, Kuroda S: Surgical therapy for adult moyamoya disease. Can surgical revascularization prevent the recurrence of intracerebral hemorrhage? *Stroke* 1996;27:1342-1346

[118]Mizoi K, Kayama T, Yoshimoto T, Nagamine Y: Indirect revascularization for moyamoya disease: is there a beneficial effect for adult patients? *Surg. Neurol.* 1996; 45:541-548; discussion 548-549

[119]Houkin K, Ishikawa T, Yoshimoto T, Abe H: Direct and indirect revascularization for moyamoya disease surgical techniques and peri-operative complications. *Clin. Neurol. Neurosurg.* 1997;99 Suppl 2:S142-145

[120]Iwama T, Hashimoto N, Miyake H, Yonekawa Y: Direct revascularization to the anterior cerebral artery territory in patients with moyamoya disease: report of five cases. *Neurosurgery* 1998;42:1157-1161; discussion 1161-1152

[121]Kohno K, Oka Y, Kohno S, Ohta S, Kumon Y, Sakaki S: Cerebral blood flow measurement as an indicator for an indirect revascularization procedure for adult patients with moyamoya disease. *Neurosurgery* 1998;42:752-757; discussion 757-758

[122]Mikulis DJ, Krolczyk G, Desal H, Logan W, Deveber G, Dirks P, Tymianski M, Crawley A, Vesely A, Kassner A, Preiss D, Somogyi R, Fisher JA: Preoperative and postoperative mapping of cerebrovascular reactivity in moyamoya disease by using blood oxygen level-dependent magnetic resonance imaging. *J. Neurosurg.* 2005;103: 347-355

[123]Oya S, Tsutsumi K, Ueki K: Adult-onset moyamoya disease with repetitive ischemic attacks successfully treated by superficial temporal-middle cerebral artery bypass--case report. *Neurol. Med. Chir (Tokyo).* 2003;43:138-141

[124]Takeuchi S, Kikuchi H, Karasawa J, Yamagata S, Nagata I: Regional cortical blood flow during extra-intracranial bypass surgery in young patients with moyamoya disease. *Neurol. Med. Chir (Tokyo).* 1989;29:10-14

[125]Choi JU, Kim DS, Kim EY, Lee KC: Natural history of moyamoya disease: comparison of activity of daily living in surgery and non surgery groups. *Clin. Neurol. Neurosurg.* 1997;99 Suppl 2:S11-18

[126]Hallemeier CL, Rich KM, Grubb RL, Jr., Chicoine MR, Moran CJ, Cross DT, 3rd, Zipfel GJ, Dacey RG, Jr., Derdeyn CP: Clinical features and outcome in North American adults with moyamoya phenomenon. *Stroke* 2006;37:1490-1496

[127]Han DH, Nam DH, Oh CW: Moyamoya disease in adults: characteristics of clinical presentation and outcome after encephalo-duro-arterio-synangiosis. *Clin. Neurol. Neurosurg.* 1997;99 Suppl 2:S151-155

[128]Hirotsune N, Meguro T, Kawada S, Nakashima H, Ohmoto T: Long-term follow-up study of patients with unilateral moyamoya disease. *Clin. Neurol. Neurosurg.* 1997;99 Suppl 2:S178-181

[129]Kawano T, Fukui M, Hashimoto N, Yonekawa Y: Follow-up study of patients with "unilateral" moyamoya disease. *Neurol. Med. Chir (Tokyo).* 1994;34:744-747

[130]Kelly ME, Bell-Stephens TE, Marks MP, Do HM, Steinberg GK: Progression of unilateral moyamoya disease: A clinical series. *Cerebrovasc. Dis.* 2006;22:109-115

[131]Kuroda S, Ishikawa T, Houkin K, Nanba R, Hokari M, Iwasaki Y: Incidence and clinical features of disease progression in adult moyamoya disease. *Stroke* 2005;36: 2148-2153

[132]Kim DS, Yoo DS, Huh PW, Kang SG, Cho KS, Kim MC: Combined direct anastomosis and encephaloduroarteriogaleosynangiosis using inverted superficial temporal artery-galeal flap and superficial temporal artery-galeal pedicle in adult moyamoya disease. *Surg. Neurol.* 2006;66:389-394; discussion 395

[133]Nakashima H, Meguro T, Kawada S, Hirotsune N, Ohmoto T: Long-term results of surgically treated moyamoya disease. *Clin. Neurol. Neurosurg.* 1997;99 Suppl 2:S156-161

[134]Okada Y, Shima T, Nishida M, Yamane K, Yamada T, Yamanaka C: Effectiveness of superficial temporal artery-middle cerebral artery anastomosis in adult moyamoya disease: cerebral hemodynamics and clinical course in ischemic and hemorrhagic varieties. *Stroke* 1998;29:625-630

[135]Wanifuchi H, Takeshita M, Izawa M, Aoki N, Kagawa M: Management of adult moyamoya disease. *Neurol. Med. Chir (Tokyo).* 1993;33:300-305

[136]Fujii K, Ikezaki K, Irikura K, Miyasaka Y, Fukui M: The efficacy of bypass surgery for the patients with hemorrhagic moyamoya disease. *Clin. Neurol. Neurosurg.* 1997;99 Suppl 2:S194-195

[137]Kobayashi E, Saeki N, Oishi H, Hirai S, Yamaura A: Long-term natural history of hemorrhagic moyamoya disease in 42 patients. *J. Neurosurg.* 2000;93:976-980

[138]Morioka M, Hamada J, Todaka T, Yano S, Kai Y, Ushio Y: High-risk age for rebleeding in patients with hemorrhagic moyamoya disease: long-term follow-up study. *Neurosurgery* 2003;52:1049-1054; discussion 1054-1045

[139]Yoshida Y, Yoshimoto T, Shirane R, Sakurai Y: Clinical course, surgical management, and long-term outcome of moyamoya patients with rebleeding after an episode of intracerebral hemorrhage: An extensive follow-Up study. *Stroke* 1999;30:2272-2276

[140]Kawaguchi S, Okuno S, Sakaki T: Effect of direct arterial bypass on the prevention of future stroke in patients with the hemorrhagic variety of moyamoya disease. *J. Neurosurg.* 2000;93:397-401

[141]Miyamoto S: Study design for a prospective randomized trial of extracranial-intracranial bypass surgery for adults with moyamoya disease and hemorrhagic onset--the Japan Adult Moyamoya Trial Group. *Neurol. Med. Chir (Tokyo).* 2004;44:218-219

In: Cerebral Ischemia in Young Adults
Editors: A. Pezzini and A. Padovani
ISBN 978-1-60741-627-2

Chapter 13

PFO/ASA and Ischemic Stroke in Young Patients

Gian Paolo Anzola**, Maria Paola Piras, Brunilda Alushi, Eustaquio Onorat and Francesco Casilli
Heart and Brain Department,
S. Orsola Hospital FBF, Brescia, Italy

Abstract

Patent foramen ovale (PFO) is a frequent finding on echocardiography and occurs in over 25% of the population. In young patients with cryptogenic stroke, the frequency is much higher suggesting paradoxical embolization may be responsible for the clinical events. There are conflicting data from studies examining the association between PFO and stroke. The combination of atrial septal aneurysm (ASA) and PFO, PFO size, the degree of functional shunting, and co-existing hypercoagulable state may add additional risk but again the data are insufficient for definite conclusions. Available information suggests no difference in subsequent stroke in patients with PFO treated with aspirin or warfarin for secondary prevention. Endovascular closure is technically feasible, but not without the possibility of periprocedural complications. The completion of ongoing, randomized clinical trials comparing percutaneous closure devices with medical management is urgently needed to clarify if the risks of invasive endovascular device placement are outweighed by a long-term reduction in recurrent vascular events.

* Correspondence: Gian Paolo Anzola, Via Vittorio Emanuele II, 27, 25100 Brescia, Italy. phone +390302971l. e-mail gpanzola@fatebenefratelli.it.

Introduction

Stroke is among the principal causes of morbidity and mortality in industrialized countries being responsible for 10-12% of all deaths and for an elevated number of permanent disabilities.

It is classically defined as a clinical syndrome characterized by rapidly developing clinical symptoms and/or signs of focal and at times global disturbance of cerebral function lasting more than 24 hours or leading to death with no apparent cause other than that of vascular origin. A more detailed definition incorporating the main pathophysiological mechanisms qualifies stroke as a "clinical syndrome characterized by an acute loss of focal cerebral function with symptoms lasting more than 24 hours or leading to death and which is thought to be due to either spontaneous haemorrhage into the brain substance or inadequate cerebral blood supply to a part of the brain as a result of low blood flow, thrombosis or embolism associated with diseases of the blood vessels, heart or blood" [1].

Stroke incidence is clearly associated with aging. Although younger adults are at lower risk, stroke in this population has a particularly high public health impact because of associated indirect costs, such as longer years of lost productivity. When it occurs in young persons, they may have a period of time to live with their disability longer than older stroke patients and this may contribute to a lifetime of medical complications which determine high socioeconomic costs.

Ischemic stroke in patients younger than 45 years of age has been considered a relatively rare event, accounting for <5% of all cerebral infarctions in the majority of studies, and few reporting figures exceeding 10% [2,3]. In one U.S. study, 8% of all strokes occurred in patients between the ages of 20 and 45 [4]. In a large Japanese study, 7% of strokes occurred in patients aged 16–50 [5]. This rate may be lower in European, and higher (20–30%) in developing countries [6].

Several studies have shown differences in stroke incidence among whites, blacks, and Hispanics, [7,8] but few specifically examining these differences in the young adult population. Kittner et al [9] described differences in stroke rates in a young white and black population and showed that young blacks had a higher incidence than whites. These findings were confirmed by the Northern Manhattan Study (NOMAS), a prospective, population based study of stroke incidence. NOMAS investigators examined stroke in a defined urban community. They found that Black and Hispanic adults had higher incidence rates of stroke in all age groups compared with whites. Annual age adjusted incidence rates were 223 per 100,000 in Black subjects; 93 in whites; and 196 in Hispanics. Although annual incidence rates were lower in younger subjects, there were still marked differences by race ethnicity. In subjects aged 35 to 44, the incidence rates were: 6 per 100,000 per year in Whites, 54 in Blacks and 53 in Hispanics [4,10].

In the various incidence studies, the incidence of all subtypes of stroke (cerebral infarction, intracerebral haemorrhage, and subarachnoid haemorrhage) is reported to be increased in the black population but especially the intracerebral and subarachnoid haemorrhage [9,11].

However, about 70% to 80% of all stroke cases in the developed countries are ischemic and only 20% haemorrhagic.

Subtypes of Ischemic Stroke

Contrary to general beliefs, ischemic stroke is not a homogeneous condition but rather a mix of clinically distinct subtypes that have different risk profiles, incidence rates, aetiological factors and management and outcomes [12]. Despite modern diagnostic methods and an extensive evaluation, a high proportion of infarcts is difficult to classify because no cause can be found or a most likely cause cannot be determined because more than one plausible cause has been found.

For these reasons, according to the TOAST criteria (Trial of ORG 10172 in Acute Stroke Treatment) five major etiologic categories have been identified [13]:

1. large-artery atherosclerosis (LAA), including large-artery thrombosis and artery-to-artery embolism;
2. cardioembolism (CE);
3. small-vessel occlusion (SAO), i.e. lacunar;
4. stroke of other determined cause (OC)
5. stroke of undetermined cause (UND).

The etiologic spectrum differs considerably between ages. Atrial fibrillation or advanced atherosclerotic disease (of small and large vessels) are the main causes in most individuals older than 50 years [14].

In contrast, idiopathic cardioembolic and nonatherosclerotic arteriopathies, such as arterial dissection, and fibromuscular dysplasia or vasculitis, are the commonest causes of stroke in younger patients (particularly in those less than 35 years old) [15,16].

Often no cause for stroke is apparent, in which case the stroke is commonly described as cryptogenic.

Cases categorized as ischemic stroke of undetermined cause do not have risk factors or prior history that might suggest a cardiac embolus or large artery thrombosis.

As many as 40% of all strokes in all age groups, but especially among patients younger than 55 years, have not a clearly identified aetiology and remain cryptogenic after careful evaluation [17].

For example, a large population-based study including adult patients of all ages indicated that the fraction of ischemic strokes that remains unknown in patients under 45 years of age is 31%, whereas it is 23% in patients between 45 to 70 years and 21% in those aged over 70 years [4]. In a study of patients <55 years of age, no cause for stroke was apparently found in as many as 64% of patients [18].

There are very few data regarding the real risk factors for cryptogenic ischemic stroke. Nevertheless emerging technologies have led to the suggestion that some of the cryptogenic infarct cases may be explained by haematologic disorders causing hypercoagulable states from protein C, free protein S, lupus anticoagulant, or anticardiolipin antibody abnormalities. Others have suggested a causal relationship with atrial septal abnormalities such as patent foramen ovale, atrial septal aneurysm, a Chiari network and prominent Eustachian valve [19].

Based on these results, especially in young patients, a correct weighting of the risk factors and adequate neurovascular investigations are needed.

However, the mix of causes and the proportion with 'no cause' depend on referral bias, investigation intensity, diagnostic criteria differences and fashion over time; all these can change as more putative causes are discovered [1].

Patent Foramen Ovale: Embryo-Anatomy and Prevalence

Patent foramen ovale (PFO), a remnant of the fetal circulation, develops when an anatomical interatrial communication remains after birth allowing the persistence of a potential shunt between the right and left atria of the heart. Anatomically, foramen ovale is an opening between the atrial septum primum and secundum at the site of their overlapping. The foramen ovale is necessary for blood flow across the fetal atrial septum. Oxygenated placental blood enters the right atrium via the inferior vena cava and crosses the valve of the foramen ovale to enter the systemic arterial circulation.

Beginning at four weeks of pregnancy the primordial single atrium divides into right and left sides by formation and fusion of two septa: the septum primum and septum secundum. The septum primum is at first crescent-shaped, creating a large window connecting the left and right atrium. It grows from the primordial atrial roof toward the endocardial cushions, partially dividing the common atrium into right and left halves.

The endocardial cushions are formed on the dorsal and ventral walls of the atrioventricular canal, approach each other, and fuse, dividing the atrioventricular canal into right and left sides. The foramen primum results, allowing oxygenated blood flow from the right to the left atrium. As the septum primum grows toward the endocardial cushions, perforations develop. These perforations form a large central window, through programmed cell death, before the septum primum and endocardial cushions fuse.

The window made as these perforations fuse is the foramen secundum, which also supplies shunt blood flow from the right to the left atrium. On the right side of the septum primum, another crescent-shaped membrane grows from the ventrocranial atrial wall: the septum secundum. It gradually grows and overlaps part of the foramen secundum, forming an incomplete septal partition as an oval-shaped window. It is this window that becomes the foramen ovale. The remaining septum primum forms a flap-like valve over the foramen ovale, which typically closes by fusing with the growing septum secundum after birth.

As oxygenated blood flow in utero from the inferior vena cava enters the right atrium, it crosses the patent foramen ovale and reaches the systemic circulation. Most blood flow from the superior vena cava is routed through the tricuspid valve and enters the right ventricle. At birth, right heart pressure and pulmonary vascular resistance drop as pulmonary arterioles open in reaction to oxygen filling the alveolus. Left atrial pressure may also rise as the amount of blood returning from the lungs increases. Either or both of these mechanisms may cause flap closure against the septum secundum. The flap of the foramen ovale (septum primum) closes against the atrial septum (septum secundum), with fusion usually occurring within the first two years of life in about 75 percent of individuals, but patency occurs in the other 25 percent [20] (Figure 1). It is a residual, oblique, slit-shaped defect resembling a tunnel.

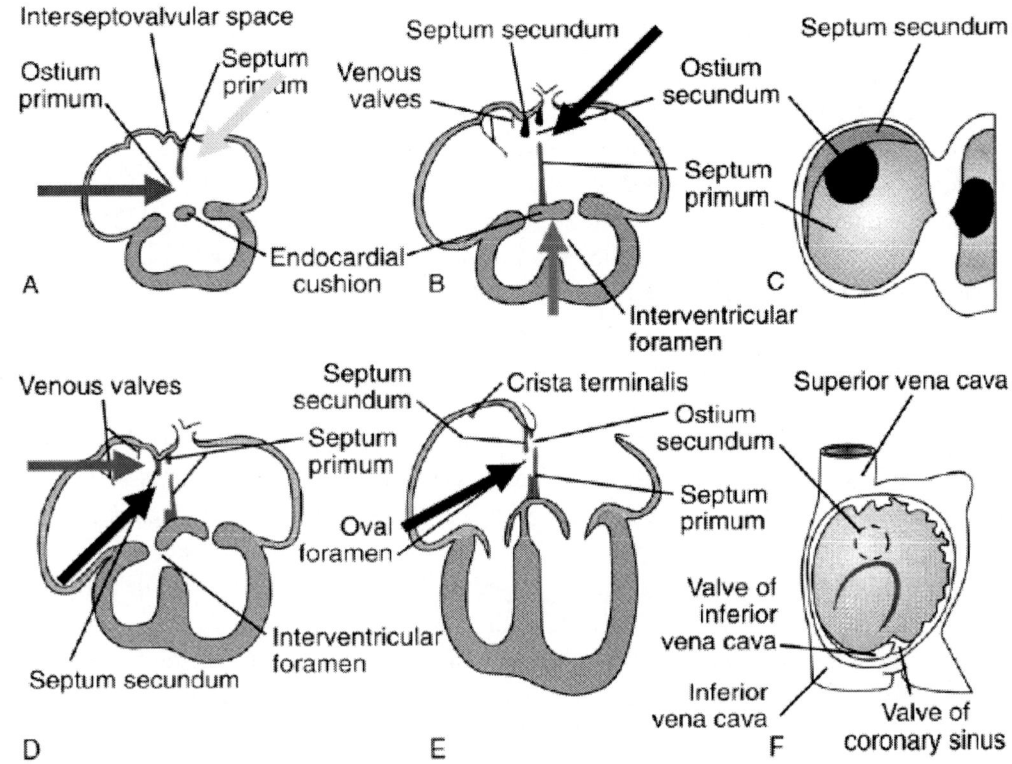

Figure 1. Embryological development of patent foramen ovale.

The reasons PFOs fail to close are unknown, but they likely relate to multifactorial inheritance [21].

Post mortem studies [22] have confirmed a PFO prevalence of overall 27% in the general population, with no gender difference (men, 26.8%, women, 27.6%) but with a trend for a reduction with advancing age (approximately 30%, 25%, and 20% for age groups 1-29 years, 30-79 years, and 80 years, respectively). In the Mayo Clinic study PFO size varied between 1 and 19 mm, with a average diameter of 4.9 mm [22].

On the other hand, the presence of PFO detected by echocardiography in normal subjects varies between 10 and 22% [23-26].

This suggests that echocardiography has a lower sensitivity in identifying PFO as compared to anatomical inspection.

Patent Foramen Ovale in Stroke Patients

An important role of patent foramen ovale in the pathogenesis of ischemic stroke was first suggested in a couple of seminal papers that appeared in the late ‘80s. Lechat et al. used transthoracic echocardiography (TTE) with contrast micro-bubble injection to study a cohort of <55 year old stroke patients and they showed a markedly higher frequency of PFO in patients with stroke of unknown causes than in patients with stroke of known cause and in age matched controls: 54%, 21% and. 10% respectively. [25]. Webster and colleagues, likewise, reported a PFO frequency of 50% in cryptogenic stroke patients vs. 15% in controls in < 30 year old subjects [24].

Numerous studies have since confirmed the high absolute frequency of PFO in young cryptogenic stroke patients [27] or the statistically higher prevalence of PFO in young cryptogenic as compared to known cause strokes or non stroke control subjects [19].

In nine studies including young stroke patients aged 55 years or less [18,24,25,28-33], PFO was present in 40.3% of the subjects as compared with 17.8% of controls, giving a significant odds ratio (OR) of 3.1 (95% CI 2.29-4.21). In studies when cryptogenic stroke patients were compared with known cause strokes the prevalence was 55.7vs. 17.1% with an OR of 6.0 95% CI (3.72-9.6) [34].

In contrast to this finding the metanalysis performed by Overell et al [34] of the three studies performed in patients aged over 55 years [29,31,32], showed no difference in the prevalence of PFO between cryptogenic stroke cases (16.3%) and controls (13.4%) or a nonsignificant trend between cryptogenic stroke (27.1%) and stroke of known origin (14.0%) [31,35,36].

In the study of Di Tullio et al. the increased higher prevalence of PFO in patients with cryptogenic stroke (compared with patients with an identifiable cause of stroke) was however observed in both the younger (<55 years; 48% compared with 4%) and the older (>=55 years; 38% versus 8%) age groups. These differences remained significant even after analysis for the presence of other known risk factors. More recently, a prospective study on a hospital based cohort of stroke patients showed a significantly higher prevalence of PFO in cryptogenic (28.3%) than in known cause (11.9%) strokes in patients $\geq$ 55 years of age. [37] Multivariate analysis adjusted for age, plaque thickness, and presence or absence of coronary artery disease and hypertension showed that the presence of patent foramen ovale was independently associated with cryptogenic stroke with an odds ratioof 3.00 (95% CI, 1.73 to 5.23; P<0.001) [37]. This observation suggests that PFO may be a risk factor for cryptogenic stroke regardless of patient age.

In conclusion, the current evidence clearly shows a significant association of PFO with ischemic stroke in general, and with cryptogenic stroke especially, among patients younger than 55 years. Because of the limited data no firm conclusions can be made among older patients even though increasing evidence tends to emphasize the relevance of the association even in older stroke patients [37,38].

PFO and Stroke Risk

A large epidemiological study of healthy adults, (the Stroke Prevention: Assessment of Risk in a Community - SPARC study), was designed to estimate the prevalence of potential risk factors for stroke in the population. It consisted of a random sample of 585 residents of Olmsted County, Minnesota, who were older than 45 years. All subjects underwent transesophageal echocardiography (TEE) and carotid ultrasonography to identify potential risk factors that included the presence of PFO, atrial septal aneurysm (ASA), valve strands, and atherosclerosis of the aorta or carotid arteries [14]. A PFO was identified in 140 (24.3%)

subjects, ASA in 11 (1.9%) subjects. Overall PFO prevalence was similar for men and women. In contrast to the findings from autopsy studies, PFO prevalence was stable across all age groups [39].

Of the 140 subjects with PFO, 6 (4.3%) had an ASA; of the 437 subjects without PFO, 5 had an ASA (1.1%, two-sided Fisher exact test, p = 0.028). During a median follow-up of 5.1 years, cerebrovascular events (cerebrovascular disease-related death, ischemic stroke, transient ischemic attack) occurred in 41 subjects. After adjustment for age and comorbidity, PFO was not a significant independent predictor of stroke (hazard ratio 1.46, 95% CI 0.74 to 2.88, p = 0.28). The risk of a cerebrovascular event among subjects with ASA was nearly four times higher than that in those without ASA (hazard ratio 3.72, 95% CI 0.88 to 15.71, p = 0.074) [39] .

In another population based prospective study Di Tullio and associates sought to assess the risk of ischemic stroke from a patent foramen ovale in the multiethnic prospective cohort of northern Manhattan [40]. The presence of PFO was assessed at baseline by using transthoracic 2-dimensional echocardiography with contrast injection in 1100 stroke-free subjects older than 39 years of age (mean age 68.7 ± 10.0 years) from the Northern Manhattan Study (NOMAS). The presence of atrial septal aneurysm also was recorded. Subjects were followed annually for outcomes. PFO was detected in 164 subjects (14.9%); ASA was present in 27 subjects (2.5%) and associated with PFO in 19 subjects. During a mean follow-up of 79.7 ± 28.0 months, an ischemic stroke occurred in 68 subjects (6.2%). After adjustment for demographics and risk factors, PFO was not found to be significantly associated with stroke (hazard ratio 1.64, 95% CI 0.87 to 3.09). The same trend was observed in all age, gender, and race-ethnic subgroups. The coexistence of PFO and ASA did not increase the stroke risk (adjusted hazard ratio 1.25, 95% CI 0.17 to 9.24). Isolated ASA was associated with elevated stroke incidence (2 of 8, or 25%; adjusted hazard ratio 3.66, 95% CI 0.88 to 15.30) [40].

The SPARC and the NOMAS studies obtained strikingly similar results: they both indicated that PFO does not increase the risk of first in a lifetime stroke even when associated with ASA whereas isolated ASA does so. However these conclusions are based on a small number of outcome events, which partially may explain the paradox of the increased risk of ASA in isolation but not in association with PFO, the follow-up period was relatively short, the mean age of the studied population was around 67 years in both studies, and the outcome events (stroke or TIA) were not qualified as cryptogenic or from known cause. Therefore, it is still uncertain in our opinion, whether PFO or the association of PFO with ASA are able to increase the risk for cryptogenic stroke in the young population in the long run.

In any case, a conclusion seems warranted: since the absolute risk of stroke in the young population is low (probably between 0.5% and 1% per year) the coexistence of PFO does not increase it substantially in absolute terms. Most patients with isolated PFO are asymptomatic and will remain so for the rest of their lives. In fact, while 27% of the population has a PFO, only 0.1% will have a cryptogenic stroke, clearly indicating that the majority of PFOs remain benign. Therefore there is no justification for a systematic search of PFO in young people and the fortuitous detection of a PFO does not justify prophylactic medical or invasive treatments.

The presence of right-to-left shunt can however be included in the list of weak risk factors for cryptogenic stroke.

Stroke Recurrence in PFO Patients

A number of studies have investigated stroke recurrence in patients with atrial septal abnormalities and some of them have compared stroke recurrence in patients with an and without PFO.

In 1996 The Lausanne Study showed that interatrial communication, a history of recent migraine, posterior cerebral artery territory infarct, and a coexisting cause of stroke were associated with recurrence, whereas ASA and treatment type (anticoagulant or antiplatelet therapy, surgical closure of PFO) were not. The overall recurrence rate in patients with PFO was 3.8% per year [41].

Cujec et al. (1999) found a high recurrence rate for stroke or TIA (12% per year) in patients having PFO after a cryptogenic stroke, while the recurrence rate in patients without PFO was 5% per year [42].

A group of investigators at the University of Rome "La Sapienza" prospectively followed 86 cryptogenic stroke patients without atrial septal abnormalities and 74 cryptogenic stroke patients with a PFO found on TEE. Patients with PFO were deemed at high risk for cerebrovascular disease if they had PFO at rest and membrane mobility >6.5 mm and at low risk if they had PFO (either at rest or during the Valsalva maneuver) and membrane mobility ≤6.5 mm, or membrane mobility >6.5 mm with PFO during the Valsalva maneuver only. The cutoff of 6.5 mm was chosen because it represented the median value of membrane mobility for the total PFO population.

The overall cumulative estimate of risk of stroke or TIA recurrence, at 3 years of follow-up, in the whole cohort of patients with PFO was 7.2% (95% CI, 1% to 13.5%), as opposed to 16.3% (95% CI, 7.2% to 25.4%) for patients with cryptogenic stroke ($p = 0.3$).When PFO patients were analyzed separately, the risk of stroke or TIA recurrence, at 3 years of follow-up, was 4.3% (95% CI, 0% to 10.2%) for those with the low-risk pattern and 12.5% (95% CI, 0% to 26.1%) for those with the high-risk profile ($p = 0.05$) [43].

Mas et al., investigating adult patients with PFO and a prior cerebrovascular ischemic event, detected a 6.7% risk rate for stroke or TIA at 2 years, with an increased rate to 9.0% in patients with both PFO and an atrial septal aneurysm [44].

Similarly, the French PFO-ASA study [45] failed to document an association between isolated PFO and increased recurrent stroke. A total of 581 patients aged less than 55 years with cryptogenic stroke were consecutively enrolled after their index event. All patients were treated with aspirin (300 mg per day) except those patients who had a deep vein thrombosis or pulmonary embolism who received 3 to 6 months of warfarin. After 4 years there was no increased risk for recurrent events among patients with a PFO alone compared with patients with no atrial septal defect, but a significantly increased risk was found among patients with both PFO and ASA (15.2 % - 95 % CI, 1.8 to 28.6 % among the patients with both patent foramen ovale and atrial septal aneurysm, and 4.2 % - 95 % C I, 1.8 to 6.6 % among the patients with neither of these cardiac abnormalities). The presence of both cardiac abnormalities was a significant predictor of an increased risk of recurrent stroke (hazard ratio for the comparison with the absence of these abnormalities, 4.17; 95 % C I, 1.47 to 11.84), whereas isolated patent foramen ovale, whether small or large, was not. In this study, PFO shunt size was not significantly associated with the risk of recurrent cerebrovascular events [45].

The PFO in Cryptogenic Stroke Study (PICSS) sought to define the rate of recurrent stroke or death in stroke patients with or without PFO who were participating in the Warfarin-Aspirin Recurrent Stroke Study (WARSS), a randomized prospective study aimed at assessing the effect of warfarin as opposed to aspirin in preventing recurrent non cardioembolic ischemic strokes [46]. All patients randomly assigned to warfarin or aspirin in WARSS who had received a TEE as part of their evaluation and those who had had a cryptogenic stroke and would agree to a TEE were eligible to participate in the PICSS trial. This study enrolled 630 stroke patients. Of this cohort, 265 patients (42%) had a cryptogenic stroke and 365 patients (58%) had a stroke from a known aetiology. A PFO was found on TEE in 203 patients (33.8%), and an ASA was present in 69 (11.5%). Among cryptogenic stroke patients, 39% had a PFO, compared to 30% in patients with a known cause of stroke ($p = 0.02$). There was no significant difference in the time to primary end points between those with and those without PFO in the overall population ($p = 0.84$; hazard ratio 0.96; 95% CI 0.62 to 1.48; 2-year event rates 14.8% versus 15.4%) or in the cryptogenic subset ($p=0.65$; hazard ratio 1.17; 95% CI 0.60 to 2.37; 2-year event rates 14.3% versus 12.7%). There was no significant difference among those with no, small, or large PFO ($p = 0.41$ for small PFO and $p=0.16$ for large PFO; 2-year event rates for no, small, and large PFO, 15.4%, 18.5%, and 9.5%, respectively). There was no significant difference between patients with isolated PFO and those with PFO in association with atrial septal aneurysm ($p = 0.84$; 2-year event rates 14.5% versus 15.9%). In patients with PFO, there was no significant difference in the time to primary end points between those treated with warfarin and those treated with aspirin ($p = 0.49$; hazard ratio 1.29; 95% CI 0.63 to 2.64; 2-year event rates 16.5% versus 13.2%).

Based on the data obtained, this study showed that, on medical therapy, neither PFO diameter nor the degree of shunt or concomitant ASA were associated with an increased risk of stroke recurrence or death on 2-year follow-up. It failed to document an increased risk of recurrent stroke in patients with PFO compared with patients without atrial septal defects but the cohort included all age patients (mean ± SD age, 59 ± 12 years), cryptogenic and non cryptogenic strokes and patients with overall more cerebrovascular risk factor as compared to the French study [45]. This probably explains the discrepancy of the results from the French study in which only cryptogenic < 55 years old patients were included (see above). Other atherosclerotic or vascular mechanisms may have represented important confounding variables [46].

Subsequent analysis of PICSS, however, showed that larger PFOs were associated with cryptogenic stroke (20% versus 9.7%, $p = 0.001$) and in cryptogenic stroke patients aged 65 years or older, the risk of adverse events (death and recurrent ischemic stroke) was significantly higher in the patients with PFO ($p = 0.01$; hazard ratio = 3.21; 95% CI, 1.33 to 7.75; 2-year event rates 37.9% versus 14.5%) [47].

Messe et al. in their review concluded that both PFO and ASA possibly increase the risk of subsequent stroke (but not death) in medically treated patients younger than 55 years. [48], but the evidence collected since then suggests that also in older patients PFO represents a risk factor for recurrent stroke [37,47].

Factors Associated with PFO and Risk of Stroke

From the evidence summarized in the previous sections of this chapter it is clear that not so much PFO per se, but rather the co-occurrence of other abnormalities or some features of PFO are required to increase the risk of recurrent stroke. In addition to the association with ASA, further PFO features have been suspected to increase the risk of stroke: PFO diameter, a tunnel-like conformation of PFO, spontaneous right-to-left shunt observable at bubble contrast-TEE in basal conditions, larger right-to-left shunt magnitude, the presence of prominent Eustachian valve orientating blood flow toward PFO, pelvic deep venous thrombosis and a coexisting hypercoagulable state.

In the next sections a detailed review of the associated conditions is presented such as those sustained by clotting factors mutations.

Atrial Septal Aneurysm

Atrial septal aneurysm (ASA) is a redundancy of the interatrial septum detected most commonly by TTE and TEE studies. PFO is commonly associated with ASA in up to 70 percent of cases, and has emerged as potentially increasing the risk of stroke occurrence or relapse; the association between PFO and ASA has been observed both in large cohort populations and in patients with suspected cardiac source of embolization [49].

ASA was defined according to criteria previously published by Hanley et al. [50]: (a) diameter of the base of the aneurysmatic portion of the interatrial septum (IAS) measuring ≥ 15 mm and either (b) protrusion of the IAS, or part of it, ≥ 15 mm beyond the plane of the IAS or (c) phasic excursion of the IAS during the cardiorespiratory cycle ≥ 15 mm in total amplitude.

Although the definition varies somewhat in different series, the prevalence of ASA in the general population is estimated with the TT imaging to be only 0.23 percent. Up to 4.6 percent is noted among those referred for TE echocardiography, most likely because of the higher sensitivity of the TE technique for imaging septal area and the selection bias for patients referred for TE echocardiography [51-53].

The prevalence of ASA is greater among patients with embolic events.Up to 38% of patients with cryptogenic stroke may exhibit PFO associated with ASA compared with patients with PFO unrelated stroke (10%) and healthy PFO patients (8%) [54].

In a prospective study on a consecutive series of 100 patients less than 55 years of age, Cabanes et al. found that both ASA (OR, 4.3; 95% CI, 1.3 to 14.6) and PFO (OR, 3.9; 95% CI, 1.5 to 10) were independently associated with the diagnosis of cryptogenic stroke, but the stroke odds of a patient with both abnormalities was 33.3 times (95% CI, 4.1 to 27.0) the stroke odds of a patient with neither of these cardiac disorders [18].

Likewise, as already mentioned above, The French study [45] and the study from Rome-La Sapienza [43] both disclosed the importance of the association in increasing the risk of relapse.

Furthermore, PFOs seen in the presence of ASA tend to be larger compared with those seen without ASA, which suggests that the association of ASA with embolic events is likely based on the high prevalence of a large PFO [55,56].

Because an ASA is usually highly mobile, protruding from the right to left atrium, it is unlikely that a thrombus forms in the ASA itself. This is corroborated by the rare finding of thrombus associated with ASA in a large series of patients [49].

In conclusion, the association of PFO with ASA seems established as a condition enhancing the recurrence risk by facilitating paradoxical embolism.

PFO Size

PFO size increases with each decade of life. The mean diameter in the first decade is 3.4 mm and in the tenth decade it is 5.8 mm, perhaps reflecting size-based selection over time where larger PFOs remain patent and smaller defects close [22].

Several reports [30,57-60] have shown significantly larger PFOs in cryptogenic stroke patients (0.6 - 2 mm.) as compared with healthy controls (2.1 - 4 mm) demonstrating a more significant association of a large PFO than a small one with stroke, and it has been reported that stroke patients with a large PFO show more brain imaging features of embolic infarcts than those with a small PFO [58,60].

In PICSS study it has been shown that large PFOs were significantly more prevalent among cryptogenic stroke patients compared with those with known cause of stroke [46].

The presence of spontaneous RLS at rest has also been associated with stroke [61]. In the Patent Foramen Ovale in Cryptogenic Stroke Study (PICSS), large PFOs — defined as at least 2 mm separation of septa or at least 10 microbubbles in the left atrium — were seen significantly more frequently among patients with cryptogenic stroke than among those with known causes of stroke [46]. In addition, the magnitude of RLS through a PFO is a significant risk factor for recurrent cerebrovascular events (odds ratio 14.8 for large PFO [defined as >10 bubbles recorded in the cerebral vessels using single gated transcranial] versus small PFO, $p = 0.01$) [62].

These results suggest a "dose-response" relationship and support a causality link between PFO and ischemic stroke [34].

Chiari's Network and Eustachian Valve

The Eustachian Valve (EV) (so called "valvula venae cavae inferioris") is a remnant of the embryonic valve of the sinus venosus. At 3 weeks of gestation, the sinus venosus is external to the primitive right atrium and its right horn gives rise to the hepatic and cardinal anterior veins, precursors respectively of the inferior vena cava (IVC) and the superior vena cava (SVC). The left horn is the future coronary sinus.

Embryologically, the Eustachian valve directs the oxygenated blood flow from the inferior vena cava to the fossa ovalis and across the patent foramen ovale into the systemic circulation.

The right valve of the sinus venosus usually regresses between the 9th and the 15th week of gestation. Its persistence has been reported to have an incidence of 1.4 percent and may develop in two different patterns: 1) "Chiari's network" defined as reticolous membrane with attachment to the upper wall of the right atrium or atrial septum; and 2) "Eustachian Valve" characterized by mobile and fenestrated membrane without any anatomical connection [63].

Therefore, the persistence of the right valve of the sinus venosus can result in various degrees of obstruction to blood flow in the right atrium, ranging from partial septation by a prominent Eustachian Valve to a complete partition of the right atrium in the so-called "cor triatriatum dexter".

All these anomalies may be associated with congenital cardiac malformations, including ASD, pulmonary atresia or stenosis, hypoplastic right ventricle, tricuspid atresia, or hypoplasia.

Limacher et al. [64] reported an incidence of persistent Eustachian valve in about 70 percent in children of various age.

Differential diagnosis is usually made with intracardiac mass , thrombus, vegetation , and the other types of persistence of right valve of sinus venosus.

Chiari's network and filamentous strands in the right atrium as well as Eustachian valve represents a not uncommon finding in patients with patent foramen ovale and in association with a RLS through an atrial septal defect [65].

In these cases, the large valve subdividing totally or partially the right atrium causes a right-to-left shunt by favouring the IVC blood flow into the left atrium via the septal defect, without changes in right heart pressure. Persistent Eustachian valve is frequently found in adult patients with septal abnormalities and mainly PFO. A persistent Eustachian valve may participate in the mechanism of a paradoxical embolism. Therefore, the presence of such anatomical variants that can direct flow from the inferior vena cava toward the PFO may increase the chance of paradoxical embolization beyond that associated with PFO size.

Increased Pulmonary Pressure

All conditions potentially causing an increase in pulmonary pressure may facilitate the opening of the virtual interatrial valve and thus promoting shunting of blood to the left heart chambers with further desaturation of arterial blood. It is therefore not surprising that RLS has been found in 70% of patients with chronic obstructive pulmonary disease and increased pulmonary pressure [66] and in the same proportion of patients with obstructive sleep apnoea, a condition that ultimately may result in pulmonary hypertension [67].

In patients with pulmonary embolism paradoxical embolization is often reported [68,69]. Similarly, patients with right ventricular infarction [70] or severe tricuspid regurgitation [71] have an increased RLS through a PFO.

Bracey and colleagues [72] described a case of a 29-year-old male that developed a fatal stroke after successful thrombolysis for massive pulmonary embolism with autoptical evidence of a large thrombus protruding through the patent foramen ovale (PFO) and extending up to the left common carotid artery. A TTE/TEE with a saline contrast agent has been proposed in case of pulmonary embolism (and pulmonary hypertension) to exclude the presence of PFO [73].

Platypnea-orthodeoxia and Aortic Root Enlargement

Platypnea-orthodeoxia is a rare clinical entity characterized by dyspnoea due to arterial oxygen desaturation induced by the upright position and relieved by recumbency. Patients typically have normal right heart pressures and the mechanism for RLS remains unknown. Most typically, platypnea-orthodeoxia develops after pneumonectomy (usually the right lung), but it has been found in a number of other conditions, such as aortic elongation, aortic aneurysm, dorsal kyphosis, pericardial effusion or constrictive pericarditis, pulmonary emphysema, arteriovenous malformation [74].

Recently Bertaux et al. demonstrated that an enlarged aortic root is likely related to size and mobility of the atrial septum. Enlargement of the aortic root may decrease the size of the atrial septum and proportionally increase its mobility. In PFO patients atrial septal mobility is directly related to the extent of right-to-left shunt that may favour platypnea-orthodeoxia syndrome [75].

It has been hypotesized that in PFO patients a reasonable interaction exists between PFO size, RLS amount and body position (standing or recumbent position). This interaction may be considered not only the result of dynamic changes in venous blood return to right atrium but possibly the consequence of the anatomic relationship between the interatrial septum and the great vessels, mainly the aorta.

In a consecutive series of 109 PFO-patients (M/F = 40/69, age 43 ± 12), we used contrast-enhanced transcranial Doppler (ce-TCD) to assess the bubble load in the right middle cerebral artery during normal breathing both in standing and in recumbent position with half of the patients first tested while standing and half while recumbent. A significant increase in the bubble number was found in 40 patients from the horizontal to the upright position, no difference was observed in 32, whereas the amount of shunt nonsignificantly decreased on standing in the remaining 31 patients. These findings indicate that the amount of permanent RLS is posture-dependent in as many as 40% of patients. A possible explanation for these findings may reside in the close proximity of the interatrial wall with both the aorta and the pulmonary artery, so that with the upright position the neighbour vessels might exert a traction on the components of the tunnel-like PFO in some patients thus increasing the amount of RLS [76].

Deep Vein Thrombosis

For paradoxical embolization to occur, a source of thrombus is needed. A significant stroke can result from an arterial occlusion by an embolus as small as 1 mm in diameter.

Stollberger et al. found a higher prevalence of deep vein thrombosis in patients with cryptogenic stroke as compared with a control group [77]. Although other studies did not confirm this finding [78], in the PELVIS (Paradoxical Emboli From Large Veins in Ischemic

Stroke) study pelvic vein thrombi detected by MRI venogram were found more frequently in young patients with cryptogenic stroke (20%) compared with those with more defined causes of stroke (4%) [79].

Moreover it is well known that some patients may present a deep venous thrombosis with or without pulmonary thromboembolism during or after a long trip as a result of prolonged immobilization as it happens in the "economy class syndrome" (ECS). In the presence of PFO, there may be a potential risk for ischemic stroke due to paradoxical embolism ("economy class stroke syndrome"). Few cases have been published in the literature to date.

Belvis et al. reported the case of young woman presenting with pulmonary thromboembolism and ischemic stroke after a non-stop flight from Lima (Peru) to Madrid (Spain). The transesophageal echocardiography and transcranial Doppler showed a massive right-to-left shunt through a PFO. The patient was also an heterozygous carrier of the C46T mutation of coagulation factor XII. The appearance of a stroke following a long trip is suggestive of paradoxical embolism through a PFO, mainly if it is associated with a deep venous thrombosis and/or a pulmonary thromboembolism [80].

More recently, Dixon and colleagues described the case of a young woman with PFO and right-to-left shunt detected by TEE who suffered from deep vein thrombosis complicated by massive pulmonary and right femoral artery embolism. She was managed with intra-arterial thrombolytics, right lower extremity arterial embolectomy and anticoagulation [81].

However, apart from the so far limited evidence linking PFO and deep vein thrombosis in the economy class syndrome, there are a number of limitations in interpreting data linking DVT with PFO-related stroke. Most studies addressing this point have evaluated only a subset, rather than a consecutive cohort, of stroke patients. An additional limitation is that many studies have evaluated only part of the lower extremity venous system, or have used methods with limited sensitivity in portions of the lower extremity venous system. Another frequent limitation has been the absence of an appropriate control group, an important concern given the substantial increase in DVT prevalence that is found beginning with the fourth day post-stroke Further studies are therefore needed to understand the significance of calf, pelvic, and other DVT in the pathogenesis of PFO-associated cryptogenic stroke [17].

Coagulation Disorders

Patients with a tendency toward venous thrombus formation may be exposed to a higher risk of paradoxical embolization in the presence of PFO.

Several case-control studies report a higher frequency of prothrombotic states such as G20210A and factor V Leiden mutations in patients with cryptogenic stroke and PFO [82-85].

Recently, Belvìs and colleagues reported a prospective study which included cryptogenic stroke patients younger than 55 years with PFO diagnosed with simultaneous transcranial Doppler and TEE. They analyzed the following prothrombotic markers: antiphospholipid antibodies (APS), protein C and protein S deficiencies, factor V Leiden FVG1691A, prothrombin gene mutation PTG20210A and coagulation factor XII mutation FXIIC46T. In 39 cryptogenic stroke patients, PFO was detected in 17 patients (43.6%). The only prothrombotic marker related to PFO size (large PFO) was APS (p = 0.043). No differences were found between PFO and non-PFO patients regarding prothrombotic markers. Female gender was the only variable related to prothrombotic markers. Large PFO was also related to deep venous thrombosis (p = 0.040) and atrial septal aneurysm (p = 0.010). The conclusion of this study was that PFO patients do not present more prothrombotic markers than non-PFO patients, but APS are more frequent in large PFO [86].

In a recent case-control study (YAMIS - Young Adult Myocardial Infarction and Ischemic Stroke), Sastry et al. did not find any significant association between thrombophilia (activated protein C resistance; lupus anticoagulant; proteins C and S; antithrombin III; fibrinogen; Factors II, VII, VIII, IX, Factor V Leiden mutation, prothrombin gene G20210A mutation) and either myocardial infarction or ischemic stroke in patients 39 years of age or younger [87].

Again, like for DVT, a number of reasons (selection bias, accuracy in diagnosis of cryptogenic stroke, thoroughness of diagnostic workup and others) may partly explain the discrepancy between different studies. Although probably unjustified as a screening tool, the search for coagulation abnormalities in selected patients with PFO associated stroke (e.g those with associated ASA and large shunt) may help to identify those patients in whom paradoxical embolism from an occult vein thrombosis may have caused the stroke.

Mechanisms of PFO Associated Stroke: The Evolution of Thinking

Historically, in 1877 Julius Cohnheim, a German pathologist, described, for the first time, the case of a young woman that had died with cerebral arterial embolism. He hypothesized that a clot passing through the PFO must have caused ischemic stroke (paradoxical embolism).

In 1884 the term “l`embolie croisée” (crossed embolism) was proposed, and the term “paradoxale embolie” (paradoxical embolism) was introduced in 1885 [88]. Although paradoxical embolism had been described 100 years earlier, only 150 cases had been reported by the 1970`s, most of them post mortem, and only 20 cases had been detected during life [89]. Thus it was considered no more than a rare curiosity. In most cases the thrombus was found trapped in the PFO, while other possible but much rarer routes for venous to arterial embolism were an atrial or ventricular septal defect, patent ductus arteriosus or a pulmonary arteriovenous fistula.

For a long time it was difficult to make a diagnosis of paradoxical embolism during life, and it was only after the development of contrast echocardiography for the detection of PFO that Harvey et al. (1986) did their first study of young patients with cryptogenic stroke and found evidence of RLS in 73% of cases, raising the idea that paradoxical embolisation may be more common than had previously been believed. Based on these results, they recommended an echocardiographic contrast examination in all cases of young patients with arterial emboli, even if all the other cardiac findings were normal. The subsequent contemporary publication of the two reports by Lechat et al. and by Webster et al in 1988 finally boosted the interest in PFO associated stroke and opened the way to the myriad of subsequent studies.

Until recently four conditions were deemed necessary for the diagnosis of paradoxical embolism: 1) an arterial embolism – cerebral or systemic – with no apparent source in the left side of the heart or arterial circulation; 2) the presence of a venous or pulmonary embolism; 3) the existence of an abnormal communication between the right and left circulations; 4) elevation of right heart pressure: constant, as during pulmonary hypertension, or transitory, as during pulmonary embolism, cough or the Valsalva manoeuvre [90].

However since right-to-left shunting through a patent foramen ovale can usually be demonstrated also during normal breathing in the absence of pulmonary hypertension (see below) the fourth criterion is usually neglected in modern times. In addition, the venous source of emboli is often lacking and venous thrombi may pass undetected because they are clinically silent, of small size, located in unusual sites or may have dissolved early.

The practical consequence of this is the contemporary attitude to interpret as paradoxical embolism any ischemic lesion appearing in the absence of an obvious arterial embolic source provided that a PFO is detected.

The presumed mechanism is the migration of a thrombus, or less commonly fat or air from the venous side of the circulation (eg, lower extremity veins and right atrium) to the left atrium via a PFO, with subsequent systemic embolisation.

However, two further mechanism have been proposed to explain PFO associated strokes:

- The origin of thrombi in situ within the PFO and ASA.
- An increased susceptibility to develop major arrhythmias as a consequence of the abnormal anatomy of the His bundle related to PFO [91].

Imaging Modalities in the Diagnosis of PFO

Echocardiography

Since the first report in 1968 by Gramiak [92], contrast echocardiography has become an indispensable tool for cardiovascular imaging. In the normal circulation no echo-enhancing agent would appear in the left side of the heart if the bubbles of which the contrast agent is formed are larger than the capillary diameter because they would be trapped in the capillary bed of the lung. However in the presence of a shortcut from the venous to the arterial circulation (either a pulmonary fistula or an atrial septal defect) the contrast agent may image the left atrium because it has skipped the pulmonary filter. This property forms the basis of the used technique for detection of shunts especially in the current era if PFO closure is considered [93,94].

Echocardiographic examination defines patent foramen ovale as flap-like opening in the atrial septum secundum, with the septum primum serving as a one-way valve allowing for permanent or transient right-to-left shunt.

As PFO represents a tunnel-like communication of the interatrial septum where septum primum (thin, fibrous) and secundum (thick, muscular) overlap, trans-oesophageal echocardiography (TEE) may help to define this complex anatomical structure by measuring both the size of the tunnel (the largest separation between the primum and secundum septa) and the length of the tunnel itself.

TEE also provides additional information regarding the association with atrial septal aneurysm (ASA), Eustachian valve or Chiari's network, the presence or absence of intratrial thrombus or masses and it allows to rule out associated forms of congenital heart diseases requiring surgical correction.

The majority of right to left shunts (RLSs) cannot be seen during conventional TEE and TCD [23,95]. Therefore, provocative manouevres such as Valsalva or coughing are used to disclose transient RLSs. Coughing or releasing a sustained Valsalva manoeuvre results in increased filling of the right atrium and therefore a right-to-left atrial pressure gradient develops with opening of the foramen ovale. Abdominal compression may be used instead if the patient is deeply sedated during TEE; however it seems not as sensitive as a good Valsalva manoeuvre. Kronik and colleagues [95] were the first to demonstrate the effect of the Valsalva manoeuvre for the detection of RLSs. Later on, Lynch and associates [23] demonstrated that in healthy volunteers the detection of PFO increased from 5% to 18% using the Valsalva manoeuvre. Likewise, a 3–4 times increase in sensitivity for shunt detection was shown for TEE.

According to the principle of semi-quantification of shunt a PFO is judged to be present if any microbubble is seen in the left-sided cardiac chambers within three cardiac cycles from the maximal right atrial opacification. The degree of interatrial shunting across the PFO is determined by counting the maximum number of microbubbles seen in the left atrium in any single frame after intravenous contrast injection during Valsalva maneuver; "significant" shunts are categorized as > 20 bubbles in the left atrium.

However, there is no uniform definition in the literature about the number of microbubbles that should appear in the left atrium; either 1 [58], 3 [45,96] or 5 [60] microbubbles were considered positive for PFO.

Braun et al. [97], considered the RLS as "small", "moderate" and "large" when 3 to 10 bubbles, 10 to 20 bubbles and > 20 bubbles respectively were detected in the left atrium. Windecker et al. graded spontaneous or provoked right-to-left shunt semiquantitatively according to the amount of bubbles detected in the left atrium after crossing the interatrial septum on a still frame: grade 1 = minimal (1 to 5 bubbles), grade 2 = moderate (6 to 20 bubbles), and grade 3 = severe (> 20 bubbles) [98]. In a different way, Serena et al. graded right-to-left shunt as "moderate" when uncountable microbubbles were less echogenic in the left atrium than in the right atrium, and "severe" when the same microbubbles echogenicity was documented in both the atria [99].

A methodological study using TEE demonstrated that contrast injection via the femoral vein approach is superior to the antecubital route for PFO detection [100].

The incidence of PFO using TEE is quite similar to the incidence of PFO in pooled autopsy data and this finding has generated the concept that a properly performed TEE is the clinical gold standard for the detection of PFO during life.

A false-negative TEE may result from inadequate visualization within the oesophagus, elevated left atrial pressures preventing right-to-left passage of contrast [101], and difficulty to perform a correct Valsalva maneuver.

Use of harmonic imaging with trans-thoracic echocardiography (TTE) and contrast injection and coughing during injection may increase the sensitivity of PFO detection [35,102,103].

Although TTE may identify patients with RLS, TEE with saline contrast injection is more sensitive by allowing visualization and microbubbles count in the left atrium that would otherwise be filtered by the lung capillary [104].

Using agitated saline contrast, the sensitivities of traditional TTE for RLS detection are at most half those of TEE: in large active laboratories PFO detection by TTE was 10 to 18 percent in comparison to 18 to 33 percent incidence using TEEin one study [18].

Even though less sensitive than TEE, TTE has been used to quantify the microbubble amount by mean of Doppler signal across the mitral valve [105].

Because of its semi-invasive nature TEE has some limitations, especially in elderly patients with acute strokes. A good Valsalva manoeuvre is often more difficult to obtain from a patient during a TEE study, especially if he/or she is heavily sedated than during a TTE study. Aspiration, airway obstruction, oesophageal perforation and vocal cord dysfunction have also been reported [106,107].

More recently, three-dimensional echocardiography has been employed to provide a useful insight on the relationship between the atrial septal defect or patent foramen ovale and the other cardiac structures. It also allows a better detection of additional fenestrations in the atrial septum and a fine anatomic definition of the surrounding rim tissues.

For this reasons, three-dimensional echocardiography might become the main imaging modality to monitoring and guiding interventional procedures of PFO (and ASD) closure.

Cardiac Magnetic Resonance Imaging

Cardiac magnetic resonance imaging (CMRI) is a powerful non-invasive diagnostic tool providing detailed information on cardiac anatomy and function and on hemodynamic parameters in patients with structural heart disease [108].

In a small population (20 patients) a 100% concordance was reported between CMRI and TEE in detecting PFO and atrial septal aneurysm (ASA) [109].

On the contrary, Nusser et al. documented that both right-to-left shunt and the presence of ASA were significantly less frequently detected by CMRI compared with TEE. On the other hand, CMRI may not only give additional information on anatomical details such as the left and right atrium, the atrial septum and the left and right ventricles but may also assess the main hemodynamic parameters [110].

Furthermore, cardiac magnetic resonance imaging may be performed following a percutaneous closure of PFO, thus enabling a non-invasive evaluation of patients [111], even though with a limited diagnostic impact in terms of detection of residual right-to-left shunting.

Cardiac magnetic resonance imaging is indicated to detect anomalous venous returns, which are often associated with atrial septal defects (Task Force of the European Society of Cardiology 1998).

However, the relatively scarce availability of machines has thus far limited the use of CMRI to research.

Contrast-enhanced Transcranial Doppler

Transcranial Doppler sonography of the middle cerebral artery during contrast injection (ce-TCD) is a non invasive method to detect the presence and the amount of RLS; therefore, it has been proposed as alternative to echocardiography for detecting the presence of PFO.

However, it must be underlined that ce-TCD does not identify the site of RLS; actually the detection of microbubbles in the cerebral circulation may depend not necessarily on the presence of a PFO, but may also be the consequence of intrapulmonary shunts or pulmonary arteriovenous malformations.

A number of recent reports have emphasized the amount of right-to-left shunt (RLS) as the crucial factor underlying the likelihood of paradoxical brain embolism in stroke patients [55,59,99,112-114].

The ce-TCD test is performed by an experienced neurosonologist following the guidelines of the Consensus Conference of Venice [115] with the patient in the supine position: the right middle cerebral artery (MCA) is insonated with a 2-MHz hand-held probe at the depth where the MCA and the anterior cerebral artery are both visible. The contrast agent is prepared by mixing 10 times 1 ml air and 9 ml saline into two syringes connected through a three-way stopcock to an indwelling catheter placed in the antecubital vein. The bubble containing saline is then injected as a bolus and the patient performs a Valsalva strain for 5 seconds. High intensity signals appearing in the MCA spectrum and reflecting the passage of bubbles are automatically recorded and counted by the machine. Before accepting the automatic count each signal is visually inspected offline and checked for unidirectionality and typical sound.

RLS is graded 0 if no signal is detected within 30 seconds of Valsalva strain release, 1 (small shunt) if < 10 bubbles are recorded, 2 (large shunt) if > 10 bubbles are counted.

Assuming that the number of bubbles recorded in cerebral vessels is roughly proportional to the amount of intracardiac RLS, Serena et al. [99] performed a case control study comparing PFO characteristics in an unselected cohort of stroke patients and in a sample of normal controls, suggesting that it is only beyond the critical threshold of 10 bubbles that RLS conveys an increased risk of stroke. The author proposed a classification in small (< 10 bubbles) and large (> 10 bubbles) shunt with a further subdivision of large shunts in "shower" (> 25 bubbles) and "curtain" (uncountable signals) patterns. The "curtain" pattern was encountered only in cryptogenic stroke patients and the detection of "curtain" or "shower" patterns was associated with the highest risk of cryptogenic stroke (OR, 12,4; 95% CI, 4.08 to 38.09).

Moreover, Anzola et al. have suggested that quantifying the RLS in patients with PFO and stroke may be useful to pick up those who are at increased risk of suffering a relapse [62].

In a more recent paper published from our group [116], the extent of RLS in patients with migraine, cryptogenic stroke and in controls has been analyzed. The authors concluded that patients with migraine have overall larger shunts than non-migraineurs, particularly if they have had a stroke. RLS may be then causally related to migraine and to the increased stroke risk of migraine.

A unique advantage of ce-TCD is its ability to detect microembolic signals (MES) in the brain vessels. This allows not only to assess the amount of RLS but also the occurrence of spontaneous embolism, which is likely to occur in the presence of carotid artery disease or during invasive percutaneous procedures (i.e.: coronary and aortic angiography and carotid artery stenting) [117,118].

Spontaneous embolism may also happen during percutaneous PFO closure; at this regard our group performed a ce-TCD monitoring of the brain vessels with MES quantification in 29 consecutive patients who underwent PFO closure. Silent brain embolism occurred during the procedure particularly at the opening of the left disc in the left atrium in spite of different devices used [119].

Table 1. Comparison of different imaging techniques for RLS in comparison with TEE.

Authors	Year	Patients	Imaging Technique	Contrast Agent	TEE+	Sensitivity	Specificity
Di Tullio et al	1993	49	TCD	Saline	19	68	100
Jobat al.	1994	137	TCD	Gelifundol®	64	89	92
Klötzsch et al	1994	111	TCD	Echovist®	50	91	94
Anzola et al.	1995	40	TCD	Saline	19	90	100
Devuyst et al.	1997	37	TCD	Saline	24	100	100
Hamann et al.	1998	44	TCD	Echovist®	22	75	100
Stendel et al.	2000	92	TCD	Echovist®	24	92	97
Droste et al.	2000	64	TCD	Echovist®	20	100	65
Di Tullio et al	1993	49	TTE-FI	Saline	19	47	100
Kuhl et al.	1999	111	TTE-FI	Gelifundol®	51	62	100
			TTE-HI	Gelifundol®	51	92	100
Stendel et al.	2000	92	TTE-FI	Echovist®	24	42	83
Ha et al.	2000	136	TTE-FI	Saline	40	22	100
			TTE-HI	Saline	40	63	100
Van Camp	2000	109	TTE-FI	Saline	24	46	100
			TTE-HI	Saline	24	100	100
Daniels et al.	2004	256	TTE-HI	Saline	53	91	97

FI = fundamental imaging, HI = harmonic imaging, TCD = transcranial Doppler ultrasonography, TTE = transthoracic echocardiography, TEE+ = number of patients with TEE proven RLS.

The patient position during the test seems also important in improving the sensitivity of TCD in the detection of PFO [76,120]. It is thus recommended, in the case of a first negative test, to change the patient's position for a repeated TCD examination.

A recent simultaneous study with TCD and TEE showed an almost perfect concordance for PFO detection and RLS quantification [121].

Technical advances have led to more therapeutic options in patients with PFO associated stroke, including device closure of PFO. Therefore, optimal diagnosis of PFO has become of greater clinical importance. Contrast echocardiography with non-transpulmonary contrast agents has been the cornerstone in diagnosis of PFO with RLS for over four decades. Despite being a relatively invasive procedure, TEE is still considered the gold standard for detection of RLS. Several other imaging techniques such as TTE with second harmonic imaging and ce-TCD have shown acceptable sensitivity and specificity compared to TEE for the detection of PFO with RLS (see table 1).

For screening purposes ce-TCD represents the ideal tool for its non invasiveness, ease of execution and unambiguous findings. Direct cardiac imaging is needed only after a RLS has been established by ce-TCD to show the anatomical details of the shunt. For this purpose TTE with harmonic imaging is probably the best alternative to TEE, which, in our opinion, should be reserved for those cases only in whom an alternative cardiac or aortic arch source of emboli is suspected.

Treatment

The management of patients with PFO is controversial. Therapeutic options for secondary stroke prevention in patients with a PFO include two major strategies: 1) conservative long-term medical treatment with antithrombotic therapy (anti platelet drugs) or oral anticoagulation, and 2) invasive treatment with surgical or interventional closure of the interatrial communication.

No prospective randomized controlled trial comparing invasive vs. medical treatments or antiplatelet vs. anticoagulant drugs has been so far completed. Therefore, the evidence on which the therapeutical decision is to be based is at best circumstantial inasmuch as the published studies have been observational, with disparate definitions of the qualifying or recurrent cerebrovascular event, non uniform criteria for interatrial septal abnormalities, absence of blinding during examination of echocardiograms or ascertainment of end points, and incomplete accounting of associated risk factors or the use of adjunctive therapies.

One difficulty in assessing the relative merits of various therapeutical options stems from the fact that the risk of stroke recurrence in patients 60 years of age or younger who have unexplained cerebral ischemia and PFO appears to be low, regardless of the therapy used.

In a prospective study of 140 medically or surgically treated patients (according to their physicians' discretion), the annual rate of stroke recurrence was 1.9 percent, and the strategy of treatment had no detectable influence [41].

Likewise, the French Study found similarly low rates of stroke recurrence at four years among patients with PFO (2.3%; 95% CI, 0.3 to 4.3%) and those without PFO (4.2%; 95 % CI, 1.8 to 6.6 %). Patients who had both PFO and atrial septal aneurysm (ASA), however, had a 15.2 (95% CI, 1.8 to 28.6%) percent rate of recurrence despite the use of aspirin therapy – a rate nearly fourfold that observed among patients who did not have either abnormality [45].

Medical Therapy

Conventional therapy for prevention of recurrent events in patients with cryptogenic stroke includes both antiplatelet therapy (aspirin, dipyridamole, or clopidogrel as single agents or in combination) and anticoagulation with warfarin.

In a retrospective study of 90 patients younger than 60 years of age with cerebral ischemia, 52 of whom had PFO, an almost three-fold rate of recurrence was found in those receiving aspirin or no therapy compared to those treated with warfarin [42]. However, the small number of patients prevented statistically meaningful comparisons between the groups, treatment assignments were at the discretion of the consulting neurologist, treatment crossover was frequent and ascertainment of end points, which included multiple events, was not blinded.

For similar reasons, it is difficult to draw firm conclusions from the data derived from a meta-analysis in which warfarin, as compared with antiplatelet therapy, lowered the risk of recurrence (odds ratio, 0.37; 95% confidence interval, 0.23 to 0.60) among patients with cerebral ischemia and patent foramen ovale [122].

In a randomized trial (PICSS), a subgroup analysis of 98 patients with cryptogenic stroke and patent foramen ovale revealed a trend for a better performance of warfarin compared with aspirin in the two-year incidence of recurrent stroke or death (9.5% vs. 17.9%; hazard ratio, 0.52; 95% confidence interval, 0.16 to 1.67), although the difference was not statistically significant, perhaps for the relatively small sample size. Although the incidence of major haemorrhage did not differ between warfarin and aspirin (1.78 vs. 1.91 events per 100 patient-years, $p= 1.0$), warfarin increased the rate of minor haemorrhage (22.9 vs. 8.66 events per 100 patient-years, $p < 0.001$) [46].

The high recurrent event rate seen in this randomized trial raises some concerns about the real effectiveness of medical therapy in PFO patients for prevention of cryptogenic stroke.

From the analysis of these studies there is clearly neither expert consensus nor sufficient quality evidence to determine which approach, antiplatelet or antithrombotic, is superior.

Also in spite of medical therapy, up to 25 percent of patients with cryptogenic stroke may experience recurrent stroke or transient ischemic attack within 4 years from the initial event.

Surgical Therapy

The traditional approach to foraminal closure involves open thoracotomy. Reported case series are small, but the rate of postoperative stroke ranges from 0 to 3.5 percent at two years [123-125]. The mortality associated with closure of an uncomplicated atrial septal defect is less than 1.5 percent [126]. Perioperative risks also include atrial fibrillation, pericardial sequelae, and the need for reexploration because of bleeding. Minimally invasive surgery is an alternative approach [127].

In one follow-up study of young patients with cryptogenic stroke and PFO, surgical closure was performed if there were at least two of four "high-risk" features for paradoxical embolism: major shunt > 50 bubbles, atrial septal aneurysm, infarcts in multiple territories, and Valsalva–provoking activity preceding the onset of stroke. There were no recurrences after 23 months, but the study did not include a control group [123].

A decision analysis modelling different therapeutic approaches in a 55-year-old patient with patent foramen ovale concluded that, for a yearly risk of stroke recurrence of 0.8 percent, surgical closure or warfarin were the best options (percutaneous closure was not considered) [126]. Surgery became the treatment of choice when the annual risk of recurrence reached 1.4 percent. These conclusions, however, rest on the questionable assumptions that paradoxical embolism underlies the risk of stroke and that anticoagulation lowers the risk of recurrence to the same degree as it does in persons with venous thromboembolism or atrial fibrillation.

Percutaneous Closure

Percutaneous PFO closure is a catheter-based technique using atrial septal occlusion devices. It was initially advocated for prevention of recurrent stroke in 1992 [128]. Since then, safety and feasibility have been addressed in several subsequent studies.

The efficacy of catheter PFO closure in fixing RLS ranges between 86 and 100 percent. Recurrent neurological and peripheral embolic events are reported as 0 to 3.8 percent per year.

A systematic review found that among 1355 patients undergoing percutaneous closure, the rate of recurrent stroke or transient ischemic attack was 0 to 4.9 percent at one year. Even though cerebrovascular recurrence rate appeared to be higher among 895 patients receiving medical therapy (3.8 to 12%), several considerations preclude meaningful comparison: the nonrandomized treatment assignment, differences in the clinical characteristics of the patients treated by the various techniques, and inconsistent criteria for ascertainment of outcomes.

Serious complications of percutaneous closure (major haemorrhage, cardiac tamponade, the need for surgery, pulmonary embolism, and death) were reported in 1.5 percent of the patients, and minor complications (arrhythmia, device fracture or embolization, air embolism, femoral hematoma, and fistula) in 7.9 percent [129].

Careful analysis of this apparently plain operation reveals that nickel toxicity, thrombus formation, residual shunt, malpositioning, and erosions are still active and real problems, whereas the pathophysiology of right-to-left shunt, the role of coagulation abnormalities, the significance of atrial septal aneurysm and other sources of shunt remain unresolved issues.

Aspirin and/or clopidogrel are recommended for a period of three to six months to prevent thrombus formation on the device, until the endothelialization process is fairly completed. Antibiotic prophylaxis for six months is highly recommended.

Krumsdorf and colleagues [130] reported 1000 consecutive patients undergoing ASD and PFO closure using different transcatheter devices (nine different technologies). The study reported thrombus formation in the left atrium (n= 11), right atrium (n= 6) or both (n= 3) in 1.2 percent of ASD patients and in 2.5 percent of PFO patients (p= NS). Thrombus was diagnosed in 14 of 20 patients at four weeks and in 6 of 20 patients later than four weeks. The most frequent thrombus formation occurred on the CardioSEAL device (NMT Medical, Boston, Massachusetts) (7.1%), whereas a 5.7 percent incidence of thrombus formation was observed on the STARFlex device (NMT Medical), 6.6 percent on the PFO-Star device (Applied Biometrics Inc., Burnsville, Minnesota), 3.6 percent on the ASDOS device (Osypka Corp., Grenzach-Wyhlen, Germany), 0.8 percent on the Helex device (WL Gore, Flagstaff, Arizona) and no thrombus formation on the Amplatzer device (AGA Medical, Golden Valley, Minnesota). Limitations of this retrospective review include the observation that the effect of heparin was often reversed by protamine immediately after the procedure. It is worth noticing that hematologic screening was not performed before device implant. The authors concluded that thrombus formation on closure devices is low and usually resolves with anticoagulation therapy.

Indicators for Percutaneous Closure

A recent systematic review comparing medical vs. interventional treatment for preventing recurrent PFO associated strokes found that "*For both comparisons, percutaneous closure gives lower event rates compared with medical therapy (P≤0.0001). However, very importantly, indirect comparison of medical treatment and percutaneous closure is very difficult to interpret. Inclusion criteria for the studies reviewed are not uniform, and definitions of what constitutes a cryptogenic stroke or TIA vary widely among studies. The age of subjects is variable, which may significantly affect the observed event rates. Many of the studies are also subject to potential selection bias and do not use independent blinded adjudication of events. There also is prolonged time from the index event to percutaneous closure in some studies and the use of medical therapy in patients undergoing PFO closure is not accounted for in some studies. Devices may also carry a placebo effect and the number of events is small, particularly for percutaneous closure, resulting in estimates with broad CIs. As such, results of ongoing randomized studies are needed to provide convincing evidence with regard to treatment options*" [131].

Pending the results of the ongoing trials (see Homma and Sacco 2005 for a complete list), major scientific societies have issued their own guidelines, that reflect the substantial uncertainty on which treatment may perform better.

The American College of Chest Physicians Conference on Antithrombotic and Thrombolytic Therapy [132] and the American Heart Association (AHA)/American Stroke Association Council on Stroke Practice Guidelines [133] recommend antiplatelet therapy after cryptogenic stroke in the majority of patients. Warfarin use is suggested in the setting of known deep venous thrombosis or documented hypercoagulable state (Table 2). Scientific societies have commented on the use of closure devices as a therapy for cryptogenic stroke in the presence of a PFO. The American Academy of Neurology (AAN) [48] found "insufficient evidence regarding the effectiveness of either surgical or endovascular closure of PFO" and promotes the enrolment of cryptogenic stroke patients with PFO in randomized controlled studies. The AHA/American Stroke Association concluded that insufficient data exist to make a recommendation about PFO closure in patients with a first stroke and a PFO; however PFO closure may be considered for patients with recurrent cryptogenic stroke despite medical therapy (Class IIb, Level of Evidence C).

Table 2. Summary of guidelines for PFO closure

Association	Recommendations
American College of Chest Physicians	Antiplatelet therapy after cryptogenic stroke should include 1 of the following: (1) aspirin 50 to 325 mg daily; (2) aspirin 25 mg and extended-release dipyridamole 200 mg twice daily; or (3) clopidogrel 75 mg daily. Antiplatelet agents are recommended instead of oral anticoagulation unless a patient has a well-documented prothrombotic disorder. After cryptogenic ischemic stroke, in the presence of a PFO, antiplatelet therapy is recommended instead of warfarin unless a patient has evidence of deep venous thrombosis.
American Academy of Neurology	After cryptogenic stroke, evidence indicates the risk of recurrent stroke or death does not vary between patients with and without PFOs who are treated medically. There is insufficient evidence to determine the superiority of antiplatelet agents vs warfarin. There is insufficient evidence regarding the effectiveness of PFO closure.
AHA/American Stroke Association	After noncardioembolic ischemic stroke or TIA, antiplatelet agents rather than oral anticoagulation are recommended to reduce the risk of recurrent stroke and other cardiovascular events (class I, level of evidence A). Aspirin (50 to 325 mg/d), aspirin and extended-release dipyridamole in combination, and clopidogrel are all acceptable options for initial therapy (class IIa, level of evidence A). After ischemic stroke or TIA in patients with a PFO, antiplatelet therapy is reasonable to prevent a recurrent event (class IIa, level of evidence B). Warfarin is reasonable for high-risk patients who have other indications for oral anticoagulation, such as underlying hypercoagulable state or evidence of venous thrombosis (class IIa, level of evidence C). Insufficient data exist to make a recommendation about PFO closure in patients with a first stroke and a PFO. PFO closure may be considered for patients with recurrent cryptogenic stroke despite optimal medical therapy (class IIb, level of evidence C).

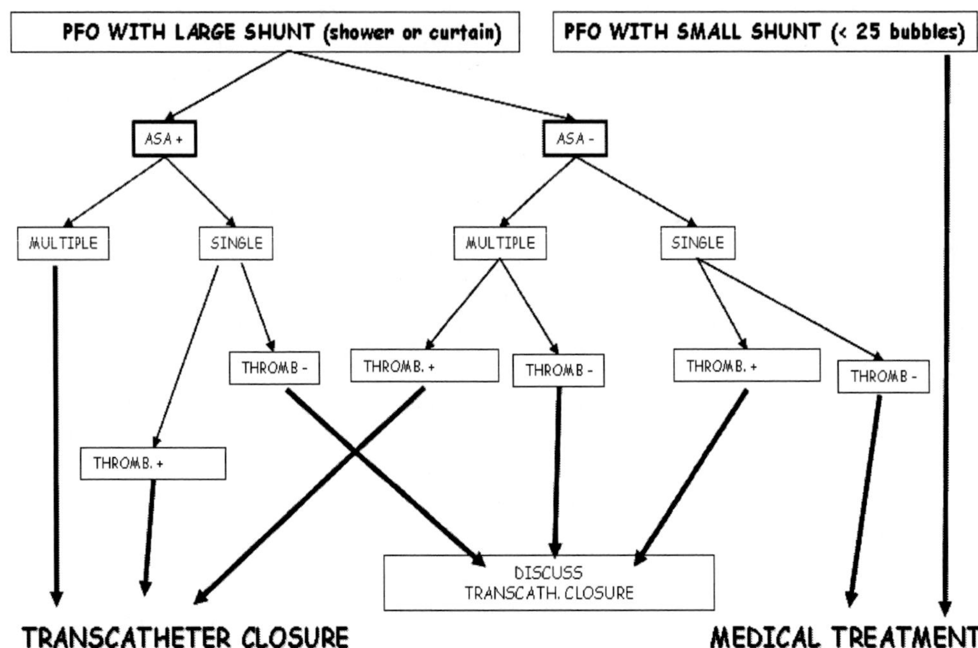

MULTIPLE-SINGLE = multiple lesions on neuroimaging or multiple clinical events.
ASA= atrial septal aneurysm.
THROMB. = thrombophilic disorder and/or evidence of venous thrombosis.

Figure 2. Proposal of decision making strategy for PFO closure.

General agreement exists about the need of randomized trials to determine the efficacy of percutaneous occluders in preventing recurrent cryptogenic stroke.

As long as we are waiting for the results of randomized trials (results probably not to be expected soon), evidence based medicine has to be replaced by common sense. In the meanwhile, our group, according with actual international evidences, suggests to stratify symptomatic PFO patients with presumed PFO-related stroke in different risk classes to different therapeutic options (medical vs transcatheter treatment) with a rigorous "decision making strategy" that includes ce-TCD (figure 2). Indeed, while TEE is paramount to assess the cardiac location of the shunt and its volume and the co-occurrence of ASA and other subtle cardiac abnormalities (Eustachian valve or Chiari network) that can facilitate the passage of venous blood into the systemic circulation, ce-TCD can directly assess the shunt at the level of the brain vessels and quantify more specifically the degree of cerebral RLS.

With this combined diagnostic workup, which tries to capitalize the currently available evidence on the weight of different factors (shunt amount, ASA and other associate abnormalities, DVT, coagulation abnormalities and neuroimaging) as summarized by Desai and associates [134] it may become easier to stratify patients in different risk classes with different therapeutic options. The proposed flowchart may lead to three therapeutical "boxes". On one extreme stand those cases in whom PFO is most likely to be responsible for he clinical event and in whom the only reasonable alternative to closure is life-long anticoagulation, which may be unacceptable in young patients. On the other end are those cases in whom the mechanism of stroke is likely non embolic, PFO is detected as an innocent bystander and antiplatelet treatment is probably protective. In the middle are the cases belonging to the truly grey area of uncertainty in whom the final treatment may depend more on the patients expectations and life style than on firm evidence of efficacy of whatever treatment is considered.

Conclusion

PFO as a cause of cryptogenic stroke is a diagnosis of exclusion and is completely dependent on appropriately ruling out all potential causes. Despite the lack of certainty of causation, the main hypothesis involved for potential stroke in PFO is paradoxical embolism of venous emboli to the arterial circulation. At this regard deep venous thrombosis and pelvic vein thrombosis have been reported by several authors to be observed more frequently in young patients who suffered from cryptogenic stroke than in those who had stroke from other more defined causes. The association between PFO and paradoxical embolism and the greater frequency of cryptogenic strokes in patients with PFO and prothrombotic states have suggested the potential benefit of antiplatelet therapy with aspirin and possibly clopidogrel, or anticoagulant therapy with warfarin. However, there is neither expert consensus nor sufficient quality evidence to determine which approach, antiplatelet or antithrombotic, is superior.

Also in spite of medical therapy, up to 25 percent of patients with cryptogenic stroke experience recurrent stroke or transient ischemic attack within 4 years of the initial event. Because PFO represents a lesion which may be repaired a number of expert clinicians believe that mechanical closure should be the primary treatment modality for patients with PFO after cryptogenic stroke; interest has grown on percutaneous devices and in the last years there has been great technological advancement of percutaneous techniques for PFO closure.

Cryptogenic stroke by definition needs thorough investigation in order to rule out all potential causes of stroke. Our goal is to differentiate patients in whom the culprit PFO has to be closed from those who do not necessitate to close a bystander PFO. Various factors need to be considered such as atrial anatomic variation (PFO size, ASA, Eustachian valve anatomy), hemodynamic parameters, presence of venous thrombus identified through higher sensitivity tests such as lower extremity/ abdominal/pelvic MRI, and the presence of hypercoagulable genetic variables. At the same time, efforts to develop safer and more effective closure devices are under way. These devices include those with little or no metal component and those with biodegradable discs. Ideally, we should be able to identify at-risk patients before they sustain a stroke and to prevent stroke by closing the PFO with a device that should result in complete closure, be made of material that conforms to both sides of the septum, and have no risk of erosion, infection, arrhythmia, or thrombogenicity.

Randomized trials comparing medical and percutaneous closure approaches are underway, but large patient enrollment is necessary because of the low event rate in the younger patients. Meanwhile, as the complication rate from device implantation decreases and simpler devices are developed with reliability further demonstrated, the threshold for percutaneous closure is likely to decline.

References

[1] Warlow CP, Dennis MS, van Gijn J, Hankey GJ, Sandercock PAG, Bamford JM, Wardlaw J. Stroke: a practical guide to management. 2001. Blacwell Science Ltd.

[2] Kristensen B, Malm J, Carlberg B, Stegmayr B, Backman C, Fagerlund M, Olsson T. Epidemiology and etiology of ischemic stroke in young adults aged 18 to 44 years in northern Sweden. *Stroke* 1997;28:1702-1709.

[3] Nencini, P, Inzitari D, Baruffi MC, Fratiglioni L, Gagliardi R, Benvenuti L, Buccheri AM, Cecchi L, Passigli A, Rosselli A, et al. Incidence of stroke in young adults in Florence, Italy. *Stroke* 1988;19:977-981.

[4] Jacobs BS, Boden-Albala B, Lin IF, Sacco RL. Stroke in the young in the northern Manhattan stroke study. *Stroke* 2002;33:2789-2793.

[5] Yonemura K, Kimura K, Hasegawa Y, Yokota C, Minematsu K, Yamaguchi T. Analysis of ischemic stroke in patients aged up to 50 years. Rinsho Shinkeigaku. 2000; 40:881-886.

[6] Al Rajeh S, Awada A. Stroke in Saudi Arabia. *Cerebrovasc. Dis.* 2002;13:3-8.

[7] Sacco RL, Boden-Albala B, Gan R, Chen X, Kargman DE, Shea S, Paik MC, Hauser WA. Stroke incidence among white, black, and Hispanic residents of an urban community: the Northern Manhattan Stroke Study. *Am. J. Epidemiol.* 1998;147:259-268.

[8] Bruno A, Carter S, Qualls C, Nolte KB. Incidence of spontaneous intracerebral hemorrhage among Hispanics and non-Hispanic whites in New Mexico. *Neurology* 1996;47:405-408.

[9] Kittner SJ, McCarter RJ, Sherwin RW, Sloan MA, Stern BJ, Johnson CJ, Buchholz D, Seipp MJ, Price TR. Black-white differences in stroke risk among young adults. *Stroke* 1993;24:13-15.

[10] Chong JY, Sacco R. Epidemiology of Stroke in Young Adults: Race/Ethnic Differences *J. Thromb Thrombolysis* 2005;20:77–83.

[11] Qureshi AI, Safdar K , Patel M, Janssen RS, Frankel MR. Stroke in young black patients. Risk factors, subtypes, and prognosis. *Stroke* 1995;26:1995-1998.

[12] Thrift AG, Dewey HM, Macdonell RA, McNeil JJ, Donnan GA. Incidence of the major stroke subtypes: initial findings from the North East Melbourne stroke incidence study (NEMESIS). *Stroke* 2001;32:1732-1738.

[13] Adams HP Jr, Bendixen BH, Kappelle LJ, Biller J, Love BB, Gordon DL, Marsh EE 3rd. Classification of subtype of acute ischemic stroke: definitions for use in a multicenter clinical trial. *Stroke* 1993;24:35-41.

[14] Meissner I, Whisnant JP, Khandheria BK, Spittell PC, O'Fallon WM, Pascoe RD, Enriquez-Sarano M, Seward JB, Covalt JL, Sicks JD, Wiebers DO. Prevalence of potential risk factors for stroke assessed by transesophageal echocardiography and carotid ultrasonography: the SPARC study. Stroke Prevention: Assessment of Risk in a Community. *Mayo Clin. Proc.* 1999;74:862-869.

[15] Levy, D. E. Transient CNS deficits: a common, benign syndrome in young adults. *Neurology* 1988;38:831-836.

[16] Bogousslavsky J, Regli F. Ischemic stroke in adults younger than 30 years of age. Cause and prognosis. *Arch Neurol.* 1987;44:479-482.

[17] Cramer, S. C. Patent foramen ovale and stroke: prognosis and treatment in young adults. *J. Thromb. Thrombolysis* 2005;20:85-91.

[18] Cabanes, L, Mas JL, Cohen A, Amarenco P, Cabanes PA, Oubary P, Chedru F, Guérin F, Bousser MG, de Recondo J. Atrial septal aneurysm and patent foramen ovale as risk factors for cryptogenic stroke in patients less than 55 years of age. A study using transesophageal echocardiography. *Stroke* 1993;24:1865-1873.

[19] Amarenco P. Patent foramen ovale and the risk of stroke: smoking gun guilty by association? *Heart* 2005;91:441–443.

[20] Moore KL. The Developing Human: Clinically Oriented Embryology. 2nd ed. Philadelphia, PA: W.B. Saunders. 1997.

[21] Clark EB. Pathogenetic mechanisms of congenital cardiovascular malformations revisited. *Semin. Perinatol.* 1996;20:465-472.

[22] Hagen PT, Scholz DG, Edwards WD. Incidence and size of patent foramen ovale during the first 10 decades of life: an autopsy study of 965 normal hearts. *Mayo Clin. Proc.* 1984;59:17-20.

[23] Lynch JJ, Schuchard GH, Gross CM, Wann LS,. Prevalence of right-to-left atrial shunting in a healthy population: detection by Valsalva maneuver contrast echocardiography. *Am. J. Cardiol.* 1984;53:1478-1480.

[24] Webster MW, Chancellor AM, Smith HJ Swift DL, Sharpe DN, Bass NM, Glasgow GL. Patent foramen ovale in young stroke patients. *Lancet* 1988;2:11-12.

[25] Lechat P, Mas JL, G. Lascault P, Loron P, Theard M, Klimczac M, Drobinski G, Thomas D, Grosgogeat Y. Prevalence of patent foramen ovale in patients with stroke. *N. Engl. J. Med.* 1988;318:1148-1152.

[26] Hausmann, D, Mugge A, Becht I, Daniel WG. Diagnosis of patent foramen ovale by transesophageal echocardiography and association with cerebral and peripheral embolic events. *Am. J. Cardiol.* 1992;70:668-672.

[27] Lamy C, Giannesini C, Zuber, Arquizan C, Meder JF, Trystram D, Coste J, Mas JL. Clinical and imaging findings in cryptogenic stroke patients with and without patent foramen ovale: the PFO-ASA Study. Atrial Septal Aneurysm. *Stroke* 2002;33:706-711.

[28] Chen WJ, Lin SL, Cheng JJ, Lien WP. The frequency of patent foramen ovale in patients with ischemic stroke: a transesophageal echocardiographic study. *J. Formos Med. Assoc.* 1991;90:744–748.

[29] De Belder MA, Tourikis L, Leech G, Camm AJ. Risk of patent foramen ovale for thromboembolic events in all age groups. *Am. J. Cardiol.* 1992;69:1316-1320.

[30] Job FP, Ringelstein EB, Grafen Y, Flachskampf FA, Doherty C, Stockmanns A, Hanrath P. Comparison of transcranial contrast Doppler sonography and transesophageal contrast echocardiography for the detection of patent foramen ovale in young stroke patients. *Am. J. Cardiol.* 1994;74:381-384.

[31] Jones EF, Calafiore P, Donnan GA, Tonkin AM. Evidence that patent foramen ovale is not a risk factor for cerebral ischemia in the elderly. *Am. J. Cardiol.* 1994;74:596-599.

[32] Zahn R, Lehmkuhl S, Lotter R. Cardiac sources of et al. Cerebral ischemic events with special regard to a patent foramen ovale. *Herz Kreislauf* 1995;27:279–284.

[33] Del Sette M, Angeli S, Lenadri M, Ferriero G, Bruzzone GL, Finocchi C, Gandolfo C. Migraine with aura and right-to-left shunt on transcranial Doppler: a case-control study. *Cerebrovasc. Dis.* 1998;8:327-330.

[34] Overell JR, Bone I , Lees KR. Interatrial septal abnormalities and stroke: a meta-analysis of case-control studies. *Neurology* 2000;55:1172-9.

[35] Di TullioM , Sacco RL, Venketasubramanian N, Sherman D, Mohr JP, Homma S. Comparison of diagnostic techniques for the detection of a patent foramen ovale in stroke patients. *Stroke* 1993;24:1020-1024.

[36] Yeung M, Khan KA, Shuaib A. Transcranial Doppler ultrasonography in the detection of venous to arterial shunting in acute stroke and transient ischaemic attacks. *J. Neurol. Neurosurg. Psychiatry* 1996;61:445-449.

[37] Handke M, Harloff A, Olschewski M, Hetzel A, Geibel A. Patent Foramen Ovale and Cryptogenic Stroke in Older Patients *N. Engl. J. Med.* 2007;357:2262-2268.

[38] Yahia AM, Shaukat A , Kirmani JF , Qureschi AI. Age is not a predictor of patent foramen ovale with right-to-left shunt in patients with cerebral ischemic events. *Echocardiography* 2004;21:517-522.

[39] Meissner I, Khandheria K, Heit JA, Petty GW, Sheps SG, Schwartz GL, Whisnant JP, Wiebers DO, Covalt JL, Petterson TM, Christianson TJ, Agmon Y. Patent Foramen Ovale: Innocent or Guilty? Evidence From a Prospective Population-Based Study. *J. Am. Coll. Cardiol.* 2006;47:440-445.

[40] Di Tullio MR, Sacco RL, Sciacca RR, Jin Z, Homma S. Patent Foramen Ovale and the Risk of Ischemic Stroke in a Multiethnic Population. *J. Am. Coll. Cardiol.* 2007;49: 797-802.

[41] Bogousslavsky J, Garazi S, Jeanrenaud X, Aebischer N, Van Melle G. Stroke recurrence in patients with patent foramen ovale: the Lausanne Study. Lausanne Stroke with Paradoxal Embolism Study Group. *Neurology* 1996;46:1301-1305.

[42] Cujec, B,. Mainra R, Johnson DH. Prevention of recurrent cerebral ischemic events in patients with patent foramen ovale and cryptogenic strokes or transient ischemic attacks. *Can. J. Cardiol.* 1999;15:57-64.

[43] De Castro S, Cartoni D, Fiorelli M, Rasura M, Anzini A, Zanette EM, Beccia M, Colonnese C, Fedele F, Fieschi C, Pandian NG. Morphological and functional characteristics of patent foramen ovale and their embolic implications. *Stroke* 2000;31: 2407-2413.

[44] Mas JL, Zuber M. Recurrent cerebrovascular events in patients with patent foramen ovale, atrial septal aneurysm, or both and cryptogenic stroke or transient ischemic attack. French Study Group on Patent Foramen Ovale and Atrial Septal Aneurysm. *Am. Heart J.* 1995;130:1083-1088.

[45] Mas, JL, Arquizan C, Lamy C, Zuber M, Cabanes L, Derumeaux G, Coste J; Patent Foramen Ovale and Atrial Septal Aneurysm Study Group. Recurrent cerebrovascular events associated with patent foramen ovale, atrial septal aneurysm, or both. *N. Engl. J. Med.* 2001;345:1740-1746.

[46] Homma S, Sacco RL, Di Tullio MR, Sciacca RR, Mohr JP; PFO in Cryptogenic Stroke Study (PICSS) Investigators. Effect of medical treatment in stroke patients with patent

foramen ovale: patent foramen ovale in Cryptogenic Stroke Study. *Circulation* 2002; 105:2625-31.

[47] Homma S, Di Tullio MR, Sacco RL, Sciacca RR, Mohr JP; PICSS Investigators. Age As a Determinant of Adverse Events in Medically Treated Cryptogenic Stroke Patients With Patent Foramen Ovale. *Stroke* 2004;35:2145-2149.

[48] Messé SR, Silverman IE, Kizer JR Homma S, Zahn C, Gronseth G, Kasner SE; Quality Standards Subcommittee of the American Academy of Neurology. Practice parameter: recurrent stroke with patent foramen ovale and atrial septal aneurysm: report of the Quality Standards Subcommittee of the American Academy of Neurology. *Neurology* 2004;62:1042-1050.

[49] Marazanof M, Roudaut R, Cohen A, Tribouilloy C, Malergues MC, Halphen C, Bussiere JL, Schultz R, Marcaggi X, Lardoux H, et al. Atrial septal aneurysm. Morphological characteristics in a large population: pathological associations. A French multicenter study on 259 patients investigated by transoesophageal echocardiography. *Int. J. Cardiol*. 1995;52:59–65.

[50] Hanley PC, Tajik AJ, Hynes JK, Edwards WD, Reeder GS, Hagler DJ, Seward JB. Diagnosis and classification of atrial septal aneurysm by two-dimensional echocardiography: Report of 80 consecutive cases. *J. Am. Coll. Cardiol.* 1985;6:1370-1382.

[51] Mügge A, Daniel WG, Angermann C, Spes C, Khandheria BK, Kronzon I, Freedberg RS, Keren A, Denning K, Engberding R, et al. Atrial septal aneurysm in adult patients: a multicenter study using transthoracic and transesophageal echocardiography. *Circulation* 1995; 91:2785-2792.

[52] Rodriguez CJ, Homma S, Sacco RL, Di Tullio MR, Sciacca RR, Mohr JP; PICSS Investigators. Race-ethnic differences in patent foramen ovale, atrial septal aneurysm, and right atrial anatomy among ischemic stroke patients. *Stroke* 2003;34:2097-2102.

[53] Agmon Y, Khandheria BK, Meissner I, Gentile F, Whisnant JP, Sicks JD, O'Fallon WM, Covalt JL, Wiebers DO, Seward JB. Frequency of atrial septal aneurysms in patients with cerebral ischemic events. *Circulation* 1999;99:1942-1944.

[54] Hanna JP, Sun JP, Furlan AJ, Stewart WJ, Sila CA, Tan M. Patent foramen ovale and brain infarct. Echocardiographic predictors, recurrence, and prevention. *Stroke* 1994; 25:782-786.

[55] Homma S, Sacco RL, Di Tullio MR, Sciacca RR, Mohr JP. Atrial anatomy in non-cardioembolic stroke patients: effect of medical therapy. *J. Am. Coll. Cardiol.* 2003; 42:1066-1072.

[56] Fox ER, Picard MH, Chow CM, Levine RA, Schwamm L, Kerr AJ. Interatrial septal mobility predicts larger shunts across patent foramen ovale: an analysis with transmitral Doppler scanning. *Am. Heart J.* 2003;145:730-736.

[57] Homma S, Di Tullio MR, Sacco RL, Mihalatos D, Li Mandri G, Mohr JP. Characteristics of patent foramen ovale associated with cryptogenic stroke. A biplane transesophageal echocardiographic study. *Stroke* 1994;25:582-586.

[58] Steiner MM, Di Tullio MR, Rundek T, Gan R, Chen X, Liguori C, Brainin M, Homma S, Sacco RL. Patent foramen ovale size and embolic brain imaging findings among patients with ischemic stroke. *Stroke* 1998;29:944-948.

[59] Hausmann, D, Mugge A, Daniel WG. Identification of patent foramen ovale permitting paradoxic embolism. *J. Am. Coll. Cardiol.* 1995;26:1030-1038.

[60] Schuchelnz HW, Weihs W, Horner S, Quehenberger F. The association between the diameter of a patent foramen ovale and the risk of embolic cerebrovascular events. *Am. J. Med.* 2000;109:456-462.

[61] De Castro S, Cartoni D, Fiorelli M, Rasura M, Beni S, Urani C, Papetti F, Fedele F. Patent foramen ovale and its embolic implications. *Am. J. Cardiol.* 2000;86:51G-52G.

[62] Anzola GP, Zavarize P, Morandi E, Rozzini L, Parrinello G. Transcranial Doppler and risk of recurrence in patients with stroke and patent foramen ovale. *Eur. J. Neurol.* 2003;10:129-35.

[63] De Dominicis E, Ometto R, Frigiola A, Menicanti L, Arfiero S, Vincenzi M. Echocardiographic patterns of persistence of the right sinus venosus valve. *G. Ital. Cardiol.* 1985;15:80-83.

[64] Limacher MC, Gutgesell HP, Vick GW, Cohen MH, Huhta JH. Echocardiographic anatomy of the Eustachian valve. *Am. J. Cardiol.* 1986;57:363-365.

[65] Bashour T, Kabbani S, Saalouke M, Cheng TO. Persistent Eustachian valve causing severe cyanosis in atrial septal defect with normal right heart pressures. *Angiology* 1983;34:79-83.

[66] Soliman A, Shanoudy H, Liu J, Russell DC, Jarmukli NF. Increased prevalence of patent foramen ovale in patients with severe chronic obstructive pulmonary disease. *J. Am. Soc. Echocardiogr.* 1999;12:99-105.

[67] Shanoudy H, Soliman A, Raggi P, Liu JW, Russell DC, Jarmukli NF. Prevalence of patent foramen ovale and its contribution to hypoxemia in patients with obstructive sleep apnoea. *Chest* 1998;113:91-96.

[68] Lapostolle F, Borron SW, Surget V, Sordelet D, Lapandry C, Adnet F. Stroke associated with pulmonary embolism after air travel. *Neurology* 2003;60:1983-1985.

[69] Kasper W, Geibel A, Tiede N, Just H. Patent foramen ovale in haemodynamically significant pulmonary embolism. *Lancet* 1992;340:561-564.

[70] Bansal RC, Marsa RJ, Holland D, Beehler C, Gold PM. Severe hypoxemia due to shunting through a patent foramen ovale: a correctable complication of right ventricular infarction. *J. Am. Coll. Cardiol.* 1985;5:188-192.

[71] Harpaz D, Motro M, Kaplinsky E, Vered Z. Right-to-left shunt through a patent foramen ovale caused by severe tricuspid regurgitation detected with color Doppler echocardiography. *J. Am. Soc. Echocardiogr.* 1992;5:77-80.

[72] Bracey TS, Langrish C, Darby M, Soar J. Cerebral infarction following thrombolysis for massive pulmonary embolism. *Resuscitation* 2006;68:135-137.

[73] Serra W, De Iaco G, Reverberi C, Gherli T. Pulmonary embolism and patent foramen ovale thrombosis: the key role of TEE. *Cardiovasc. Ultrasound* 2007;24:5-26.

[74] Cheng TO. Platypnea-orthodeoxia syndrome: etiology, differential diagnosis, and management. *Catheter Cardiovasc. Interv.* 1999;47:64–66.

[75] Bertaux G, Eicher JC, Petit A, Dobsák P, Wolf JE. Anatomic interaction between the aortic root and the atrial septum: a prospective echocardiographic study. *J. Am. Soc. Echocardiogr.* 2007;20:409-414.

[76] Caputi L, Carriero MR, Parati EA, Onorato E, Casilli F, Berti M, Anzola GP. Postural Dependency of Right to Left Shunt. Role of Contrast-Enhanced Transcranial Doppler and Its Potential Clinical Implications. *Stroke* 2008;39:2380-2381.
[77] Stollberger C, Slany J, Schuster I, Leitner H, Winkler WB, Karnik R. The prevalence of deep venous thrombosis in patients with suspected paradoxical embolism. *Ann. Intern. Med.* 1993;119:461-465.
[78] Lethen H, Flachskampf FA, Schneider R, Sliwka U, Köhn G, Noth J, Hanrath P. Frequency of deep vein thrombosis in patients with patent foramen ovale and ischemic stroke or transient ischemic attack. *Am. J. Cardiol.* 1997;80:1066-1069.
[79] Cramer SC, Rordorf G, Maki JH, Kramer LA, Grotta JC, Burgin WS, Hinchey JA, Benesch C, Furie KL, Lutsep HL, Kelly E, Longstreth WT Jr. Increased pelvic vein thrombi in cryptogenic stroke: results of the Paradoxical Emboli From Large Veins in Ischemic Stroke (PELVIS) Study. *Stroke* 2004;35:46-50.
[80] Belvís R, Masjuan J, García-Barragán N, Cocho D, Martí-Fàbregas J, Santamaría A, Leta RG, Martínez-Castrillo JC, Fernández-Ruiz LC, Gilo F, Martí-Vilalta JL. Stroke and pulmonary thromboembolism after a long flight. *Eur. J. Neurol.* 2005;12:732-734.
[81] Dixon T, Panda M, Desbiens N. The simultaneous occurrence of deep vein thrombosis and pulmonary and arterial embolization. *J. Gen. Intern. Med.* 2007;22:1040-1041.
[82] Chaturvedi S. Coagulation abnormalities in adults with cryptogenic stroke and patent foramen ovale. *J. Neurol. Sci.* 1998;160:158-160.
[83] Lichy C, Reuner KH, Buggle F, Litfin F, Rickmann H, Kunze A, Brandt T, Grau A. Prothrombin G20210A mutation, but not factor V Leiden, is a risk factor in patients with persistent foramen ovale and otherwise unexplained cerebral ischemia. *Cerebrovasc. Dis.* 2003;16:83-87.
[84] Pezzini A, Del Zotto E, Magoni M, Costa A, Archetti S, Grassi M, Akkawi NM, Albertini A, Assanelli D, Vignolo LA, Padovani A. Inherited thrombophilic disorders in young adults with ischemic stroke and patent foramen ovale. *Stroke* 2003;34:28–33.
[85] Karttunen V, Hiltunen L, Rasi V, Vahtera E, Hillbom M. Factor V Leiden and prothrombin gene mutation may predispose to paradoxical embolism in subjects with patent foramen ovale. *Blood Coagul. Fibrinolysis* 2003;14:261-268.
[86] Belvis R, Santamaria A, Martì-Fàbregas J, Leta RG, Cocho D, Borrell M, Fontcuberta J, Martí-Vilalta JL. Patent foramen ovale and prothrombotic markers in young stroke patients. *Blood Coagul. Fibrinolysis* 2007;18:537-542.
[87] Sastry S, Riding G, Morris J. Young Adult Myocardial Infarction and Ischemic Stroke: The Role of Paradoxical Embolism and Thrombophilia (The YAMIS Study). *J. Am. Coll. Cardiol.* 2006;48:686-691.
[88] Johnson BI. Paradoxical embolism. *J. Clin. Path* 1951;4:316-332.
[89] Cheng TO. Paradoxical embolism. A diagnostic challenge and its detection during life. *Circulation* 1975;53:565-568.
[90] Meister SG, Grossman W, Dexter L, Dalen JE. Paradoxical embolism. Diagnosis during life. *Am. J. Med.* 1972;53:292-298.
[91] Berthet K, Lavergne T, Cohen A, Guize L, Bousser MG, Le Heuzey JY, Amarenco P. Significant association of atrial vulnerability with atrial septal abnormalities in young patients with ischemic stroke of unknown cause. *Stroke* 2000;31:398-403.

[92] Gramiak R, Shah PM, Kramer DH. Ultrasound cardiography: contrast studies in anatomy and function. *Radiology* 1969;92:939-48.

[93] Schneider B, Zienkiewicz T, Jansen V, Hofmann T, Noltenius H, Meinertz T. Diagnosis of patent foramen ovale by transesophageal echocardiography and correlation with autopsy findings. *Am. J. Cardiol.* 1996;77:1202-1209.

[94] Stendel R, Gramm HJ, Schroder K, Lober C, Brock M. Transcranial Doppler ultrasonography as a screening technique for detection of a patent foramen ovale before surgery in the sitting position. *Anesthesiology* 2000;93:971-975.

[95] Kronik G, Slany J, Moesslacher H. Contrast M-mode echocardiography in diagnosis of atrial septal defect in acyanotic patients. *Circulation* 1979;59:372-378.

[96] Martin F, Sanchez PL, Doherty, Colon-Hernandez PJ, Delgado G, Inglessis I, Scott N, Hung J, King ME, Buonanno F, Demirjian Z, de Moor M, Palacios IF. Percutaneous transcatheter closure of patent foramen ovale in patients with paradoxical embolism. *Circulation* 2002;106:1121-1126.

[97] Braun MU, Fassbender D, Schoen SP, Haass M, Schraeder R, Scholtz W, Strasser RH. Transcatheter closure of patent foramen ovale in patients with cerebral ischemia. *J. Am. Coll. Cardiol.* 2002;39:2019-2025.

[98] Windecker S, Wahl A, Nedeltchev K, Arnold M, Schwerzmann M, Seiler C, Mattle HP, Meier B. Comparison of medical treatment with percutaneous closure of patent foramen ovale in patients with cryptogenic stroke. *J. Am. Coll. Cardiol.* 2004;44: 750-758.

[99] Serena J, Segura T, Perez-Ayuso MJ. The need to quantify right-to-left shunt in acute ischemic stroke: a case-control study. *Stroke* 1998;29:1322-1328.

[100] Gin KG, Huckell VF, Pollick C. Femoral vein delivery of contrast medium enhances transthoracic echocardiographic detection of patent foramen ovale. *J. Am. Coll. Cardiol.* 1993;22:1994-2000.

[101] Movsowitz, HD, Movsowitz C, Jacobs LE, Kotler MN. Negative air-contrast test does not exclude the presence of patent foramen ovale by transesophageal echocardiography. *Am. Heart J.* 1993;126:1031-1032.

[102] Ha JW, Shin MS, Kang S, Pyun WB, Jang KJ, Byun KH, Rim SJ, Huh J, Lee BI, Chung N. Enhanced detection of right-to-left shunt through patent foramen ovale by transthoracic contrast echocardiography using harmonic imaging. *Am. J. Cardiol.* 2001; 87:669-671.

[103] Madala D, Zaroff JG, Hourigan L, Foster E. Harmonic imaging improves sensitivity at the expense of specificity in the detection of patent foramen ovale. *Echocardiography* 2004;21:33-36.

[104] Schneider B, Hanrath P, Vogel P, Meinertz T. Improved morphologic characterization of atrial septal aneurysm by transesophageal echocardiography: relation to cerebrovascular events. *J. Am. Coll. Cardiol.* 1990;16:1000-1009.

[105] Kerr AJ, Buck T, Chia K, Chow CM, Fox E, Levine RA, Picard MH. Transmitral Doppler: a new transthoracic contrast method for patent foramen ovale detection and quantification. *J. Am. Coll. Cardiol.* 2000;36:1959-1966.

[106]Daniel WG, Erbel R, Kasper W, Visser CA, Engberding R, Sutherland GR, Grube E, Hanrath P, Maisch B, Dennig K, et al. Safety of transesophageal echocardiography. A multicenter survey of 10,419 examinations. *Circulation* 1991;83:817-821.

[107]Urbanowicz JH, Kernoff RS, Oppenheim G, Parnagian E, Billingham ME, Popp RL. Transesophageal echocardiography and its potential for esophageal damage. *Anesthesiology* 1990;72:40-43.

[108]Hombach, V, Grebe O, Merkle N, Waldenmaier S, Höher M, Kochs M, Wöhrle J, Kestler HA. Sequelae of acute myocardial infarction regarding cardiac structure and function and their prognostic significance as assessed by magnetic resonance imaging. *Eur. Heart J.* 2005;26:549-557.

[109]Mohrs OK, Petersen SE, Erkapic D, Rubel C, Schräder R, Nowak B, Fach WA, Kauczor HU, Voigtlaender T. Diagnosis of patent foramen ovale using contrast-enhanced dynamic MRI: a pilot study. *AJR- Am. J. Roentgenol.* 2005;184:234-240.

[110]Nusser T, Höher M, Merkle N, Grebe OC, Spiess J, Kestler HA, Rasche V, Kochs M, Hombach V, Wöhrle J. Cardiac magnetic resonance imaging and transesophageal echocardiography in patients with transcatheter closure of patent foramen ovale. *J. Am. Coll. Cardiol.* 2006;48:322-329.

[111]Grebe O, Giesler M, Kestler HA, Hombach V, Höher M. Magnetic resonance imaging after percutaneous closure of a patent foramen ovale. *Circulation* 2001;104:E117-E118.

[112]Stoddard MF, Keedy DL , Dawkins PR. The cough test is superior to the Valsalva maneuver in the delineation of right-to-left shunting through a patent foramen ovale during contrast transesophageal echocardiography. *Am. Heart J.* 1993;125:185-189.

[113]Droste D, Silling K, Stypmann J Grude M, Keméy V, Wichter T, Kühne K, Ringelstein EB. Contrast transcranial doppler ultrasound in the detection of right-to-left shunts : time window and threshold in microbubble numbers. *Stroke* 2000;31:1640-1645.

[114]Stone DA, Godard J, Corretti MC, Kittner SJ, Sample C, Price TR, Plotnick GD. Patent foramen ovale: association between the degree of shunt by contrast transesophageal echocardiography and the risk of future ischemic neurologic events. *Am. Heart J.* 1996;131:158-161.

[115]Jauss M, Zanette E. Detection of right-to-left shunt with ultrasound contrast agent and transcranial Doppler sonography. *Cerebrovasc. Dis.* 2000;10:490-496.

[116]Anzola GP, Morandi E, Casilli F, Onorato E. Different degrees of right-to-left shunting predict migraine and stroke: data from 420 patients. *Neurology* 2006;66:765-767.

[117]Hamon M, Gomes S, Oppenheim, Morello R, Sabatier R, Lognoné T, Grollier G, Courtheoux P, Hamon M. Cerebral microembolism during cardiac catheterization and risk of acute brain injury: a prospective diffusion-weighted magnetic resonance imaging study. *Stroke* 2006;37:2035-2038.

[118]Hamon M, Burzotta F, Oppenheim C, Morello R, Viader F, Hamon M; SCIPION Investigators. Silent cerebral infarct after cardiac catheterization as detected by diffusion weighted Magnetic Resonance Imaging: a randomized comparison of radial and femoral arterial approaches. *Trials* 2007;8:15.

[119]Morandi E, Anzola GP, Casilli F, Onorato E. Silent brain embolism during transcatheter closure of patent foramen ovale: a transcranial Doppler study. *Neurol. Sci.* 2006;27:328-331.

[120]Telman G, Kouperberg E, Sprecher E, Yarnitsky D. The positions of the patients in the diagnosis of patent foramen ovale by transcranial Doppler. *J. Neuroimaging* 2003; 13:356-358.

[121]Belvis R, Leta RG, Marti-Fabregas J, Cocho D, Carreras F, Pons-Lladó G, Martí-Vilalta JL. Almost perfect concordance between simultaneous transcranial Doppler and transesophageal echocardiography in the quantification of right-to-left shunts. *J. Neuroimaging* 2006;16:133-138.

[122]Orgera MA, O'Malley PG, Taylor AJ. Secondary prevention of cerebral ischemia in patent foramen ovale: systematic review and meta-analysis. *South Med. J.* 2001;94: 699-703.

[123]Devuyst G, Bogousslavsky J, Ruchat P, Jeanrenaud X, Despland PA, Regli F, Aebischer N, Karpuz HM, Castillo V, Guffi M, Sadeghi H. Prognosis after stroke followed by surgical closure of patent foramen ovale: a prospective follow-up study with brain MRI and simultaneous transesophageal and Transcranial Doppler ultrasound. *Neurology* 1996;47:1162-1166.

[124]Homma S, Di Tullio MR, Sacco RL, Sciacca RR, Smith C, Mohr JP. Surgical closure of patent foramen ovale in cryptogenic stroke patients. *Stroke* 1997;28:2376-2381.

[125]Dearani JA, Ugurlu BS, Danielson GK, Daly RC, McGregor CG, Mullany CJ, Puga FJ, Orszulak TA, Anderson BJ, Brown RD Jr, Schaff HV. Surgical patent foramen ovale closure for prevention of paradoxical embolism-related cerebrovascular ischemic events. *Circulation* 1999;100(Suppl II):171-175.

[126]Nendaz MR, Sarasin FP, Junod AF, Bogousslavsky J. Preventing stroke recurrence in patients with patent foramen ovale: antithrombotic therapy, foramen closure, or therapeutic abstention? A decision analytic perspective. *Am. Heart J.* 1998;135:532-541.

[127]Deeik RK, Thomas RM, Sakiyalak P, Botkin S, Blakeman B, Bakhos M. Minimal access closure of patent foramen ovale: is it also recommended for patients with paradoxical emboli? *Ann. Thorac. Surg.* 2002;74:S1326-S1329.

[128]Bridges ND, Hellenbrand W, Latson L, Filiano J, Newburger JW, Lock JE. Transcatheter closure of patent foramen ovale after presumed paradoxical embolism. *Circulation* 1992;86:1902-1908.

[129]Khairy P, O'Donnell CP, Landzberg MJ. Transcatheter closure versus medical therapy of patent foramen ovale and presumed paradoxical thromboemboli: a systematic review. *Ann. Intern. Med.* 2003;139:753-760.

[130]Krumsdorf U, Ostermayer S, Billinger K, Trepels T, Zadan E, Horvath K, Sievert H. Incidence and clinical course of thrombus formation on atrial septal defect and patient foramen ovale closure devices in 1.000 consecutive patients. *J. Am. Coll. Cardiol.* 2004;43:302–309.

[131]Homma S, Sacco RL. Patent Foramen Ovale and Stroke. *Circulation* 2005;112:1063-1072.

[132]Albers GW, Amarenco P, Easton JD, Sacco RL, Teal P. Antithrombotic and thrombolytic therapy for ischemic stroke: the Seventh ACCP Conference on Antithrombotic and Thrombolytic Therapy. *Chest* 2004;126:483S–512S.

[133]Sacco RL, Adams R, Albers G, Alberts MJ, Benavente O, Furie K, Goldstein LB, Gorelick P, Halperin J, Harbaugh R, Johnston SC, Katzan I, Kelly-Hayes M, Kenton EJ, Marks M, Schwamm LH, Tomsick T; American Heart Association; American Stroke Association Council on Stroke; Council on Cardiovascular Radiology and Intervention; American Academy of Neurology. Guidelines for prevention of stroke in patients with ischemic stroke or transient ischemic attack: a statement for healthcare professionals from the American Heart Association/American Stroke Association Council on Stroke: co-sponsored by the Council on Cardiovascular Radiology and Intervention: the American Academy of Neurology affirms the value of this guideline. *Stroke* 2006;37:577-617.

[134]Desai AJ , Fuller CJ, Jesurum JT, Reisman M. Patent foramen ovale and cerebrovascular diseases. *Nature Clin. Pract. Cardiovasc. Med.* 2006;3:446-455.

In: Cerebral Ischemia in Young Adults
Editors: A. Pezzini and A. Padovani

ISBN 978-1-60741-627-2

Chapter 14

Other Causes of Cardioembolism in Young Adults

Riccardo Raddino*[•], *Giorgio Caretta and Enrico Vizzardi
Section of Cardiovascular Diseases, Department of Experimental and Applied Medicine, University of Brescia, Brescia, Italy

Abstract

Embolism of cardiac origin accounts for about one fifth of ischemic strokes in general population. Embolism from the heart usually results from thrombosis in the cardiac chambers because of local blood stasis (e.g. atrial fibrillation) or release of material, not necessarily a thrombus, from an abnormal surface (e.g. vegetations, valvular calcification, turmors). Cardioembolic causes of ischemic strokes and transient ischemic attacks are not much different in the young and in the elderly. The most important sources of emboli are atrial fibrillation, mitral stenosis, prostethic heart valves, recent myocardial infarction, infective endocarditis, intracardiac thrombus and cardiac tumors. Other less relevant conditions considered sources of cardiac emboli include aortic stenosis, mitral valve prolapse, mitral annulus calcification, ventricular non-compaction and ventricular aneurism.

This chapter reviews the epidemiology, pathophysiology and therapeutical strategies of commonly recognized causes of cardioembolism (Tabale 1). Paradoxical embolism, which requires the passage of a venous thrombus into arterial circulatory system through an abnormal intracardiac defect, is not discussed in this chapter.

Table 1. Commonly recognized cardioembolic sources

[•] Correspondence: Riccardo Raddino, Brescia University Medical School, P.le Spedali Civili, 1, 25123 Brescia, Italy. e-mail: riccardo.raddino@libero.it.

Major embolic sources	Minor embolic sources
Atrial Fibrillation	Patent foramen ovale *
Mitral stenosis	Atrial septal aneurism *
Endocarditis	Aortic stenosis
Mechanical valvular prosthesis	Mitral valve prolapse
Left ventricular thrombus	Papillary fibroelastoma
Recent myocardial infarction	
Atrial myxoma	

Major sources are at high embolic risk, minor source are at low or uncertain risk.
*Discussed in the respective chapter.

Atrial Fibrillation

Atrial fibrillation (AF) is the most common sustained arrhytmia with clinical relevance among adults. It is associated with increased morbidity and mortality, particularly due to stroke and thromboembolism [1]. In fact, AF is the most potent common risk factor for ischemic stroke. It is associated with a fourfold to fivefold increase in the risk of stroke and it is estimated that 15% of all strokes are caused by atrial fibrillation [2]. AF is present in approximately 20-25% of all stroke patients, and stroke associated with AF carries higher mortality, morbidity and health care costs [3]. The risk of stroke in patients with paroxysmal, persistent or thyrotoxic AF is similar to the risk in patients with permanent AF [4].

The mechanisms underlying the strong association between AF and stroke are multiple and complex, but they appear primarily to be related to thrombus formation into the left atrium. Loss of atrial contraction leads to blood stasis especially in the left atrial appendage [5]. Moreover, stasis is associated with increased concentrations of fibrinogen, D-dimer and Von-Willebrand factor thus determining a prothrombotic state [6]. Finally, recent data showed abnormalities in atrial wall of patients with AF, characterized by endocardial damage and inflammatory infiltrations that may further contribute to thrombogenesis [7,8]. Therefore, all the criteria of Virchow's triad (i.e. stasis, wall abnormalities and abnormalities of coagulation) appear to be fulfilled in AF, thus favoring thrombosis.

Among patients with AF the annual risk of stroke is in the range of 1% to 12% [1]. The considerable variation of cerebrovascular risk in patients with AF is related to several factors such as age, sex (older women are at high risk [9]), comorbidities and underlying heart diseases. Thromboembolic risk assessment is critical in determining the best therapeutical approach for stroke prevention. The most important risk factors for stroke in AF are well indentified and includes previous TIA or stroke, older age (>65y), hypertension, diabetes mellitus, valvular heart disease, left ventricular dysfunction (moderate to severe) and coronary artery disease [1,10]. Several risk-stratification models have been developed from pooled data of antithrombotic treatment trials in AF [11].

Although AF is considered the most common cause of cardioembolism to the brain, it has a minor relevance among young patients. It is well documented that the prevalence of AF considerably increases with age: it rises to a peak of 10% in patients over the age of 80 years and is less than 1% in patients younger than 60 years. The attributable risk of stroke due to AF increases from 1.5% at the age of 50 to 24% at the age of 80% [12]. Several risk factors for stroke in AF such as hypertension, coronary artery disease and heart failure are more common at older ages.

Lone AF in young patients, with no risk factors or cardiac diseases, has a low risk of stroke. In a retrospective, population based study over 3 decades, the cumulative 15-years risk for stroke in patients with lone AF and younger than 60 years was 1.3% [13]. The coexistence of hypertension, diabetes, left ventricular dysfunction, atrial enlargement and valvular or coronary diseases adds substantial risk [1].

Treatment of AF consists in restore sinus rhythm, control ventricular rate and antithrombotic therapy [14]. Surprisingly, strategy for the control of ventricular rate of permanent or persistent arrhythymias is not inferior to a strategy for restoration of sinus rhythm in preventing stroke. Two large randomized trials, AFFIRM [15] and RACE [16] trials, showed that ischemic events occurred with equal frequency regardless of whether a rate control or rhythm control strategy was followed. A possible explanation of the failure of rhythm control to reduce the risk of stroke is that the rate of recurrence of AF despite antiarrhythmic drug therapy at 1 year after successful cardioversion is 40% to 60% [17,18]. For this reason antithrombotic therapy remains a fundamental strategy in preventing stroke in AF.

In young patients with lone AF, antiplatelet therapy with aspirin is suggested. These patients should be periodically checked for risk factors to assess need of anticoagulation. In young patients with risk factors such as hypertension, left ventricular dysfunction, diabetes mellitus and vascular disease, long-term anticoagulation with vitamin K antagonist targeted with an INR (International Normalized Ratio) between 2 and 3 is recommended. Patients with AF who had a prior TIA or stroke are those at higher risk of stroke (or stroke recurrence), therefore long-term anticoagulation in this population is mandatory [9,19].

Valvular Diseases

Mitral Stenosis

Mitral stenosis is a condition in which the mitral valve leaflets become thickened and the commissures fused along with thickening and shortening of the chordae tendineae. Mitral stenosis is almost always the result of rheumatic fever. Before the surgical era the outlook for patients with this disease was unfavourable.

From 1925 Rowe et al [20] studied 250 patients with mitral stenosis. By 10 years 39% of patients had died, 22% had become more dyspneic, and 16% had developed at least one thromboembolic complication. By 20 years, 79% had died 8% had become more symptomatic, and 26% had developed at least one thromboembolic event. Progression of disease is the rule at least in the symptomatic group. The younger patients follow a more benign course then their old counter parts [20].

The risk of systemic embolism is increased in patients with rheumatic mitral stenosis, even in the absence of documented atrial fibrillation. Systemic, especially cerebral, embolism is one of the major causes of illness and death in patients with mitral stenosis (2-6)[21-25]. The incidence of embolism in large groups of such patients is 4%/year [25,26]. The Framingham Study [26] reported an 18-fold increase in the incidence of stroke in patients who had mitral stenosis and atrial fibrillation compared with matched control subjects.

Several workers [27-29] have demonstrated that the mural thrombi in mitral stenosis are situated predominantly in the atria, particularly in the left atrium. Rarely do mural thrombi occur in the ventricles in mitral stenosis.

In a prospective cohort study of 534 consecutive patients with a mitral valve area of 2.0 cm^2 or less was evaluated the predictors of systemic embolism. Among these patients followed for just over three years, 60 had an embolic event. Independent risk factors for embolic events among the 132 patients in sinus rhythm were older age, mitral valve area, left atrial thrombus, and significant aortic regurgitation. Among the 402 patients in AF, the only two independent predictors of embolic events were not having had a percutaneous balloon mitral commissurotomy and a history of previous systemic embolism [30].

Other retrospective studies have shown that atrial fibrillation [21,22,31], age [21,31] and previous embolism [23] correlate with increased incidence of systemic embolism in patients with mitral stenosis and that age is closely related to the prevalence of atrial fibrillation [32] and to a history of embolization [21,22,31]. Several studies have shown that anticoagulation reduces the incidence of systemic embolism in patients with mitral stenosis and atrial fibrillation [33-35].

Previous retrospective studies have reported that the presence of left atrial smoky echoes by transesophageal echocardiography might favor the occurrence of systemic embolism in patients with mitral stenosis [36-39].

There are some data in literature that show an activation of coagulation system in the left atrium of patients with mitral stenosis even during anticoagulation [40,41].

Mitral annulus calcification has been cited as a possible source of cerebral embolism on the basis of anecdotal reports. However, one study that addressed this possibility concluded that mitral annulus calcification was more of a marker for generalized calcific atherosclerosis than a clear source of embolus [42].

Long term anticoagulation (INR 2.0-3.0) is indicated in patients with mitral stenosis, even in sinus rhythm [43] and is often used for primary prevention, especially for patients with left atrium enlarged or presence of thrombus, and is strongly indicated after a stroke or over embolic event.

Mechanical Prosthesis

Stroke is a devastating complication that may occur early or late after operation in patients with prosthetic heart valves and result from embolism, intracranial hemorrhage, or both. Although intracranial hemorrhage is a relatively rare event except in elderly anticoagulated patients, an embolic stroke may occur in virtually any patient and with any type of valve prosthesis.

The frequency of thromboembolic complications in mechanical heart valve patients is 1% to 4% per patient-year despite optimal anticoagulation [44,45]. The majority of these thromboembolic events involve the cerebral circulation, resulting in an increased frequency of transient ischemic attacks and ischemic strokes [46].

Thrombotic prosthetic valve occlusion is an uncommon but serious complication that has been reported to occur in 0.5% to 8% of the left-sided mechanical prosthetic valves and in up to 20% of tricuspid prostheses. Mechanical prosthetic heart valves are complicated by thrombosis followed by embolism.

Mechanical prosthetic valves offer satisfactory hemodynamic functioning and long-term durability, but they are thrombogenic and patients who receive them require long-term anticoagulation with warfarin. The frequency of thromboembolism is twice as high in patients with a valve implanted in the mitral compared with the aortic position [47,48]. The majority of these thromboembolic events involve the central nervous system [49], and their incidence is related to valve type [47,49,50] and the presence of atrial fibrillation [50]. Most valves appear to show the highest risk for thromboembolic events in the first 6 to 12 months after implantation [47,51].

In 1994, Reddy et al. [50] published the series with lowest embolization rate and suggested that advanced age and atrial fibrillation may be the risk factors for embolic complications. Roudaut et al. [52], however, found that class IV clinical status was the only predictor of embolic complications (and death).

Asymptomatic emboli, detected by transcranial Doppler, are surprisingly frequent, but probably made by gaseous cavitation bubbles; solid fragments of thrombi are considered to be the cause of TIAs, and the risk of embolism in patients on anticoagulation is 2% per year.

The majority of literature studies have indirectly suggested that most cerebral cerebral microembolic signals in mechanical heart valve patients are gaseous [53,54]. Gaseous emboli are probably cavitation bubbles produced by local high-pressure gradients during valve closure, causing "cavitation," with the release of dissolved blood gases. Advances in Doppler technology have made it possible to detect not only gaseous emboli [55,56] but also emboli composed of solid elements that are frequently involved in cerebral embolism [57]. Solid cerebral microemboli were detected by multifrequency transcranial Doppler ultrasonography in 35% of a mechanical heart valve population, and the frequency was higher in patients who experienced cerebrovascular events during the first year after valve replacement [58].

The clinical significance of microemboli in prosthetic heart valve patients remains unclear. Some authors have found evidence that suggests an increased risk of ischemic injury to the brain [59,60] whereas others have not [61,62].

Valve strands (it appear as highly mobile linear echodense structures attached to the valve or sewing ring) are common on the left-sided heart valves of normal subjects and patients regardless of gender and age; they persist unchanged over time and in some studies do not appear to be a primary source of cardioembolism [63] but in others represent a potential cardiac source of embolism [64].

Prevention of embolic events in patients with mechanical valvular prosthesis is an evidence-based indication for the use of combined oral anticoagulants and aspirin. It should be considered adding low dose aspirin to anticoagulation in presence of mechanical prosthesis when the risk of thromboembolism is high: prior embolism despite adequate INR, left ventricular dysfunction, hypercoagulable state and when the risk of bleeding are deemed to be low [65,66].

Aortic Stenosis

Aortic valve calcification is a complex pathological process that starts at the base of the aortic cusp, primarily in response to endothelial damage caused by blood flow shear stress, and is followed by inflammatory cell infiltration, lipid and calcium deposition, and activation of osteoblast-like cells.

Abnormalities of the aortic valve, without (aortic sclerosis) or with obstruction to left ventricular outflow (aortic stenosis) are particularly frequent in the general population, are associated to a high incidence of cardiovascular events, are related to risk factors for atherosclerosis and share similarities with atherosclerotic plaques.

Heart valve calcifications are rarely recognized as a potential source for cerebral embolism. Previous studies have identified aortic valve calcifications to be risk factors for stroke.

Calcified cerebral emboli secondary to aortic valve disease have been previously reported [67-69]. According to the literature, aortic stenosis seems to be the source of calcific microemboli to the brain, the retinal artery, and other small vessels in some rare cases [70,71].

Calcific emboli from a calcific aortic stenosis is an uncommon event, usually following local trauma, as from cardiac surgery or left heart catheterization or as a sequel to bacterial endocarditis and may be more common in patients with chronic atrial fibrillation and thromboembolic stroke or in patients with bicuspid valves [72-74].

Evidence that an ischemic stroke in a patient with aortic valve calcification is cardioembolic may be suggested indirectly from an association of aortic valve calcification with territorial rather than small deep infarcts, because small deep infarcts are unlikely to be caused by cardiogenic embolism [75,76]; an others argument in favor of cardiac embolism could come from the finding of silent brain infarcts in patients with aortic valve calcification [76-80]. However, a prospective study in a large cohort of patients with aortic valve calcification demonstrated that the risk of embolic stroke was not increased and this supports the idea that aortic valve calcification is not a potential stroke source [81].

The mechanisms of spontaneous migration of calcific deposits from a calcified valve may be ulceration, friability, and disintegration combined with hemodynamic forces acting on the aortic cusps, such as violent ventricular contraction, tightness of the aortic orifice, high systolic blood pressure, and a high systolodiastolic pressure gradient.

However patients with aortic stenosis who experience ischemic stroke should be carefully evaluated for coexistent cerebrovascular disease or other cardiac sources of emboli before attributing the stroke to aortic valve disease.

Mitral Valve Prolapse

Mitral valve prolapse (MVP) is generally defined as the displacement of an abnormally thickened, redundant mitral leaflet into the left atrium during systole [82]. MVP is one of the most prevalent cardiac valvular abnormalities. In the past, a wide range of prevalence was reported, probably due to the lack of standard diagnostic criteria. Recent studies based on rigorous echocardiographic criteria showed a prevalence of 2-3% in the general population [83,84]. The disease is characterized by a myxomatous proliferation of the spongiosa component (i.e. the central layer of the leaflet) resulting in cusp expansion and elongation. The leaflets become redundant and prolapsed thus determining different grade of mitral regurgitation. Foci of endothelial disruptions are common and may lead to formation of thrombus, vegetation, and calcification of valve that may serve as a source for thromboembolism.

The hypothesis that mitral valve prolapse may be a cause of thromboembolic events, especially among young adults, has been widely debated in the past decades.

Strokes and transient ischemic attacks have been reported to occur more frequently in patients with MVP in the past, suggesting that cerebral emboli are unusually common in this condition. Some small cohort studies based on in-hospital populations described an association between mitral valve prolapse and stroke in young adults [85-87]. However, such studies often used echocardiographic diagnostic criteria now considered inappropriate [88,89] and the presence of confounding risk factors for stroke was frequent.

Although it has been proposed that embolization secondary to MVP may be a significant cause for unexplained strokes in young people without cerebrovascular disease, a large case-controlled study [83] and a recent cohort study [90], performed with rigorous diagnostic criteria, showed no association between MVP and ischemic neurological events in persons under 45 years of age [83].

MVP is a heterogeneous condition, and its natural history may vary from benign with normal life to adverse with significant morbidity and mortality. Important predictors of cardiovascular mortality are moderate to severe mitral regurgitation (MR), reduced left ventricular ejection fraction, atrial fibrillation and evidence of thickened MV leaflets (5 mm or greater) at echocardiography (guidelines). When these conditions occur, an increased risk of cardiovascular events (including stroke) has been reported [91,92]. Currently, uncomplicated and asymptomatic MVP, with no additional disorders, should no longer be considered an embolic source for stroke [92].

In patients with MVP and history of TIA or stroke aspirin therapy is recommended if there is no evidence of high-risk condition (i.e. atrial fibrillation, MR, atrial thrombus, heart failure, echocardiographyc thickening > 5mm of leaflets) [93,94]. When these conditions are present warfarin therapy is recommended. Young adults with MVP and atrial fibrillation with no evidence of MR, hypertension or heart failure can be treated with aspirin alone; anticoagulation is reasonable if TIA occurs [94,95].

Infective Endocarditis

Embolism represents one of the most frequent and severe complications of infective endocarditis (IE) and has been reported to occur in 13% to 49% of patients with IE [96]. If the total risk of embolism associated with IE is very high, the risk of new embolism occurring after initiation of therapy is much lower, from 6% to 21% [97]. The risk of embolism seems particularly high during the first 2 weeks after diagnosis [98].

Embolic events could explicate with stroke (65%) involving in 90% cases medium cerebral artery, retina ischemia or haemorrhage, liver or splenic ischemia or abscesses or pulmonary embolism or abscesses (if endocarditis is localized on tricuspid valve) [99].

The exact role of echocardiography (Transthoracic-TTE and Transaesophageal-TEE) in predicting embolism has been largely debated [100-102] but is well recognized that it is essential for the correct diagnosis and for the risk stratification. The sensitivity and specificity of TEE for identifying valve vegetations vary in the studies from 82–100% and 91–100%, respectively, to 10–63% and 91–98% [103,104] for transthoracic echocardiography.

The main result is that the echocardiographic characteristics of vegetation are clearly associated with the embolic risk. The presence of large vegetations (vegetation length >10 mm) or severe vegetation mobility or both are associated with an increased embolic risk. Conversely, new embolic events (EE) are infrequent in low-risk subgroup patients with both vegetation length <10 mm and no severe mobility [101,106].

Predictors other than vegetation characteristics were identified by several studies. For example, antiphospholipid antibodies, coagulation parameters, and endothelial cell activation have been associated with an increased embolic risk [106]. Bacteriologic factors and localization of IE have also been previously reported to influence the incidence of EE. For example, *Staphylococcus aureus*[107] and *S.bovis* [108] have been associated with an increased embolic risk. However, in regard to the occurrence of new-EE, vegetation length and mobility remained the only predictors after adjustment for these microbiological variables. The higher incidence of EE in mitral valve IE is debated [99,105].

Even though the antibiotic treatments for infective endocarditis are well-documented [109], the indications for and the timing of surgery still pose problems. The principal dilemma is whether to operate early to limit the risk of emboli and/or to avoid eventual severe cardiac insufficiency, or to delay surgical intervention after the episode of infection to reduce the risks of surgery. Moreover, replacement of valves implies anticoagulation for life as well as the risk of a further infective episode involving the mechanical valve.

The identification of factors associated with increased mortality is a crucial challenge because it will allow the identification of high-risk patients in whom an aggressive strategy will be potentially useful.

In the literature, the development of the size of the vegetation over time seemed to be a prognostic factor for the severity of infective endocarditis and the increased risk in embolic events [102].

A correlation was identified between a higher mortality rate and increased vegetation size.

Antibiotic treatment seemed to influence the size of the vegetation [110]. Embolization became less frequent with longer duration of therapy, as previously reported [105].

It appears that early diagnosis with initiation of adequate antibiotic therapy is still the best way to prevent embolic complications.

Ventricular Thrombus

Ventricular thrombi are visually define as a distinct masses of echoes in the left ventricular cavity, they appear as irregular sessile or mobile structures that are contiguous with the endocardium in the area of abnormal wall motion, such as ischemic or infracted myocardium.

Left ventricular thrombus (LVT) is a frequent complication in patients with acute anterior myocardial infarction (MI) and in those with dilated cardiomyopathy (DCM).

Ventricular thrombi should be associated with a wall motion abnormality in the same location; rarely thrombi may form in ventricles with normal wall motion like setting of transient ischemia or coronary spasm. Thrombi also are seen in patients with dilated cardiomyophaties secondary to ischemic or non-ischemic genesis. Thrombi that are protruding and mobile are most likely to embolize.

The clinical importance of left ventricular thrombus lies in its potential to embolize.

If LVT is detected during the course of MI or DCM, therapeutic anticoagulation is usually indicated with the expectation that the majority of thrombi will resolve without clinical evidence of systemic embolism.

Recent Myocardial Infarction

Before the advent of thrombolysis, stroke complicated 0,8% to 5,5% of acute myocardial infarction (MI) [111,112]. Stroke after MI were almost uniformly ischemic and generally though to be embolic. An embolic mechanism is supported by pathological studies demostring left ventricular mural thrombi in 38 to 67% of cases, typically in the apex of left ventricle with anteroapical infarction [113,115].

Acute myocardial infarction (MI) is associated with a 2% absolute risk of stroke in the first 30 days, resulting from multiple mechanism including acute atrial fibrillation, hypotension, simultaneous coronary and carotid plaque inflammation, reduced left ventricular function and left ventricular mural thrombosis [116].

Most mural thrombi occur within the first 2 weeks of an anterior myocardial infarction (12% incidence) and nearly all in the setting of a large infarct that results in reduced left ventricular function and or apical akinesis [117,118].

The incidence of early embolism is high, possible up to 22%, and is most likely when the thrombus is mobile or protrude into the ventricle [119], but the embolism is rare after first 4 months [113,114]. The risk varies from 6% for anterior wall myocardial infarctions to approximately 1% for inferior wall infarctions.

Left ventricular thrombus (LVT) can develop in 20% of patients after a large anterior acute myocardial infarction (LV ejection fraction<35%); however, with thrombolytic therapy the incidence has decreased to 4% or less [120]. The peak incidence of development of LV thrombus is 48 to 72 hours after a large infarction.

Factors that enhance the risk of stroke include severe left ventricular dysfunction with low cardiac output, left ventricular aneurysm or thrombus, and associated arrhythmias such as AF [121]. History of arterial hypertension and prior stroke also increase the stroke risk [122].

In the Survival and Ventricular Enlargement (SAVE) trial [121], patients that had left ventricular enlargement after an acute myocardial infarction were found to have a 5-year rate of stroke of 8.1%. Patients with an ejection fraction less than 28% had a relative risk of stroke of 1.86 compared with patients with an ejection fraction greater than 35%. Furthermore, for every absolute decrease of 5% in ejection fraction, the risk of stroke increases by 18%.

Transthoracic echocardiography should be performed during in the first few days following infarction to evaluate regional and global left ventricular function and to detect LVT. For patients with anterior infarction, echocardiographic evaluation also should be performed before discharge or near the end of the first postinfarct week specifically to detect LVT and evaluate for change in left ventricular regional and global function.

Flow patterns in the left ventricle can predict thrombus formation after myocardial infarction. An abnormal Doppler flow pattern is highly associated with the formation of thrombus. In a study of 62 patients, no patients with a normal Doppler flow pattern seen within 24 hours of myocardial infarction went to on develop a thrombus [122]. Furthermore, Celik et al showed that the incidence of LVT formation is higher in patients with restrictive LV filling pattern [123].

Before the widespread use of primary percutaneous coronary intervention and glycoprotein IIb/IIIa inhibitors left ventricular thrombus formation had been reported to complicate up to 20% of acute myocardial infarctions (MI). The incidence of LV thrombus formation after acute MI, in the current era of rapid reperfusion, is lower than what has been historically reported [124].

Therapeutic anticoagulation during acute MI reduces the incidence of LVT, and long-term anticoagulation has been associated with a reduction in recurrent infarction and ischemic stroke, but carries hemorrhagic risk.

Strategies to prevent stroke following infarction include risk stratification for development of LVT and embolism. For patients with anterior MI, particularly those with apical akinesis or dyskinesis, therapeutic anticoagulation reduces the number of LVT and cardioembolic strokes. However, the absolute number of ischemic strokes prevented with this strategy may only be marginal, given the anticoagulation risk, particularly if antiplatelet agents are used concurrently.

Therapeutic anticoagulation with high-dose subcutaneous heparin or low molecular heparin weight reduces the incidence of LVT in patients with acute anterior MI [125-127]. It is assumed that prevention of LVT in this high-risk group reduces the incidence of cardioembolic stroke. Limiting therapeutic anticoagulation to this high-risk group is appealing but has not been tested in a large clinical trial. Recent clinical trials have demonstrated a reduction in the incidence of systemic stroke following MI for those receiving therapeutic anticoagulation, but these studies enrolled patients regardless of infarct site, used high levels of long-term anticoagulation (international normalized ratio [INR] targets of 2.5 to 4.8) and did not include aspirin [128,129]. We prefer a strategy that combines serial echocardiographic evaluation during the course of infarction with long-term therapeutic anticoagulation (INR of 2.0 to 3.0) reserved for patients showing LVT. In a single large clinical trial, fixed low-dose warfarin in addition to aspirin (325 mg/d) was not more effective than aspirin alone (325 mg/d) in preventing stroke following acute MI [130].

There are no randomized data and the guidelines differ in the treatment recommendation for acute left ventricular mural thrombosis. A minimum of 3 months anticoagulation is suggested in any case but ACC/AHA guidelines suggest lifelong in patients with low bleeding risk [131] whereas American Stroke Association guidelines suggest a maximum of 12 months anticoagulation only in the patients where the thrombus has caused a stroke or systemic embolism [65].

Ventricular Aneurysm

Left ventricular aneurysm (LVA) has been strictly defined as a distinct area of a segment of the ventricular wall that exhibits paradoxical systolic expansion [132], another authors define LVA more loosely as any large area of left ventricular akinesia or dyskinesia that reduces left ventricular ejection fraction [133-135].

The incidence of LVA in patients suffering myocardial [136] infarction (MI) has varied between 10 and 35% depending on the definition and the methods used. Of patients undergoing cardiac catheterization in the Coronary Artery Surgery Study (CASS), 7.6% had angiographic evidence of LVAs [137]. The absolute incidence of LVAs may be declining due to the increased use of thrombolytics and revascularization after MI [138,139].

Over 95% of left ventricular aneurysms reported in the literature result from coronary artery disease and myocardial infarction. Another causes also are trauma Chagas' disease [140], or sarcoidosis [141]. A very small number of congenital left ventricular aneurysms also have been reported and have been termed diverticular of the left ventricle [142].

At least 88% of dyskinetic ventricular aneurysms result from anterior infarction, while the remainder follows inferior infarction [143]. Posterior infarctions that produce a distinct dyskinetic left ventricular aneurysm are relatively unusual.

In term of embolic risk a chronic left ventricular aneurysm can be evaluated as a special case of chronic left ventricular mural thrombus. About a 50% of left ventricular aneurysm, principally in the antero-apical position develop thrombi [144], but these observational and retrospective data suggest that the incidence of systemic embolism is low [145-147]. Dyskinetic segments that remodel into aneurysms remain chronic foci for potential thrombosis [145-147].

The excellent prognosis of asymptomatic patients with dyskinetic ventricular aneurysms who were treated medically was demonstrated in a series of 40 patients followed for a mean of 5 years [148].

Factors that influence survival with medically managed left ventricular aneurysm include age, heart failure score, extent of coronary disease, duration of angina, prior infarction, mitral regurgitation, ventricular arrhythmias, aneurysm size, function of residual ventricle, and left ventricular end-diastolic pressure [148]. Early development of aneurysm within 48 hours after infarction also diminishes survival [149].

In general, the risk of thromboembolism is low for patients with aneurysms (0.35% per patient-year) [149], and long-term anticoagulation is not usually recommended. However, in the 50% of patients with mural thrombus visible by echocardiography after myocardial infarction, 19% develop thromboembolism over a mean follow-up period of 24 months

[124,150]. In these patients, anticoagulation and close echocardiographic follow-up may be indicated. AF and large aneurysmal size are additional risk factors for thromboembolism.

Therefore, an antiembolic approach similar to that for left ventricular mural thrombi should probably be used. Long-term anticoagulation must be used in presence of additional embolic risk factors (recent stroke, persistent apical diskinesis or persistently mobile thrombus). Aneurismectomy may be appropriate in patients with left ventricular aneurism and recurrent embolism despite anticoagulation.

Ventricular Non-compaction

Non-compaction of the left ventricle (LVNC) is a disorder of endomyocardial morphogenesis that results in multiple trabeculations in the left ventricular myocardium. This rare disorder is characterised by an excessively prominent trabecular meshwork and deep intratrabecular recesses. This idiopathic cardiomyopathy is characterised by an altered structure of the myocardial wall as a result of intrauterine arrest of compaction of the myocardial fibres in the absence of any coexisting congenital lesion. It can be associated with neuromuscular disorders and can co-exist with other cardiac malformations and it is accompanied by depressed ventricular function, systemic embolism and ventricular arrhythmia. Echocardiography is the method of choice to diagnose LVNC but the correct diagnosis is often missed or delayed because of lack of knowledge about this uncommon disease and its similarity to other diseases of the myocardium and endocardium. There is a two-layered structure of the myocardial wall consisting of a thin compacted epicardial layer and a thick noncompacted endocardial layer with prominent trabeculations and deep recesses.

The current literature suggests that LVNC in adults is rare and associated with a poor prognosis [151-154]. In the largest series to date, 48% of patients died or underwent cardiac transplantation over a period of 44 months [151]. Prognosis in the asymptomatic patients in their study was clearly better than the prognosis in the symptomatic patients [155]. The prognosis depends upon the severity and is generally grim due to cardiovascular complications like congestive failure (heart failure was caused by systolic and diastolic dysfunction), shock, arrhythmias and fatal thromboembolic events. The high prevalence of thromboembolic events (24% of patients) was consistent and was independent of LV size or function [156]. The deep recesses may aggravate the risk of thrombus formation and be an additional factor for this serious complication.

The occurrence of thromboembolic events, including cerebrovascular accidents, transient ischemic attacks, pulmonary embolism, and mesenteric infarction, ranged from 21% to 38% [151,157-159]. Embolic complications may be related to development of thrombi in the extensively trabeculated ventricle, depressed systolic function, or the development of AF [157]. Stasis of blood in the deep intratrabecular recesses is thought to be responsible of embolic events but also depressed left ventricular systolic function; or the development of atrial fibrillation.

The frequency of thromboembolic was as high as 24% in the Oechslin's study [151], manifesting as cerebrovascular accidents, transient ischaemic attacks, mesenteric infarction, and pulmonary embolism. Subsequent studies have suggested a lower prevalence of thromboembolism, but most available data corroborate its occurrence in sinus rhythm and its importance as a cause of morbidity in both adults and children [155]. Of interest, no systemic embolic events were reported in the largest pediatric series with LVNC [160]. The prevalence of thromboembolic events is independent of LV size or function [156]. Most patients with LVNC develop embolic events after 40 years of age unless they have associated coagulation abnormalities [156,157,160,161].

In a detailed review of 62 patients by Stollberger and Finsterer suggested that LVNC by itself was not a risk factor for stroke or embolism and in the absence of LV dysfunction [161].

Prophylactic anticoagulation may be warranted because of the higher risk of thrombus formation within the intratrabecular recesses and should be considered in patients who have been given in the presence of LV dysfunction with or without atrial fibrillation and is imperative after an episode of systemic embolism.

Cardiac Tumors

Intracardiac Myxoma

Cardiac myxoma is the most frequent primary cardiac tumor and may be a rare cause of cerebrovascular disease. It is usually benign and it is thought to derive from multipotential mesechimal cells of the endocardium [162]. The incidence of cardiac myxoma is about 0.5 per million population per year [163]. There is a female 2:1 preponderance and the age at the time of diagnosis is usually between 20 and 60 years. Myxomas may originate in any of the cardiac chambers, however 75% of cases occur in the left atrium [160,164]. Cardiac myxomas are usually sporadic but in about 7% of cases are familial and may be associated to cutaneous myxomas and endocrinopathies [165]. When situated in the left side of the heart cardiac myxomas can lead to systemic embolization. The clinical presentation of often comprises the classic diagnostic triad consisting in cardiac (60%), embolic (30-40%) and constitutional symptoms [166,167]. As many as 10% of patients with cardiac myxoma present with no symptoms [166]. Cardiac symptoms are generally related to mitral valve obstruction and often include dizziness, syncope, exertional dyspnea and pulmonary edema [164,168]. Constitutional symptoms may be mediated by secretion of inflammatory cytokines by the tumor itself and may include muscular weakness, fever, myalgia, arthralgia and fatigue [167]. Neurologic symptoms have been reported in about 26% to 45% of patients, with cerebral infarct being the most frequently observed event [166,169,170]. Embolization is typical of left sided tumors, but even right-sided ones may embolize through an atrial septal defect or patent foramen ovale [171,172]. Systemic embolization is the first clinical manifestation in 16% of patients with atrial myxoma and may occur at any time in up to one third of cases [166,173,174]. Strokes are often recurrent [175] and the presentation may range from multi-infarct dementia to massive embolic stroke causing death [176]. Involvement of multiple vascular territory is frequent and left middle cerebral artery territory appear to be the most common site of embolization [177,178].

Emboli may consist in both thrombi and turmor fragments. Since histological studies found surface thrombi in 41% of cardiac myxomas, the systemic embolization is most likely related to myxoma surface thrombus [179]. Embolic tumors usually have a surface thrombus and frondlike mixomatous projections [179]. In older patients, non-thrombotic and fibrotic turmos are more likely to be found.

Irregular and friable surface can also be a source of myxomatous emboli [166]. Myxomatous emboli may lead both to ischemic acute events and secondary delayed cerebral hemorrages. In fact, intracranial aneurims are a rare complication of cardiac myxoma. Myxomatous tumor cell can penetrate the artery wall after embolization, infiltrating and growing in subintimal space. The result is a weakening in vessel wall with subsequent aneurismal formation [180,181]. Since aneurism formation associated with atrial myxoma is not related to blood-flow dynamics, such aneurisms have the angiographyc pattern similar to those of septic emboli, characterized by multiplicity, peripheral localization and fusiform shape [182]. Bilateral fusiform aneurisms are a common finding in patients with cardiac myxomas [181,183], and may predispone to cerebral hemorrage. A recent review reported that 12% of patient with cardiac myxoma had an intracranial hemorrage as neurological presentation [178].

Patients with neurological manifestation of cardiac myxoma appear to be younger [184]. Furthermore, cardiac tumors are found more commonly in young adults with stroke or transient ischemic attack (1 in 250) than in older patients with acute cerebrovascular ischemic events (1 in 750) [163]. These findings taken together suggest that cardiac myxoma, even if rare, should be considered an important cardiogenic cause of stroke in young adults. Therefore, young patients with neurological symptoms suspected for embolic phenomena should always be investigated for presence of atrial myxoma, especially when other clinically evident causes have been reasonably excluded.

Echocardiography represents the diagnostic test of choice [167,173]. It is accurate, reliable and readily available. Transthoracic echocardiography is not invasive, and it has been reported to have a sensitivity up to 95% [185], reaching 100% in experienced echo-laboratories [185]. Transesophageal echocardiography (TEE) is more invasive, but gives a complete view of the atria with higher resolution and can detect small tumors (< 3 mm) [167]. TEE may also be useful in detecting PFO, atrial septal aneurism and other major cardioembolic source such as vegetations, intracardiac thrombus, complicated aortic plaques [186]. Cardiac MRI and CT represent valid alternative to echocardiography and can better differentiate tissue composition [50]. However they are more expensive and less accessible.

The treatment of choice of cardiac myxoma is surgical resection [174,187]. Recurrence rate is low, about 5% in literature [188], most commonly due to incomplete excision or multifocal tumor. Perioperative mortality is low (2-4%)[160,166] when there is not concomitant cerebral insult. After diagnosis has been defined, surgery should be performed as soon as possible due to high risk of recurrent embolism and mechanical complications [160,167]. Anticoagulants and antiplatelet agents may not be protective because they are ineffective in preventing embolization of myxomatous fragments. In a case series of patients with stroke and atrial myxoma, cerebral embolization recurred in 40% of patients before surgical resection, despite anticoagulation therapy [169]. Moreover anticoagulation may increase risk of cerebral hemorrage in patients with fusiform aneurisms. Currently, the effectiveness of pre-operation anticoagulation has not been established.

Valvular Papillary Fibroelastoma

Papillary fibroelastoma is the third most common cardiac tumor, accounting to 5-10% of all primary cardiac tumors [189]. Although rare, it is reported to be associated to stroke and transient ischemic attacks [190-194] secondary to embolization. Papillary fibroelastomas are classified as endocardial tumors and may originate in any part of endocardial surface, but they usually arise in the valvular endothelium. In fact, they account for 70-80% of all valvular tumors [189,195]. The valvular distribution predominates the left side of the heart: 29% of case involves the aortic valve and 25% the mitral valve [196]. Fibroelastomas are usually described as "sea anemone" and appear like small, avascular, usually peduncolate, solid tumors with multiple and friable papillary fronds [189,197,198].

Most of fibroelastomas are asymptomatic and are usually found incidentally during echocardiography or cardiac surgery and post-mortem [199]. Although it is often diagnosed incidentally, it can result in life-threatening complications such as stroke, myocardial infarction and sudden death [200]. The clinical presentation is related to location and mobility of the tumor. Left-sided and highly mobile tumors have a high risk of embolization [189,201]. Most common sites of embolization are cerebral, coronary, and systemic circulation. In a series of 71 patients who underwent surgery for valvular fibroelastoma, 38 cases with of cerebral embolization were observed [202]. A review of echocardiografic evolution of patients with fibroelastoma showed that neurological events (stroke, transitory ischemic attacks) were the most frequent clinical presentations [203]. Motility appears to be the most important and independent factor for embolization and is a death predictor [197].

The two mechanisms that could explain embolic complications consist in either embolization of tumor itself or from the thrombus on its surface [190]. However, unlike myxomas, pathologic studies only rarely found fragments of fibroelastoma in the site of embolism [204]. Therefore, embolism from thrombin formed on the uneven surface of the tumor has been proposed as the main underlying mechanism of embolization [197,204-206]. For this reason, fusiform aneurisms and cerebral hemmorage (typical of myxomas) appear not to be associated to fibroelsatomas. Embolus composition may have important therapeutical implications since anticoagulation could be effective in preventing thrombotic embolization. However, the efficacy of anticoagulation has not been studied.

Surgical excision with or without valve repair is considered the first-choice treatment for papillary fibroelastoma. Gowda et al [189] analyzed 725 cases of cardiac fibroelastoma and documented a 50% mortality rate in patients who did not undergo curative resection. Its complete resection is curative and the long-term prognosis is excellent [189]. Since the tumors are usually pedunculate their removal is usually easy. Recent improvements in surgical techniques including video-assisted surgery [207] and robotic surgery [208] reduced morbity and permits valve-sparing surgery in selected cases. Surgical removal of fibroelastoma is mandatory for symptomatic patients [189,195]. Asymptmoatic patients should be surgically treated if the turmor is large or mobile [189]. Asymptomatic patients with small and non-mobile tumors could be monitored with a close echocardiographic follow-up until they become mobile or symptoms occur [189,197,209]. Oral anticoagulation is recommended in patients not eligible for surgery or in follow up [189]. However, no data from clinical trial are available on efficacy of anticoagulation.

In conclusion valvular fibroelastoma represent a potentially treatable cause of embolic stroke in young adults [210]. A young individual with embolic stroke with no evidence of cerebrovascular disease and in sinus rhythm should always be investigated for the presence of a cardiac turmor.

References

[1] Lip GY, Lim HS. Atrial fibrillation and stroke prevention. *Lancet Neurol.* 2007;6(11): 981-993.

[2] Wolf PA, Abbott RD, Kannel WB. Atrial fibrillation as an independent risk factor for stroke: the Framingham Study. *Stroke* 1991;22(8):983-988.

[3] Marini C, De Santis F, Sacco S, Russo T, Olivieri L, Totaro R, Carolei A. Contribution of atrial fibrillation to incidence and outcome of ischemic stroke: results from a population-based study. *Stroke* 2005;36(6):1115-1119.

[4] Hart RG, Pearce LA, Rothbart RM, McAnulty JH, Asinger RW, Halperin JL. Stroke with intermittent atrial fibrillation: incidence and predictors during aspirin therapy. Stroke Prevention in Atrial Fibrillation Investigators. *J. Am. Coll. Cardiol.* 2000;35(1): 183-187.

[5] Goldman ME, Pearce LA, Hart RG, Zabalgoitia M, Asinger RW, Safford R, Halperin JL. Pathophysiologic correlates of thromboembolism in nonvalvular atrial fibrillation: I. Reduced flow velocity in the left atrial appendage (The Stroke Prevention in Atrial Fibrillation [SPAF-III] study). *J. Am. Soc. Echocardiogr.* 1999; 12(12):1080-1087.

[6] Hamer ME, Blumenthal JA, McCarthy EA, Phillips BG, Pritchett EL. Quality-of-life assessment in patients with paroxysmal atrial fibrillation or paroxysmal supraventricular tachycardia. *Am. J. Cardiol.* 1994;74(8):826-829.

[7] Frustaci A, Chimenti C, Bellocci F, Morgante E, Russo MA, Maseri A. Histological substrate of atrial biopsies in patients with lone atrial fibrillation. *Circulation* 1997; 96(4):1180-1184.

[8] Goldsmith I, Kumar P, Carter P, Blann AD, Patel RL, Lip GY. Atrial endocardial changes in mitral valve disease: a scanning electron microscopy study. *Am. Heart J.* 2000;140(5):777-784.

[9] Lip GY, Watson T, Shantsila E. Anticoagulation for stroke prevention in atrial fibrillation: is gender important? *Eur. Heart J.* 2006;27(16):1893-1894.

[10] Go AS, Hylek EM, Phillips KA, Borowsky LH, Henault LE, Chang Y, Selby JV, Singer DE. Implications of stroke risk criteria on the anticoagulation decision in nonvalvular atrial fibrillation: the Anticoagulation and Risk Factors in Atrial Fibrillation (ATRIA) study. *Circulation* 2000;102(1):11-13.

[11] Independent predictors of stroke in patients with atrial fibrillation: a systematic review. *Neurology* 2007;69(6):546-554.

[12] Ferro JM. Cardioembolic stroke: an update. *Lancet Neurol.* 2003;2(3):177-188.

[13] Kopecky SL, Gersh BJ, McGoon MD, Whisnant JP, Holmes DR, Jr., Ilstrup DM, Frye RL. The natural history of lone atrial fibrillation. A population-based study over three decades. *N. Engl. J. Med.* 1987;317(11):669-674.

[14] Fuster V, Ryden LE, Cannom DS, Crijns HJ, Curtis AB, Ellenbogen KA, Halperin JL, Le Heuzey JY, Kay GN, Lowe JE, Olsson SB, Prystowsky EN, Tamargo JL, Wann S, Smith SC, Jr., Jacobs AK, Adams CD, Anderson JL, Antman EM, Hunt SA, Nishimura R, Ornato JP, Page RL, Riegel B, Priori SG, Blanc JJ, Budaj A, Camm AJ, Dean V, Deckers JW, Despres C, Dickstein K, Lekakis J, McGregor K, Metra M, Morais J, Osterspey A, Zamorano JL. ACC/AHA/ESC 2006 Guidelines for the Management of Patients with Atrial Fibrillation: a report of the American College of Cardiology/American Heart Association Task Force on Practice Guidelines and the European Society of Cardiology Committee for Practice Guidelines (Writing Committee to Revise the 2001 Guidelines for the Management of Patients With Atrial Fibrillation): developed in collaboration with the European Heart Rhythm Association and the Heart Rhythm Society. *Circulation* 2006;114(7):e257-354.

[15] Wyse DG, Waldo AL, DiMarco JP, Domanski MJ, Rosenberg Y, Schron EB, Kellen JC, Greene HL, Mickel MC, Dalquist JE, Corley SD. A comparison of rate control and rhythm control in patients with atrial fibrillation. *N. Engl. J. Med.* 2002;347(23):1825-1833.

[16] Van Gelder IC, Hagens VE, Bosker HA, Kingma JH, Kamp O, Kingma T, Said SA, Darmanata JI, Timmermans AJ, Tijssen JG, Crijns HJ. A comparison of rate control and rhythm control in patients with recurrent persistent atrial fibrillation. *N. Engl. J. Med.* 2002;347(23):1834-1840.

[17] Antonielli E, Pizzuti A, Palinkas A, Tanga M, Gruber N, Michelassi C, Varga A, Bonzano A, Gandolfo N, Halmai L, Bassignana A, Imran MB, Delnevo F, Csanady M, Picano E. Clinical value of left atrial appendage flow for prediction of long-term sinus rhythm maintenance in patients with nonvalvular atrial fibrillation. *J. Am. Coll. Cardiol.* 2002;39(9):1443-1449.

[18] Zarembski DG, Nolan PE, Jr., Slack MK, Caruso AC. Treatment of resistant atrial fibrillation. A meta-analysis comparing amiodarone and flecainide. *Arch Intern. Med.* 1995;155(17):1885-1891.

[19] Singer DE, Albers GW, Dalen JE, Fang MC, Go AS, Halperin JL, Lip GY, Manning WJ. Antithrombotic therapy in atrial fibrillation: American College of Chest Physicians Evidence-Based Clinical Practice Guidelines (8th Edition). *Chest* 2008;133(6 Suppl): 546S-592S.

[20] Rowe JC, Bland EF, Sprague HB, White PD. The course of mitral stenosis without surgery: ten- and twenty-year perspectives. *Ann. Intern. Med.* 1960;52:741-749.

[21] Casella L, Abelmann WH, Ellis LB. Patients with Mitral Stenosis and Systemic Emboli; Hemodynamic and Clinical Observations. *Arch Intern. Med.* 1964;114:773-781.

[22] Coulshed N, Epstein EJ, McKendrick CS, Galloway RW, Walker E. Systemic embolism in mitral valve disease. *Br. Heart J.* 1970;32(1):26-34.

[23] Easton JD, Sherman DG. Management of cerebral embolism of cardiac origin. *Stroke* 1980;11(5):433-442.

[24] Horstkotte D, Niehues R, Strauer BE. Pathomorphological aspects, aetiology and natural history of acquired mitral valve stenosis. *Eur. Heart J.* 1991;12 Suppl B:55-60.

[25] Fleming HA, Bailey SM. Mitral valve disease, systemic embolism and anticoagulants. *Postgrad. Med. J.* 1971;47(551):599-604.

[26] Wolf PA, Dawber TR, Thomas HE, Jr., Kannel WB. Epidemiologic assessment of chronic atrial fibrillation and risk of stroke: the Framingham study. *Neurology* 1978; 28(10):973-977.

[27] Garvin F. Mural thrombi in heart. . *Am. Heart J.* 1941;21:713.

[28] Graef G, Berger A, J B. Auricular thrombosis in rheumatic heart disease. . *Arch Path* 1937;24:344.

[29] Harvey E, S L. A study of uninfected mural thrombi of the heart. . *Am. J. M. Sc.* 1930.

[30] Chiang CW, Lo SK, Ko YS, Cheng NJ, Lin PJ, Chang CH. Predictors of systemic embolism in patients with mitral stenosis. A prospective study. *Ann. Intern. Med.* 1998; 128(11):885-889.

[31] Chiang CW, Lo SK, Kuo CT, Cheng NJ, Hsu TS. Noninvasive predictors of systemic embolism in mitral stenosis. An echocardiographic and clinical study of 500 patients. *Chest* 1994;106(2):396-399.

[32] Benjamin EJ, Levy D, Vaziri SM, D'Agostino RB, Belanger AJ, Wolf PA. Independent risk factors for atrial fibrillation in a population-based cohort. The Framingham Heart Study. *JAMA.* 1994;271(11):840-844.

[33] Roy D, Marchand E, Gagne P, Chabot M, Cartier R. Usefulness of anticoagulant therapy in the prevention of embolic complications of atrial fibrillation. *Am. Heart J.* 1986;112(5):1039-1043.

[34] Petersen P, Boysen G, Godtfredsen J, Andersen ED, Andersen B. Placebo-controlled, randomised trial of warfarin and aspirin for prevention of thromboembolic complications in chronic atrial fibrillation. The Copenhagen AFASAK study. *Lancet* 1989;1(8631):175-179.

[35] Petersen P, Godtfredsen J. Embolic complications in paroxysmal atrial fibrillation. *Stroke* 1986;17(4):622-626.

[36] Black IW, Hopkins AP, Lee LC, Walsh WF. Left atrial spontaneous echo contrast: a clinical and echocardiographic analysis. *J. Am. Coll. Cardiol.* 1991;18(2):398-404.

[37] Daniel WG, Nellessen U, Schroder E, Nonnast-Daniel B, Bednarski P, Nikutta P, Lichtlen PR. Left atrial spontaneous echo contrast in mitral valve disease: an indicator for an increased thromboembolic risk. *J. Am. Coll. Cardiol.* 1988;11(6):1204-1211.

[38] Chimowitz MI, DeGeorgia MA, Poole RM, Hepner A, Armstrong WM. Left atrial spontaneous echo contrast is highly associated with previous stroke in patients with atrial fibrillation or mitral stenosis. *Stroke* 1993;24(7):1015-1019.

[39] Gonzalez-Torrecilla E, Garcia-Fernandez MA, Perez-David E, Bermejo J, Moreno M, Delcan JL. Predictors of left atrial spontaneous echo contrast and thrombi in patients with mitral stenosis and atrial fibrillation. *Am. J. Cardiol.* 2000;86(5):529-534.

[40] Yamamoto K, Ikeda U, Seino Y, Mito H, Fujikawa H, Sekiguchi H, Shimada K. Coagulation activity is increased in the left atrium of patients with mitral stenosis. *J. Am. Coll. Cardiol.* 1995;25(1):107-112.

[41] Asakura H, Hifumi S, Jokaji H, Saito M, Kumabashiri I, Uotani C, Morishita E, Yamazaki M, Shibata K, Mizuhashi K, et al. Prothrombin fragment F1 + 2 and thrombin-antithrombin III complex are useful markers of the hypercoagulable state in atrial fibrillation. *Blood Coagul. Fibrinolysis* 1992;3(4):469-473.

[42] Furlan AJ, Craciun AR, Salcedo EE, Mellino M. Risk of stroke in patients with mitral annulus calcification. *Stroke* 1984;15(5):801-803.

[43] Bonow RO, Carabello BA, Chatterjee K, de Leon AC, Jr., Faxon DP, Freed MD, Gaasch WH, Lytle BW, Nishimura RA, O'Gara PT, O'Rourke RA, Otto CM, Shah PM, Shanewise JS, Smith SC, Jr., Jacobs AK, Adams CD, Anderson JL, Antman EM, Fuster V, Halperin JL, Hiratzka LF, Hunt SA, Nishimura R, Page RL, Riegel B. ACC/AHA 2006 guidelines for the management of patients with valvular heart disease: a report of the American College of Cardiology/American Heart Association Task Force on Practice Guidelines (writing Committee to Revise the 1998 guidelines for the management of patients with valvular heart disease) developed in collaboration with the Society of Cardiovascular Anesthesiologists endorsed by the Society for Cardiovascular Angiography and Interventions and the Society of Thoracic Surgeons. *J. Am. Coll. Cardiol.* 2006;48(3):e1-148.

[44] Edmunds LH, Jr. Thromboembolic complications of current cardiac valvular prostheses. *Ann. Thorac. Surg.* 1982;34(1):96-106.

[45] Kontos GJ, Jr., Schaff HV, Orszulak TA, Puga FJ, Pluth JR, Danielson GK. Thrombotic obstruction of disc valves: clinical recognition and surgical management. *Ann. Thorac. Surg.* 1989;48(1):60-65.

[46] Thorburn CW, Morgan JJ, Shanahan MX, Chang VP. Long-term results of tricuspid valve replacement and the problem of prosthetic valve thrombosis. *Am. J. Cardiol.* 1983; 51(7):1128-1132.

[47] Karp R, Sand M. Mechanical prosthesis: old and new. In Heart Valve Replacement and Reconstruction. *Chicago IL: Year Book Medical Publisher Inc.* 1987:235-253.

[48] Akins CW. Mechanical cardiac valvular prostheses. *Ann. Thorac. Surg.* 1991;52(1): 161-172.

[49] Burchfiel CM, Hammermeister KE, Krause-Steinrauf H, Sethi GK, Henderson WG, Crawford MH, Wong M. Left atrial dimension and risk of systemic embolism in patients with a prosthetic heart valve. Department of Veterans Affairs Cooperative Study on Valvular Heart Disease. *J. Am. Coll. Cardiol.* 1990;15(1):32-41.

[50] Reddy DB, Jena A, Venugopal P. Magnetic resonance imaging (MRI) in evaluation of left atrial masses: an in vitro and in vivo study. *J. Cardiovasc. Surg. (Torino).* 1994; 35(4):289-294.

[51] Kuntze CE, Ebels T, Eijgelaar A, Homan van der Heide JN. Rates of thromboembolism with three different mechanical heart valve prostheses: randomised study. *Lancet* 1989; 1(8637):514-517.

[52] Roudaut R, Labbe T, Lorient-Roudaut MF, Gosse P, Baudet E, Fontan F, Besse P, Dallocchio M. Mechanical cardiac valve thrombosis. Is fibrinolysis justified? *Circulation* 1992;86(5 Suppl):II8-15.

[53] Telman G, Kouperberg E, Sprecher E, Yarnitsky D. The nature of microemboli in patients with artificial heart valves. *J. Neuroimaging* 2002;12(1):15-18.

[54] Georgiadis D, Baumgartner RW, Karatschai R, Lindner A, Zerkowski HR. Further evidence of gaseous embolic material in patients with artificial heart valves. *J Thorac Cardiovasc. Surg.* 1998;115(4):808-810.

[55] Braekken SK, Russell D, Brucher R, Svennevig J. Incidence and frequency of cerebral embolic signals in patients with a similar bileaflet mechanical heart valve. *Stroke* 1995; 26(7):1225-1230.

[56] Fuster V, Pumphrey CW, McGoon MD, Chesebro JH, Pluth JR, McGoon DC. Systemic thromboembolism in mitral and aortic Starr-Edwards prostheses: a 10-19 year follow-up. *Circulation* 1982;66(2 Pt 2):I157-161.

[57] Lindblom D, Lindblom U, Qvist J, Lundstrom H. Long-term relative survival rates after heart valve replacement. *J. Am. Coll. Cardiol.* 1990;15(3):566-573.

[58] Skjelland M, Michelsen A, Brosstad F, Svennevig JL, Brucher R, Russell D. Solid cerebral microemboli and cerebrovascular symptoms in patients with prosthetic heart valves. *Stroke* 2008;39(4):1159-1164.

[59] Deklunder G, Roussel M, Lecroart JL, Prat A, Gautier C. Microemboli in cerebral circulation and alteration of cognitive abilities in patients with mechanical prosthetic heart valves. *Stroke* 1998;29(9):1821-1826.

[60] Uekermann J, Suchan B, Daum I, Kseibi S, Perthel M, Laas J. Neuropsychological deficits after mechanical aortic valve replacement. *J. Heart Valve Dis.* 2005;14(3):338-343.

[61] Chung E, Fan L, Degg C, Evans DH. Detection of Doppler embolic signals: psychoacoustic considerations. *Ultrasound Med. Biol.* 2005;31(9):1177-1184.

[62] .Jesty J, Yin W, Perrotta P, Bluestein D. Platelet activation in a circulating flow loop: combined effects of shear stress and exposure time. *Platelets* 2003;14(3):143-149.

[63] Roldan CA, Shively BK, Crawford MH. Valve excrescences: prevalence, evolution and risk for cardioembolism. *J. Am. Coll. Cardiol.* 1997;30(5):1308-1314.

[64] Orsinelli DA, Pearson AC. Detection of prosthetic valve strands by transesophageal echocardiography: clinical significance in patients with suspected cardiac source of embolism. *J. Am. Coll. Cardiol.* 1995;26(7):1713-1718.

[65] Sacco RL, Adams R, Albers G, Alberts MJ, Benavente O, Furie K, Goldstein LB, Gorelick P, Halperin J, Harbaugh R, Johnston SC, Katzan I, Kelly-Hayes M, Kenton EJ, Marks M, Schwamm LH, Tomsick T. Guidelines for prevention of stroke in patients with ischemic stroke or transient ischemic attack: a statement for healthcare professionals from the American Heart Association/American Stroke Association Council on Stroke: co-sponsored by the Council on Cardiovascular Radiology and Intervention: the American Academy of Neurology affirms the value of this guideline. *Stroke* 2006;37(2):577-617.

[66] Salem DN, Stein PD, Al-Ahmad A, Bussey HI, Horstkotte D, Miller N, Pauker SG. Antithrombotic therapy in valvular heart disease--native and prosthetic: the Seventh

ACCP Conference on Antithrombotic and Thrombolytic Therapy. *Chest* 2004;126(3 Suppl):457S-482S.

[67] Kapila A, Hart R. Calcific cerebral emboli and aortic stenosis: detection of computed tomography. *Stroke* 1986;17(4):619-621.

[68] Vernhet H, Torres GF, Laharotte JC, Tournut P, Bierme T, Froment JC, Duquesnel J. Spontaneous calcific cerebral emboli from calcified aortic valve stenosis. *J. Neuroradiol.* 1993;20(1):19-23.

[69] Rancurel G, Marelle L, Vincent D, Catala M, Arzimanoglou A, Vacheron A. Spontaneous calcific cerebral embolus from a calcific aortic stenosis in a middle cerebral artery infarct. *Stroke* 1989;20(5):691-693.

[70] Holley KE, Bahn RC, McGoon DC, Mankin HT. Spontaneous Calcific Embolization Associated with Calcific Aortic Stenosis. *Circulation* 1963;27:197-202.

[71] Brockmeier LB, Adolph RJ, Gustin BW, Holmes JC, Sacks JG. Calcium emboli to the retinal artery in calcific aortic stenosis. *Am. Heart J.* 1981;101(1):32-37.

[72] Aronow WS, Gutstein H, Hsieh FY. Risk factors for thromboembolic stroke in elderly patients with chronic atrial fibrillation. *Am. J. Cardiol.* 1989;63(5):366-367.

[73] Oliveira-Filho J, Massaro AR, Yamamoto F, Bustamante L, Scaff M. Stroke as the first manifestation of calcific aortic stenosis. *Cerebrovasc. Dis.* 2000;10(5):413-416.

[74] Salka S, Almassi GH, Leitschuh ML. Spontaneous coronary artery embolus associated with calcific aortic stenosis. *Chest* 1994;105(4):1289-1290.

[75] Ringelstein EB, Koschorke S, Holling A, Thron A, Lambertz H, Minale C. Computed tomographic patterns of proven embolic brain infarctions. *Ann. Neurol.* 1989;26(6): 759-765.

[76] Kittner SJ, Sharkness CM, Price TR, Plotnick GD, Dambrosia JM, Wolf PA, Mohr JP, Hier DB, Kase CS, Tuhrim S. Infarcts with a cardiac source of embolism in the NINCDS Stroke Data Bank: historical features. *Neurology* 1990;40(2):281-284.

[77] Feinberg WM, Seeger JF, Carmody RF, Anderson DC, Hart RG, Pearce LA. Epidemiologic features of asymptomatic cerebral infarction in patients with nonvalvular atrial fibrillation. *Arch Intern. Med.* 1990;150(11):2340-2344.

[78] Bogousslavsky J, Cachin C, Regli F, Despland PA, Van Melle G, Kappenberger L. Cardiac sources of embolism and cerebral infarction--clinical consequences and vascular concomitants: the Lausanne Stroke Registry. *Neurology* 1991;41(6):855-859.

[79] Cardiogenic brain embolism. The second report of the Cerebral Embolism Task Force. *Arch Neurol.* 1989;46(7):727-743.

[80] Broderick JP, Phillips SJ, O'Fallon WM, Frye RL, Whisnant JP. Relationship of cardiac disease to stroke occurrence, recurrence, and mortality. *Stroke* 1992;23(9):1250-1256.

[81] Boon A, Lodder J, Cheriex E, Kessels F. Risk of stroke in a cohort of 815 patients with calcification of the aortic valve with or without stenosis. *Stroke* 1996;27(5):847-851.

[82] Devereux RB, Kramer-Fox R, Shear MK, Kligfield P, Pini R, Savage DD. Diagnosis and classification of severity of mitral valve prolapse: methodologic, biologic, and prognostic considerations. *Am. Heart J.* 1987;113(5):1265-1280.

[83] Gilon D, Buonanno FS, Joffe MM, Leavitt M, Marshall JE, Kistler JP, Levine RA. Lack of evidence of an association between mitral-valve prolapse and stroke in young patients. *N. Engl. J. Med.* 1999;341(1):8-13.

[84] Freed LA, Levy D, Levine RA, Larson MG, Evans JC, Fuller DL, Lehman B, Benjamin EJ. Prevalence and clinical outcome of mitral-valve prolapse. *N. Engl. J. Med.* 1999; 341(1):1-7.

[85] Barnett HJ, Boughner DR, Taylor DW, Cooper PE, Kostuk WJ, Nichol PM. Further evidence relating mitral-valve prolapse to cerebral ischemic events. *N. Engl. J. Med.* 1980;302(3):139-144.

[86] Scharf RE, Hennerici M, Bluschke V, Lueck J, Kladetzky RG. Cerebral ischemia in young patients: it is associated with mitral valve prolapse and abnormal platelet activity in vivo? *Stroke* 1982;13(4):454-458.

[87] Kouvaras G, Bacoulas G. Association of mitral valve leaflet prolapse with cerebral ischaemic events in the young and early middle-aged patient. *Q. J. Med.* 1985; 56(219): 387-392.

[88] Levine RA, Triulzi MO, Harrigan P, Weyman AE. The relationship of mitral annular shape to the diagnosis of mitral valve prolapse. *Circulation* 1987;75(4):756-767.

[89] Levine RA, Stathogiannis E, Newell JB, Harrigan P, Weyman AE. Reconsideration of echocardiographic standards for mitral valve prolapse: lack of association between leaflet displacement isolated to the apical four chamber view and independent echocardiographic evidence of abnormality. *J. Am. Coll. Cardiol.* 1988;11(5):1010-1019.

[90] Orencia AJ, Petty GW, Khandheria BK, Annegers JF, Ballard DJ, Sicks JD, O'Fallon WM, Whisnant JP. Risk of stroke with mitral valve prolapse in population-based cohort study. *Stroke* 1995;26(1):7-13.

[91] Avierinos JF, Gersh BJ, Melton LJ, 3rd, Bailey KR, Shub C, Nishimura RA, Tajik AJ, Enriquez-Sarano M. Natural history of asymptomatic mitral valve prolapse in the community. *Circulation* 2002;106(11):1355-1361.

[92] St John Sutton M, Weyman AE. Mitral valve prolapse prevalence and complications: an ongoing dialogue. *Circulation* 2002;106(11):1305-1307.

[93] Bonow RO, Carabello BA, Chatterjee K, de Leon AC, Jr., Faxon DP, Freed MD, Gaasch WH, Lytle BW, Nishimura RA, O'Gara PT, O'Rourke RA, Otto CM, Shah PM, Shanewise JS. 2008 focused update incorporated into the ACC/AHA 2006 guidelines for the management of patients with valvular heart disease: a report of the American College of Cardiology/American Heart Association Task Force on Practice Guidelines (Writing Committee to revise the 1998 guidelines for the management of patients with valvular heart disease). Endorsed by the Society of Cardiovascular Anesthesiologists, Society for Cardiovascular Angiography and Interventions, and Society of Thoracic Surgeons. *J. Am. Coll. Cardiol.* 2008;52(13):e1-142.

[94] Bonow RO, Carabello BA, Kanu C, de Leon AC, Jr., Faxon DP, Freed MD, Gaasch WH, Lytle BW, Nishimura RA, O'Gara PT, O'Rourke RA, Otto CM, Shah PM, Shanewise JS, Smith SC, Jr., Jacobs AK, Adams CD, Anderson JL, Antman EM, Fuster V, Halperin JL, Hiratzka LF, Hunt SA, Nishimura R, Page RL, Riegel B. ACC/AHA 2006 guidelines for the management of patients with valvular heart disease: a report of the American College of Cardiology/American Heart Association Task Force on Practice Guidelines (writing committee to revise the 1998 Guidelines for the Management of Patients With Valvular Heart Disease): developed in collaboration with

the Society of Cardiovascular Anesthesiologists: endorsed by the Society for Cardiovascular Angiography and Interventions and the Society of Thoracic Surgeons. *Circulation* 2006;114(5):e84-231.

[95] Vahanian A, Baumgartner H, Bax J, Butchart E, Dion R, Filippatos G, Flachskampf F, Hall R, Iung B, Kasprzak J, Nataf P, Tornos P, Torracca L, Wenink A. Guidelines on the management of valvular heart disease: The Task Force on the Management of Valvular Heart Disease of the European Society of Cardiology. *Eur. Heart J.* 2007; 28(2):230-268.

[96] Habib G. Embolic risk in subacute bacterial endocarditis: determinants and role of transesophageal echocardiography. *Curr. Cardiol. Rep.* 2003;5(2):129-136.

[97] Vilacosta I, Graupner C, San Roman JA, Sarria C, Ronderos R, Fernandez C, Mancini L, Sanz O, Sanmartin JV, Stoermann W. Risk of embolization after institution of antibiotic therapy for infective endocarditis. *J. Am. Coll. Cardiol.* 2002;39(9):1489-1495.

[98] Steckelberg JM, Murphy JG, Ballard D, Bailey K, Tajik AJ, Taliercio CP, Giuliani ER, Wilson WR. Emboli in infective endocarditis: the prognostic value of echocardiography. *Ann. Intern. Med.* 1991;114(8):635-640.

[99] Bayer AS, Bolger AF, Taubert KA, Wilson W, Steckelberg J, Karchmer AW, Levison M, Chambers HF, Dajani AS, Gewitz MH, Newburger JW, Gerber MA, Shulman ST, Pallasch TJ, Gage TW, Ferrieri P. Diagnosis and management of infective endocarditis and its complications. *Circulation* 1998;98(25):2936-2948.

[100] De Castro S, Magni G, Beni S, Cartoni D, Fiorelli M, Venditti M, Schwartz SL, Fedele F, Pandian NG. Role of transthoracic and transesophageal echocardiography in predicting embolic events in patients with active infective endocarditis involving native cardiac valves. *Am. J. Cardiol.* 1997;80(8):1030-1034.

[101] Di Salvo G, Habib G, Pergola V, Avierinos JF, Philip E, Casalta JP, Vailloud JM, Derumeaux G, Gouvernet J, Ambrosi P, Lambert M, Ferracci A, Raoult D, Luccioni R. Echocardiography predicts embolic events in infective endocarditis. *J. Am. Coll. Cardiol.* 2001;37(4):1069-1076.

[102] Thuny F, Di Salvo G, Belliard O, Avierinos JF, Pergola V, Rosenberg V, Casalta JP, Gouvernet J, Derumeaux G, Iarussi D, Ambrosi P, Calabro R, Riberi A, Collart F, Metras D, Lepidi H, Raoult D, Harle JR, Weiller PJ, Cohen A, Habib G. Risk of embolism and death in infective endocarditis: prognostic value of echocardiography: a prospective multicenter study. *Circulation* 2005;112(1):69-75.

[103] Shively BK, Gurule FT, Roldan CA, Leggett JH, Schiller NB. Diagnostic value of transesophageal compared with transthoracic echocardiography in infective endocarditis. *J. Am. Coll. Cardiol.* 1991;18(2):391-397.

[104] Birmingham GD, Rahko PS, Ballantyne F, 3rd. Improved detection of infective endocarditis with transesophageal echocardiography. *Am. Heart J.* 1992;123(3):774-781.

[105] Hill EE, Herijgers P, Claus P, Vanderschueren S, Peetermans WE, Herregods MC. Clinical and echocardiographic risk factors for embolism and mortality in infective endocarditis. *Eur. J. Clin. Microbiol. Infect. Dis.* 2008;27(12):1159-1164.

[106] Kupferwasser LI, Hafner G, Mohr-Kahaly S, Erbel R, Meyer J, Darius H. The presence of infection-related antiphospholipid antibodies in infective endocarditis determines a major risk factor for embolic events. *J. Am. Coll. Cardiol.* 1999;33(5):1365-1371.

[107] Erbel R, Liu F, Ge J, Rohmann S, Kupferwasser I. Identification of high-risk subgroups in infective endocarditis and the role of echocardiography. *Eur. Heart J.* 1995;16(5): 588-602.

[108] Pergola V, Di Salvo G, Habib G, Avierinos JF, Philip E, Vailloud JM, Thuny F, Casalta JP, Ambrosi P, Lambert M, Riberi A, Ferracci A, Mesana T, Metras D, Harle JR, Weiller PJ, Raoult D, Luccioni R. Comparison of clinical and echocardiographic characteristics of Streptococcus bovis endocarditis with that caused by other pathogens. *Am. J. Cardiol.* 2001;88(8):871-875.

[109] Wilson WR, Karchmer AW, Dajani AS, Taubert KA, Bayer A, Kaye D, Bisno AL, Ferrieri P, Shulman ST, Durack DT. Antibiotic treatment of adults with infective endocarditis due to streptococci, enterococci, staphylococci, and HACEK microorganisms. American Heart Association. *JAMA* 1995;274(21):1706-1713.

[110] Rohmann S, Erhel R, Darius H, Makowski T, Meyer J. Effect of antibiotic treatment on vegetation size and complication rate in infective endocarditis. *Clin. Cardiol.* 1997; 20(2):132-140.

[111] Johannessen KA, Nordrehaug JE, von der Lippe G. Left ventricular thrombosis and cerebrovascular accident in acute myocardial infarction. *Br. Heart J.* 1984;51(5):553-556.

[112] Komrad MS, Coffey CE, Coffey KS, McKinnis R, Massey EW, Califf RM. Myocardial infarction and stroke. *Neurology* 1984;34(11):1403-1409.

[113] Keating EC, Gross SA, Schlamowitz RA, Glassman J, Mazur JH, Pitt WA, Miller D. Mural thrombi in myocardial infarctions. Prospective evaluation by two-dimensional echocardiography. *Am. J. Med.* 1983;74(6):989-995.

[114] Weinreich DJ, Burke JF, Pauletto FJ. Left ventricular mural thrombi complicating acute myocardial infarction. Long-term follow-up with serial echocardiography. *Ann. Intern. Med.* 1984;100(6):789-794.

[115] Meltzer RS, Visser CA, Fuster V. Intracardiac thrombi and systemic embolization. *Ann. Intern. Med.* 1986;104(5):689-698.

[116] Szummer KE, Solomon SD, Velazquez EJ, Kilaru R, McMurray J, Rouleau JL, Mahaffey KW, Maggioni AP, Califf RM, Pfeffer MA, White HD. Heart failure on admission and the risk of stroke following acute myocardial infarction: the VALIANT registry. *Eur. Heart J.* 2005;26(20):2114-2119.

[117] Chiarella F, Santoro E, Domenicucci S, Maggioni A, Vecchio C. Predischarge two-dimensional echocardiographic evaluation of left ventricular thrombosis after acute myocardial infarction in the GISSI-3 study. *Am. J. Cardiol.* 1998;81(7):822-827.

[118] Porter A, Kandalker H, Iakobishvili Z, Sagie A, Imbar S, Battler A, Hasdai D. Left ventricular mural thrombus after anterior ST-segment-elevation acute myocardial infarction in the era of aggressive reperfusion therapy--still a frequent complication. *Coron Artery Dis.* 2005;16(5):275-279.

[119] Stratton JR, Resnick AD. Increased embolic risk in patients with left ventricular thrombi. *Circulation* 1987;75(5):1004-1011.

[120]Vecchio C, Chiarella F, Lupi G, Bellotti P, Domenicucci S. Left ventricular thrombus in anterior acute myocardial infarction after thrombolysis. A GISSI-2 connected study. *Circulation* 1991;84(2):512-519.

[121]Loh E, Sutton MS, Wun CC, Rouleau JL, Flaker GC, Gottlieb SS, Lamas GA, Moye LA, Goldhaber SZ, Pfeffer MA. Ventricular dysfunction and the risk of stroke after myocardial infarction. *N. Engl. J. Med.* 1997;336(4):251-257.

[122]Delemarre BJ, Visser CA, Bot H, Dunning AJ. Prediction of apical thrombus formation in acute myocardial infarction based on left ventricular spatial flow pattern. *J. Am. Coll. Cardiol.* 1990;15(2):355-360.

[123]Celik S, Baykan M, Erdol C, Gokce M, Durmus I, Orem C, Kaplan S. Doppler-derived mitral deceleration time as an early predictor of left ventricular thrombus after first anterior acute myocardial infarction. *Am. Heart J.* 2000;140(5):772-776.

[124]Rehan A, Kanwar M, Rosman H, Ahmed S, Ali A, Gardin J, Cohen G. Incidence of post myocardial infarction left ventricular thrombus formation in the era of primary percutaneous intervention and glycoprotein IIb/IIIa inhibitors. A prospective observational study. *Cardiovasc. Ultrasound* 2006;4:20.

[125]Turpie AG, Robinson JG, Doyle DJ, Mulji AS, Mishkel GJ, Sealey BJ, Cairns JA, Skingley L, Hirsh J, Gent M. Comparison of high-dose with low-dose subcutaneous heparin to prevent left ventricular mural thrombosis in patients with acute transmural anterior myocardial infarction. *N. Engl. J. Med.* 1989;320(6):352-357.

[126]Randomised controlled trial of subcutaneous calcium-heparin in acute myocardial infarction. The SCATI (Studio sulla Calciparina nell'Angina e nella Trombosi Ventricolare nell'Infarto) Group. *Lancet* 1989;2(8656):182-186.

[127]Kontny F, Dale J, Abildgaard U, Pedersen TR. Randomized trial of low molecular weight heparin (dalteparin) in prevention of left ventricular thrombus formation and arterial embolism after acute anterior myocardial infarction: the Fragmin in Acute Myocardial Infarction (FRAMI) Study. *J. Am. Coll. Cardiol.* 1997;30(4):962-969.

[128]Smith P. Long-term anticoagulant treatment after acute myocardial infarction. The Warfarin Re-Infarction Study. *Ann. Epidemiol.* 1992;2(4):549-552.

[129]Effect of long-term oral anticoagulant treatment on mortality and cardiovascular morbidity after myocardial infarction. Anticoagulants in the Secondary Prevention of Events in Coronary Thrombosis (ASPECT) Research Group. *Lancet* 1994;343(8896): 499-503.

[130]Randomised double-blind trial of fixed low-dose warfarin with aspirin after myocardial infarction. Coumadin Aspirin Reinfarction Study (CARS) Investigators. *Lancet* 1997; 350(9075):389-396.

[131]Antman EM, Anbe DT, Armstrong PW, Bates ER, Green LA, Hand M, Hochman JS, Krumholz HM, Kushner FG, Lamas GA, Mullany CJ, Ornato JP, Pearle DL, Sloan MA, Smith SC, Jr., Alpert JS, Anderson JL, Faxon DP, Fuster V, Gibbons RJ, Gregoratos G, Halperin JL, Hiratzka LF, Hunt SA, Jacobs AK. ACC/AHA guidelines for the management of patients with ST-elevation myocardial infarction--executive summary: a report of the American College of Cardiology/American Heart Association Task Force on Practice Guidelines (Writing Committee to Revise the 1999 Guidelines

for the Management of Patients With Acute Myocardial Infarction). *Circulation* 2004; 110(5):588-636.

[132]Morrow D, Gersh B, Braunwald E. Chronic ischemic heart disease, in Braunwald E (ed): Heart Disease: A textbook of cardiovascular Medicine. Philadelphia. Saunders. 2004:1332.

[133]Buckberg GD. Defining the relationship between akinesia and dyskinesia and the cause of left ventricular failure after anterior infarction and reversal of remodeling to restoration. *J. Thorac. Cardiovasc. Surg.* 1998;116(1):47-49.

[134]Dor V, Sabatier M, Di Donato M, Montiglio F, Toso A, Maioli M. Efficacy of endoventricular patch plasty in large postinfarction akinetic scar and severe left ventricular dysfunction: comparison with a series of large dyskinetic scars. *J. Thorac. Cardiovasc. Surg.* 1998;116(1):50-59.

[135]Di Donato M, Sabatier M, Dor V, Toso A, Maioli M, Fantini F. Akinetic versus dyskinetic postinfarction scar: relation to surgical outcome in patients undergoing endoventricular circular patch plasty repair. *J. Am. Coll. Cardiol.* 1997;29(7):1569-1575.

[136]Grieco JG, Montoya A, Sullivan HJ, Bakhos M, Foy BK, Blakeman B, Pifarre R. Ventricular aneurysm due to blunt chest injury. *Ann. Thorac. Surg.* 1989; 47(2):322-329.

[137]Cooley DA, Frazier OH, Duncan JM, Reul GJ, Krajcer Z. Intracavitary repair of ventricular aneurysm and regional dyskinesia. *Ann. Surg.* 1992;215(5):417-423; discussion 423-414.

[138]Faxon DP, Ryan TJ, Davis KB, McCabe CH, Myers W, Lesperance J, Shaw R, Tong TG. Prognostic significance of angiographically documented left ventricular aneurysm from the Coronary Artery Surgery Study (CASS). *Am. J. Cardiol.* 1982;50(1):157-164.

[139]Cosgrove DM, Lytle BW, Taylor PC, Stewart RW, Golding LA, Mahfood S, Goormastic M, Loop FD. Ventricular aneurysm resection. Trends in surgical risk. *Circulation* 1989;79(6 Pt 2):I97-101.

[140]de Oliveira JA. Heart aneurysm in Chagas' disease. *Rev. Inst. Med. Trop. Sao Paulo.* 1998;40(5):301-307.

[141]Silverman KJ, Hutchins GM, Bulkley BH. Cardiac sarcoid: a clinicopathologic study of 84 unselected patients with systemic sarcoidosis. *Circulation* 1978;58(6):1204-1211.

[142]Davila JC, Enriquez F, Bergoglio S, Voci G, Wells CR. Congenital aneurysm of the left ventricle. *Ann. Thorac. Surg.* 1965;1(6):697-710.

[143]Mills NL, Everson CT, Hockmuth DR. Technical advances in the treatment of left ventricular aneurysm. *Ann. Thorac. Surg.* 1993;55(3):792-800.

[144]Reeder GS, Lengyel M, Tajik AJ, Seward JB, Smith HC, Danielson GK. Mural thrombus in left ventricular aneurysm: incidence, role of angiography, and relation between anticoagulation and embolization. *Mayo Clin. Proc.* 1981;56(2):77-81.

[145]Lapeyre AC, 3rd, Steele PM, Kazmier FJ, Chesebro JH, Vlietstra RE, Fuster V. Systemic embolism in chronic left ventricular aneurysm: incidence and the role of anticoagulation. *J. Am. Coll. Cardiol.* 1985;6(3):534-538.

[146]Cabin HS, Roberts WC. Left ventricular aneurysm, intraaneurysmal thrombus and systemic embolus in coronary heart disease. *Chest* 1980;77(5):586-590.

[147]Simpson MT, Oberman A, Kouchoukos NT, Rogers WJ. Prevalence of mural thrombi and systemic embolization with left ventricular aneurysm. Effect of anticoagulation therapy. *Chest* 1980;77(4):463-469.

[148]Grondin P, Kretz JG, Bical O, Donzeau-Gouge P, Petitclerc R, Campeau L. Natural history of saccular aneurysms of the left ventricle. *J. Thorac. Cardiovasc. Surg.* 1979; 77(1):57-64.

[149]Meizlish JL, Berger HJ, Plankey M, Errico D, Levy W, Zaret BL. Functional left ventricular aneurysm formation after acute anterior transmural myocardial infarction. Incidence, natural history, and prognostic implications. *N. Engl. J. Med.* 1984;311(16): 1001-1006.

[150]Keren A, Goldberg S, Gottlieb S, Klein J, Schuger C, Medina A, Tzivoni D, Stern S. Natural history of left ventricular thrombi: their appearance and resolution in the posthospitalization period of acute myocardial infarction. *J. Am. Coll. Cardiol.* 1990; 15(4):790-800.

[151]Oechslin EN, Attenhofer Jost CH, Rojas JR, Kaufmann PA, Jenni R. Long-term follow-up of 34 adults with isolated left ventricular noncompaction: a distinct cardiomyopathy with poor prognosis. *J. Am. Coll. Cardiol.* 2000;36(2):493-500.

[152]Dusek J, Ostadal B, Duskova M. Postnatal persistence of spongy myocardium with embryonic blood supply. *Arch Pathol.* 1975;99(6):312-317.

[153]Tong KL, Ding ZP. Isolated non-compaction of ventricular myocardium: a report of three cases. *Ann. Acad. Med. Singapore* 2001;30(5):539-541.

[154]Shah CP, Nagi KS, Thakur RK, Boughner DR, Xie B. Spongy left ventricular myocardium in an adult. *Tex. Heart Inst. J.* 1998;25(2):150-151.

[155]Ichida F, Hamamichi Y, Miyawaki T, Ono Y, Kamiya T, Akagi T, Hamada H, Hirose O, Isobe T, Yamada K, Kurotobi S, Mito H, Miyake T, Murakami Y, Nishi T, Shinohara M, Seguchi M, Tashiro S, Tomimatsu H. Clinical features of isolated noncompaction of the ventricular myocardium: long-term clinical course, hemodynamic properties, and genetic background. *J. Am. Coll. Cardiol.* 1999;34(1): 233-240.

[156]Chin TK, Perloff JK, Williams RG, Jue K, Mohrmann R. Isolated noncompaction of left ventricular myocardium. A study of eight cases. *Circulation* 1990;82(2):507-513.

[157]Ritter M, Oechslin E, Sutsch G, Attenhofer C, Schneider J, Jenni R. Isolated noncompaction of the myocardium in adults. *Mayo Clin. Proc.* 1997;72(1):26-31.

[158]Kenton AB, Sanchez X, Coveler KJ, Makar KA, Jimenez S, Ichida F, Murphy RT, Elliott PM, McKenna W, Bowles NE, Towbin JA, Bowles KR. Isolated left ventricular noncompaction is rarely caused by mutations in G4.5, alpha-dystrobrevin and FK Binding Protein-12. *Mol. Genet. Metab.* 2004;82(2):162-166.

[159]Skowasch D, Lentini S, Kubini R, Luderitz B, Bauriedel G. [Noncompaction of the left ventricular myocardium. Case report and review of the literature]. *Z. Kardiol.* 2002; 91(6):503-507.

[160]MacGowan SW, Sidhu P, Aherne T, Luke D, Wood AE, Neligan MC, McGovern E. Atrial myxoma: national incidence, diagnosis and surgical management. *Ir. J. Med. Sci.* 1993;162(6):223-226.

[161]Stollberger C, Finsterer J. Left ventricular hypertrabeculation/noncompaction and stroke or embolism. *Cardiology* 2005;103(2):68-72.

[162]Johansson L. Histogenesis of cardiac myxomas. An immunohistochemical study of 19 cases, including one with glandular structures, and review of the literature. *Arch Pathol. Lab. Med.* 1989;113(7):735-741.

[163]Hart R, Albers G, Koudstaal P. Cardioembolic stroke. In: Gisberg MD, Bogousslavsky J, editors. . *Cerebrovascualr disease: pathophysiology, diagnosis and management.* . 1998;London: Blackwell Science.:1932-1429.

[164]Reynen K. Frequency of primary tumors of the heart. *Am. J. Cardiol.* 1996;77(1):107.

[165]Kirschner LS, Sandrini F, Monbo J, Lin JP, Carney JA, Stratakis CA. Genetic heterogeneity and spectrum of mutations of the PRKAR1A gene in patients with the carney complex. *Hum. Mol. Genet.* 2000;9(20):3037-3046.

[166]Pinede L, Duhaut P, Loire R. Clinical presentation of left atrial cardiac myxoma. A series of 112 consecutive cases. *Medicine (Baltimore).* 2001;80(3):159-172.

[167]Reynen K. Cardiac myxomas. *N. Engl. J. Med.* 1995;333(24):1610-1617.

[168]Sellke FW, Lemmer JH, Jr., Vandenberg BF, Ehrenhaft JL. Surgical treatment of cardiac myxomas: long-term results. *Ann. Thorac. Surg.* 1990;50(4):557-561.

[169]Knepper LE, Biller J, Adams HP, Jr., Bruno A. Neurologic manifestations of atrial myxoma. A 12-year experience and review. *Stroke* 1988;19(11):1435-1440.

[170]Sandok BA, von Estorff I, Giuliani ER. CNS embolism due to atrial myxoma: clinical features and diagnosis. *Arch Neurol.* 1980;37(8):485-488.

[171]Butler MJ, Adams HP, Jr., Hiratzka LF. Recurrent cerebral embolism from a right atrial myxoma. *Ann. Neurol.* 1986;19(6):608-609.

[172]McWhirter WR, Tetteh-Lartey EV. A case of atrial myxoma. *Br. Heart J.* 1974;36(8): 839-840.

[173]St John Sutton MG, Mercier LA, Giuliani ER, Lie JT. Atrial myxomas: a review of clinical experience in 40 patients. *Mayo Clin. Proc.* 1980;55(6):371-376.

[174]Bjessmo S, Ivert T. Cardiac myxoma: 40 years' experience in 63 patients. *Ann. Thorac. Surg.* 1997;63(3):697-700.

[175]Hutton JT. Atrial myxoma as a cause of progressive dementia. *Arch Neurol.* 1981; 38(8):533.

[176]Bienfait HP, Moll LC. Fatal cerebral embolism in a young patient with an occult left atrial myxoma. *Clin. Neurol. Neurosurg.* 2001;103(1):37-38.

[177]Lee VH, Connolly HM, Brown RD, Jr. Central nervous system manifestations of cardiac myxoma. *Arch Neurol.* 2007;64(8):1115-1120.

[178]Ekinci EI, Donnan GA. Neurological manifestations of cardiac myxoma: a review of the literature and report of cases. *Intern. Med. J.* 2004;34(5):243-249.

[179]Burke AP, Virmani R. Cardiac myxoma. A clinicopathologic study. *Am. J. Clin. Pathol.* 1993;100(6):671-680.

[180]Furuya K, Sasaki T, Yoshimoto Y, Okada Y, Fujimaki T, Kirino T. Histologically verified cerebral aneurysm formation secondary to embolism from cardiac myxoma. Case report. *J. Neurosurg.* 1995;83(1):170-173.

[181]Josephson SA, Johnston SC. Multiple stable fusiform intracranial aneurysms following atrial myxoma. *Neurology* 2005;64(3):526.

[182]Jean WC, Walski-Easton SM, Nussbaum ES. Multiple intracranial aneurysms as delayed complications of an atrial myxoma: case report. *Neurosurgery* 2001;49(1):200-202; discussion 202-203.

[183]Roeltgen DP, Weimer GR, Patterson LF. Delayed neurologic complications of left atrial myxoma. *Neurology* 1981;31(1):8-13.

[184]Gee GT, Bazan C, 3rd, Jinkins JR. Imaging of cerebral infarction caused by atrial myxoma. *Neuroradiology* 1994;36(4):271-272.

[185]Nomeir AM, Watts LE, Seagle R, Joyner CR, Corman C, Prichard RW. Intracardiac myxomas: twenty-year echocardiographic experience with review of the literature. *J. Am. Soc. Echocardiogr.* 1989;2(2):139-150.

[186]Kapral MK, Silver FL. Preventive health care, 1999 update: 2. Echocardiography for the detection of a cardiac source of embolus in patients with stroke. Canadian Task Force on Preventive Health Care. *CMAJ* 1999;161(8):989-996.

[187]Castells E, Ferran V, Octavio de Toledo MC, Calbet JM, Benito M, Fontanillas C, Granados J, Obi CL, Saura E. Cardiac myxomas: surgical treatment, long-term results and recurrence. *J. Cardiovasc. Surg. (Torino).* 1993;34(1):49-53.

[188]Blondeau P. Primary cardiac tumors--French studies of 533 cases. *Thorac. Cardiovasc. Surg.* 1990;38 Suppl 2:192-195.

[189]Gowda RM, Khan IA, Nair CK, Mehta NJ, Vasavada BC, Sacchi TJ. Cardiac papillary fibroelastoma: a comprehensive analysis of 725 cases. *Am. Heart J.* 2003;146(3):404-410.

[190]Gagliardi RJ, Franken RA, Protti GG. Cardiac papillary fibroelastoma and stroke in a young man--etiology and treatment. *Cerebrovasc. Dis.* 2008;25(1-2):185-187.

[191]Salcedo EE, Cohen GI, White RD, Davison MB. Cardiac tumors: diagnosis and management. *Curr. Probl. Cardiol.* 1992;17(2):73-137.

[192]Graca A, Nunes R, Costeira A, Almeida J, Bastos P. Cardiac papillary fibroelastoma of a mitral valve chordae revealed by stroke. *Rev. Port Cardiol.* 1999;18(10):937-939.

[193]Klarich KW, Enriquez-Sarano M, Gura GM, Edwards WD, Tajik AJ, Seward JB. Papillary fibroelastoma: echocardiographic characteristics for diagnosis and pathologic correlation. *J. Am. Coll. Cardiol.* 1997;30(3):784-790.

[194]Giannesini C, Kubis N, N'Guyen A, Wassef M, Mikol J, Woimant F. Cardiac papillary fibroelastoma: aA rare cause of ischemic stroke in the young. *Cerebrovasc. Dis.* 1999; 9(1):45-49.

[195]Sun JP, Asher CR, Yang XS, Cheng GG, Scalia GM, Massed AG, Griffin BP, Ratliff NB, Stewart WJ, Thomas JD. Clinical and echocardiographic characteristics of papillary fibroelastomas: a retrospective and prospective study in 162 patients. *Circulation* 2001;103(22):2687-2693.

[196]Mc Allister H, Fenoglio J. Tumors of the cardiovascular system. In: Mc Allyster HA, Fenoglio JJ, editors. Atlas of tumor pathology. *Washigton DC: Armed Forces Institute of Pathology* 1978.

[197]Kanarek SE, Wright P, Liu J, Boglioli LR, Bajwa AS, Hall M, Kort S. Multiple fibroelastomas: a case report and review of the literature. *J. Am. Soc. Echocardiogr.* 2003;16(4):373-376.

[198] Kasarskis EJ, O'Connor W, Earle G. Embolic stroke from cardiac papillary fibroelastomas. *Stroke* 1988;19(9):1171-1173.

[199] Edwards FH, Hale D, Cohen A, Thompson L, Pezzella AT, Virmani R. Primary cardiac valve tumors. *Ann. Thorac. Surg.* 1991;52(5):1127-1131.

[200] Pomerance A. Papillary "tumours" of the heart valves. *J. Pathol. Bacteriol.* 1961;81: 135-140.

[201] Matsumoto N, Sato Y, Kusama J, Matsuo S, Kinukawa N, Kunimasa T, Ichiyama I, Takahashi H, Kimura S, Orime Y, Saito S. Multiple papillary fibroelastomas of the aortic valve: case report. *Int. J. Cardiol.* 2007;122(1):e1-3.

[202] Grinda JM, Couetil JP, Chauvaud S, D'Attellis N, Berrebi A, Fabiani JN, Deloche A, Carpentier A. Cardiac valve papillary fibroelastoma: surgical excision for revealed or potential embolization. *J. Thorac. Cardiovasc. Surg.* 1999;117(1):106-110.

[203] Hicks KA, Kovach JA, Frishberg DP, Wiley TM, Gurczak PB, Vernalis MN. Echocardiographic evaluation of papillary fibroelastoma: a case report and review of the literature. *J. Am. Soc. Echocardiogr.* 1996;9(3):353-360.

[204] Roberts WC. Papillary fibroelastomas of the heart. *Am. J. Cardiol.* 1997;80(7):973-975.

[205] Nawaz MZ, Lander AR, Schussler JM, Grayburn PA, Hamman BL, Roberts WC. Tumor excision versus valve replacement for papillary fibroelastoma involving the mitral valve. *Am. J. Cardiol.* 2006;97(5):759-764.

[206] Veinot JP. Fibroelastoma and embolic stroke. *Circulation* 1999;99(20):2709-2712.

[207] Espada R, Talwalker NG, Wilcox G, Kleiman NS, Verani MS. Visualization of ventricular fibroelastoma with a video-assisted thoracoscope. *Ann. Thorac. Surg.* 1997; 63(1):221-223.

[208] Woo YJ, Grand TJ, Weiss SJ. Robotic resection of an aortic valve papillary fibroelastoma. *Ann. Thorac. Surg.* 2005;80(3):1100-1102.

[209] Brown RD, Jr., Khandheria BK, Edwards WD. Cardiac papillary fibroelastoma: a treatable cause of transient ischemic attack and ischemic stroke detected by transesophageal echocardiography. *Mayo Clin. Proc.* 1995;70(9):863-868.

[210] Saw W, Nicholls S, Trim G, Thomson D, Hughes C, Mitchell S, Leitch J. Papillary fibroelastoma, a rare but potentially treatable cause of embolic stroke: report of three cases. *Heart Lung Circ.* 2001;10(2):105-107.

In: Cerebral Ischemia in Young Adults
Editors: A. Pezzini and A. Padovani

ISBN 978-1-60741-627-2

Chapter 15

Thrombophilic Disorders

Francesco Guercini, Stefano Radicchia, Maurizio Paciaroni and Valeria Caso
Division of Internal and Cardiovascular Medicine, Stroke Unit,
Santa Maria della Misericordia Hospital, University of Perugia, Italy

Abstract

Thrombophilia is defined as an enhanced tendency to form intravascular thrombi, which may be arterial or venous. Of the inherited thrombophilias, factor V Leiden and the prothrombin 20210 mutation have been associated with stroke, but the strength of this association appears to be higher in children and young adults. The risk of stroke in patients with these mutations is substantially increased by concomitant exposure to oral contraceptives. The diagnosis of thrombophilia should be considered in stroke patients who are young, have a family history of thrombosis, or have recurrent strokes, or no obvious cause of infarction. Various strategies have been developed that can guide the selection of patients (based on specific characteristics) and tests in the evaluation of thrombophilias. Although the diagnosis of thrombophilia could explain the potential stroke etiology, the best regimen for secondary prevention treatment for the majority of thrombophilias is still unknown.

Introduction

The pathogenesis of both arterial and venous diseases is complex and involves multiple genetic and environmental factors related to atherosclerosis and thrombosis plus interactions among these factors. In addition to well-established risk factors such as diabetes, dyslipidemia, hypertension, obesity, family history and smoking, an increasing number of haemostatic factors have been recently reported to be implicated in arterial disease. Over the last two decades, considerable gains have been made in the understanding of various thrombophilia defects.

However, it is still not known whether information obtained from thrombophilia screening can be considered relevant enough for treatment decision making. In fact, in the setting of arterial thrombosis, the relationship between thrombophilia and clinical events is less well documented than in venous thromboembolism.

In this chapter, coagulation cascade and its antithrombotic pathway along with a description of the principle thrombophilic defects and their roles in vascular ischemic thrombosis and ischemic stroke is outlined.

Coagulation Cascade

Haemostasis is a physiologic mechanism that contributes to blood fluidity. The coagulation of blood is mediated by cellular components and soluble plasma proteins. In response to vascular injury, circulating platelets adhere, aggregate, and provide cell-surface phospholipid for the assembly of blood-clotting enzyme complexes.

Primary haemostasis is the name given to the process of platelet plug formation at injury sites. This occurs within seconds of injury and is necessary for stopping capillary, small arteriole and venule haemorrhages. *Secondary haemostasis* is characterized by reactions of the plasma coagulation system that result in fibrin formation, which requires several minutes for completion. The fibrin strands that are produced strengthen the primary haemostatic plug. This process is particularly important in the larger vessels to avoid re-bleeding hours or days after injury. Although they are commonly described as two distinct events, primary and secondary hemostasis are closely linked. For example, activated platelets accelerate plasma coagulation and products of the plasma coagulation reaction, such as thrombin, inducing platelet activation. Effective primary haemostasis requires three clinical events: platelet adhesion, granule release, and platelet aggregation. Within a few seconds of injury, platelets adhere to collagen fibrils in the vascular sub-endothelium by at least two collagen receptors, glycoprotein (Gp)Ia/IIa, a member of integrin family, and GpVI. This interaction with collagen is stabilized by the von Willebrand factor (vWF), an adhesive glycoprotein that allows platelets to remain attached to the vessel wall despite the high shear forces generated within the vascular lumen. vWF accomplishes this task by creating a link between a platelet receptor site on Gp Ib/IX and collagen fibrils. The adherent activated platelets release preformed granule constituents and generate de novo mediators. The binding of agonists such as epinephrine, collagen or thrombin to platelet surface receptors activates two membrane enzymes: phospholipase C and phospholipase A2. These enzymes catalyse the release of arachidonic acid from two of the major membrane phospholipids, phosphatidylinositol and phospahtidylcoline. Initially, a small quantity of the released arachidonic acid is converted into thromboxane A2 (TXA2), which, in turn, can activate phospholipase C. The formation of TXA2 from arachidonic acid is mediated by enzyme ciclooxigenase. This enzyme is inhibited by aspirin and non-steroidal anti-inflammatory drugs. Platelet signal transduction pathways are complex. Potential platelet-activating agents bind to a surface receptor that initiate a cascade of signalling events. The four principle classes of receptors are: GpIb/IX complex that binds vWF; integrin family receptors GpIIB/IIIa binds fibrinogen; GpIa/IIa binds collagen and finally GpVI/FcγRII binds collagen. Following activation, platelets secrete their granule contents into plasma. Endoglycosidases and heparin-cleaving enzymes are released from lysosomes, as calcium, serotonin, and ADP are released from the dense granules. At the same time, several proteins, including vWF, fibronectin, fibrinogen, thrombospondin and platelet-derived growth factor (PDGF) are released from α granules.

Once the primary haemostatic plug is formed, plasma coagulation proteins are activated to initiate secondary haemostasis. The coagulation process consists of four reactions that culminates in the production of sufficient quantities of thrombin to convert a small amount of plasma fibrinogen into fibrin. Each of the four reactions requires the formation of surface-bound complexes and the conversion of inactive precursor proteins into active proteases by limited proteolysis and each of these is regulated by both plasma and cellular cofactors and calcium. In reaction 1, the intrinsic or contact phase of coagulation, three plasma proteins, Hageman factor (factor XII), high-molecular-weight kininogen (HMWK), and prekallikrein (PK), form a complex on vascular subendothelial collagen. After binding to HMWK, factor XII is slowly converted into an active protease (XIIa), which then activates PK into kallikrein and factor XI into XIa.

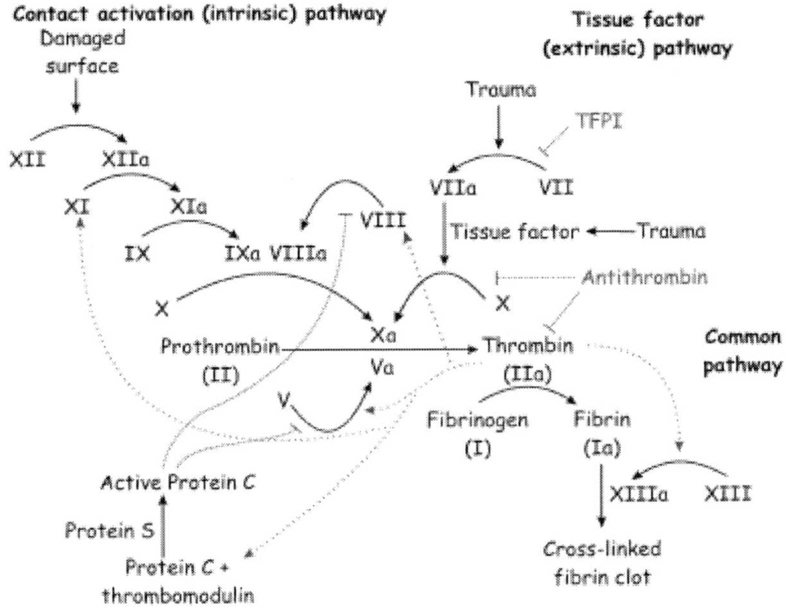

TFPI: Tissue factor pathway inhibitor; red lines: antithrombotics mechanism or negative feedback; green lines: positive feedback.

Figure 1. The pathways of blood coagulation and antithrombotics mechanism.

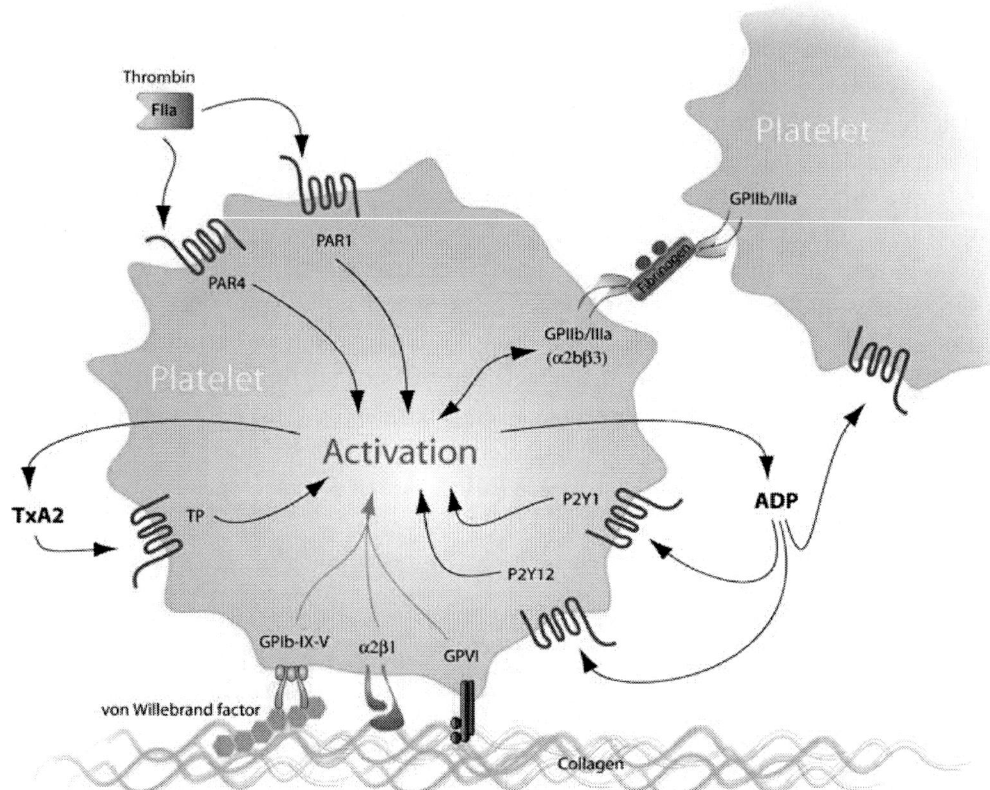

PAR: protease activated receptor; TxA2: Thromboxane A2; ADP: adenosine diphosphate.

Figure 2. Platelet activation.

Reaction 2 provides a second pathway to initiate coagulation by turning factor VII into a protease. In this extrinsic, or tissue factor-dependent pathway, a complex forms among factor VII, calcium, and the tissue factor, an ubiquitous lipoprotein present in cellular membranes and exposed because of cellular injury. Furthermore, factor VII and three other coagulation proteins-factors II (prothrombin), IX, and X require calcium and vitamin K for biological activity. These proteins are synthesized in the liver, where a vitamin K-dependent carboxylase catalyses a unique post-translational modification that adds a second carboxyl group to certain glutamic acid residues. Pairs of these digamma-carboxyglutamic acid residues bind to calcium, which in turn alter protein formation which then bind to phospholipid surfaces and produce biologic activity. Inhibition of this process, using vitamin K antagonists, is the rationale of one of the most common forms of anticoagulant therapy.

In reaction 3, factor X is activated by the proteases generated in two previous reactions. In the first, a calcium and lipid-dependent complex is formed between factors VIII, IX and X. Within this complex, factor IX is first converted into IXa by factor XIa that had already been generated within the intrinsic pathway. Factor X is then activated by factor IXa together with factor VIII. Alternatively, both factors IX and X can be activated more directly by factor VIIa, generated by extrinsic pathway. Reaction 4, the final step, converts prothrombin into thrombin in the presence of cofactor V, calcium and phospholipid Although prothrombin conversion can take place on various natural and artificial phospholipd-rich surfaces, it proceeds several thousand times faster on either activated platelet or endothelial cell surfaces. Thrombin has multiple functions in haemostasis. Although its principal role in haemostasis is the conversion of fibrinogen into fibrin, it also activates factors V, VIII, XI and XIII, and stimulates platelet aggregation. Following the release of fibrinopeptides A and B from α and β chains of fibrinogen, the modified molecule, now called fibrin monomer, polymerizes into an insoluble gel. The fibrin polymer is then stabilized by the cross-linking of individual chains by factor XIIIa, a plasma transglutaminase. Clot lysis and vessel repair begin immediately after the formation of the definitive haemostatic plug. Three potential activators of the fybrinolitic system are Hageman fragments; urinary plasminogen activator (uPA) or urokinase and tissue plasminogen activator (tPA). The principle physiologic activators, tPA and uPA, released from endothelial cells convert the plasminogen, present inside the fibrin clot, into plasmin. Then, plasmin degrades fibrin polymer into small fragments. Although plasmin can also degrade fibrinogen, the reaction remains localized because tPA and some forms of uPA activate plasminogen more effectively when they are absorbed inside the fibrin clots. The circulating plasmin is rapidly bound and neutralized by the alfa2 plasmin inhibitor and endothelial cells release a plasminogen activator inhibitor (PAI) 1, which blocks the action of tPA. Only a small quantity of each coagulation enzyme is converted into an active form. Consequently, the haemostatic plug does not propagate beyond the injury site. These regulation processes are important, since each millimetre of blood contains enough clotting material to clot all the fibrinogen in the body in about 10 to 15 seconds [1]. Blood fluidity is maintained by blood flow, the absorption of coagulation factors to surfaces, their trapping in the emerging clot and by multiple inhibitors in plasma [2]. These latter factors reduce the concentration of the above potent enzymes and cofactors reduce reaction rates. Antithrombin, proteins C and S, and tissue factor pathway inhibitor (TFPI) are important inhibitors that maintain blood fluidity. These inhibitors have distinct modes of action. Antithrombin forms complexes with all serine protease coagulation factors except factor VII. Rates of complex formation are accelerated by heparin and heparin-like molecules on the surface of endothelial cells. Protein C is converted into an active protease by thrombin after it is bound to an endothelial protein called thrombomodulin. Activated protein C then inactivates the two plasma cofactors V and VIII by limited proteolysis, which slows down two critical coagulation reactions. Protein C also stimulates the release of tPA from endothelial cells. The inhibitory function of protein C is enhanced by protein S. Finally, TFPI blocks the pathway of the extrinsic way. Reduced levels of these inhibitors or dysfunctional forms of these molecules result in a hypercoagulable or prothrombotic state. In addition, a particularly common inheritable defect associated with a hypercoagulable state is the presence of a form of factor V (factor V Leiden) that is resistant to protein C inhibition.

Thrombophilia

Thrombophilia may be defined as an increased risk of developing thrombosis, may be congenital or acquired, and may affect the venous side, the arterial side, or both. Nonetheless, the term thrombophilia is usually used for venous thromboembolism (VTE).

A seminal step forward toward understanding the pathophysiology of venous VTE was made in the second half of the 19th century by a work of Rokitansky and later confirmed by Virchow [3,4]. On the basis of pathologic observations, carried out mainly on fatal cases of postpartum VTE, the two abovementioned pathologists independently identified the time-honored triad of pathogenetic factors: damage to the vein, slowing of venous blood flow, and changes in the blood leading to an increased tendency to form the clots (hypercoagulability). The biochemical and molecular bases of the third component of the triad, hypercoagulability, were later identified.

History of Thrombophilia

The existence of inherited factors which increase the risks of VTE through the induction of hypercoagulability was first described by Egeberg [5] in a Norwegian family. These family members presented venous thrombosis at a young age along with a high tendency of recurrence. In fact, several family members had a reduction in plasma antithrombin of up to half-normal levels, and this insufficiency was closely related to thrombotic tendency. These findings can be considered biologically plausible, as antithrombin is a naturally occurring anticoagulant protein that inactivates the main coagulation enzymes (thrombin, activated factor IX, activated factor X and activated factor XI). However, the antithrombin deficiency has been reported to be responsible of only few congenital VTE cases (0.1% or less of the patients with a first-ever thrombotic episode).

In the early 1980s, Griffin and Esmon et al., [6-8] independently proved that protein C and protein S deficiencies were inherited risk factors for VTE, accounting for approximately 0.5% of first-ever episodes of thrombosis. The active enzymatic form of protein C (activated protein C [APC]) with its cofactor protein S deactivates coagulation cofactors V and VII, thus explaining why the deficiency of protein C and S leads to a decreased inactivation of these cofactors and finally to a hypercoagulable state. In heterozygote subjects, the reductions in proteins C and S (and antithrombin) can lead to half normal plasma levels, which can then increase the risk of venous thrombosis [6-8]. In homozygotes, very low levels of protein C or protein S are associated with more severe thrombotic symptoms which are life threatening and often occur in the neonatal period [9,10]. However, it is still believed that homozygosis for antithrombin is incompatible with life. Despite this evidence on the genetic basis of hypercoagulability, most cases of VTE, particularly those occurring in the absence of acquired risk factors remain unexplained. In 1993, Dahlbäck [11], et. al, demonstrated an association between the inherited resistance of plasma to the anticoagulant action of APC and the development of VTE. This finding was confirmed Griffin et al [12], Koster et al [13], and Faioni et. al, in the same year [14].

The genetic basis of APCR remained unclear until 1994, when Rogier Bertina et al [15] from Leiden, demonstrated APCR to be associated with a missense mutation in the gene encoding coagulation factor V (G1691A). This mutation, called factor V Leiden, slows the cleavage of the activated form of this cofactor by APC and leads to an increased function in activated factor V, that in turn, causes a hypercoagulable state [16]. The clinical relevances of APCR and factor V Leiden were subsequently corroborated by the findings that these changes are present in approximately 20% of patients who have a first-ever episode of VTE [13] and that in populations of European descent, the background frequency of this mutation is at least 2-3% higher. The high frequency of the factor V Leiden mutation, which originates from a single founder, has led to interesting evolutionary hypotheses. During the so-called fight or flight pattern of primitive life, hypercoagulability that is associated with this mutation may have conferred advantages to humans, especially favouring women by reducing blood loss during delivery. The discoveries of APCR and factor V Leiden were breakthroughs in clinical medicine. After the original description of the factor V Leiden, Bertina's research group [17] added further understanding to the pathogenesis of inherited thrombophilia. This group identified a gain-of-function mutation in the gene which encodes the coagulation zymogen, factor II or prothrombin, leading to hypercoagulability and thrombosis. The substitution of guanine by adenine at the position 20210 in the 3' noncoding region of the gene promotes high prothrombin plasma levels and thereby produces a hypercoagulability. Overall, the two above mentioned gain-of-function mutations, alone or in association with acquired risk factors, are responsible for approximately 20 to 30% of first-ever unselected cases of VTE and 60 to 70% of recurrent cases along with thrombosis occurring in young patients.

Inherited Thrombophilia

The main causes of congenital or inherited thrombophilia may be broadly classified as a function loss such as antithrombin (AT), protein C (PC), and protein S (PS) deficiencies, or a function gain such as activated PC resistance (APCR) due to factor V Arg506Gln mutation (factor V Leiden), hyperprothrombinemia due to the presence of the prothrombin mutation G20210A, or dysfibrinogenemia and possibly moderate hyperhomocystinemia due to alterations of the relevant metabolic pathways.

Acquired Deficiencies

Acquired AT, protein C and protein S deficiencies have been reported to produce a prothrombotic state related to brain infarction. Although extensive epidemiological studies have not been performed as of yet, acquired anticoagulant protein deficiencies have been associated with stroke in particular clinical settings. Many of these clinical situations are reported in the Table.

Reduced levels of the anticoagulant proteins have been found prior to surgery in pregnant women or in women taking oral contraceptives and in patients with malignancies, hepatic failures or nephrotic syndromes. Acute anticoagulant protein level fluctations can also be observed after plasmapheresis or hemodialysis. When transient ischemic attacks (TIA), stroke, or amaurosis fugax are encountered in the above patients, a thorough examination must be carried out to uncover any possible prothrombotic states.

Antithrombin Deficiency

Antithrombin complexes with activated coagulation proteins block their biologic activity. The rate of this reaction is enhanced by heparin and heparin-like molecules within the vessel walls or endothelial cells. Plasma antithrombin III content is 5 to 15 mg/L and if its values are only slightly below normal, they increase thrombosis risk. The antithrombin III concentration is measured by immunoassay and the plasma antithrombin and heparin cofactor activities are assessed by functional assay. The results of this assay is measured as a percentage of normal activity. “Normal” or 100% is considered the average activity in plasma samples from at least 30 healthy persons. The range is considered between 80 and 120%. The most common defect (1:2,000 individuals) is classified as mild (heterozygous) antithrombin deficiency. Dysfunctional antithrombin molecules having mutations on either the serine protease or heparin-binding site or the activation of heparin inhibitor have also been described. Furthermore, two distinct types of antithrombin deficiency have been identified. Their definitions are based on whether plasma levels are reduced (type I), or whether plasma levels are essentially normal but antithrombin functionality compromised (type II). Acquired antithrombin deficiency is a consequence of different conditions: 1) acute thrombosis and disseminated intravascular coagulation, which leads to increased consumption, 2) liver disease causing lower synthesis, 3) nephrotic syndrome resulting in renal loss; and 4) the use of oral contraceptives and heparin. Antithrombin deficiency is a recognized cause of inherited VTE. Among patients with first-ever VTE, antithrombin deficiency is found in around 0.5 to 1%. This means that it is rarer than other causes of thrombophilia [18]. In a large study of 150 families with thrombophilia, antithrombin deficiency was associated with a relative VTE risk of 8.1 (95% CI, 3.4 to 19.6) [19]. To date, only few case reports and small studies have examined the antithrombin deficiency and myocardial infarction risk association [20-22]. In a Greek study among patients with myocardial infarction younger than 36 years, the frequency of antithrombin deficiency did not differ between cases and controls [20]. In another antithrombin deficiency was not reported among 75 patients with myocardial infarction, 45 years or younger [22].

Table. Acquired thrombophilia

Disseminated intrvascular coagulation (shock, sepsis)	Heparin
Surgery	Vaculitis
Pre-eclampsia	Infection
Liver disfunction	Hemodialysis
Acute hepatic failure, cirrhosis	Plasmapheresis
Renal disease, nephritic syndrome, hemolythic uremic syndrome	Cancer
Inflammatory bowel disease	Leukemia
Drugs	Malnutrition and gastrointestinal loss
Estrogens-progestins	Vascular reconstruction (diabetes, age)
	Other

Furthermore, several case reports have suggested that antithrombin deficiency may be associated with IS risk, especially among low atheroslcerotic burden patients [23,24]. Even so, IS studies [25] have not convincingly revealed any evidence of a significant association between antithrombin deficiency and IS. Among children with IS or cerebral venous thrombosis, 13% had evidence of antithrombin deficiency. However, in this study there was no control group [26]. Antithrombin deficiency was not evidenced in neonates with IS, children with IS or in young adult stroke patients [27].

Protein C Deficiency

Protein C is a vitamin K-dependent hepatic protein that binds to the endothelial cell surface of thrombomodulin and is converted into an active protease by thrombin. Activated protein C, in conjunction with protein S, proteolyses factors Va and VIIIa, which shuts down fibrin formation. Furthermore, the cleavage reaction of factor V is increased an additional 50-fold in the presence of calcium ions and phospholipids. The binding of thrombin to thrombomodulin has long been thought to result in a simultaneous loss in thrombin procoagulant activity. Activated protein C may also stimulate fibrinolysis and accelerate clot lysis. Protein C and S deficiencies are autosomal dominant disorders.

Protein C is present in plasma concentrations ranging from 3 to 5 mcg/mL with a half-life of approximately 7h. These concentrations yield activity ranges between 60 and 130% of a normal plasma pool (defined as 100% activity or approximately 4 mcg/mL). Quantitative analysis is generally performed by either Laurell rocket electrophoresis or enzyme-linked immunosorbement assays (ELISA). Functional protein C assays are of two types: amidolytic (fluorescent) or clotting assay. Utilizing both quantitative and functional tests, it is possible to evidence the two principle deficiency states. Type I protein C deficiency, the most common type, is defined as a decreased PC antigen with a concomitant decrease in functional activity. Most patients with type I deficiency are heterozygous for a wide variety of mutations in the affected protein C allele and typically have protein C levels which are 30 to 60% of normal ones. In type II deficiency there is adequate PC antigen production but an abnormal protein is produced which exhibits decreased activity in functional assay. Protein C deficiency is inherited in an autosomal dominant manner with incomplete penetrance. Genetic protein C deficiency was first described in a case-report by Griffin et. al, in 1981. The patient was a 21-year-old male, whose father and paternal uncle had had lower extremity thrombophlebitis and pulmonary emboli and their protein C levels were 41%, 35%, and 45%, respectively. Acquired protein C deficiency can be attributed to either consumption or decreased or defective production. Common consumptive etiologies include disseminated intravascular coagulation, recent thrombosis, haemolitic uremic syndrome, and thrombotic thrombocytopenia purpura. Production defects are typically due to vitamin K-dependent factors, including protein C deficiency with oral anticoagulation, vitamin K deficiency, and liver disease.

The relationship between protein C deficiency and the risk of IS has been studied. In fact, a large study among an unselected group of patients with IS found that protein C deficiency was not significantly associated with stroke risk [25]. On the other hand, several studies have focused on patient populations with a low atheroslcerotic burden, especially in young adults and children. Positive associations have been reported mainly in small studies and case reports [28,29], but larger studies have not been able to confirm a significant association [30,31]. Among 127 young adults with IS, the rarely detected cases of protein C deficiency were either acquired or transient [30]. Among 120 adults who suffered from IS, three were found to have low levels of protein C, but these abnormalities appeared to be transient, as they could not be confirmed at follow-up testing [32]. In a study among children with stroke, none presented protein C deficiency [31]. Another study among children with IS or cerebral venous thrombosis detected protein C deficiency in 7%, but this study had no control group [26].

In myocardial infarction, as well, few large studies have investigated the relationship between coagulation inhibitors and IS. Prospective studies have provided conflicting data. An early prospective study revealed no case of IS occurrence among nine patients with hereditary AT deficiency, and 36 patients with hereditary PC deficiency and 36 patients with PS deficiency over 160 patient-years of follow-up[33]. Two prospective studies found that lower baseline PC levels, but not AT levels, had a borderline significant association for the risk of IS over a 6- to 9-year follow-up [33] and that lower baseline PC levels were significantly associated with silent cerebral infarctions as identified by magnetic resonance imaging (MRI) performed over a 6-year follow-up. However, baseline MRIs were not performed for comparison [34]. In these two studies, it was not stated whether patients had hereditary or acquired PC or AT deficiency. In a case control study of 219 hospital cases with a first-ever IS and 205 randomly selected community control subjects, no significant differences in the prevalence of PC, PS, and AT deficiencies between cases and control subjects or between pathogenic subtype of IS were reported [25]. Retrospective studies have also examined the risk of stroke in patients with AT, PC and PS deficiencies. In a Japanese study of 26,800 cardiovascular inpatients, age at IS presentation among patients with hereditary PC deficiencies was significantly lower compared to those with normal PC statuses [35] in a retrospective study of 150 families. Here, it was revealed that 0% of AT, 1.6% of PC, and 4.8% of PS-deficient subjects experienced IS, compared to 0.6% of relatives without any of these three deficiencies [19]. In this study, the overall rate of arterial thrombosis events (either IS or MI) was not significantly different between subjects with and without deficiency subjects.

Protein S Deficiency

In 1977, Seattle investigators discovered a vitamin K-dependent protein which they designated “S” for Seattle. Three years later, Walker demonstrated that the same protein enhanced activated protein C inactivation of factor Va. Furthermore, it was demonstrated that protein S is inherited in an autosomal dominant manner. Two genes for protein S reside in chromosome 3. PS α, which codes for protein S and a pseudogen, PS β which contains multiple base changes, which codes for termination codons and frameshifts. Protein S circulates tightly but is reversibly bound to C4b-binding protein (C4b-BP). Only free PS has APC cofactor activity and circulating free PS comprises approximately 40% of the total.

Therefore, the amount of C4b-BP, as well as protein S, may account for observed thrombophilia. C4b-BP is an acute-phase reactant; being so, any process that induces its production may decrease free PS levels. Additionally, the level of free PS is influenced by hormones, and, therefore is usually lower in both pre-menopausal and pregnant women, and in those taking oral contraceptions.

The deficiency states are classified as type I and type II. The former is determined by quantitative assay while the latter is based upon functional activity. Type I PS deficiency is characterized by decreased total protein S and above all decreased free PS levels. The activity is also decreased in the free protein S, which is the active form of PS. Type I is the most commonly diagnosed form of deficiency. Type II deficiency has two subclasses: type IIa and type IIb. In type IIa deficiency there are normal levels of total protein S with decreased free protein S and decreased activity. Type IIb deficiency is characterized by normal total and free protein S with decreased activity. Protein S assessment should be performed after the discontinuation of oral anticoagulation and not during the oral anticoagulation treatment. Laboratory assessment can be achieved with quantitative tests and/or clot based quantitative tests that rely on the functional activity of protein S. Normal levels of total protein S are 60 to 130% of normal reference plasma with 40% found free and 60% bound to C4b-PB. Methodologies employed to quantitatively measure both total and free PSs are: radioimmunoassay, enzyme-linked immunosorbment assays (ELISA) and Laurell rocket electrophoresis..Finally, the functional activity of protein S can be evaluated by a quantitative clotting assay.

Acquired protein S deficiencies are similar to acquired protein C deficiency and may be conveniently classified into consumptive or productive acquired deficiency states. Production defects are attributed to warfarin therapy, vitamin K deficiency or liver disease. Consumptive disorders are identical to those described above for protein C. Additionally, conditions which are described above such as estrogen therapy will increase the protein S binding protein, C4b-BP, thereby decreasing the free protein S.

Several small studies and case reports have suggested that an association may exist between protein S deficiency and the risk of IS [23]. However, larger studies have not be able to confirm this relationship. To this end, a large study examined an unselected group of patients with IS and it was reported that protein S deficiency was not significantly associated [25]. Research that has focused on patient populations with low atheroslcerotic burdens and evidence for a strong relationship between protein S deficiency and stroke in these populations was not found. Among 127 patients younger than 45 years who suffered an IS, inherited protein S deficiency was not observed. [30]. While in another study examining 120 young patients with an IS or transient ischemic attack, many patients had decreased plasma levels of protein S shortly after the index event, but only two patients were found to have consistently low protein S plasma levels at follow-up [32]. In a study carried out on children with arterial or venous cerebrovascular disease, 12% had evidence of protein S deficiency, but this study reported no control group [36]. Protein S deficiency was not detected among 91 neonates with IS [27].

Equally, to date, prospective studies have also provided conflicting data on the role of Proteins S and C and AT as risk factors for vascular disease. One of these prospective studies was not able to reveal any IS occurrence in nine patients with hereditary AT deficiency, 36 patients with hereditary protein C deficiency and 36 patients with hereditary protein S deficiency over 160 patient-years of follow-up. [33] Two further prospective studies found that lower baseline PC levels, but not AT levels, had significant associations which were only borderline regarding IS risk over a 6- to 9-year follow-up [37]. Additionally in another prospective study, lower baseline protein C levels were significantly associated with silent cerebral infarctions identified by MRI. This study was performed over a 6-year follow-up. Unfortunately, in this study baseline MRIs were not performed for comparison [38]. Finally, in these two last studies, it was not specified whether patients had either hereditary or acquired protein C or hereditary or acquired AT deficiencies.

Activated Protein C Resistance (APCR)

Worldwide, Factor V Leiden mutation is the most commonly reported risk factor for venous thromboembolism. The molecular basis for Factor V Leiden mutation is due to the fact that arginine substitutes glutamine at position 506 in F V. This mutation abolishes a cleavage site for activated protein C, leading to a reduced inactivation and thereby fostering a prothrombotic phenotype. Globally, roughly 3-6% of the general population is thought to be heterozygous for this mutation. Heterozygosity can increase an individual's risk 7-fold for venous thromboembolism. This relative risk further increases in the presence of risk factors such as oral contraceptive use, pregnancy and smoking habit. The association between FV Leiden mutation and the risk of developing stroke has been studied extensively. In fact, large studies have not found any significant association in unselected ischemic stroke patients [25,39,40]. Furthermore, several studies on FV Leiden and stroke risk have focused on patient populations deemed to have low atheroslcerotic burdens which is an approach often used in studying myocardial infarction and thrombophilia association. In three meta-analyses, the possible association between FV Leiden and IS has been studied. In fact, in 2002, Juul et. al, [41] published a meta-analysis of eight studies which included a total of 1,270 adult patients and 2,269 control subjects. FV Leiden was present in 5.3% of patients compared to 7.2% of control subjects. Thus, the OR for IS was 1.05% (95% CI, 0.73 to 1.50). When including the Copenhagen City Heart Study (one case control study of 231 patients and 7,907 control subjects and one prospective study of 410 patients and 8,835 control subjects), the OR was 1.00 (95% CI, 0.75 to 1.34)[41]. In 2003, Kim and Becker [42] published another meta-analysis of 15 case control studies having 3,039 patients and 12,200 control subjects. It was reported that IS risk was OR 1.27 (95% CI, 0.86 to 1.87). Additionally, patients younger than 55 were at a higher risk for arterial ischemic event (both MI an IS) compared to older patients with FV Leiden (OR 1.37; 95% CI, 0.96 to 1.97). In 2004, Casas et al [43] published a third meta-analysis of 26 case-control studies that included 4,588 cases and 13,798 controls. Statistically significant associations with IS were identified for FV Leiden (OR 1.33; CI 95%, 1.12 to 1.58). However, a significant inter-study OR heterogeneity was observed due to one study that had had a wide heterogeneity. After removing this study from meta-analysis, OR was attenuated and no longer significant: OR 1.18 (95% CI, 0.98 to 1.42). Since the publication of these three meta-analyses, few studies have been carried out. In one of these few, Aznar et al [44] reported no association between FV Leiden and IS in a group of 49 young patients with cryptogenic stroke (OR 2.62; CI, 95% 0.49 to 13.95). However, in the same study, oral contraceptives seemed to be significant risk factors for cryptogenic stroke (OR 3.59; CI 95%, 1.28 to 10.05) and this risk was increased when genetic thrombophilic defects were present.

Prothrombin G20210A Mutation

Prothrombin (factor II) is the precursor for thrombin, which is the key enzyme of the coagulation cascade. The prothrombin gene contains a common guanine to adenine mutation at nucleotide 20210 in the 3'-untraslated region. This molecular defect represents a gain-of-function mutation that causes enhanced cleavage site recognition, increased 3'-end processing, increased mRNA accumulation and protein synthesis. Therefore, G20210A mutation carriers tend to have higher plasma prothrombin levels than non-carriers and have an approximately 3-fold increased risk of VTE. The relationship between the prothrombin G20210A mutation and risk of stroke has also been studied. In a large study of an unselected group of patients with IS, prothrombin mutation was not significantly associated with stroke risk [25]. In the Physician's Health Study, where the endpoint was unselected ischemic stroke, no such association was observed [34]. Also the Cardiovascular Health Study detected no significant association between either prothrombin plasma levels or the G20210A mutation and risk of cerebrovascular disease [45]. However, several studies investigating the risk of stroke at a young age have reported significant associations with stroke risk. In fact, patients younger than 50 with documented IS and without cardiovascular risk factors were more likely to carry the G20210A mutation than controls [46]. A study of 468 patients younger than 60 having cerebrovascular disease found an elevated risk of stroke among male prothrombin mutation carriers (OR, 6.1% CI 95% 1.3 to 28.3) but not among women [47]. In contrast, two other large studies observed no significant association between the G20210A mutation and risk of developing stroke at a young age [28, 48]. A meta-analysis by Kim and Baker [42] included 10 case-control studies with 1,625 patients and 5,050 controls. The observed risk of this mutation with IS was 1.30 (CI 95%, 0.91 to 1.87). When the analysis was limited to patients younger than 55, the association was statistically significant (OR 1.66 CI 95%, 1.13 to 2.46) for myocardial infarction and IS together; though no subgroup analysis was reported. In a meta-analysis by Casas et. al, [43], 10 case-control studies including 3,028 cases and 7,131 controls were reviewed. A statistically significant association between F II G2021A and ischemic stroke was identified (OR 1.44; 95% CI, 1.11 to 1.86) without any significant inter-study heterogeneity. Since the publication of these two meta-analyses, few other studies have been published. Of these studies, Aznar et. al, [44] found a weak relationship between FI G20210A mutation and IS in a group of 49 patients with cryptogenic stroke (OR 3.75; 95% CI, 1.05 to 13.34). In contrast, Rubattu et al, carried out a case control study [49], which showed no statistically significant difference between the two groups.

Pezzini and colleagues [50] performed a case-control study and showed that, in the PFO subgroup, the PTG20210A variant and to a lesser extent the FV G1691A mutation were both associated with the risk of stroke. This suggests that the roles of such mutations in the pathogeneses of stroke could be related to PFO. To confirm this hypothesis, a large prospective study is required to investigate the possible stroke risk association between PFO and systemic thrombophilia.

Hyperhomocysteinemia

Over the past 30 years, homocysteine has been identified as an independent risk factor that contributes to vascular occlusive disease. In 1969, McCully first described the relationship between severely elevated homocysteine levels found in patients with homocysteinuria and premature vascular disease [51]. In 1976, Wilcken and Wilcken were the first to report on an association between mildly elevated homocysteine levels and coronary artery disease [52]. Subsequently, numerous reports have supported the hypothesis that mild hyperomocysteinemia is an independent risk factor for cerebrovascular, carotid, coronary, peripheral arterial and veno-occlusive disease. Homocysteine is a thiol-containing amino acid, which readily undergoes auto-oxidation in the plasma resulting in oxidized forms of homocysteine. Plasma homocysteine levels are typically determined by utilizing methods that reduce all forms of protein-bound homocysteine to free homocysteine in order to measure the total homocyst(e)ine (tHcy) level. Homocysteine levels can be determined either after an overnight fast or 4 to 8 hours following a 100mg/Kg methionine load. Both fasting and post-methionine load hyperhomocysteinemia have been associated with an increased risk for vascular occlusive disease. The methionine load test has the advantage of detecting a mildly to moderately impaired methionine metabolism, which leads to transient homocysteine increase. Hyperhomocysteinemia results when homocysteine metabolism is impaired. Homocysteine is metabolised by either transsulfuration to cystathionine or remethylation to methionine. Enzyme mutations that catabolize homocysteine are known to result in hyperomocysteinemia. Similarly, deficiencies of enzymes cofactors or cosubstrates that catalyse the transsulfuration and remethylation pathways can result in an homocysteine plasma level increase. In the remethylation pathway, homocysteine is converted into methionine; in this series of reactions. 5,10-methylene tetrahydrofolate is converted into 5-methyltetrahydrofolate by the folate–dependent enzyme methylene tetrahydrofolate reductase (MTHFR). Methyltetrahydrofolate is a methyl donor for homocysteine which forms methionine and tetrahydrofolate. This biochemical reaction, catalized by 5-methyl tetrahydrofolate-homocysteine methyltransferase (methionine syntase) requires B12 as its cosubstrate. In the transsulfuration pathway, methionine is converted into homocysteine through the intermediaries S-adenoylmethionine (SAM) and S-adenosyl-homocysteine. Finally, homocysteine irreversibly condenses with serine to form cystathionine. This reaction is catalysed by cystathionine-beta-synthase (CBS) which is a vitamin B6-dependent enzyme. Cystathionine is hydrolysed to cysteine, by the gamma-cystathioninase, and is also a vitamin B6-dependent reaction.

Factors contributing to hyperhomocysteinemia include nutrition, age, medications, systemic illness, and genetics. It is worth noting that hyperomocysteinemia has been associated with hypotyroidism, diabetes and renal disease. Genetic mutations of MTHFR and CBS have also been associated with hyperhomocysteinemia. To date, about 18 CBS mutations and 10 MTHFR points of mutation have been identified. Specifically, regarding the MTHFR gene, nine thermolabile mutations have been found on chromosome 1p36.3. The two most common forms of these mutations are: C559T transition which converts an arginine codon into termination codon and G482a transition that converts an arginine into a glutamine residue. The most common MTHFR mutation gene, is the C677T transition which results in a thermolabile variant of the enzyme. This autosomal recessive mutation substitutes an alanine for a valine residue in the MTHFR protein. The homozygous thermolabile MTHFR polymorphism is characterized by an enzyme activity of about 50% compared to normal. Homozygous CBS mutations are the most common causes of homocystinuria. These homozygotic CBS carriers have an altered phenotype characterized by mental retardation, dislocated ocular lenses, osteoporosis, skeletal abnormalities and premature atheroslcerotic disease while heterozygotic CBS carriers, possess normal phenotypes. Heterozygotes tend to have variable, but less than 50% of CBS enzyme activity. As residual enzyme activity commonly overlaps with the normal range, it is difficult to predict enzyme activity in the CBS genotype. Worldwide, homozygous CBS point mutations are present in 1/20,000 to 1/200,000 persons, while heterozygous are in 1/70 to 1/225. This means that 30 to 40% of individuals with premature vascular disease are heterozygous for CBS point mutations [54].

Presently, available data provide insight into potential homocysteine-driven mechanisms that result in endothelial damage, platelet activation and a prothrombotic state. These data have been obtained from in-vitro experiments where homocysteine concentrations were significantly higher compared to patients with mild hyperhomocysteinemia and vascular occlusive disease. Homocysteine is postulated to disrupt the normal procoagulant-anticoagulant balance of the endothelium and create a prothrombotic micro-environment. In-vitro studies have shown that homocysteine may be directly damage the endothelium. It has been demonstrated that hyperhomocysteinemia interferes with nitric oxide (NO) leading to a reduced NO bioavailability. In addition, homocysteine induces proliferation and migration of vascular smooth muscle cells which is one of the major factors in development of atherosclerosis.

In 1994, Verhoef et.al, [54] reported on the results from the Physician's Health Study. Here, homocysteine was measured in 109 subjects who had ischemic stroke and in 427 controls. Increased Hcy levels were associated with a low, but not significant increased risk of IS. Another study demonstrated that hyperhomocysteinemia is a predictor of carotid artery disease. In 1993, Malinow [55] reported on a study of 287 case-control pairs of asymptomatic adults. In this study, the intimal wall thickness of the carotid artery was measured by ultrasound. These study subjects were between 45 and 64 years old and had no reported history of atheroslcerotic disease. The OR for a thickened carotid wall was 3.15 ($P = 0.001$) for patients in the top quintile of plasma homocysteine levels (> 10 μMol) compared to those in the lowest quintile (< 5.88 μMol). This study showed that carotid artery thickening was correlated with plasma homocysteine levels. In 1998, Voutilainen et al, reported that in men, but not in women, total plasma homocysteine concentrations > 11.5 μMol were associated with increased common carotid artery intima-media thickness. This study concluded that increased plasma homocysteine levels were associated with early atherosclerosis. Furthermore, the Framingham Study also found non-fasting total homocysteine levels to be an independent risk factor for the incidence of stroke in the elderly [56].

Thrombophilia and Stroke Related to Paradoxical Embolism (PFO)

Karttunen et al, [57] studied 57 adult patients with cryptogenic stroke and patent foramen ovale (PFO) compared to104 matched controls. FV Leiden was found more often in cases than in controls, but the difference was not statistically significant (OR 7.8; CI 95%, 0.8 to71.3). There were only four subjects with heterozygous FV Leiden among the stroke/PFO cohort and only one among the controls. FII G20210A was found in two PFO cases and one in the control group. Using multivariate analysis, the presence of any type of coagulation abnormality along with the presence of any predisposing event for deep vein thrombosis within 3 months resulted in a significantly and independently associated risk of stroke in PFO patients. It also appeared that both mutations and migraine with aura were significantly associated with cryptogenic stroke brain infarction. Pezzini et al, [50] investigated 125 consecutive young patients with IS and 149 age and sex matched control subjects. FII G20210A was more frequent in the group of patients in which the pathogenic role of PFO was presumed (n = 36) compared to controls (11.1% vs 2.0%; OR 0.19; CI 95%, 0.04 to 0.94) and the group of patients in which the stroke was considered unrelated with right-to-left shunt (n = 89) (11.1% vs 1.1%; OR 10.09; CI 95%, 1.09 to 109). There was no statistically significant difference seen among these three groups in relation to FV Leiden. The Young Adult Myocardial Infarction and Ischemic Stroke (YAMIS) study investigated 101 young adults for the frequency of venous-to-arterial circulation shunts, which are usually caused by PFO, and thrombophilia in young adults suffering from IS compared to matched controls [58]. Thrombophilia (FV Leiden, FII G20210A, AT, Pc, Ps, Lupus anticoagulant) was not significantly associated with ischemic stroke recurrence. While only "major" venous-to-arterial circulation shunts were associated with stroke in young adults.

Stroke in Children and Neonates

In their meta-analysis, Juul et al, [41] also investigated hemostatic markers in infants and children with IS. Seven studies including a total of 453 patients and 1,180 controls were reviewed. The prevalence of FV Leiden among controls was 6.7% (range 3.3% to 13.8%) and 18.5% (range 5.4% to 34.9%) among cases. The OR for IS in this meta-analysis was 4.79 (95% CI, 3.26 to 7.03). In 2005, Haywood et al, [59] performed a systematic review of case-control studies reporting the prevalence of thrombophilia in children with a first-ever arterial IS. Eighteen studies met the chosen criteria with a total of 3,235 patients and 9,019 controls. The pooled ORs (and 95% CIs) were: FV Leiden 1.22 (0.80 to 1.87); FII G20210A, 1.10 (0.51 to 2.34); AT deficiency, 1.02 (0.28 to 3.67); PC deficiency, 6.49 (2.96 to 14.27), and PS deficiency, 1.14 (0.34 to 3.80).

In another prospective study, 301 children with a history of IS and familial inhibitor deficiency confirmed by repeated testing for thrombofilia in both the patient and family members were followed up. Here, the reported risk of a subsequent stroke was significantly increased in those with familial PC deficiency but not in those with familial PS or AT deficiencies [60]. Several other studies have found a possible association between PC deficiency and IS in children, but generally an exclusion of acquired causes, confirmatory family testing, and repeated testing were not performed.

Concerning neonates, a retrospective, case-control study of 91 neonates [27] with IS found an association with FV Leiden. In a case series of 24 neonates with cerebral infarction, five (21%) had FV Leiden [61]. Follow-up on these patients at age 2 or older revealed that all five patients (100%) with FV Leiden had hemiplegia, whereas only 21% without FV Leiden had hemiplegia.

Inherited Thrombophilia: To Test or not to Test?

Currently, the most debated issue concerning thrombophilia is the value of screening patients and their family members [62,63]. Generally speaking, laboratory tests should be undertaken whenever it is thought that the results will help clinicians to make better decisions related to primary prevention, treatment or secondary prevention of disease. However, in the field of thrombophilia none of these goals are completely achieved by testing. In fact, the treatment of acute thrombotic events is essentially the same whatever the cause. Exceptions are related to rare cases of congenital AT deficiency with poor response to heparinization, or homozygous PC o PS deficiency with purpura fulminans. However, these instances can be revealed by other non-thrombophilic tests or from a knowledge of the patient's clinical history. The duration of anticoagulation for the prevention of recurrences is still a debated issue in thrombophilia, and testing might be useful for selecting those patients who may benefit from a long-term antithrombotic prophylaxis. Regarding this, to date, study results have been contradictory. Even so, there has been evidence from many centers treating thrombophilic patients that congenital AT deficiency could very likely be a severe risk factor. Thus, taking this into consideration, patients with a previous history of thrombosis along with congenital AT deficiency should be treated indefinitely [64].

Nonetheless, it is highly unlikely that a randomized study will one day be undertaken as this condition is extremely rare and the follow-up period needed to draw valid conclusions would be terribly long.

The same consideration may apply to PC or PS deficiency, although the severity of these risk factors seems to be lower. Besides this, numerous case-control and prospective studies have been carried out over the last decade in an attempt to discover any possible associations having a recurrence risk after a first venous or arterial event which include risk factors such as: APC resistance due to factor V Arg506Gln polymorphism or hyperprothrombinemia due to the presence of the prothrombin mutation G20210A [65-67]. Notwithstanding the considerable number of these latter studies that have been carried out, their conclusions remain contradictory. Roughly, half of the studies have supported the hypothesis that the above thrombophilic deficiencies may influence the recurrence risk. However, even if the detection of heterozygous factor V Leiden or prothrombin mutation is discovered not to be helpful, the detection of homozygosity for the same defects would probably be of use. This is because these conditions are associated with a higher risk [68].

Finally, the last consideration is to decide whether to test family members of the proband [62,63]. Family members are very often asymptomatic and their carrier status does not require any kind of treatment. [62]. Furthermore, knowledge of their carrier status for such a mild risk factor such as factor V Leiden, in the absence of clinical symptoms may create an unnecessary fear of disease. Conversely, the detection of congenital defects, even if mild, may help to prevent thrombotic events at times when carriers are exposed to transient risk factors such as surgery and pregnancy.

In conclusion, although it is difficult to formulate accepted guidelines, testing for congenital thrombophilia should be carried out after thoroughly examining clinical history. Young patients who experience either unprovoked thrombotic events or recurrences should be deemed candidates for laboratory investigation. Current evidence does not support laboratory investigation for congenital thrombophilia in the general population before exposure to circumstantial risk factors or in asymptomatic women prior to starting oral contraceptives. Laboratory testing, at least for the phenotypes, should be performed at least 6 months after the acute thrombotic event to avoid any misinterpretations of the results. Furthermore, testing, at least PC and PS, should be done at least 2 weeks after oral anticoagulation has been discontinued. Finally, if testing is done, screening should be comprehensive and include all of the above parameters, given that the identification of patients having combined defects may help clinicians to make better decisions because these defects are known to be associated with higher risks for thrombosis [69-71].

References

[1] Colman RW. Overview of haemostasis, in Haemostasis and Thrombosis, 5th ed. Philadelphia, Lippincott Williams and Wilkins, 2006 pp 3-6.

[2] Bauer KA. Management of thrombophilia. *JTH* 2003;1:1429-34

[3] Rokitansky C. Pathological Anatomy, IV. London Sydenham Society; 1852.

[4] Virchow R. Cellular Pathology. London : Churchill; 1860

[5] Egeberg O. Inherited antithrombin deficiency causing thrombophilia. *Thromb Death Haemorrh*. 1965; 13 :516-520

[6] Griffin JH, Evatt B, Zimmerman T, Kleiss A, Wideman C. Deficiency of protein C in congenital thrombotic disease. *J. Clin. Invest* 1981;68:1370-73

[7] Comp PC, Esmon CT. recurrent venous thromboembolism in patients with a partial deficiency of protein S. *NEJM* 1984;311:1525-28

[8] Schwartz HP, Fischer M, Hopmeier P, Batard M, Griffin J. Plasma protein S deficiency in familial thrombotic disease. *Blood* 1984;63:1297-1300

[9] Branson HE, Katz J, Marble R, Griffin JH. Inherited protein C deficiency and coumarin-responsive chronic relapsing purpura fulminans in a newborn infant. *Lancet* 1983;2:1165-68.

[10] Mahasandana C, suvatte V, Marlar RA, Manco-Johnson MJ, Jacobson LJ, Hathaway WE. Neonatal purpura fulminans associated with homozygous protein S deficiency. *Lancet* 1990;335:61-62.

[11] Dahlbäck B, Carlsson M, Svensson PJ. Familial thrombophilia due to a previously unrecognised mechanism characterized by poor anticoagulant response to activated

protein C: prediction of a cofactor to activated protein C. *Proc. Natl. Acad. Sci. USA* 1993;90:1004-08.

[12] Griffin JH, Evatt B, Wideman C, Fernandez JA. Anticoagulant protein C pathway defective in majority of thrombophilic patients. *Blood* 1993;82:1989-93.

[13] Koster T, Rosendaal FR, de Ronde H, Briet E, Vandebrucke JP, Bertina RM. Venous thrombosis due to poor anticoagulant response to activated protein C: Leiden Thrombophilia study. *Lancet* 1993; 342:1503-1506.

[14] Faioni EM, Franchi F, Asti D, sacchi E, Bernardi F, Mannucci PM. Resistance to activated protein C in nine thrombophilic families: interferences in a protein S functional assay. *Thromb Haemost.* 1993;70:1067-71

[15] Bertina RM, Koeleman BPC, Koster T. Mutation in blood coagulation factor V associated with resistance to activated protein C. *Nature* 1994;369:64-67.

[16] Kalafatis M, Bertina RM, Rand MD, Mann KG. Characterization of the molecular defect in factor V R506Q. *J. boil. chem.* 1995; 270:4053-57..

[17] Poort SR, Rosendaal FR, Reitsma PM, Bertina RM. A common genetic variation in the 3'-untraslated region of the prothrombin gene is associated with elevated plasma protrhombin levels and an increase in venous thrombosis. *Blood* 1996; 88:3698-3703.

[18] Mateo J, Oliver A, Borrel M, Sala N, Fonteuberta J. Laboratory evaluation and clinical characteristics of 2,132 consecutive unselected patients with venous thromboembolism results of the Spanish Multicentric study on Thromboembolia (EMET-study). *Thromb Haemost.* 1997;77:444-4451.

[19] Martinelli I, Mannucci PM, De Stefano V, Taioli E, Rossi V, Crosti F, Paciaroni K, Leone G, Faioni EM. Different risks of thrombosis in four coagulations defects associated with inherited thrombophilia: a study of 150 families. *Blood* 1998;92:2353-2358.

[20] Rallidis LS, Belesi CI, Manioudaki HS, Chatziioakimidis VK, Fakitsa VC, Sinos LE, Laoutaris NP, Apostolou TS. Myocardial infarction under the age of 36: prevalence of thrombophilic disorders. *Thromb Haemost.* 2003; 90:272-278.

[21] Peeters S, Vandenplas Y, Jochmans K, Bougatef A, De Waele M, De Wolf D. Myocardial infarction in a neonate with hereditary antithrombin III deficiency. *Acta Pediatr.* 1993;82:610-613.

[22] Dacosta A, Tardy-Poncet B, Isaaz K, Cerisier A, Mismetti P, Simitsidis S, Reynaud J, Tardy B, Piot M, Decousus H, Guyotat D. Prevalence of factor V Leiden and other inherited thrombophilias in young patients with myocardial infarction and normal coronary arteries. *Heart* 1998;80:338-340.

[23] Green D, Otoya J, Oriba H, Rovner R. Protein S deficiency in middle aged women with stroke. *Neurology* 1992;42:1029-33.

[24] Arima T, Motomura M, Nishiura Y, Tsujihata M, Okajima K, Abe H, Nagataki S. Cerebral infarction in a heterozygotes with variant antithrombin III. *Stroke* 1992;23: 1822-25.

[25] Hankey GJ, Eikelboom JW, van Bockxmeer FM, Lofthouse E, Staples N, Baker RI. Inherited thrombophilia in ischemic stroke and its pathogenic subtypes. *Stroke* 2001; 32:1793-1799.

[26] deVeber G, Monagle P, Chan A, MacGregor D, Curtis R, Lee S, Vegh P, Adams M, Marzinotto V, Leaker M, Massicotte MP, Lillicrap D, Andrew M. Prothrombotic disoerders in infants and children with cerebral thromboembolism. *Arch Neurol.* 1998; 55:1539-1543.

[27] Günther G, Junker R, Sträter R, Schobess R, Kurnik K, Heller C, Kosch A, Nowak-Göttl U; Childhood Stroke Study Group. Symptomatic ischemic stroke in full term neonates: role of acquired and genetic prothrombotic risk factors. *Stroke* 2000;31:2437-2441.

[28] Austin H, Chimowitz MI, Hill HA, Chaturvedi S, Wechsler LR, Wityk RJ, Walz E, Wilterdink JL, Coull B, Sila CA, Mitsias P, Evatt B, Hooper WC; Genetics and Stroke in the Young Study Group. Cryptogenic stroke in relation to genetic variation in clotting factors and other genetic polymorphism among young men and women. *Stroke* 2002;33:2762-2768.

[29] Martinez HR, Rangel-Guerra RA, Marfil LJ. Ischemic stroke due to deficiency of coagulation inhibitors. Report of 10 young adults. *Stroke* 1993;24:19-25.

[30] Douay X, Lucas C, Caron C, Goudemand J, Leys D. Antithrombin, protein C and protein S levels in 127 consecutive young adults with ischemic stroke. *Acta Neurol. Scand.* 1998;98:124-27.

[31] Ganesan V, McShane MA, Liesner R, Cookson J, Hann I, Kirkham FJ. Inherited prothrombotic states and ischemic stroke in childhood. *J. Neurol. Neurosurg. Psychiatry* 1998;65:508-511.

[32] Munts AG, van Genderen PJ, Dippel DW, van Kooten F, Koudstaal PJ. Coagulation disorders in young adults with acute cerebral ischaemia. *J. Neurol.* 1998;245:21-25.

[33] Finazzi G, Barbui T. Different incidence of venous thrombosis in patients with inherited deficiencies of antithrombin III, protein C and protein S. *Thromb Haemost.* 1994;71:15-18.

[34] Ridker PM, Hennekens CH, Miletich JP. G20210A mutation in prothrombin gene and risk of myocardial infarction, stroke, and venous thrombosis in a large cohort of US men. *Circulation* 1999;99:999-1004.

[35] Sakata T, Kario K, Katayama Y, Matsuyama T, Kato H, Miyata T. Studies on congenital protein C deficiency in japanese: prevalence, genetic analysis and relevance to thr onset of arterial occlusive disease. *Semin. Thromb Haemost.* 2000; 26:11-16.

[36] Segev A, Ellis MH, Segev F, Friedman Z, Reshef T, Sprakes JD. High prevalence of thrombophilia among young patients with myocardial infarction and few conventional risk factors. *Int. J. Cardiol.* 2005;98:421-424.

[37] Folson AR Rosamond WD, Shar E, Cooper LS, Aleksic N, Nieto FJ. Prospective study of markers of hemostatic function with risk of ischemic stroke. The Atherosclerosis Risk in Communities (ARIC) Study Investigators. *Circulation* 1999;100:736-742.

[38] Knuiman MW, Folson AR, Chambless LE, Liao D, Wu KK. Association of hemostatic variables with MRI-detected cerebral abnormalities. The Atherosclerosis Risk in Communities Study. *Neuroepidemiology* 2001;20:96-104.

[39] Ridker PM, Hennekens CH, Lindpaintner K, Stampfer MJ, Eisenberg PR, Miletich JP. Mutation in the gene coding for coagulation factor V and the risk of myocardial

infarction, stroke, and venous thrombosis in apparently healthy men. *NEJM* 1995; 932: 912-17.

[40] Cushman M, Rosendaal FR, Psaty BM, Cook EF, Valliere J, Kuller LH, Tracy RP. Factor V Leiden is not a risk factor for arterial vascular disease in the elderly: results from the Cardiovascular Health Study. *Thromb Haemost.* 1998;79:912-15.

[41] Juul K, Tybjaerg-Hansen A, Steffensen R, Kofoed S, Jensen G, Nordestgaard BG. Factor V Leiden: The Copenhagen city Heart Study and 2 meta-analyses. *Blood* 2002; 100:3-10.

[42] Kim RJ, Becker RC. Association between factor V Leiden, prothrombin G20210A, and methylentetrahydrofolate reductase C677T mutations and events of the arterial circolatory system: a meta-analysis of pubplished studies-. *Am. Heart J.* 2003;146:948-957.

[43] Casas JP, Hingorani AD, Bautista LE, Sharma P. Meta-analysis of genetic studies in ischemic stroke: Thirty-two genes involving approxymately 18,000 cases and 58,000 controls. *Arch Neurol.* 2004;61:1652-1661.

[44] Aznar J, Mitra Y, Vaya A, Corella D, Ferrando F, Villa P, Estelles A. Factor V Leiden and prothrombin G20210A mutations in young adults with cryptogenic ischemic stroke. *Thromb Haemost.* 2004;911031-1034.

[45] Smiles AM, Jenny NS, Tang Z, Arnold A, Cushman M, Tracy RP. No association of plasma prothrombin concentration or the G20210A mutation with incident cardiovascular disease: results from the Cardiovascular Health Study. *Thromb Haemost.* 2002;87:614-621.

[46] De Stefano V, Chiusolo P, Paciaroni K, Casorelli I, Rossi E, Molinari M, Servidei S, Tonali PA, Leone G. Prothrombin G20210A mutant genotype is a risk factor for cerebrovascular ischemic disease in young patients. *Blood* 1998;91-3562-65.

[47] Lalouschek W, Schillinger M, Hsieh K, Endler G, Tentschert S, Lang W, Cheng S, Mannhalter C. Matched case-control study on factor V Leiden and the prothrombin G20210A mutation in patients with ischemic stroke/transient ischemic attack up to the age of 60 years. *Stroke* 2005 Jul;36:1405-9.

[48] Pezzini A, Grassi M, Del Zotto E, Archetti S, Spezi R, Vergani V, Assanelli D, Caimi L, Padovani A. Cumulative effect of predisposing genotypes and their interaction with modifiable factors on the risk of ischemic stroke in young adults. *Stroke* 2005 Mar;36:533-9.

[49] Rubattu S, Di Angelantonio E, Nitsch D, Gigante B, Zanda B, Stanzione R, Evangelista A, Pirisi A, Rosati G, Volpe M. Polymorphisms in prothrombotic genes and their impact on ischemic stroke in a Sardinian population. *Thromb Haemost.* 2005 Jun;93(6):1095-100.

[50] Pezzini A, Del Zotto E, Magoni M, Costa A, Archetti S, Grassi M, Akkawi NM, Albertini A, Assanelli D, Vignolo LA, Padovani A. Inherited thrombophilic disorders in young adults with ischemic stroke and patent foramen ovale. *Stroke* 2003 Jan;34(1):28-33.

[51] McCully KS. Hyperhomocysteinemia and arteriosclerosis: historical perspectives *Clin. Chem. Lab. Med.* 2005;43(10):980-6

[52] Wilcken DE, Wilcken B. The pathogenesis of coronary artery disease. A possible role for methionine metabolism. *J. Clin. Invest.* 1976 Apr;57(4):1079-82.
[53] Tsai MY, Bignell M, Yang F, Welge BG, Graham KJ, Hanson NQ. Polygenic influence on plasma homocysteine: association of two prevalent mutations, the 844ins68 of cystathionine beta-synthase and A(2756)G of methionine synthase, with lowered plasma homocysteine levels. *Atherosclerosis* 2000 Mar;149:131-7.
[54] Verhoef P, Hennekens CH, Malinow MR, Kok FJ, Willett WC, Stampfer MJ. A prospective study of plasma homocyst(e)ine and risk of ischemic stroke *Stroke* 1994 Oct;25(10):1924-30.
[55] Malinow MR, Nieto FJ, Szklo M, Chambless LE, Bond G. Carotid artery intimal-medial wall thickening and plasma homocyst(e)ine in asymptomatic adults. The Atherosclerosis Risk in Communities Study. *Circulation* 1993 Apr;87(4):1107-13
[56] Halil M, Yavuz B, Yavuz BB, Cankurtaran M, Dede DS, Ulger Z, Barak A, Karabulut E, Aytemir K, Kabakci G, Ariogul S, Oto A. Novel cardiovascular risk factors in the elderly and their correlation with the Framingham risk score. *J. Cardiovasc. Med.* (Hagerstown). 2008 Jul;9(7):683-7
[57] Karttunen V, hiltunen L, Rasi V, Vahtera E, Hillbom M. Factor V Leiden and prothrombin gene mutation may predispose to paradoxical embolism in subjects with patent foramen ovale. *Blood coagul. Fibrinolysis* 2003;14:261-268.
[58] Sastry S, Riding G, Morris J, Taberner D, Cherry N, Heagerty A, McCollum C. Young Adult Myocardial Infarction and Ischemic Stroke: the role of paradoxical embolism and thrombophilia (The YAMIS Study). *J. Am. Coll. Cardiol.* 2006 Aug 15;48(4):686-91
[59] Haywood S, Liesner R, Pindora S, Ganesan V. Thrombophilia and first arterial ischemic stroke: a systematic review. *Arch Dis. Child* 2005;90:402-405.
[60] Sträter R, Becker S, von Eckardstein A, Heinecke A, Gutsche S, Junker R, Kurnik K, Schobess R, Nowak-Göttl U. Prospective assessment of risk factors for recurrent stroke during childhood--a 5-year follow-up study. *Lancet* 2002 Nov 16;360:1540-5
[61] Mercuri E, Cowan F, Gupte G, Manning R, Laffan M, Rutherford M, Edwards AD, Dubowitz L, Roberts I. Prothrombotic disorders and abnormal neurodevelopmental outcome in infants with neonatal cerebral infarction. *Pediatrics* 2001;107:1400-4
[62] Greaves M, Baglin T. Laboratory testing for heritable thrombophilia: impact on clinical management of thrombotic disease. *Br. J. Haematol.* 2000;109:699-703.
[63] Mannucci PM. Genetic hypercoagulopaty: prevention suggests testing family members. *Blood* 2001;98:21-22.
[64] De Stefano V, Finazzi G, Mannucci PM. Inherited thrombophilia: pathogenesis, clinical syndromes and management. *Blood* 1996;87:3531-3544.
[65] Eichinger S, Pabinger I, Stümpflen A, Hirschl M, Bialonczyk C, Schneider B, Mannhalter C, Minar E, Lechner K, Kyrle PA. The risk of recurrent venous thromboembolism in patients with and without factor V Leiden. *Thromb Haemost.* 1997 Apr;77(4):624-8
[66] Ridker PM, Miletich JP, Stampfer MJ, Goldhaber SZ, Lindpaintner K, Hennekens CH. Factor V Leiden and risks of recurrent idiopathic venous thromboembolism *Circulation* 1995 Nov 15;92(10):2800-2.

[67] Miles JS, Miletich JP, Goldhaber SZ, Hennekens CH, Ridker PM G20210A mutation in the prothrombin gene and the risk of recurrent venous thromboembolism. *J. Am. Coll. Cardiol.* 2001 Jan;37(1):215-8

[68] Rosendaal FR, Koster T, Vandenbroucke JP, Reitsma PH. High risk of thrombosis in patients homozygous for factor V Leiden (activated protein C resistance). *Blood* 1995; 85:1504-1508.

[69] Koeleman BPC, Reitsma PH, Allaart CF, Bertina RM. Activated protein C resistance as an additional risk factor for thrombosis in protein C deficient families. *Blood* 1994; 84:1031-35.

[70] Zoller B, Berntsdotter A, Garcia de Frutos P, Dahlback B. Resistance to activated protein C as an additional genetic risk factor in hereditary deficiency of protein S. *Blood* 1995;85:3518-3523.

[71] Ridcker PM, Hennekens CH, Selhub J, Miletich JP, Malinow MR, Stampfer MJ. Interrelation of hyperhomocysteinemia, factor V Leiden and the risk of future venous thromboembolism. *Circulation* 1997;95:1777-1782.

In: Cerebral Ischemia in Young Adults
Editors: A. Pezzini and A. Padovani

ISBN 978-1-60741-627-2

Chapter 16

Ischaemic Stroke in Young People and Antiphospholipid Syndrome

Pietro Offelli and Vittorio Pengo[2]
Department of Cardiothoracic and Vascular Sciences, Clinical Cardiology,
Thrombosis Centre, University of Padua, Italy

Abstract

The Antiphospholipid Syndrome (APS) is characterized by the occurrence of vascular thrombosis or pregnancy loss, and by the presence of pathogenic antiphospholipid antibodies (aPL). The diagnosis of APS requires definite clinical and laboratory criteria to be met; laboratory positivity to aPL doesn't *per se* define APS, as not all aPL are associated with clinical events, and positivity to aPL tests is also a common finding in healthy people. Screening for aPL acquires importance when there is a clinical suspicion of APS.

In young patients cerebral ischemia is often cryptogenic, and the presence of aPL is of etiological value only if the diagnostic criteria for APS are met, thus preventing over-diagnosis; laboratory tests pattern also define thrombotic risk. In these patients stroke seems to be caused by cardioembolism from valvular deposits of thrombotic nature (Libman-Sacks endocarditis).

Secondary prevention of APS, consistently with the stroke mechanism, is based on anticoagulant therapy. Although the intensity of anticoagulation is still a matter of debate, present data suggest that patients benefit from a target INR of 2.0 - 3.0.

[2] Correspondence: Vittorio Pengo, Ospedale 'Ex Busonera',Via Gattamelata 64, 35128 Padova, Italy. Tel and fax +39 049 8215658, Mobile 3298324844. E-mail: vittorio.pengo@unipd.it.

Introduction

The story of antiphospholipid (aPL) antibodies saw its birth at the beginning of the past century when Wasserman and Michaelis set up complement fixation and flocculation tests able to identify 'reagins' present in sera of patients suffering from syphilis. It soon became apparent that the 'reagins' were not directed against the pathogen responsible for that disease but instead against lipids obtained by extracts from various normal tissues and organs. It was found that the heart is largely composed of this compound which was thus termed 'cardiolipin', and that is constituted by anionic phospholipids whose phosphate residues are negatively charged at a physiological pH. Two important discoveries were made in the 1950's: a) it was found that 'reagins' were also present in the sera of patients not affected by syphilis and b) that they were sometime found in subjects who also presented a particular coagulation inhibitor. To describe this entity, originally associated with systemic lupus erythematosus (SLE), in 1972 Feinstein and Rapaport coined the term 'Lupus Anticoagulant' (LAC). In 1980 it was demonstrated that an IgM paraprotein with LAC activity reacted in immunodiffusion with anionic but not zwitterionic PL. Based on these findings, a radioimmunoassay and then an ELISA were developed to detect antibodies against anionic PL using cardiolipin as antigen [1]. 'Antiphospholipid' was the term commonly used at that time to indicate immunoglobulins detectable by PL-dependent coagulation tests or immunological assays using anionic PL as antigens. After initial descriptions of isolated cases of thrombosis and pregnancy loss in patients with LAC were made, the more sensitive anticardiolipin (aCL) assay led to the identification of numerous patients. The concurrence of aCL antibodies, LAC, false positive VDRL and thrombosis or pregnancy loss occurred frequently enough to merit this clinical entity's recognition as the 'antiphospholipid syndrome' (APS) [2-4] The denomination was kept but it is now evident that aPL are not directed towards PL but to PL-binding proteins, the most relevant of which appear to be β2-Glycoprotein I (β2GPI) and prothrombin.

β2GPI and Anti-β2GPI Antibodies

β2GPI is a 50-kDa glycoprotein that is present in plasma at a concentration of approximately 200 μg/mL. This protein is a member of the complement control proteins (CCPs) [5]. β2GPI consists of 5 CCP repeats in which the first 4 domains are regular repeats consisting of 60 amino acids. The fifth domain is different from the other 4 domains as it consists of 82 amino acids, 4 conserved hydrophobic amino acids, 3 disulfide bonds instead of 2, and a cluster of positively charged amino acids, which is responsible for binding of β2GPI to phospholipids [6-9] The surface of domain I also contains a hydrophilic patch, which is described to be highly immunogenic.

Not all anti–β2GPI IgG antibodies have the same epitope specificity; a substantial number of antibodies recognize an epitope around G40-R43 on domain I, and these antibodies seem to be the pathogenic ones because their presence was highly related with a history of thrombosis [10]; the anti–β2GPI IgG antibodies against epitope G40-R43 in domain I are antibodies that cause LAC activity. Anti–β2GPI IgG antibodies that do not recognize G40-R43 in domain I are not related to a history of thrombosis.

The primary event inducing generation of aPL is not known. Peptides based on the linear structure of β2GPI were shown to have molecular mimicry with cytomegalovirus [11], thus a cross-reaction may be involved in aPL production. Given the identification of the true autoantigen (β2GPI) and the fact that its injection in animals reproduces the disease [12], APS might be considered a specific autoimmune disorder.

Two possible explanations for the mechanism of action of β2GPI/anti-β2GPI Ab complexes were suggested in the literature. First, β2GPI undergoes conformational changes when it interacts with PL exposing neoepitopes recognized by anti-β2GPI Abs [13-17]. Second, β2GPI is able to form bivalent complexes when it interacts with an anti-β2GPI Ab increasing antibody affinity [18,19].

Several hypothesis have been proposed to explain the pathophysiology of anti phospholipids antibodies. An increased resistance against the anticoagulant capacity of annexin A5 is one of them [20]. An increased resistance to protein C, independent of factor V Leiden (a factor known to cause hypercoagulation), has also been postulated to explain APS [21]. Aβ2GPI are also associated with increased levels of activated von Willebrand factor. As β2GPI-dependent LAC (and hence antidomain I antibodies) causes increased resistance to annexin A5 and activated protein C, it could be hypothesized that the clinical symptoms of APS are caused by different pathogenetic mechanisms rather than by one mechanism [22].

Definition

A syndrome is a collection or group of signs and symptoms that occur together and characterize a particular abnormality. APS is characterized by the association of at least one clinical (vascular thrombosis and pregnancy loss) and one laboratory (circulating aPL antibodies, with a specific pattern of positivity) finding. Half of the patients have no underlying disorder while the remaining are mainly affected by SLE or other connective tissue diseases [23].

Clinical and laboratory criteria for APS diagnosis were first stated at Sapporo preliminary report [24], and recently updated on the Sydney Consensus Conference [25].

Clinical Suspicion of APS

Thrombosis-related events are extremely common being the main cause of morbidity and mortality in Western countries. In the case of an indiscriminate search for aPL in these patients, the above definition may be applied to a large number of patients depending on the sensitivity and cut-off values used by the particular laboratory. The risk of overdiagnosis and its related costs should be limited by screening only those patients who present signs inducing clinical suspicion. For example screening is not indicated in a 75 years old patient with stroke and atrial fibrillation, while is highly recommended in a young woman with cryptogenic stroke; presence of other certain or presumptive stroke causes doesn't exclude

APS diagnosis, but decreases clinical significance of aPL. Moreover screening is recommended when vascular thrombosis is recurrent or occurs in uncommon sites or in both venous and arterial circulation. Suspicion may be reinforced when there is a coexistence of accompanying features such as epilepsy, migraine-like headaches, livedo reticularis and thrombocytopenia. Although testing for aPL should not be carried out close to the index event, an exception should be made for acutely ill patients when a catastrophic APS is suspected. Finally, laboratory tests should necessarily be carried out when unprovoked vascular thrombosis and fetal loss occur in patients affected from other autoimmune diseases.

Clinical Criteria

It was recently stated that the index clinical event should not precede positive laboratory results of more than 5 years and less than 12 weeks for APS diagnosis [25].

Vascular Thrombosis

The most frequent event in APS is venous thromboembolism. Objective criteria must be used for its diagnosis, namely venography or compression ultrasonography for deep vein thrombosis and spiral tomography, ventilation-perfusion lung scan or pulmonary angiography for pulmonary embolism. Likewise arterial thrombosis needs to be assessed using appropriate imaging (i.e. angiography, ultrasonography, standard computed tomography, angiography, magnetic resonance angiography). Assessment of thrombosis in cerebral vessels may be more difficult requiring computed tomography scan or magnetic resonance. As the criteria of the Sapporo preliminary report [24] were too indefinite ("imaging") and included a non-objective technique ("Doppler"), the Sydney update of the classification criteria [25] better defined that both venous and arterial thrombosis must be confirmed by objective validated criteria. Moreover, it was confirmed that thrombosis should be present without significant evidence of inflammation in the vessel wall for histopathologic detection. At variance with the Sapporo criteria, thrombophlebitis, a typical inflammatory disease of the superficial veins was correctly excluded. A further step forward in the Sydney update was the classification of APS into two subgroups according to the absence or presence of additional risk factors for thrombosis. The latter situation is intriguing as, for example, older age is a risk factor for thrombosis and is normally associated with higher aCL antibody values [26,27]. The relative importance of each component to the thromboembolic event remains disputable. On the contrary, if we consider a group of patients in whom aPL antibodies constitute the only appreciable risk factor for the disease we can better evaluate its natural history and appropriate treatment.

Obstetric Complications

Diagnosis of obstetric APS applies to women with otherwise unexplained obstetric complications. Other possible causes of miscarriage such as chromosomal, infectious, hormonal or anatomical abnormalities must therefore be excluded. Pregnancy morbidity has been classified in three groups: a) death of a normal fetus beyond the 10th week of gestation; b) premature birth due to of severe eclampsia or preeclampsia, or severe placental insufficiency before the 34th week of gestation; c) three or more spontaneous abortions prior to 10th week of gestation. The first group appears to be the most specific type of pregnancy loss in APS, resulting from placental insufficiency due to intravillous thrombosis and infarction [28]. It is interesting that thrombosis may be the main pathogenic mechanism in these subjects as we have recently demonstrated a statistically significant association between late obstetric complications and previous thromboembolic events in women with obstetric APS [11]. Some problems may be encountered with the second group in relation to the definitions used for specific pregnancy morbidity and the timing of delivery which is often based on the obstetrician's judgement [25]. The third group, characterized by early pregnancy loss, remains an obstetric criterion for APS although thrombosis is not commonly recognized as a pathogenic mechanism in these cases [29].

Other Features

One clinical and one laboratory criteria are required for diagnosis of APS, but this syndrome is also characterized by other features that often are present in these patients [25], including heart valve disease (see above), livedo reticularis, thrombocytopenia, nephropathy, neurological manifestations, IgA aCL, IgA anti-b2GPI, antiphosphatidylserine antibodies, antiphosphatidylethanolamine antibodies, antibodies against prothrombin alone, and antibodies to the phosphatidylserine–prothrombin complex. Some of these features are undoubtedly frequent but not specific in patients with APS.

Laboratory Criteria

Laboratory tests used to evaluate presence of aPL are LAC, aCL, and aβ_2GPI. We remark that aPL positivity is only a laboratory finding, that does not constitute *per se* a syndrome. In contrast APS is defined in presence of clinical findings, and a definite laboratory pattern of aPL. The crucial problem in APS diagnosis is the identification the presence of *pathogenic aPL* (autoantibodies directed against β2GPI causing LAC): we don't dispose a direct laboratory test for such antibodies, but we can determinate their presence by the combination of the three aPL tests, that taken isolated are also positive in many other conditions.

Positive of laboratory testing should be persistent if diagnosis of APS is to be formulated. Recently, the interval of at least 6 weeks between two positive test results was brought to 12 weeks [25].

Testing aCL and β2GPI, medium high titre positivity is required for diagnosis of APS.

Lupus Anticoagulant

The currently utilized criteria for the diagnosis of LAC are those proposed by Brandt in 1995 [30]: prolongation of at least 1 PL-dependent coagulation assay out of 2 or more screening tests (activated Partial Thromboplastin Time, aPTT, Kaolin Clotting Time, KCT, diluted Russell Viper Venom Time, dRVVT, diluted Prothrombin Time, dPT or other less popular ones). To exclude factors' deficiency test plasma is mixed with pooled normal plasma at a ratio of 1:1. A confirmatory test using an excess of phospholipids or activated platelets or hexagonal PL neutralizes the anticoagulant effect demonstrating that the inhibitor is actually sensitive to PL. The presence of heparin, which interferes with most LAC assays, in the test plasma is neutralized by including a heparin neutralizer in the reagent or excluded by performing the thrombin time (TT) [31].

In the case of positivity, it is essential that a new test be performed at least twelve weeks later in order to rule out preanalytical or analytical problems or a transient positivity. It is important to underline that apparently only some antibodies to a specific domain of β2-GPI express LAC activity [18,32] and are strongly correlated to thromboembolic events [10].

Anticardiolipin (aCL) Antibodies

Anticardiolipin antibodies, IgG and IgM isotypes, are measured by standardized ELISA [33-35]; medium high titer is defined as > 40 GPL or MPL, or > the 99th percentile. Positivity must be confirmed by a second test, performed 12 weeks apart.

Anti β2-glycoprotein I (aβ2GPI) Antibodies

aβ2GPI antibodies, IgG and IgM isotypes, are assessed by standardized ELISA [36]; medium-high titer is defined as > 99th percentile. As for LAC and aCL a second test, performed at least 12 weeks apart, is required for diagnosis of APS.

On the basis of laboratory findings patients are classified into one of the following categories:

I more than one laboratory criteria present (any combination);
II a LAC present alone;
II b aCL antibody present alone;
II c anti-b2 glycoprotein-I antibody present alone.

Interpretation of aPL Antibody Pattern

When aPL positivity is part of the Syndrome? As described above among the multitude of antibodies and conditions that lead to positive aPL tests, the sole involved in APS are *persistent auto-antibodies (IgG) anti-human β2-GPI causing LAC*, most likely directed against *domain I* of β2-GPI. These antibodies, which represent a small part of all aPL, are known to be associated to thrombosis, and they can be individuated by performing all three aPL tests. aPL test positivity due to any other antibody does not configure an antiphospholipid syndrome, and the trombotic event cannot be attributed to these antibodies.

The report of the Sydney consensus conference clearly states that a single positive test among the three laboratory criteria allows diagnosis of APS to be made. In this way laboratories performing a single test could diagnose APS without knowing results of the other two tests. In addition to the fact that the amount of false positive results of a single test is not negligible, the possibility of classifying patients in category I (multiple positivity – high risk patients) is not met. Therefore all the three tests must be performed and pathologists and clinicians should draw conclusion on the basis of laboratory profiles and clinical events.

Profiles with a Single Positive Test

- [positive LAC; negative aCL; negative aβ2GPI] In patients with positive LAC and normal aCL and aβ2GPI, a false positive LAC should be taken into consideration. If LAC positive only is confirmed, these patients may be considered at low risk of thrombosis [37,38].
- [negative LAC; positive aCL; negative aβ2GPI] aCL ELISA suffer from interpretation problems especially when it is the only positive test out of those determining the presence of aPL antibodies. Moreover, when isotypes from ELISAs obtained for aCL positive patients were considered, we have shown that only the IgG isotype was associated with the presence of a previous thromboembolic event or obstetric complications [37]. Autoimmune anticardiolipin antibodies are directed against β2-glycoprotein I which is the relevant autoantigen in APS. When aCL is positive but the same aβ2GPI isotype is negative then the aCL test may be false positive or the aCL may bind to bovine β2GPI or directly to cardiolipin. In 8 patients with suspected APS in which aCL was the only positive test, we found that 5 individuals had antibodies to bovine instead of to human β2GPI [39]. These subjects may be incorrectly classified as APS patients in the absence of autoimmune antibodies (i.e. anti human β2GPI). It would seem from these data that human β2GPI-dependency of aCL should be assayed using the combined testing by ELISA of aCL and anti human β2GPI antibodies. This approach would avoid overdiagnosing APS by identifying only patients with an autoimmune disease. Nevertheless, the Sydney consensus statement [25] confirmed that positivity of aCL, based on a single positive test result, remains a criterion for the diagnosis of APS and did not specify how to test for autoimmune aCL. Though a better definition of the threshold for positive aCL (>40 GPL or MPL units, or >99th percentile) was introduced [25], the role of aCL as the sole positive test to diagnose APS was not discussed. We have recently shown that when individual tests (LAC, aCL, aβ2GPI) were considered in a multivariate analysis taking age, gender, the presence of SLE or other autoimmune diseases and established risk factors for venous and arterial

thromboembolism into account, aCL antibodies were not an independent risk factor for thrombosis [37].

- [negative LAC; negative aCL; positive aβ2GPI] As suggested at the 48th SSC/ISTH meeting held in Boston in June, 2002 [40], positivity of anti-human β2GPI antibodies should be included in the laboratory criteria of APS, as it identifies LAC-positive patients at risk for thrombosis [10,41] and autoimmune aCL [39]. In the Sydney consensus statement [25] it was indeed decided (by the majority) that IgG and IgM aβ2GPI (in title > 99th percentile) should be included as part of the modified Sapporo criteria. There is evidence that aβ2GPI antibodies are an independent risk factor for thrombosis and pregnancy loss [42-44] but a recent metanalysis of available studies was unable to reach a clear conclusion [45]. It is important to underline that apparently only some antibodies to a specific domain of β2GPI express LAC activity and correlate strongly with thromboembolic events. Therefore, IgG aβ2GPI are associated with thrombosis only in a subset of patients. Other autoantibodies to β2GPI may not be pathogenic and this might explain why studies on their detection have not produced uniform results [45]. In those cases (from 2% to 10%) in which aβ2GPI is the only positivity detected in patients with clinical manifestations of the antiphospholipid syndrome [46,47], aβ2GPI may not be pathogenic as these antibodies do not recognize β2GPI bound to an anionic PL surface. To homogenize test results from various laboratories aβ2GPI antibodies should be tested following the indications of the Standardization Group of the European Forum on antiphospholipid antibodies [48].

Profiles with Multiple Positive Tests

- [negative LAC; positive aCL; positive aβ2GPI] The simultaneous positivity of aCL and aβ2GPI of the same isotype is very helpful as it excludes the presence of infective antibodies and confirms the presence of relevant autoimmune antibodies. We have found that this aPL profile (IgG isotype for both tests) is associated with thrombosis but the association is much stronger with pregnancy morbidity [37]. Titre of aβ2GPI antibodies is significantly lower than that of triple positive patients and this probably explains the absence of LAC activity in plasma samples.
- [positive LAC; positive aCL; positive aβ2GPI] A full positive pattern appears to reflect the presence of significant amounts of autoantibodies to human β2GPI with a consequent increased risk of thrombosis-related events or obstetric complications [49]. When anti-phospholipid antibody profiles were analyzed in multivariate model triple positivity was a strong independent risk factor (Odds Ratio 33.3, Confidence Interval 7.0–157.6) for thrombosis-related events, retaining its significance when only venous (Odds Ratio 8.5, Confidence Interval 3.6–20.2) or arterial thromboembolism (Odds Ratio 4.5, Confidence Interval 2.0–10.3) was considered [37]. These patients should be classified as a high risk, homogeneous group of APS for whom treatment efficacy should be documented by specific clinical trials and new therapeutic procedures should be considered [50].

Cerebral Ischaemia

Epidemiology

Low titre and habitually non-pathogenic aPL are found in 5–10% of healthy people [51] and may be transiently elevated after viral infections and drug exposures [52,53]. Persistent high titre aPL antibodies are detected in less than 2% of healthy adults. aPL are found in 30% of adult and over 50% of paediatric lupus patients [53,54].

aPL have been fairly well-established as risk factors for first juvenile ischemic stroke, but their role in recurrent stroke is less clear, and the association becomes weaker in older people [55]. Hughes suggests that up to one in five of all juvenile strokes (under 45 years) may be associated with APS [56]. Case-control and prospective studies that evaluated aPL in young adults, primarily in patients without SLE, found an increased risk for incident ischemic stroke [57-61]. One study [58] evaluating the risk for recurrent stroke and aPL in young adults (age 18-44 years) found that patients with antiphospholipid antibodies had significantly more prior cerebral events, and, by survival analysis, higher probability of cerebral ischemic or systemic thrombotic events during follow-up than patients without.

Our group tested aPL in a selected cohort of 76 young patient with cryptogenic stroke and patent foramen ovale [62], and 20 aPL positivity were found (none LAC, 8 aCL and 12 ab2GPI); confirmatory testing performed more than 12 weeks later showed that only two patients had persistent positivity of aPL, in a single test (1 aCL persistent positive patient and 1 aβ2GPI persistent positive patient). This is a paradigm of aPL transient positivity, don't causing APS.

Several studies have shown that strokes and transient ischemic attacks (TIAs) are the most common arterial thrombotic events in patients with APS [63-66]. The Euro-Phospholipid Project Group is studying the clinical and immunologic manifestations and patterns of disease expression of APS in a cohort of 1,000 patients [63] satisfying Sapporo criteria for APS [67]; at study entry stroke was the most common arterial thrombotic manifestation occurring in 13.1% patients, transient ischemic attack 7.0% and amaurosis fugax in 2.8% patients. Amaurosis fugax, transient paresthesias, ataxia, motor weakness, vertigo, and transient global ischemia can all be expressions of TIAs [68]. Cerebral ischemia is common in SLE patients. In 323 consecutive patients cerebrovascular disease occurred in 14.5% patients; multivariate analysis showed that aPL were independently strongly associated with cerebrovascular disease, and also with headache and seizure; LAC was independently associated with white matter hyperintensity lesions on MRI [69]. The clinical spectrum ranges from transient ischaemic attacks and focal lesions to widespread cerebral infarction, ataxia, bladder, and gait disturbance and – in extreme cases – multi-infarct dementia [56]. Stroke patients with aPL are younger and more likely to be women in comparison with stroke patients without aPL [70,71].

Pathology and Pathophysiology

Pathogenesis of cerebral ischaemia is still unclear, but many findings suggest an embolic mechanism. At autoptical examination, thrombus histology was similar in both aPL-positive and aPL-negative subjects, with no evidence of vasculitis in the aPL-positive individuals [72].

Cerebral ischaemia, often due to middle cerebral artery occlusion, may affect any cerebral arterial territory [73]; cerebral angiography typically demonstrates intracranial branch or trunk occlusion or is normal in about one third of patients [74]. Large artery disease is uncommon in young patients with APS and stroke [58]. Cortical magnetic resonance imaging findings are consistent with large vessel occlusion [53,75]. aPL patients often present small foci of high signal in the brain white matter at MRI, which are often defined as consistent with the presence of small vessel disease. Not only are these lesions non-specific but their aetiology is unclear. Larger size and atypical topographic distribution of these lesions in aPL patients may be also consistent with demyelination and sometimes difficult to differentiate from MRI pictures in multiple sclerosis [76,77].

Embolic Sources

Cardiac valve lesions are common in APS, and they are potential sources of emboli. Transthoracic echocardiography is abnormal in one third of patients, typically demonstrating non-specific left-sided valvular (predominantly mitral) lesions characterized by valve thickening [63,78-80]. Such thickening is due to Libman-Sacks nonbacterial endocarditis. Lockshin et al. [81] reviewed literature about cardiac manifestation of APS.

Valve Abnormalities

Heart valves are frequently affected in patients with APS with or without SLE and in patients with aPL alone [63,82,83]. Echocardiographic valvular involvement is characterized by thickening of the leaflets (Libman–Sacks endocarditis) and it can be associated with valvular dysfunction; the mitral valve is more commonly involved than the aortic valve [84]. Several studies have reported high prevalence of valvular heart disease in APS; there is, however, a wide variability in the reported prevalence of this phenomenon, ranging from 32%–82% [84,85]. This variability is probably related to the differences in the examined populations, aPL test performance, and different echocardiographic techniques. A prevalence of 32%–38% was reported by transthoracic echocardiography (TTE) studies [84], while higher rates (82%) were reported in a study using transesophageal echocardiography (TEE) [85]; such difference in result impose a TEE evaluation of APS patients affected by stroke. Valve involvement is associated with increased risk of central nervous system manifestations, mainly stroke and epilepsy [86]. An high aCL titer (> 40 GPL) was also suggested to be a risk factor for thromboembolism [85].

Several studies on APS patients reported a strong association between valvular abnormalities and arterial thromboses, especially those involving the central nervous system [87-90]. Cervera et al. [87] reported that 52% of primary APS patients with valvulopathy suffered from strokes or transient ischemic attacks compared with only 15 % of patients without valvulopathy ($P < 0.01$). Erdogan and colleagues [89] recently, reported valve lesions in all stroke patients and in most with other arterial or venous thrombosis. Roldan et al. [90] showed that lupus anticoagulant positivity and valvular lesions (vegetation, thickening and regurgitation) were independent predictors of MRI-proven cerebrovascular disease in lupus patients (OR 5.3–10.6, $p < 0.03$).

Unpublished work from our group compared stroke patients with and without APS. We considered 12 patients with triple aPL positivity, and 12 sex and age-matched controls with triple negativity for aPL. At TEE examination we found a statistically significant increase of mitral valve thickening (cases 4.45 ± 1.26 mm, controls 3.01 ± 1.24 mm, $p < 0.01$).

The deformed valves of the APS patients show aCL and complement deposits in the subendothelial connective tissue. There is positive staining for IgG and complement along the surface of the cusps. Histologically, there is endothelial cell proliferation with focal inflammatory changes, edema or fibrosis, focal calcifications, resulting in valve thickening, rigidity and dysfunction [91]. Although the pathogenesis of the valve lesions is not clear, several studies have tried to elucidate the precipitating event that triggers the inflammatory response; deposition of aPL [92,93] and anti-β2GPI [94] seem to be involved in the process. The anti-β2GPI deposition raises the possibility that bacterial antigens induce a crossreactivity immune response leading to Libman-Sacks nonbacterial endocarditis.

Qaddoura and colleagues [95] published four cases of primary APS patients with valve disease. The pathologic appearance of the valves paralleled TEE: focal, symmetric, nodular abnormalities resulting from thrombi at the coapting edges of the valve leaflets or cusps.

Several studies [91,96,97] showed that these thrombi are resistant to antithrombotic or antiaggregant therapy.

Although frequent, the valve lesions in aPL-positive patients rarely require surgical treatment [98].

Intracardiac Thrombi

Contrary to the valve abnormalities in case of primary APS which involve the left side of the heart, intracardiac thrombi formation prevails in the right side, having an etiologic role in pulmonary embolism events [92]. Even if less common than valve abnormalities, left atrial appendage thrombus may represent a cardiac source for stroke [96], and its presence must be evaluated with TEE.

The only neurological manifestation that is considered to have sufficient evidence to justify it being a part of the criteria for the diagnosis of (APS) is cerebral ischemia. Other neurological manifestations of APS are dementia and cognitive dysfunction, migraine, seizure, chorea, transverse myelopathy, optic neuropathy and multiple sclerosis [99]. Ischaemic lesions are also observed in these patients, but relation between thrombosis and such neurologic manifestation is uncertain. However, the possible effects of aPL are unlikely to be exclusively thrombotic and cross-reactivity with cerebral structures, inflammation, vasculopathy and accelerated atherosclerosis are all potential mechanisms [100].

Treatment

Don't treat aPL, treat APS

Evidence-based guidelines for treatment of APS, as defined by new more specific classification criteria, are still lacking, and need randomized clinical trials that keep in consideration difference between high risk category I APS and middle-low risk single positivity. In the meantime, treatment is based on available data, and should be guided by pathogenesis of cerebral ischaemia. In transient, single test positive patients aPL can be considered as a non specific marker of modestly increased risk of incident stroke, largely present in healthy people and without an established causative role. On the opposite side triple positivity shows an high risk condition needing treatment appropriate to thrombosis mechanism. Treatment must also be directed by evaluation of bleeding risk.

Primary Prevention

Transient aPL positivity without prior thrombosis doesn't require any treatment. Among 552 randomly selected blood donors, no thrombotic events were observed after 12 months of follow-up in the patients found to have aCL [101]. Neither persistent aPL positivity need treatment, even if in patient with SLE low-dose aspirin con be employed, especially when other risk factors for thrombosis coexist [102,103]. Another condition that requires a separate evaluation is occasional finding of triple positivity, although this situation is unusual, and doesn't constitute an APS.

Secondary Prevention

Thrombosis, associated to a specific laboratory pattern, is a required clinical criterion for diagnosis of APS, thus by definition the treatment of APS is based on secondary prevention.

A systematic review of secondary thromboprophylaxis in patients with aPL was recently published by Ruiz-Irastorza et al. [104].

Nine cohort studies were included in this review [64,105-112]. Patients included fulfilled laboratory criteria for APS, except that for two studies [64,105]. Untreated patients had high recurrence rates (19% - 29% per year), making evident a dose-effect of oral anticoagulation, with fewer recurrent thrombotic events among patients treated with high-intensity anticoagulation (INR of 3.0 – 4.0) as compared with those with a target INR of 2.0 – 3.0. Only 1 study analyzed arterial and venous events separately [64], and found an higher risk of recurrences for arterial than for venous events in all therapeutic groups.

Five studies were classified as subgroup analyses of cohort studies [113-115] and randomized controlled trials [116,117] designed to investigate the relationship between aPL positivity and recurrent thrombotic events; so these studies were not focused on therapy. The frequencies of recurrent events seen in both treated and untreated patients were lower than those found in cohort studies. Only one study in this group recruited patients fulfilling laboratory criteria for definite APS [113]. Only APASS [117] included patients with arterial and/or venous thrombosis, the others investigated only patients with venous thromboembolism.

The APL and Stroke Study (APASS) [117] is a prospective cohort study within the Warfarin Aspirin Recurrent Stroke Study (WARSS) [118], a randomized double-blind trial comparing warfarin (INR 1.4 – 2.8) and aspirin 325 mg/day for preventing recurrent stroke or death. The study group had an average age of 60 years (much higher than the average for APS population), the aPL determination was performed only once at the study entry, and the cut-off for assigning a patient to the positive aCL group was very low, with the consequence that most patients were not affected by APS. Only patients with noncardioembolic stroke were included, while in APS cardioembolism is the most likely mechanism. So results from this study can not be generalized to APS patients.

Two randomized controlled trials (one Canadian [119] and one European [120]) compared standard anticoagulant treatment (target INR of 2.5) with high-intensity anticoagulant treatment (target INR of 3.5) for the secondary prophylaxis of thrombosis in APS. Patients included fulfilled classification criteria for APS. Main APS manifestation was venous thromboembolism, present in 76% and 63%, respectively, of the individuals enrolled. Patients with recent stroke were excluded from the Canadian trial. Both studies demonstrated no advantage of high-intensity anticoagulation (target INR of 3.0 – 4.0) versus standard anticoagulation (target INR of 2.0 – 3.0) in terms of preventing recurrent events.

These studies also showed management problems of high intensity anticoagulation, as patients in this group frequently failed to achieve the target INR. In the Canadian study, these patients were below the therapeutic range 43% of the time, and in the European study the mean INR in the high-intensity group was only 3.2 (implying that an important number of measurements were below the threshold of 3.0). It is possible that a greater oscillation in INR values in high intensity warfarin treatment expose patients to transient low anticoagulant efficacy, giving a non-significant increase in recurrent events in this group.

Before instituting an anticoagulant treatment, bleeding risk should be assessed for each patient. Published data show that the frequency and severity of bleeding complications is not high in patients with APS treated with oral anticoagulation, even at target INRs >3.0 [108, 119,121], maybe due in part to the lower age of this population as compared, for example, with patients affected by chronic atrial fibrillation.

In presence of a thrombotic event it is essential to establish if it is part of the Syndrome or not. In case of single low titre aPL positivity we cannot impute cerebral ischaemia to pathogenic aPL, and the stroke must be accredited to other causes, or if no cause is found classified as cryptogenic stroke and treated with aspirin as aPL negative subjects [117,122]. Even in presence of a single persistent high titre positivity, that realizes a middle-low risk APS, causative relation between aPL and stroke is in doubt, so considering aPL positivity as a marker it is reasonable to treat patients with aspirin [53,117,123] in absence of potential cardioembolic sources after complete evaluation including TEE; moderate warfarin should be considered in presence of associated venous thrombosis or other features of APS, and when a cardioembolic source is found.

By contrast a triple positivity identifies the presence of pathogenic auto-antibodies (IgG) anti-human β2-GPI causing LAC, configuring a high risk antiphospholipid syndrome; in such contest there is a causative relation between aPL and stroke, through a cardioembolic mechanism. Such causative relations is reinforced by findings of embolic sources at TEE. Even if there is a general consensus about the indication of warfarin therapy in these patients (according to cardioembolic mechanism), intensity of treatment is subject to debate [124-127]. Due to the often devastating consequences of stroke and the young age of individuals we are considering, appears justifiable the strategy that best avoid such outcomes. While recurrent thromboses are exceptional with INRs >3.0, many cases have been documented within the usual therapeutic range of 2.0–3.0 [108,109]. However recent randomized controlled trials [119,120] demonstrated a non-significative increased recurrent rate in patients treated with high-intensity oral anticoagulation, apparently related to management of the therapy, frequently presenting wide INR excursions in these patients.

Therefore, specific therapy must be determined on an individual basis, taking into account the severity of the initial thrombotic event, the concurrent presence of other vascular risk factors or additional thromboses and the estimated bleeding risk according to age, bleeding history and polypharmacy [128,129]. Accordingly, moderate-intensity oral anticoagulation (INR range 2-3) would be justified in patients with triple positivity APS and stroke [53].

During pregnancy women must discontinue warfarin because of its teratogenic effect, and bridging treatment with heparin (LMWH) associated to aspirin is recommended [130].

Finally, there are no data to recommend additional antithrombotic treatment such as aspirin for patients who experience recurrent events while receiving oral anticoagulants achieving a 3.0 – 4.0 target INR [104].

Cerebral Venous Thrombosis

Cerebral venous sinus thrombosis (CVT) is a rare disorder that may result from a number pathologic processes including hypercoagulable states [131] such as the syndrome of activated protein C resistance due to factor V Leiden mutation [132]. The presence of aPL has been associated with an increased incidence of CVT [131]; the presence of aPL predisposes the patients to experience CVT at a younger age and with a broader superficial and deep cerebral venous system involvement. The clinical presentation of CVT includes headache, long tract signs, cognitive disturbances, papilloedema and visual dysfunction, seizures, focal deficits and coma [133]. The presence of aPL predisposes patients to a higher rate of post CVT migraine and higher incidence of infarctions on brain imaging studies [131].

Sneddon's Syndrome

This syndrome was described in 1965 by the dermatologist Sneddon, who first observed the development of cerebrovascular disease (stroke or TIA) in the presence of widespread livedo reticularis [134]. The neuropathologic findings are multiple small, predominantly cortical, infarcts, with focal hyperplasia and fibrotic occlusion of arterial vessels in the superficial white matter, cortex, and leptomeninges, suggesting a noninflammatory occlusive arteriopathy as underlying mechanism [135]. aPL are a common finding in Sneddon's syndrome [136], and livedo reticularis is a frequent cutaneous manifestation in patients with APS, affecting tipically females with SLE. Toubi and colleagues [137] found livedo reticularis in 16% of 308 APS patients; they also found a strong association with cerebrovascular disease, migraines, epilepsy, cardiac valve thickening, and vegetations, suggesting that patients with APS and livedo reticularis are at higher risk for thrombosis.

Catastrophic APS

This term, coined in 1972, indicates a clinical pattern characterized by small vessel thrombosis, occurring within a short time period (days or weeks), fatal in 50% cases. It can appear 'de novo', or following infective event, and represent about 1% of APS manifestation. The catastrophic APS can present with an acute organic brain syndrome characterized by fulminant encephalopathy [98,138]. Microthrombotic occlusive disease of multiple small vessels ('thrombotic microangiopathy') has been reported in a large number of patients [139].

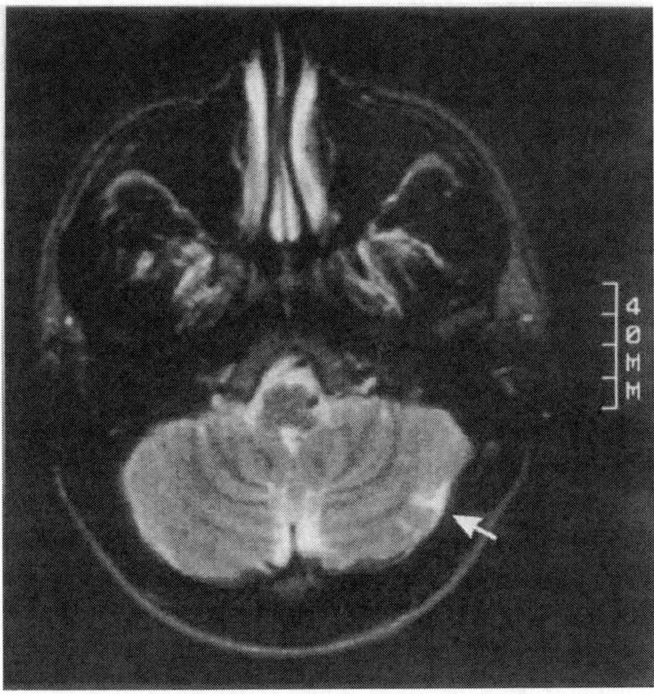

Figure 1. Transient ischemic attack associated with a cerebellar lesion at MRI in a patients with APS.

Conclusion

The diagnosis of APS requires the presence of both clinical and laboratory criteria that explain the association between the thrombotic event and the aβ2GPI autoantibodies that cause LAC. If these criteria are not satisfied the latter association is weak and not only the presence of aPL does not confer a high thromboembolic risk to the patient but also is considered a nonspecific finding, which is quite frequent.

In young patients the cerebral ischemia is often cryptogenic, as a result the presence of aPL is of etiological value only if the diagnostic criteria for APS are met, thus preventing over-diagnosis. Stroke in these patients seems to result from cardioembolism from valvular deposits of thrombotic nature (Libman-Sacks endocarditis); in fact autopsy reports reveal occlusion of large arteries with no signs of inflammation, and in patients with APS and stroke it is frequent a valvular thrombotic involvement.

The secondary prevention of APS, parallel to the stroke mechanism, is based on anticoagulant therapy. The anticoagulant therapy is of imperative importance especially in patients with triple positivity for APS who are subject to the highest thrombotic risk of all APS. Although the intensity of anticoagulation is still a matter of debate, present data suggest that patients benefit from target INR 2.0 – 3.0.

References

[1] Shapiro SS. Lupus anticoagulants and anticardiolipin antibodies: personal reminiscences, a little history, and some random thoughts. *J. Thromb Haemost.* 2005;3: 831–833.

[2] Harris EN, Gharavi AE, Boey ML et al. Anticardiolipin antibodies: detection by radioimmunoassay and association with thrombosis in systemic lupus erithematosus. *Lancet* 1983;2:1211-1214.

[3] Hughes GRV, Harris EN, Gharavi AE. The anticardiolipin syndrome. *J. Rheumatol.* 1986;13;486-9.

[4] Harris EN. Syndrome of the black swan. *Br. J. Rheumatol.* 1987;26:324-6.

[5] Steinkasserer A, Estaller C, Weiss EH, Sim RB, Day A. Complete nucleotide and deduced amino acid sequence of human b2-glycoprotein I. *Biochem. J.* 1991;227:387-391.

[6] Steinkasserer A, Barlow PN, Willis AC, et al. Activity, disulphide mapping and structural modelling of the fifth domain of human b2-glycoprotein I. *FEBS Lett.* 1992; 313:193-197.

[7] Hunt J, Krilis S. The fifth domain of b2-glycoprotein I contains a phospholipid binding site (Cys 281-Cys 288) and a region recognized by anticardiolipin antibodies. *J. Immunol.* 1994;152:653-659.

[8] Mehdi H, Naqvi A, Kamboh MI. A hydrophobic sequence at position 313-316 (Leu, Ala, Phe, Trp) in the fifth domain on apolipoprotein H (b2-glycoprotein I) is crucial for cardiolipin binding. *Eur. J. Biochem.* 2000;267:1770-1776.

[9] Sheng Y, Sali A, Herzog H, Lahnstein J, Krilis SA. Site-directed mutagenesis of recombinant human b2-glycoprotein I identifies a cluster of lysine residues that are critical for phospholipid binding and anti-cardiolipin antibody activity. *J. Immunol.* 1996; 157:3744-3751.

[10] de Laat B, Derksen RH, Urbanus RT, de Groot PG. IgG antibodies that recognize epitope Gly40- Arg43 in domain I of beta2-glycoprotein I cause LAC, and their presence correlates strongly with thrombosis. *Blood* 2005;105:105:1540-1545.

[11] Gharavi AE, Pierangeli SS, Espinola RG, Liu X, Colden-Stanfield M, Harris EN: Antiphospholipid antibodies induced in mice by immunization with a cytomegalovirus-derived peptide cause thrombosis and activation of endothelial cells in vivo. *Arthritis Rheum.* 2002;46:545–552.

[12] Blank M, Faden D, Tincani A et al. Immunization with anticardiolipin cofactor (beta-2-glycoprotein I) induces experimental antiphospholipid syndrome in naive mice. *J. Autoimmun.* 1994;7:441–455.

[13] Matsuura E, Igarashi Y, Yasuda T, Triplett DA, Koike T: Anticardiolipin antibodies recognize beta 2-glycoprotein I structure altered by interacting with an oxygen modified solid phase surface. *J. Exp. Med.* 1994;179:457–462.

[14] Wagenknecht DR, McIntyre JA: Changes in beta 2-glycoprotein I antigenicity induced by phospholipid binding. *Thromb Haemost.* 1993;69:361–365.

[15] Ichikawa K, KhamashtaMA,KoikeT, Matsuura E, Hughes GR: Beta2-glycoprotein I reactivity of monoclonal anticardiolipin antibodies from patients with the antiphospholipid syndrome. *Arthritis Rheum.* 37:1453–1461, 1994.

[16] Wang SX, Sun YT, Sui SF: Membrane-induced conformational change in human apolipoprotein H. *Biochem. J.* 348(Pt 1):103–106, 2000.

[17] Pengo V, Biasiolo A, Fior MG. Autoimmune antiphospholipid antibodies are directed against a cryptic epitope expressed when b2-Glycoprotein-I is bound to a suitable surface. *Thromb Haemost.* 1995; 73:29–34.

[18] Arnout J, Wittevrongel C, Vanrusselt M, Hoylaerts M, Vermylen J: Beta-2-glycoprotein I dependent lupus anticoagulants form stable bivalent antibody beta-2-glycoprotein I complexes on phospholipids surfaces. *Thromb Haemost.* 79:79–86, 1998.

[19] Sheng Y, Kandiah DA, Krilis SA: Anti-beta 2-glycoprotein I autoantibodies from patients with the "antiphospholipid" syndrome bind to beta 2-glycoprotein I with low affinity: Dimerization of beta 2-glycoprotein I induces a significant increase in anti-beta2-glycoprotein I antibody affinity. *J. Immunol.* 161:2038–2043,1998.

[20] Rand JH et al. Pregnancy loss in the antiphospholipid-antibody syndrome – a possible thrombogenic mechanism. *N. Engl. J. Med.* 1997;337: 154–160.

[21] De Laat B et al. Correlation between the potency of a β2-glycoprotein I dependent lupus anticoagulant and the level of resistance to activated protein C [abstract]. Abstract P-S-539, XXIst congress of the ISTH, Geneva 2007.

[22] de Laat B, Mertens K, de Groot PG. Mechanisms of disease: antiphospholipid antibodies-from clinical association to pathologic mechanism. *Nat. Clin. Pract. Rheumatol.* 2008 Apr;4(4):192-9.

[23] Asherson RA, Cervera R, Piette JC, Shoenfeld Y. The antiphospholipid syndrome. Boca Raton: CRC Press Inc.; 1996:3-12.

[24] Wilson WA, Gharavi AE, Koike T, et al. International Consensus Statement On Preliminary Classification Criteria for Definite Antiphospholipid Syndrome: Report of an International Workshop. *Arthritis Rheum*. 1999;2(7):1309–1311.

[25] Miyakis S, Lockshin MD, Atsumi T, Branch DW, Brey RL, Cervera R, Derksen RHWM, de Groot PG, Koike T, Meroni PL, Reber G, Shoenfeld Y, Tincani A, Vlachoyiannopoulos PG, Krilis SA. International consensus statement on an update of the classification criteria for definite antiphospholipid syndrome (APS). *J. Thromb Haemost*. 2006;4:295-306.

[26] Manoussakis MN, Tzioufas AG, Silis MP, Pange PJ, Goudevenos J, Moutsopoulos HM. High prevalence of anti-cardiolipin and other autoantibodies in a healthy elderly population. *Clin. Exp. Immunol.* 1987;69:557-65.

[27] Ruffatti A, Rossi L, Calligaro A, Del Ross T, Lagni M, Marson P, Todesco S. Autoantibodies of systemic rheumatic diseases in the healthy elderly. *Gerontology* 1990; 36:104-111.

[28] Branch DW, Scott JR, Kochenour NK, Hershgold E. Obstetric complications associated with the Lupus Anticoagulant. *N. Engl. J. Med*. 1985;313:1322-6.

[29] Branch DW. Antiphospholipid antibodies and foetal compromise. *Thromb Res*. 2004; 114:415-8.

[30] Brandt JT, Triplett DA, Alving B, Scharrer I. Criteria for the diagnosis of lupus anticoagulants: an update. On behalf of the Subcommittee on Lupus Anticoagulant/Antiphospholipid Antibody of the Scientific and Standardisation Committee of the ISTH. *Thromb Haemost*. 1995;74:1185-90.

[31] Tripodi A, Biasiolo A, Chantarangkul V, Pengo V. Lupus anticoagulant (LA) testing: performance of clinical laboratories assessed by a national survey using lyophilized affinity-purified immunoglobulin with LA activity. *Clin. Chem.* 2003;49:1608-14.

[32] Takeya H, Mori T, Gabazza EC, Kuroda K, Deguchi H, Matsuura E, IchikawaK, Koike T, Suzuki K. Anti-β2-Glycoprotein I monoclonal antibodies with lupus anticoagulant activity enhance the β2-Glycoprotein I binding to phospholipids. *J. Clin. Invest* 1997; 99:2260-8.

[33] Tincani A, Allegri F, Sanmarco M, Cinquini M, Taglietti M, Balestrieri G, Koike T, Ichikawa K, Meroni P, Boffa MC. Anticardiolipin antibody assay: a methodological analysis for a better consensus in routine determinations – a cooperative project of the European Antiphospholipid Forum. *Thromb Haemost.* 2001; 86: 575–83.

[34] Harris EN, Pierangeli SS. Revisiting the anticardiolipin test and its standardization. *Lupus* 2002; 11: 269–75.

[35] Wong RC, Gillis D, Adelstein S, Baumgart K, Favaloro EJ, Hendle MJ,Homes P, Pollock W, Smith S, SteeleRH, Sturgess A, Wilson RJ. Consensus guidelines on anti-cardiolipin antibody testing and reporting. *Pathology* 2004; 36: 63–8.

[36] Reber G, Tincani A, Sanmarco M, de Moerloose P, Boffa MC. Proposals for the measurement of anti-beta2-glycoprotein I antibodies. Standardization group of the European Forum on Antiphospholipid Antibodies. *J. Thromb Haemost.* 2004; 2: 1860–2.

[37] Pengo V, Biasiolo A, Pegoraro C, Cucchini U, Noventa F, Iliceto S. Antibody profiles for the diagnosis of antiphospholipid syndrome. *Thromb Haemost*. 2005;93:1147-52.

[38] Pengo V, Biasiolo A, Gresele P, Marongiu F, Erba N, Veschi F, et al. A Survey on lupus anticoagulant diagnosis by central evaluation of positive plasma samples. *J. Thromb Haemost*. 2007; 5: 925-30.

[39] Pengo V, Biasiolo A. The risk of overdiagnosis of antiphospholipid antibody syndrome. *Thromb Haemost*. 2001;86:933.

[40] Pengo V. Communication, 48th Annual SSC meeting, Boston, MA, USA, July 18, 2002. See annual SSC reports at the ISTH website: http://www.med.unc.edu/isth.

[41] Zoghlami-Rintelen C, Vormittag R, Sailer T, Lehr S, Quehenberger P, Rumpold H, et al. I. The presence of IgG antibodies against β2-glycoprotein I predicts the risk of thrombosis in patients with the lupus anticoagulant. *J. Thromb Haemost.* 2005; 3: 1160-5

[42] Cabiedes J, Cabral AR, Alarcon-Segovia D. Clinical manifestations of the antiphospholipid syndrome in patients with systemic lupus erythematosus associate more strongly with anti-β2-Glycoprotein-I than with antiphospholipid antibodies. *J. Rheumatol.* 1995;22:1899-1906.

[43] Balestrieri G, Tincani A, Spatola L, et al. Anti-β2- Glycoprotein-I antibodies: a marker of antiphospholipid syndrome? *Lupus* 1995;4:122-130.

[44] Martinuzzo ME, Forastiero RR, Carreras LO. Anti-β2-Glycoprotein-I antibodies detection and association with thrombosis. *Br. J. Haematol*. 1995;89:397-402.

[45] Galli M, Luciani B, Bertolini G, Barbui T. Anti-β2-Glycoprotein I, anti-prothrombin antibodies and the risk of thrombosis in the antiphospholipid sindrome. *Blood* 2003; 102:2717-23.

[46] Ebelin F, Pettersson T, Muukkonen L, Vahtera E, Rasi V. β2-Glycoprotein I antibodies in patients with thrombosis. *Scand. J. Clin. Lab.* 2003;63:11-8.

[47] Myers B, Gould J. The place of β2-Glycoprotein I in the assessment of antiphospholipid syndrome. *Blood Coag. Fibrinolysis* 2003;14:1-2

[48] Reber G, Schousboe I, Tincani A, Sanmarco M, Kveder T, de Moerloose P, et al. Interlaboratory variabilità of anti-β2-glycoprotein I measurement. *Thromb Haemost.* 2002; 88: 66-73

[49] Ruffatti A, Tonello M, Del Ross T, Cavazzana A, Grava C, Noventa F, et al. Antibody profile and clinical course in primary antiphospholipid syndrome with pregnancy morbidity. *Thromb Haemost*. 2006; 96: 337-41.

[50] Ruffatti A, Marson P, Pengo V, Favaro M, Tonello M, Bortolati M, et al. Plasma exchange in the management of high risk pregnant patients with primary antiphospholipid syndrome. A report of 9 cases and a review of the literature. *Autoimmun. Rev*. 2007; 6: 196-202.

[51] Muscal E, Brey RL, Neurological manifestations of the antiphospholipid syndrome: risk assessments and evidence-based medicine. *Int. J. Clin. Pract.* 2007 Sep;61(9): 1561-8.

[52] Hanly JG. Antiphospholipid syndrome: an overview. *CMAJ* 2003; 168: 1675–82.

[53] Lim W, Crowther MA, Eikelboom JW. Management of the antiphospholipid antibody syndrome: a systemic review. *JAMA* 2006; 295: 1050–7.

[54] Kamat AV, D'Cruz DP, Hunt BJ. Managing antiphospholipid antibodies and antiphospholipid syndrome in children. *Haematologica* 2006; 91: 1674–80.

[55] Brey RL. Antiphospholipid Antibodies in Young Adults with Stroke. *Journal of Thrombosis and Thrombolysis* 20(2), 105–112, 2005.

[56] Hughes GR. Migraine, memory loss, and ''multiple sclerosis.'' Neurological features of the antiphospholipid (Hughes') syndrome. *Postgrad. Med. J.* 2003;79:81–3.

[57] Brey RL, Hart RG, Sherman DG, Tegeler CT. Antiphospholipid antibodies and cerebral ischemia in young people. *Neurology* 1990;40:1190–1196.

[58] Nencini P, Baruffi MC, Abbate R, Massai G, Amaducci L, Inzitari D. Lupus anticoagulant and anticardiolipin antibodies in young adults with cerebral ischemia. *Stroke* 1992;23:189–193.

[59] Toschi V, Motta A, Castelli C, Paracchini ML, Zerbi D, Gibelli A. High prevalence of antiphosphatidylinositol antibodies in young patients with cerebral ischemia of undetermined cause. *Stroke* 1998;29:1759–1764.

[60] Singh K, Gaiha M, Shome DK, Gupta VK, Anuradha S. The association of antiphospholipid antibodies with ischemic stroke and myocardial infarction in young and their correlation: a preliminary study. *J. Assoc. Physicians India* 2001;49:537–529.

[61] Brey RL, Stallworth CL, McGlasson DL, et al. Antiphospholipid antibodies and stroke in young women. *Stroke* 2002;33:2396–2400.

[62] Offelli P, Zanchetta M, Pedon L, Marzot F, Cucchini U, Pegoraro C, Iliceto S, Pengo V. Thrombophilia in young patients with cryptogenic stroke and patent foramen ovale (PFO). *Thromb Haemost.* 2007 Oct;98(4):906-7.

[63] Cervera R, Piette JC, Font J, Khamashta MA, Shoenfeld Y, Camps MT, Jacobsen S, Lakos G, Tincani A, Kontopoulou-Griva I, Galeazzi M, Meroni PL, Derksen RH, de Groot PG, Gromnica-Ihle E, Baleva M, Mosca M, Bombardieri S, Houssiau F, Gris JC, Quere I, Hachulla E, Vasconcelos C, Roch B, Fernandez-Nebro A, Boffa MC, Hughes GR, Ingelmo M. Antiphospholipid syndrome: clinical and immunologic manifestations and patterns of disease expression in a cohort of 1000 patients. *Arthritis Rheum.* 2002; 46: 1019–27.

[64] Krnic-Barrie S, O'Connor CR, Looney SW, et al.Aretrospective review of 61 patients with antiphospholipid syndrome. Analysis of factors influencing recurrent thrombosis. *Arch Intern. Med.* 1997;157:2101–8.

[65] Shah NM, Khamashta MA, Atsumi T, et al. Outcome of patients with anticardiolipin antibodies: a 10 year follow-up of 52 patients. *Lupus* 1998;7:3–6.

[66] Sastre-Garriga J, Montalban X. APS and the brain. *Lupus* 2003;12:877–82.

[67] Wilson WA, Gharavi AE, Koike T, et al. International Consensus Statement On Preliminary Classification Criteria for Definite Antiphospholipid Syndrome: Report of an International Workshop. *Arthritis Rheum.* 1999;2(7):1309–1311.

[68] Asherson RA, Khamashta MA, Gil A, et al. Cerebrovascular disease and antiphospholipid antibodies in systemic lupus erythematosus, lupus-like disease, and the primary antiphospholipid syndrome. *Am. J. Med.* 1989;86:391–9.

[69] Sanna G, Bertolaccini ML, Cuadrado MJ, et al. Neuropsychiatric manifestations in sistemi lupus erythematosus: prevalence and association with antiphospholipid antibodies. *J. Rheumatol.* 2003;30:985–92.

[70] Hilker R, Thiel A, Geisen C, et al. Cerebral blood flow and glucose metabolism in multiinfarct-dementia related to primary antiphospholipid antibody syndrome. *Lupus* 2000;9:311–6.

[71] Terashi H, Uchiyama S, Hashimoto S, et al. Clinical characteristics of stroke patients with antiphospholipid antibodies. *Cerebrovasc. Dis.* 2005;19:384–90.

[72] Ford SE, Kennedy LA, Ford PM. Clinico-pathological correlations of antiphospholipid antibodies. *Arch Path Lab. Med.* 1994;118:491–495.

[73] Coull BM, Levine SR, Brey RL. The role of antiphospholipid antibodies and stroke. *Neurol. Clin.* 1992;10:125–143.

[74] Antiphospholipid Antibodies in Stroke Study (APASS) Group. Clinical and laboratory findings in patients with antiphospholipid antibodies and cerebral ischemia. *Stroke* 1990;21:1268–1273.

[75] Sanna G, Bertolaccini ML, Cuadrado MJ et al. Central nervous system involvement in the antiphospholipid (Hughes) syndrome. *Rheumatology* 2003; 42: 200–13.

[76] Cuadrado MJ, Khamashta MA, Ballesteros A, Godfrey T, Simon MJ, Hughes GRV. Can neurologic manifestations of Hughes (antiphospholipid) syndrome be distinguished from multiple sclerosis? Analysis of 27 patients and review of the literature. *Medicine* (Baltimore) 2000;79:57–68.

[77] Ruiz-Irastorza G, Khamashta MA. Warfarin for multiple sclerosis? *Q. J. Med.* 2000;93: 497–9.

[78] Ford SE, Lillicrap DM, Brunet D, Ford PM. Thrombotic endocarditis and lupus anticoagulant, a pathogenetic possibility for idiopathic rheumatic type valvular heart disease. *Arch Pathol. Lab. Med.* 1989;113:350–353.

[79] Khamashta MA, Cervera R, Asherson RA, et al. Association of antibodies against phospholipids with valvular heart disease in patients with systemic lupus erythematosus. *Lancet* 1990; 335(8705):1541–1544.

[80] Cervera R. Coronary and valvular syndromes and antiphospholipid antibodies. *Thromb Haemostas.* 2004;114:501–508.

[81] Tenedios F, Erkan D, Lockshin MD. Cardiac manifestations in the antiphospholipid syndrome. *Rheum. Dis. Clin. North Am.* 2006 Aug;32(3):491-507.

[82] Lockshin M, Tenedios F, Petri M, et al. Cardiac disease in the antiphospholipid syndrome: recommendations for treatment. Committee consensus report. *Lupus* 2003; 12(7):518–23.

[83] Tincani A, Biasini-Rebaioli C, Cattaneo R, et al. Nonorgan specific autoantibodies and heart damage. *Lupus* 2005;14(9):656–9.

[84] Hojnik M, George J, Ziporen L, et al. Heart valve involvement (Libman-Sacks endocarditis) in the antiphospholipid syndrome. *Circulation* 1996;93(8):1579–87.

[85] Turiel M, Muzzupappa S, Gottardi B, et al. Evaluation of cardiac abnormalities and embolic sources in primary antiphospholipid syndrome by transesophageal echocardiography. *Lupus* 2000;9(6):406–12.

[86] Krause I, Lev S, Fraser A, et al. Close association between valvar heart disease and central nervous system manifestations in the antiphospholipid syndrome. *Ann. Rheum. Dis.* 2005; 64(10):1490–3.

[87] Cervera R, Khamashta MA, Font J, et al. High prevalence of significant heart valve lesions in patients with the ''primary'' antiphospholipid syndrome. *Lupus* 1991;1(1): 43–7.

[88] Galve E, Ordi J, Barquinero J, et al. Valvular heart disease in the primary antiphospholipid syndrome. *Ann. Intern. Med.* 1992;116(4):293–8.

[89] Erdogan D, Goren MT, Diz-Kucukkaya R, et al. Assessment of cardiac structure and left atrial appendage functions in primary antiphospholipid syndrome: a transesophageal echocardiographic study. *Stroke* 2005;36(3):592–6.

[90] Roldan CA, Gelgand EA, Qualls CR et al. Valvular heart disease as a cause of cerebrovascular disease in patients with systemic lupus erythematosus. *Am. J. Cardiol.* 2005; 95: 1441–7.

[91] Espinola-Zavaleta N, Vargas-Barron J, Colmenares-Galvis T, et al. Echocardiographic evaluation of patients with primary antiphospholipid syndrome. *Am. Heart J.* 1999; 137(5):973–8.

[92] Amital H, Langevitz P, Levy Y, et al. Valvular deposition of antiphospholipid antibodies in the antiphospholipid syndrome: a clue to the origin of the disease. *Clin. Exp. Rheumatol.* 1999; 17(1):99–102.

[93] Afek A, Shoenfeld Y, Manor R, et al. Increased endothelial cell expression of alpha3beta1 integrin in cardiac valvulopathy in the primary (Hughes) and secondary antiphospholipid syndrome. *Lupus* 1999;8(7):502–7.

[94] Blank M, Shani A, Goldberg I, et al. Libman-Sacks endocarditis associated with antiphospholipid syndrome and infection. *Thromb Res.* 2004;114(5–6):589–92.

[95] Qaddoura F, Connolly H, Grogan M, et al. Valve morphology in antiphospholipid antibody syndrome: echocardiographic features. *Echocardiography* 2005;22(3):255–9.

[96] Espinola Zavaleta N, Montes RM, Soto ME, et al. Primary antiphospholipid syndrome: a 5-year transesophageal echocardiographic followup study. *J. Rheumatol.* 2004; 31: 2402–7.

[97] Turiel M, Sarzi-Puttini P, Peretti R, et al. Five-year follow-up by transesophageal echocardiographic studies in primary antiphospholipid syndrome. *Am. J. Cardiol.* 2005; 96(4):574–9.

[98] Nesher G, Ilany J, Rosenmann D, et al. Valvular dysfunction in antiphospholipid syndrome: prevalence, clinical features, and treatment. *Semin. Arthritis Rheum.* 1997; 27(1):27–35.

[99] Brey RL, Differential diagnosis of central nervous system manifestations of the antiphospholipid antibody syndrome. *J. Autoimmun.* 2000 Sep;15(2):133-8.

[100] Ferreira S, D'Cruz DP, Hughes GR. Multiple sclerosis, neuropsychiatric lupus and antiphospholipid syndrome: where do we stand? *Rheumatology* (Oxford). 2005 Apr; 44(4):434-42. Epub 2005 Jan 11.

[101] Vila P, Hernandez MC, Lopez-Fernandez MF, Batlle J. Prevalence, follow-up and clinical significance of the anticardiolipin antibodies in normal subjects. *Thromb Haemost.* 1994; 72:209–213.

[102] G Bertsias, J P A Ioannidis, J Boletis, S Bombardieri, R Cervera, C Dostal, J Font, I M Gilboe, F Houssiau, T Huizinga, D Isenberg, C G M Kallenberg, M Khamashta, J C Piette, M Schneider, J Smolen, G Sturfelt, A Tincani, R van Vollenhoven, C Gordon

and D T Boumpas. EULAR recommendations for the management of systemic lupus erythematosus. Report of a Task Force of the EULAR Standing Committee for International Clinical Studies Including Therapeutics. *Ann. Rheum. Dis*. 2008;67;195-205.

[103]Brey RL. Management of the neurological manifestations of APS - what do the trials tell us? *Thromb Res.* 2004; 114: 489–99.

[104]Ruiz-Irastorza G, Hunt BJ, Khamashta MA. A systematic review of secondary thromboprophylaxis in patients with antiphospholipid antibodies. *Arthritis Rheum.* 2007 Dec 15;57(8):1487-95.

[105]Rosove MH, Brewer PM. Antiphospholipid thrombosis: clinical course after the first thrombotic event in 70 patients. *Ann. Intern. Med.* 1992;117:303–8.

[106]Khamashta MA, Cuadrado MJ, Mujic F, Taub N, Hunt BJ, Hughes GR. The management of thrombosis in the antiphospholipid antibody syndrome. *N. Engl. J. Med.* 1995; 332:993–7.

[107]Munoz-Rodriguez FJ, Font J, Cervera R, Reverter JC, Tassies D, Espinosa G, et al. Clinical study and follow-up of 100 patients with the antiphospholipid syndrome. *Semin. Arthritis Rheum*. 1999;29:182–90.

[108]Ruiz-Irastorza G, Khamashta MA, Hunt BJ, Escudero A, Cuadrado MJ, Hughes GR. Bleeding and recurrent thrombosis in definite antiphospholipid syndrome: analysis of a series of 66 patients treated with oral anticoagulation to a target international normalized ratio of 3.5. *Arch Intern. Med.* 2002;162:1164–9.

[109]Derksen RH, de Groot PG, Kater L, Nieuwenhuis HK. Patients with antiphospholipid antibodies and venous thrombosis should receive long term anticoagulant treatment. *Ann. Rheum. Dis.* 1993;52:689–92.

[110]Wittkowsky AK, Downing J, Blackburn J, Nutescu E. Warfarin-related outcomes in patients with antiphospholipid antibody syndrome managed in an anticoagulation clinic. *Thromb Haemost.* 2006;96:137–41.

[111]Ames PR, Ciampa A, Margaglione M, Scenna G, Iannaccone L, Brancaccio V. Bleeding and re-thrombosis in primary antiphospholipid syndrome on oral anticoagulation: an 8-year longitudinal comparison with mitral valve replacement and inherited thrombophilia. *Thromb Haemost.* 2005;93:694–9.

[112]Giron-Gonzalez JA, Garcia del Rio E, Rodriguez C, Rodriguez-Martorell J, Serrano A. Antiphospholipid syndrome and asymptomatic carriers of antiphospholipid antibody: prospective analysis of 404 individuals. *J. Rheumatol.* 2004;31:1560–7.

[113]Prandoni P, Simioni P, Girolami A. Antiphospholipid antibodies, recurrent thromboembolism, and intensity of warfarin anticoagulation [letter]. *Thromb Haemost.* 1996;75:859.

[114]Rance A, Emmerich J, Fiessinger JN. Anticardiolipin antibodies and recurrent thromboembolism [letter]. *Thromb Haemost.* 1997;77:221–2.

[115]Ginsberg JS, Wells PS, Brill-Edwards P, Donovan D, Moffat K, Johnston M, et al. Antiphospholipid antibodies and venous thromboembolism. *Blood* 1995;10:3685–91.

[116]Schulman S, Svenungsson E, Granqvist S, and the Duration of Anticoagulation Study Group. Anticardiolipin antibodies predict early recurrence of thromboembolism and

death among patients with venous thromboembolism following anticoagulant therapy. *Am. J. Med.* 1998;104:332–8.

[117]Levine SR, Brey RL, Tilley BC, et al, APASS Investigators. Antiphospholipid antibodies and subsequent thrombo-occlusive events in patients with ischemic stroke. *The Journal of the American Medical Association* 2004; 291: 576–584.

[118]WARSS Study Group. A double-blind study using an anticoagulant: the design and initial progress of the Warfarin-Aspirin Recurrent Stroke Study (WARSS). *Cerebrovasc. Dis.* 1997;7:100-112.

[119]Crowther MA, Ginsberg JS, Julian J, Denburg J, Hirsch J, Douketis J, et al. A comparison of two intensities of warfarin for the prevention of recurrent thrombosis in patients with the antiphospholipid syndrome. *N. Engl. J. Med.* 2003;349:1133–8.

[120]Finazzi G, Marchioli R, Brancaccio V, Schinco P, Wisloff F, Musial J, et al. A randomized clinical trial of high-intensity warfarin vs. conventional antithrombotic therapy for the prevention of recurrent thrombosis in patients with the antiphospholipid syndrome (WAPS). *J. Thromb Haemost.* 2005;3:848–53.

[121]Castellino G, Cuadrado MJ, Godfrey T, Khamashta MA, Hughes GRV. Characteristics of patients with antiphospholipid syndrome with major bleeding after oral anticoagulant treatment. *Ann. Rheum. Dis.* 2001;60:527–30.

[122]Sacco RL, Adams R, Albers G, Alberts MJ, Benavente O, Furie K, Goldstein LB, Gorelick P, Halperin J, Harbaugh R, Johnston SC, Katzan I, Kelly-Hayes M, Kenton EJ, Marks M, Schwamm LH, Tomsick T; American Heart Association; American Stroke Association Council on Stroke; Council on Cardiovascular Radiology and Intervention; American Academy of Neurology. Guidelines for prevention of stroke in patients with ischemic stroke or transient ischemic attack: a statement for healthcare professionals from the American Heart Association/American Stroke Association Council on Stroke: co-sponsored by the Council on Cardiovascular Radiology and Intervention: the American Academy of Neurology affirms the value of this guideline. *Stroke* 2006 Feb;37(2):577-617.

[123]Erkan D, Lockshin MD. New treatments for antiphospholipid syndrome. *Rheum. Dis. Clin. North Am.* 2006;32:129-48.

[124]Scully MF. Moderate dose oral anticoagulant therapy in patients with the antiphospholipid syndrome? Yes. *J. Thromb Haemost.* 2005; 3:840–841.

[125]Rickles FR, Marder VJ. Moderate dose oral anticoagulant therapy in patients with the antiphospholipid syndrome? No. *J. Thromb Haemost.* 2005; 3:842–843.

[126]Khamashta MA, Hunt BJ. Moderate dose oral anticoagulant therapy in patients with the antiphospholipid syndrome? No. *J. Thromb Haemost.* 2005; 3:844–845.

[127]Anderson DR. Oral anticoagulation for the antiphospholipid antibody syndrome: can we now say less is more? *J. Thromb Haemost.* 2005; 3:846–847.

[128]Sairam S, Baethge BA, McNearney T. Analysis of risk factors and comorbid diseases in the development of thrombosis in patients with anticardiolipin antibodies. *Clin. Rheumatol.* 2003; 22:24–9.

[129]Ruiz-Irastorza G, Khamashta MA. Stroke and antiphospholipid syndrome: the treatment debate. *Rheumatology* 2005;44:971–974

[130]Ruiz-Irastorza G, Khamashta MA. The treatment of antiphospholipid syndrome: a harmonic contrast. *Best Pract. Res. Clin. Rheumatol.* 2007 Dec;21(6):1079-92.

[131]Carhuapoma JR, Mitsias P, Levine SR. Cerebral venous thrombosis and anticardiolipin antibodies. *Neurology* 1997;28:2363–2369.

[132]Descheins M-A, Conard J, Horellou MH, et al. Coagulations studies, factor V Leiden, and anticardiolipin antibodies in 40 cases of cerebral venous sinus thrombosis. *Stroke* 1996:1724–1730.

[133]Ameri A, BousserMG. Cerebral venous thrombosis. *Neurol. Clin.* 1992;10:87–111.

[134]Sanna G, D'Cruz D, Cuadrado MJ. Cerebral manifestations in the antiphospholipid (Hughes) syndrome. *Rheum. Dis. Clin. North Am.* 2006 Aug;32(3):465-90.

[135]Hilton DA, Footitt D. Neuropathological findings in Sneddon's syndrome. *Neurology* 2003;60:1181–2.

[136]Frances C, Piette JC. The mystery of Sneddon syndrome: relationship with antiphospholipid syndrome and systemic lupus erythematosus. J. Autoimmun. 2000; 15:139–43.

[137]Toubi E, Krause I, Fraser A, et al. Livedo reticularis is a marker for predicting multi-system thrombosis in antiphospholipid syndrome. *Clin. Exp. Rheumatol.* 2005;23:499–504.

[138]Chinnery P.F., Shaw P.I., Ince P.G., Jackson G.H., Bishop R.I. 1997. Fulminant encephalopathy due to the catastrophic primary antiphospholipid syndrome. *J. Neurol. Neurosurg. Psych.* 62: 300–301

[139]Asherson R.A. 1998. The catastrophic antiphospholipid syndrome, 1998. A review of the clinical features, possible pathogenesis and treatment. *Lupus* 7(Suppl. 2): 55–62.

In: Cerebral Ischemia in Young Adults
Editors: A. Pezzini and A. Padovani

ISBN 978-1-60741-627-2

Chapter 17

Other Hematologic Causes

Bianca Maria Ricerca[1], Giulio Giordano[2] and Sergio Storti[1*]
1. Institute of Hematology,
Università Cattolica del Sacro Cuore, Roma, Italy
2. UOC Onco-Hematolgy, Centro di Ricerca e Formazione ad Alta Tecnologia
nelle Scienze Biomediche "Giovanni Paolo II",
Università Cattolica del Sacro Cuore, Campobasso, Italy

Abstract

Hematologic causes of ischemic stroke, different from those deriving from plasma coagulation disorders, can be involved in the pathogenesis of vascular thrombosis. They can be classified as *non-neoplastic* and *neoplastic*. In the first group a primary role is played by the congenital diseases of the red blood cells with hemolytic markers, Sickle Cell Anemia and Thalassemia. They together with Paroxysmal Nocturnal Hemoglobinuria share some common pathogenetic pathways that involve platelet and blood coagulation, starting from red blood cells functional defect. In other non-neoplastic forms, such as Thrombotic Thrombocytopenic Purpura and the related disorder Heparin Induced Thrombocytopenia, it is the activation of the platelets that play a major role in determining the thrombosis. Among the chronic myeloproliferative disorders, Polycythemia Vera and Essential Thrombocytemia have a high incidence of thrombosis and cerebral ischemia. In the last few years the role of leukocytes in the pathogenesis of these events has been shown to be crucial. The thrombotic events are one of the principal characteristics of the clinical picture, with a profound influence on the duration and the quality of survival. Other hematologic malignancies, such as acute leukemia and plama cell discrasyas, can determine stroke through hyperviscosity and vascular occlusion. These can be due either to the high number of large blastic leukococyte or to the high para-protein concentration in the plasma. The strategies for stroke prevention and

* Correspondence: Sergio Storti, UOC di Onco-Ematologia, Centro di Ricerca e Formazione ad Alta Tecnologia nelle Scienze Biomediche, Università Cattolica del Sacro Cuore, "S.S. Giovanni Paolo II", Largo Gemelli 1 - Contrada Tappino, 86100 Campobasso, Italia. Tel 0874/312317 - 0874/312460 - 0874/312462, Segr dipartimento: 0874/312447 cell 3336691366, Fax 0874/312324. e-mail sstorti@rm.unicatt.it.

treatment are different according to the underlying pathology, and will be discussed in detail in the present chapter.

Introduction

Stroke or TIA can be observed in the clinical picture of patients suffering from blood diseases and sometimes they can be the presenting manifestation of the hematological disorder. Often the neurological manifestation is due to a thrombosis, less frequently is a hemorrhagic stroke. Both elderly and young patients can be interested by the event, but some hereditary non malignant hematological disorders have a high incidence of cerebral thrombosis since the pediatric age. In adults the etiology is more frequently a malignant disease. In 1997 Arboix and Besses [1], among 1099 patients observed in the period 1986-92 at the Acute Stroke Unit of the Hospitals de Barcelona for their first-ever stroke, described 14 patients (12 ischemic, 2 hemorrhagic; mean age 57 years), in whom a hematological disorder was firstly diagnosed. This group represented 1.27% (14/1,099) of the total number of patients with first-ever stroke diagnosed from 1986 to 1992 and accounted for 1.32% (12/906) of all brain infarcts and 1.03 (2/193) of all hemorrhagic strokes, and was the most common etiology (25%) of ischemic stroke of unusual cause. Hematological disorders included Essential Thrombocythaemia (n = 6), Polycythaemia Vera (n = 1), smoker's polycythaemia (n = 1), Thrombotic Thrombocytopenic Purpura (n = 1), IgA lambda Myeloma (n = 1), Acute Lymphoblastic Leukaemia (n = 1), Waldenström's macroglobulinaemia (n = 1), Chronic Granulocytic Leukaemia (n = 1) and IgG lambda Myeloma (n = 1). On the other hand, the hereditary disorders of hemoglobin synthesis, such as Sickle Cell Disease and Thalassemia, can give origin to cerebral thrombotic events in a very young population. In these cases the pathogenetic mechanism, involving at first mainly the erythrocytes, is largely common among these forms of anemia and also among other congenital hemolytic anemias (spherocytosis, erythrocyte enzyme deficiency), more rarely complicated by stroke.

The incidence of these forms has been until the last decades determined by the geographic origin of the populations affected: sickle cell anemia in Africa or North America, HbE in South Eastern region of Asia, and so on. In the last years, the worldwide movement of people, has determined a large diffusion of the affected genes also in countries not interested by the genetic defect before. As a consequence, the physicians must pay attention to the ethnic origin of the patients and be aware of the possibility of a hemoglobin defect, particularly among children and young patients suffering from stroke.

In other non-malignant diseases, disorders determining the aggregation and clumpimg of platelets are the main pathogenic determinants of cerebral thrombosis. This is the case, for example, of thrombotic thrombocytopenic purpura and heparin induced thrombocytopenia. A simple classification of the most frequent causes of young stroke is reported in Table 1. They will be treated in detail in the next paragraphs.

Table 1. Principal hematologic conditions associated with stroke

Hematologic neoplasms
Hyperviscosity
Myeloma
Waldenstrom macroglobulinemia
Acute myeloid Leucemia
Chronic Myeloid leukemia
Coagulation activation
Policytemia vera
Essential Thrombocytemia
PNH
Acute Lymphoblastic leukemia
Non Malignant Hematologic conditions
Red Blood Cell
Sickle Cell Disease
Thalassemic syndromes
Other hemolytic anemias
Vitamin B12 deficiency → hyperhomocysteinemia
Platelet disorders
Thrombotic thrombocytopenic purpura
Hemolytic Uremic Syndrome
Heparin Induced Thrombocytopenia

Stoke in Non-malignant Haematological Diseases due to Red Blood Cells Defects

Table 1 lists the non malignant hematologic diseases frequently complicated by stroke. Many of them are disorders arising from congenital defects of red blood cells (RBC). Thalassemia and Sickle Cell Disease (SCD) are the most common genetic defects worldwide [2,3]. Other congenital hereditary RBC defects are less frequent. They include other hemoglobinopathies, different from SCD, with a phenotype similar to Thalassemias or characterized by hemolysis, other hemolytic anemias such as erythrocyte membrane defects (Hereditary Spherocytosis, Ellipsocytosis, Stomatocytosis, very rare alteration of membrane lipids) and the Red Cells Enzymopathies. Among the acquired diseases we also included the Paroxysmal Nocturnal Hemoglobinuria (PNH). Although this is a clonal disorder of haematopoietic stem cells, its main clinical manifestation is hemolytic anemia, clinically characterized by acute intravascular hemolytic crisis, in particular nocturnal, often overlapped to chronic haemolysis. Thus, it has a strong analogy with the congenital disorders. A large literature can be found about stroke in Thalassemias (Major and Intermedia) and in SCD patients. In other forms of RBC congenital defects the clinical experience is restricted to small case series and to case reports.

In all these diseases, there are common pathogenetic triggers, able to generate an elevated thrombotic risk and stroke. They can be summarized in 4 fundamental issues:

1. Membrane alterations and their interaction with coagulative system, platelets and endothelium.
2. The reduction of Nitric Oxide (NO), a strong mediator of vasodilatation.
3. The role of splenectomy or functional asplenia.
4. The role of transfusion therapy.

Each of these points has a different relevance in the various clinical setting according to their pathogenesis. As already stressed before, the major part of experimental and clinical evidences regards Thalassemias and SCD. These 4 points will be discussed in detail in the following section.

1. Membrane Damage

Under normal conditions, the RBC membrane lipids have a different location in the inner and in the outer layer: in the inner layer Phosphatidylserine (PS) and phosphatidylethanolamine (PE) are the most prevalent components, while in the outer layer the choline-containing phospholipids phosphatidylcholine and sphingomyelin are those most represented. This distribution is assured by some mechanisms such as an ATP-dependent aminophospholipid translocase or flipase (it transports PS and PE from the outer to the inner membrane layer), a non-specific flopase that transports phospholipids from the inner to the outer monolayer and a scramblase (a calcium-activated enzyme) able to scramble all lipids achieving a rapid PS exposure. The programmed RBC death (eryptosis) is mediated by the exposure of PS [4].

In pathological conditions, the oxidative stress, variably generated, damages cell structures. Among the effects on erythrocyte membrane there is the abnormal exposure of PS. The activation of $Ca2+$ channel with perturbation of cation RBC content and cell shrinkage, the degradation of cytoskeletron proteins, and the formation of micro vesicles play also a pathogenic role.

All these changes trigger RBC death through the recognition of PS by macrophage and/or inducing cell lysis.

The prevalent source of oxidative stress varies in each condition and some of the most important aspects of this will be discussed in details below. In Thalassemic Syndromes, for example, the precipitation of hemoglobin chains in excess is involved. A similar mechanism is involved in some hemoglobinopathies characterized by the instability of the globin chains (e.g, Hb Lepore) or of the whole hemoglobin (Unstable Hemoglobinopaties, HbH disease). In Enzymepathies the perturbation of erythrocyte metabolism can originate oxidative stress directly (G6PD or Gluthatione deficiency) or through the impairment of energy metabolism (e.g, Piruvate Kinase deficiency). In erythrocyte membrane defects the RBCs suffer for loss of pliability (Hereditary Spherocytosis and Ellypsocytosis) and alterated content of cations and water (Dehydratated and Overhydatate Stomatocytosis). In SCD the trigger is the HbS polymerization. Moreover, the iron overload, which represents a very relevant clinical problem in Thalassemias, as well as in SCD and in many of the other conditions, when transfused, is another source of oxidative stress, for the presence of free iron in the cell [5].

The accelerated cell death results in elevated cell turn-over in hemolytic anemias, where the ineffective erythropoiesis is not the most relevant pathogenetic mechanism and a high reticulocyte response to anemia can be present. Thus, a high percentage of stress reticulocytes are present in the circulation. They maintain a large amount of fibronectin receptors which share a high tendency of adhesion to endothelium. Normally, the spleen eliminates these receptors but when its function is not sufficient or not present (massive RBC destruction with high bone marrow response; functional asplenia frequent in SCD; splenectomy) the stress reticulocytes contribute to generate thrombotic events.

Finally, when an abnormal immune response is present, the easy interaction between PS and macrophages favors the immunological destruction of the cell.

2. The Role of Nitric Oxide

Endothelial NO is a key regulator of vascular-relaxation *in vivo* and it adapts the local blood flow to the metabolic needs. It acts starting soluble guanylate cyclase production of cGMP that signals intracellular Ca2+ sequestration and cell relaxation. NO is synthesized from arginine by platelet, erythrocytes, neurons and endothelial cells. NO produced by the last cells have an autocrine function (in the site of production) and a paracrine function (underlying smooth muscle). Moreover, it is highly diffusible and it is easily scavenged by haemoglobin of red cells. These properties render it an excellent local vascular tone modulator and give to endothelial cells the role of primary defenders of vascular tone [6].

Furthermore, NO has antioxidant effects (superoxide scavenging and heme oxygenase induction), reduces adhesiveness of cells (downregulates the cell adhesion molecules) and it has antithrombotic properties. In fact, it inhibits platelet activation, the fibrin strands and platelet-fibrin aggregates formation, the TF and the release of tissue-type plasminogen activator and plasminogen activator inhibitor-1.

This list of NO actions leads to understand how crucial its reduction can be.

Intravascular hemolysis is a condition causing a strong NO reduction through various pathways. In fact, during intravascular hemolysis, haemoglobin and arginase are released. Hemoglobin reacts rapidly with NO producing nitrate and methemoglobin; the arginase destroys arginine which is necessary for the NO synthesis. It was demonstrated that arginase activity is upregulated in Thalassemias and SCD.

Thus, in all intravascular hemolytic anemias the reduction of NO is an event generating oxidative damage and endothelial dysfunction.

Among the conditions discussed in the present chapter, SCD was largely studied: the two clinical markers of the disease, hemolysis and vaso-occlusion, are both closely related to NO reduction.

3. The Role of Splenectomy and Functional Asplenia

Splenectomy is indicated in Thalassemias when, for the enlargement of this organ, a significantly higher transfusional support is needed, and when hypersplenism (thrombocytopenia and leukopenia) arises. In SCD, functional asplenia is very frequent as an effect of vaso-occlusive crisis occurring in this organ.

The absence of spleen or of its function is characterized by a higher thrombotic risk, as demonstrated by many studies (see below). The reasons of this can be summarized as follows: after splenectomy platelet count rises (it can be very high) and more damaged RBCs are in circulation. Nevertheless, platelets contribute to thrombotic risk for their chronic activation rather than for their number [7].

4. The Role of Transfusion

An appropriate transfusion support reduces the thrombotic risk through two related mechanisms: it lowers circulating pathological RBC percentage, and, when appropriate, it blocks the bone marrow activity. Moreover, the mechanism of stress reticulocytes discussed above explains the higher rate of thrombosis in TI than in TM. In fact, TI patients are, generally, less transfused than TM and they show a higher reticulocyte count.

Thalassemia

To understand the bases of thrombotic risk in Thalassemia, a brief overview of the pathogenetic aspects of the disease is necessary.

The fundamental event in the pathogenesis of the disease is the imbalance of hemoglobin chain production, which gives rise to all cellular and, finally, clinical manifestations of the disease. This is the end result of various genetic defects: mutations (in β Thalassemia), deletions (in α Thalassemias) and others less frequent. The precipitation of hemoglobin chains in excess (α or β), gives rise to the formation of hemicromes which link to cell membrane. Their degradation produces Reactive Oxygen Species (ROS) damaging all cell structures, as already mentioned. Direct effects are the enhancement of apoptosis with ineffective erythropoiesis and the hemolysis. These mechanisms alter dramatically the erythropoiesis causing a severe anemia. Bone marrow expansion with bone deformity, the enlargement of liver and spleen, the multi-organ failure are all consequences of anemic hypoxia and they are all present in full expressed disease. Nevertheless, in TM the transfusion therapy performed in order to suppress bone marrow activity leads to an improvement of the typical features of the disease. This approach was possible for the introduction of iron chelating drugs necessary to contrast the devastating effects of iron overload. These strategies improved the survival of thalassemic patients [8]. Bone Marrow

Transplantation (BMT) is another treatment option. Other new therapies are still experimental. The Thalassemia Intermedia (TI) is a very heterogenous clinical entity with less severe manifestations. Its pathogenesis is similar to TM but the variability of molecular defects gives rise to a wide spectrum of clinical presentations, some of which similar to those of TM and other similar to those of Thalassemia trait. The therapeutical approach is also heterogeneous. Those patients not or scantly transfused offer an excellent disease model to be investigated.

Hypercoagulable State in Thalassemia

A chronic platelet activation state in Thalassemia has been well documented. Nevertheless, the first laboratory data, collected by Eldor et al in 1978 and a year later by Houssain et al, seemed to prove the existence of a bleeding disorder in Thalassemia. In fact, a defective platelet aggregation was observed. After these first observations, the evidence of platelet aggregates in the circulation, confirmed by kinetic experiments labeling platelets with Indium 111, and the demonstration of elevated urinary thromboxaneA2 (TXA2) and prostacyclin (PGI2) excretion, lead to clarify the puzzle of platelet function in thalassemia. These findings are consistent with the reduction of platelet lifespan for accelerated consumption due to a chronic platelet activation state [9].

More recent studies provided further support to this evidence. An increased platelet fraction carrying activation markers, such as CD62 (P selectin) and CD63 was detected in flow cytometric studies [10,11], as well as elevated plasma Factor 3 levels, morphologic changes of platelets, and increased spontaneous whole blood platelet aggregation. All these changes are more evident in splenctomized patients [9].

As to coagulation and fibrinolysis, many studies support the hypothesis of an activation of these processes. In fact, Prothrombin fragment 1.2 (F1.2), a marker of thrombin generation [12], elevation of D-dimer [9,12,13] and thrombin-ATIII (TAT) complexes [9] are elevated in a large portion of thalassemic subjects. In addition, there is evidence that only the high RBCs membrane exposure of PS has a procoagulant role, thus promoting the thrombin generation *in vivo*, leading to platelet activation and creating a hypercoagulable state.

A high level of PS in Thalassemic RBCs was observed [14]. The PS provides a "docking site" for Factor X and prothrombinase complex starting the generation of activated Factor X and Thrombin [15]. In Thalassemias, an increased thrombin generation, measured by prothrombinase assay, was observed in comparison to normal RBCs [16,17] and this evidence was related to PS exposition. These results were confirmed also in splenectomized patients [12]. Cytofluorimetric experiments utilizing fluorescein isothiocyanate (FITC)–annexin V (which recognizes PS) showed high percentage of labeled RBCs in comparison to normal controls. Moreover, a significant correlation between number of RBC-bound annexin-V molecules and the fraction of CD62P (P selectin) or CD63 platelets was also observed. At last, Protein C and protein S are reduced in many thalassemic patients independently from their ethnic origin [9,12,18,19]. The pathogenesis of this reduction is not clear. According to Eldor, it is independent on age and it is not correlated to coagulation factor levels or liver function. The various studies are not in accordance about ATIII which is normal in some of them and low in others [9,12,19]. Data available about a genetic background of hypercoagulable state in thalassemia are, at the moment, scanty and they do not consent any conclusive remark [20,21]

Clinical Issues

In a recent survey, the prevalence of thromboembolic events was 1.65% in 8,860 Thalassemic patients examined (mean age of 30 ± 13 years) living in Egypt, Greece, Iran, Israel, Italy, Jordan, Lebanon and Saudi Arabia. A statistically significant difference between TM and TI (0.9 versus 4.0%; $p < 0.001$) was present [22]. Although the venous thromboembolic events were predominant (57%), the arterial thrombosis accounted for 40% of events and simultaneous arterial and venous thromboses for 3%. Arterial events were significantly more common than venous events in patients with TM. Stroke represented 18 % of all the events. The TM patients have a significantly greater risk for stroke (OR, 3. 72; 95% CI, 1.48 to 9.32; $p = 0.005$) and for 'other' events (OR, 3.14, 95% CI 1.33 to 7.14; $p = 0.009$), while those with TI had a significantly greater risk for Deep Venous Thrombosis (DVT) (OR, 2.13, 95% CI 1.02 to 4.46; $p = 0.045$).

In TI the clinical risk factors for thrombosis were age (> 20 years), splenectomy and an individual and family history of thrombosis, while the laboratory parameters were platelet count > 600 10^3/μl and plasminogen level <60%.

Most TI patients who had a thromboembolic event were splenectomized (94%) and had average haemoglobin levels < 9 g/dl (68%) and only one-third were receiving regular blood transfusions. Logothetis et al reported a higher prevalence of thrombotic complications (20%) but in a small group of patients (n = 138) [23]. Subsequently, a multicentric study [24] showed results similar to those of Taher et al [22]. The prevalence of stroke was 2% (16 patients out of 735), but the cerebral localization was the most frequent among all thromboembolic events (50%; 16 out of 32). The mean age of these patients was 16 years (range 6 - 28). In the group with thromboembolic complications a higher incidence of associated pathologies like dilated cardiomyopathy, diabetes and hypothyroidism in comparison to the patients without (22.9 vs 9.2%; $p < 0.05$) was present, while chronic liver disease did not influence thrombotic risk. Women undergoing hormone therapy to become pregnant had a higher risk.

Finally, asymptomatic brain lesions were detected by MRI in TI patients [25]. Damage was inversely correlated with hemoglobin levels in patients with TI and increased with age.

As far as prevention is concerned, there are no studies establishing the efficacy of primary prevention. The data of Taher et al [22] show that, among patients with thrombotic complications, 52% of patients were taking aspirin regularly and 21% (TI patients) were taking hydroxyurea which lowers platelet and leukocyte counts. Nevertheless, a prophylactic antithrombotic therapy is indicated for high-risk patients with TI who undergo surgery, or are immobilizated or during pregnancy [12]. When a thrombotic event occurs in a thalassemic patient a prolonged antithrombotic therapy, as for any patients with thrombophilia, must be considered because of the profound hemostatic anomalies. Moreover, the high risk of thrombosis recurrence in those patients who experienced the first episode indicates the need of secondary prevention. Finally, in non transfused TI patients, a thromboembolic complication should induce to start a transfusional regimen.

Sickle Cell Disease

The SCD pathogenesis is very complex. Therefore, a brief summary describes only partially a scenario where many elements have a relevant role. The subjects affected by this disease are homozygous for the variant S of β chain ($\alpha_2\beta_2$ $^{6Glu\rightarrow Val}$) or compound heterozygous for HbS and β0 thalassemia, β+ thalassemia, or other variants as HbC, with a decreasing severity from the first form to the last.

The starting event is the polymerization of deoxygenate HbS which results in the formation of a gelatinous network of fibrous polymers. At this point, a chain of events occurs inside and outside the RBCs. The latter lose their pliability, become dehydrated, and assume the typical sickle shape (Sickled Cells-SC) at first reversibly, then definitively (Irreversibly-SC: ISC). All these phenomena derive from the oxidative stress arising from the polymerization of HbS, amplified by the following events. RBC membrane and all cellular structures are damaged. ISC have also an elevated tendency of adhesion to the endothelium. For all these reasons, their passage in the microcirculation is difficult and ischemic lesions occur in all districts of the body.

These few notes introduce a fundamental concept: while in thalassemia hypoxia, derived from anemia, is the crossroad of pathogenesis, in SCD two main processes play a crucial role: the hemolytic anemia, chronic with acute crises, and the dramatic vaso-occlusion which is responsible of organ damage. Intravascular hemolysis is the common pathway of both manifestations. In fact, it induces anemia and, through the reduction of NO, endothelial dysfunction which takes part to vaso-occlusive crises. In this context, alterations of coagulation,

fibrinolysis, and platelet function play an important role.

Hypercoagulable State in SCD

Many of the issues discussed above regarding Thalassemia were also demonstrated in SCD. They were widely reviewed by Ataga et al [15] and Eldor et al [7]. Like in Thalassemia, platelet aggregation is normal or reduced as expression of platelet hyperfunction, as confirmed by high urinary excretion of thromboxane A2 and prostaglandin metabolites and high plasma levels of PF3, PF4, and β-thromboglobulin. Platelets over-express P selectin and CD63 [26] which are bound by Annexin V [27]. In addition, platelet-derived soluble CD40 ligand (sCD40L) is elevated in SCD patients compared with normal controls [28]. A long list of haemostatic abnormalities in SCD patients has been detected, including elevated plasma concentrations of TAT, F1.2, and D-dimer complexes [17,27,29,30,31]. All these changes are more evident during vaso-occlusive crises. As to thrombosis inhibitors, protein S and C are reduced. This may be explained by hyperconsumption or hypoproduction due to liver dysfunction. Moreover, Wright et al in 1997 reported that patients with SCD appear to be more resistant to activated protein C than the healthy control subjects [32]. This may result from an increase in circulating plasma levels of factor VIII coagulant activity, perhaps coupled with the observed reduction in both total and free protein S. Finally, Heparin co-factor II (HCII), a circulating inhibitor of thrombin which has an action similar to antithrombin, is also decreased in SCD [33] and increases when the patient undergoes to chronic blood transfusions [34]. Also in SCD the PS exposure creates "docking sites" with procoagulant activity. Moreover, some *in vitro* experiments demonstrated that the SC with very high expression of PS, called type II PS RBCs, are able to induce a twofold production of Tissue Factor (TF) and a great correlation was found between type II PS RBCs and blood TF and plasma free hemoglobin. The same was not observed if RBCs with low PS were considered [15]. In addition, PS favors the adhesion of SC to endothelium [13]. The enhanced adhesiveness of SC, but also of leukocytes and platelets, plays a very important role in the pathogenesis of vaso-occlusion. PS exposure is only one of many pathways. They involve other membrane components such as Band3 and sulfated glycolipids, and also numerous adhesion molecules such as the integrins (a4b1, aVb3) and their receptors, the immunoglobulin family members (VCAM-1, ICAM-4), the endothelial selectins, soluble adhesion proteins such as thrombospondin, fibrinogen, fibronectin, von Willebrand factor.

Clinical Issues

Stroke in SCD is more frequently hemorrhagic in adults, ischemic in children. A wide spectrum of brain injury can be present: from the classical acute stroke, with obvious clinical manifestations, to "silent infarcts", revealed by MRI, with normal neurological examination and without any evident clinical sign related to the lesion. Nevertheless, silent infarcts are associated with impairment of cognitive function [35,36] and with a high risk of stroke recurrence [37]. In SCD patients, the lifetime risk of stroke is 25% - 30% with a peak incidence in childhood at 7 years of age [37,38]. According to Wang et al, the incidence of stroke in SCD is ~600/100, 000 patient-years, resulting in a prevalence approaching 10% by the age of 50 [39]. Anyway, it is the main cause of morbidity in SCD [40].

Transcranial Doppler ultrasonography (TCD) a reproducible, non-invasive technique to detect narrowed internal carotid or middle cerebral arteries in asymptomatic children, and it is a reliable diagnostic test to identify patients at high and intermediate risk of stroke. Children with elevated velocities (time-averaged mean velocity, TAMV, measured in the distal internal carotid artery or middle cerebral artery, ≥ 200 cm/s) have an astonishingly high rate of stroke: ~10,000/100,000 patient-years, approximately six fold higher than those with normal TCD velocities (TAMV <170 cm/s). The risk is much higher in those with both high TCD velocity and MRI sign of silent infarct. The intermediate group of risk includes children with *conditional* TAMV (170 – 199 cm/s). The stroke risk among these patients is estimated to be 2 – 5% per year, compared to 9% per year for children with abnormal velocities [41]. Although the relative risk of primary stroke is lower among patients with conditional than abnormal TAMV, more children have conditional TCD velocities, so the absolute number of children who develop stroke in the intermediate group without therapy is comparable. Based on the data available to date, all children with SCD aged 2 - 16 should be screened using TCD. The screening must be repeated annually for children with normal studies, and every 6 months for those in the "conditional" range.

Primary stroke prevention is one of the most important innovations in sickle cell care. Children with abnormal TCD (TAMV ≥ 200 cm/s) should be considered for transfusion therapy or BMT. The chronic maintenance transfusion program should be carried out using blood matched for ABO, C, D, E, and Kell antigens, dosed to keep the [HbS] ≤ 30%. This therapy diminishes the risk of stroke by more than 90% [41]. During the transfusion treatment, most of the TCD velocities revert to normal. Moreover, transfusion protects those patients with elevated TCD and silent infarcts not only from stroke, but also from new silent lesions and from the development of neuropsychologic abnormalities. The STOP II study tried and shed light on the appropriate length of transfusion therapy [42]. Children who, after at least 30 months of transfusion therapy, joined normal TAMV values were randomized to stop or to continue the transfusions. The primary end-points of the study were stroke or reversion to abnormal TAMV. In none of the children transfused the two events were observed, while 14 out of 41 (34%) had reversion of TAMV and 2 (4.8%) had stroke among those who stopped transfusion. This study gives a strong evidence of the beneficial effects of chronic maintenance of transfusion therapy in these patients. In addition, the growth of these children is improved, and their morbidity is decreased in terms of the hemolysis and acute vaso-occlusive events. On the other hand, there are also some concerns about adverse events, related to the chronic indefinite transfusion regimen. Among these, is the allo-immunization that could act negatively on life-long transfusion treatment. Further, the predictable iron overload is probably the most serious adverse effect of chronic transfusion. At the moment, there are preliminary data about the use of new oral iron-chelating agents and they are promising [43]. The exchange transfusion regimen at least at the beginning of the treatment could help to reduce the transfusion-related iron overload. Other risks are those related to possible infectious diseases, due to the known agents but also to an unpredictable emergence of a new HIV-like pathogen in the blood supply.

Regarding the management of children with conditional velocities there is debate in the literature. Although conditional TCD velocities may normalize or remain in the conditional range, a substantial proportion of patients will convert over time to abnormal values. Within the Stroke Prevention in Sickle Cell Anemia (STOP study), the overall conversion rate to abnormal TAMV was approximately 29% among children with at least one conditional velocity study, but as high as 55% among children with two high conditional TCD examinations (TAMV 185–199 cm/s) [42]. A recent study performed at the St. Jude Children's Research Hospital, Memphis, in a series of 274 subjects demonstrated a higher rate of conversion from normal to conditional TAMV for patients aged less than 10 yrs, and this rate was even more relevant for higher TAMV. The statistical significance however was reached only for the conversion from normal to conditional TAMV. At the moment no specific therapeutic intervention is recommended for the conditional TAMV group, but the persistence of stroke risk in this category makes prospective randomized studies investigating the role of interventional therapies for prevention of conversion to abnormal TCD velocities warranted. These studies should determine if these therapies can prevent primary stroke in this at-risk population.

An alternative to transfusion is Hydroxyurea (HU) therapy. Chronic long-term HU has been widely used and has well-documented benefits and adverse effects. Several studies are ongoing or have been completed investigating HU for primary and secondary stroke prevention, and the results are encouraging. HU has been approved in the therapy of SCD as HbF-inducing agent. The increase of HbF in the RBC reduces the polymerization capacity of the deoxygenated HbS, but the drug acts in many other ways. It has a NO donor effect [44], and it down-regulates the expression of adhesion molecules by reticulocytes. Furthermore, HU may decrease coagulation activation by reducing PS expression on the surface of both RBCs and platelets [45]. In addition, HU reduces haemostatic activation by decreasing white blood cell and platelet count as far as Tissue Factor expression. Several questions remain about the possible teratogenic effects of the drug and the long-term exposure risk, in general. Less is known about the impact of BMT on stroke, but as regimens improve, the potential beneficial effect increases. An interesting decision analysis comparing BMT with chronic transfusion for stroke failed to identify either as better than the other.

In consideration of platelet and coagulation activation in SCD, both anti-platelet and anti-coagulant drugs could play a potential role in the prevention and treatment of stroke in SCD, but, at the moment, there are only a few reports in the literature, with non-conclusive results.

In adult SCD patients a relevant issue is the identification of other risk factors different from those identified by TCD. In fact, with increasing age the bone-window to the cerebral vessels closes down, making it inappropriate as a screening tool for some older children and most adults. In those adult patients, who were screened using TCD as they were children, other known risk factors such as the presence of "silent infarcts", elevated blood pressure, absence of alpha thalassemia, presence of moyamoya, and the specific genetic profile could become useful guides to therapy.

We list below the most relevant biological evidence related to stroke risk.

Chang Milbauer et al, evaluated the genetic profile of 20 SCD subjects (age, 4 - 19 years) who were either at-risk (n = 11) or non-at-risk (n = 9) for ischemic stroke on the basis of the presence of occlusive disease at the circle of Willis. Gene expression profiling identified no significant single gene differences between the 2 groups. The analysis of Biological Systems Scores, using gene sets that were predetermined to survey each of the 9 biologic systems, showed that only changes in inflammation signaling are characteristic of the at-risk subjects. Also biological evidence are consistent with a relevant role of inflammation biology. The Authors conclude that the pathobiology of circle of Willis disease in SCD could reflect a difference in genetically determined endothelial biology in response to inflammation [46]. Hoppe et al recently confirmed an association between the TNF (-308) Promoter Polymorphism and Stroke Risk in Children with SCD [47]. Recently, it has been reported that mean vWF:Ag levels were significantly elevated in children and adolescents with SCD and sleep hypoxemia when compared with SCD-normoxia and control groups ($p = 0.007$), and correlated inversely with pulse oximetry ($r = -0.54$, $p = 0.01$). Densitographic analyses of vWF multimer distribution also showed an inverse correlation between % HMW-multimers and oxygen saturation ($r = -0.62$, $p = 0.03$). The previously reported association between nocturnal desaturation and SCD vascular complications, including stroke, may be influenced by hypoxemic modulation of vWF [48]. Finally, significant decreased levels of Protein C and S were found in patients who developed thrombotic stroke [49].

The moyamoya syndrome deserves special consideration. SCD children with this syndrome present a significant high risk of ischemic stroke. A surgical approach must be considered in these cases: according to Hankinson et al, encephalo-duro-arteriosynangiosis (EDAS) or pial synangiosis in the treatment of moyamoya disease could help to durably protect children with SCD and moyamoya syndrome against cerebrovascular complications [50].

Stroke treatment in SCD patients includes all general measures for vaso-occlusive crisis (transfusion, hydratation, alkalinysation). Ischemic stroke has a strong indication to exchange transfusion. Recurrent strokes occur in 57% of patients treated during the first episode with simple transfusions and in 21% of those treated with exchange transfusion [51].

Paroxysmal Nocturnal Hemoglobinuria (PNH)

PNH is associated with a somatic mutation in the phosphatidylinositol glycan complementation class A (PIG-A) gene, mapped to the X chromosome. The consequent deficiency of glycosylphosphatidylinositol (GPI) and of GPI-anchored molecules, as the Decay Accelerating Factor (DAF or CD55) and the Membrane Inhibitor of Reactive Lysis (MIRL or CD59), cause an increased susceptibility to complement-mediated lysis of erythrocytes, leukocytes and platelets.

Thromboembolic events, as a first manifestation of PNH, are uncommon (about 5%) but 8 years after diagnosis the incidence of thrombosis is 30%, rising to 50% after 15 years [52]. The thrombotic risk is proportional to the expansion of PNH clone [53]. Cerebral vascular events are major contributors to mortality in PNH and they represent the second most common thrombotic manifestation after the Budd-Chiari Syndrome. They are more often cerebral vein and sinus thrombosis, while arterial thrombotic episodes of cerebral vessels, like in other vascular districts, are quite rare [54,55].

Other Red Blood Cells Congenital Defects

As emphasized above, the experience in this setting is anecdotic. Most reports deal with patients who underwent splenectomy [56,57], more rarely not splenectomized [58]. The pathogenetic pathways in all cases are those indicated in the general part of this chapter. The lack of splenic function plays an important role. Among these diseases, the Hereditary Stomatocytosis deserves a special consideration because, in affected individuals, thromboembolic complications are very frequent after splenectomy. Therefore, the indication to splenectomy must be carefully evaluated in these cases.

Polycythaemia Rubra Vera

Polycythemia vera (PV) is a Ph-negative myeloproliferative disorder characterized by a clonal proliferation of hematopoietic precursors, leading to an increased production of erythrocytes as well as leukocytes and platelets.

PV is the prototype and also the most common of the 4 classical myeloproliferative disorders, also including chronic myelogenous leukemia (CML), essential thrombocythemia (ET), and primary myelofibrosis (PMF). Vasquez in 1892 [59] and Osler in 1903 [60] in their original descriptions noted rubor and strokes (and other thrombotic complications) as a manifestation of this disease. PV is a primary myeloproliferative stem cell disorder causing panhyperplasia of erythrocyte, leukocyte, and megakaryocyte cell lines in the bone marrow. The discovery of the JAK2V617F mutation [61-64] has made the diagnosis of PV much easier. The pathogenesis, on the other hand, is still incompletely understood [65]. Probably the JAK-2 mutation, that has been observed not only in PV and other myeloproliferative disorders (MPD) but also myelodysplastic syndromes with ring sideroblasts, is not alone sufficient to induce a MPD in humans. Ongoing studies are investigating different hypotheses such as differences in the targeted hematopoietic stem cells (HSC), host modifier polymorphisms, intensity of JAK2V617F signaling, presence of other somatic mutations, or the presence of a pre-JAK2 event that may vary according to the MPD phenotype. At the moment none of them has enough bulk of evidence to be accepted [66].

It has been estimated that 30% to 50% of PV patients have minor and major thrombotic complications, and vascular mortality accounts for 35% to 45% of all deaths [67,68].

The efficacy of available antithrombotic strategies might be optimized by a proper stratification of the individual risk. In the Framingham Study, men with hemoglobin >15 g/dl and women with Hb > 14 g/dl had twice as many cerebral infarctions as did their cohorts with lower values [69]. Other risk factors of initial development of 82 cerebral infarctions were also antecedent blood pressure status in both sexes and cigarette habit in men. When allowance is made for associated blood pressure and cigarette habit—factors found to correlate with both blood hemoglobin values and incidence of cerebral infarction—hemoglobin level had only a modest residual effect, no longer statistically significant. Recently Italian investigators in the European Collaboration on Low-dose Aspirin in Polycythemia Vera (ECLAP) study, in a multivariate analysis of thromboses and risk factors, found the lack of correlation between hematocrit between 35 to 55 and thromboses in PV. In previously published studies in congenital polycythemic disorders the correlation was lacking too. However the Authors quote "*our data on hematocrit should be more cautiously interpreted due to possible discrepancies between hematocrit and red cell mass values in PV*". In this study, in the prospective observational branch, Landolfi et al, examining the thromboses at the inclusion in the study and those observed in the follow-up, found as significant risk factors for the event age and previous history of thrombosis [70]. The incidence rate of major events was approximately doubled in patients aged more than 65 years or with previous thrombotic history, becoming approximately 4-fold higher in subjects with both conditions. Hypertension gave only a mild non significant increase of the risk, while smoking had a hazard ratio [HR], 1.90 (95% CI, 1.15 to 3.14; $p = 0.012$). During the follow-up of 1638 PV patients of the ECLAP database 668 patients (926 events) presented thrombosis: 587 subjects (721 events) had a history of thrombosis at the moment of the diagnosis, 169 (205 events) patients had thrombotic events during the follow-up. In 2/3 of the cases the thrombosis was in the arterial district; and cerebrovascular events (stroke and TIA) constituted half of all arterial events and about one third of all thromboses. Multivariate analysis using patients' white blood cell count at baseline showed that leukocytosis was significantly associated with myocardial infarction (MI) but not with other thrombotic events. The association is not evident for peripheral arterial thrombosis, stroke, and TIA. Leukocytosis probably has a direct pro-thrombotic role in MI. It is possible that an interaction between leukocyte count and other thrombotic complications might also exist, but larger studies are required for its detection. The hypothesis of a direct causative role of leukocytes has led to the consideration of the short-term use of hydroxyurea in subjects with very high vascular risk [71,72].

Age was by far the most important predictor of thrombosis in all vascular districts, as previously reported. History of venous thrombosis significantly increased the risk of a new episode in the same district, but not associated the risk of arterial thrombosis (ie, MI, stroke, and TIA). Hematocrit and platelet variations did not influence the overall thrombotic risk. Fifty-one (30%) of the 169 patients with thrombotic events presented at least one cardiovascular risk factor. Hypertension was the most prevalent (39.5% of PV patients), but it was associated with a non-significant increase in the thrombotic risk, while smoking (12.8% of patients) was significantly associated with increased risk of arterial thrombotic events, (HR, 1.90; 95% CI, 1.15 to 3.14; $P = 0.012$) and was non-significantly associated with the risk of peripheral artery disease (HR, 2.86; 95% CI, 0.92 to 8.86; $P = 0.069$) and of stroke/TIA (HR, 1.89; 95% CI, 0.89 to 4.01; $P = 0.098$). The (ECLAP) established to test the efficacy and safety of low-dose aspirin in PV. After the ECLAP trial, the recommendations on the use of aspirin in PV will likely become more uniform but debates on hydroxyurea will probably continue for a long time. In fact, a clinical trial comparing the long-term efficacy and safety of this agent with that of alternative cytoreductive strategies would be very difficult to organize. Nowadays high-risk subjects, notwithstanding aspirin and chemotherapy, still have an incidence of vascular events above 5% per year. In these patients, more aggressive treatments may provide additional benefit, but balancing the thrombotic, neoplastic, and hemorrhagic risk of the various drug combinations remains a major challenge of PV treatment strategy. Concerning patients with recurrence of thrombosis, according to De Stefano et al [73] no difference exists between PV patients and ET subjects (see after).

Ischemic stroke is less frequently associated with secondary polycythemias than with PV, but the direct influence of hematocrit elevation is obscured by the lower mean age of, the infrequency of chronic hypertension in, and the generally lower hematocrits of patients with secondary polycythemias than of those with PV [74-77]. The risk of arterial thrombosis may not be uniform in patients with all subtypes because some secondary polycythemias are compensatory responses to low arterial oxygen tension, some are caused by reduced plasma volume and a relative increase in the number of erythrocytes, and others are familial and noncompensatory [77]. Adults with cyanotic congenital heart disease complicated by compensatory polycythemia (mean age 29 years, mean hematocrit approximately 60%) were reported to have a very low risk of clinical stroke (0% in 204 patient-years of follow-up) [75,76].

Pseudopolycythemia (also called spurious, stress, or Gaisbock's polycythemia) usually occurs in hypertensive, obese, middle-aged men who smoke tobacco and who have modest increases in hematocrit (usually <60%) due to reduced plasma volume. The relative contribution of the elevated hematocrit to stroke in the presence of other cerebrovascular risk factors has been difficult to define [78-80].

Essential Thrombocythaemia (ET)

ET is a myeloproliferative disorder in which blood platelet counts above 450 000 cells/ml occur. In addition, platelets are often large and have functional abnormalities. Although occasionally such abnormalities of platelet function result in a bleeding tendency, because of circulating Von Willebrand multimers absorbtion on platelet surface, thrombosis is far more common. In fact, as in PV, arterial thrombosis is very frequent, more than venous thrombosis. Thrombotic risk in patients under 40 years is 3 times higher than in normal subjects of the same age. Stroke is a well recognised complication but headache and transient focal and non-focal neurological disturbances are also frequent. ET must be distinguished from secondary thrombocytosis, which can occur in response to conditions including inflammation, acute bleeding, iron deficiency, splenectomy, and infection [82]. A highly increased platelet count in the absence of an identifiable cause of secondary thrombocythemia suggests a diagnosis of ET. Mutation of JAK-2 gene may confirm the diagnosis. Moreover subject with omozigote JAK2 mutation in some studies show an increased thrombotic diatesis, as female subject with clonal hemopoiesis, detected by PCR-HUMARA thecnique, and normal platelet count. In ET the megakaryocytes are large and hyperploid by contrast with secondary thrombocythaemia when they are usually increased in number and of small diameter and low ploidy [83]. The management of ET requires specialist care and hydroxyurea is often used as an initial treatment in older patient. In young patient anagrelide is the drug of first choice. The small increase in hemorragic risk in patient taking anagrelide, probably is due to the weak antiaggregating activity of this drug.

Recently Passamonti et al, evaluating a serie of 605 ET patients, observed an incidence of 15.3 thrombosis per 1000 persons per year. The cumulative risk of thrombosis during follow-up was 5% at 5 years, and 14% at 10. All patients received aspirin unless contraindicated. He found that in univariate analysis age >60 and platelet count <1000000/ul were risk factors for thrombosis, while leukocytosis did not have prognostic significance. Multivariate analysis confirmed the role of age, but showed that a previous history of thrombosis was a significant risk factor for recurrence, while cytoreductive therapy was protective. History of thrombosis was a negative prognostic factor for survival [84]. In a previous study Carobbio A et al reported that in ET, as in policythemia vera, the risk of first thrombotic event and of recurrence is related to the presence of leukocytosis (>8700/ul), particularly in individual younger than 60 and without history of thrombosis (standard low risk patients)[85]. The athogenetic role of leukocytes in the thrombotic events could be related to different causes: the activation of the neutrophils; the adhesion and the binding to platelets with reciprocal activation inducing tissue factor release and endothelial damage and activation. Furthermore the leukocytes take part to the inflammatory process of the vascular wall. Adjunctive risk factors for thrombosis could be the coexistence of hereditary thrombophilia, of antiphospholipid antibodies, and some biologic characteristics of the disease: clonal haemopoiesis, detected in the females by PCR-HUMARA technique, reduced platelet expression of c-Mpl (thrombopoietin receptor), overexpression of PRV-1 mRNA. Moreover subjects with homozygote Jak2 mutation in some studies show an increased thrombotic diathesis. Other authors did not confirm this finding (Table 2). In some series the significance was for the venous thrombosis and was not always confirmed in multivariate analysis. In fact there could be some confounding variables: age, leukocyte count, leukocyte activation, platelet activation, acquired/inherited thrombophilia, anti-platelet therapy, cytoreductive therapy. More recently the mutational burden of JAK-2 has been evaluated, considering the different grades of heterozygosity, homozygosity, and wild type present in any individual subject [86]. However, the results of this analysis were not homogeneous (Table 2); The Gimema Study published by Vannucchi et al found more thrombosis among patients homozygous for the mutation. Passamonti et in a single center study did not find any difference among JAK2 genotypes in terms of thrombosis-free survival.

The thrombosis are in 2/3 of the cases in the arterial compartment. In the series of Passamonti, 66 thrombosis (11% of the patients) were observed. The incidence of the different manifestations were: ischemic stroke (n = 17, 26%), TIA (n = 18, 27%), MI (n = 12, 18%), peripheral arterial thrombosis (n = 4, 6%), deep vein thrombosis of the extremities (n = 9, 14%), thrombosis of the abdominal veins (n = 6, 9%). More than 50% of the thrombosis in the cerebral vasculature were in female subjects with normal platelet count [84].

A rationale approach to the prevention of thrombosis requires a risk stratification. Different proposal have been presented in the last years. History of thrombosis and age > 60 years are constantly evaluated in the calculation. According to the MRC in the PT1 trial the patients can be stratified in *low*, *intermediate* and *high* risk according to the criteria reported in Table 3.

The stratification is not different from that of the Italian Guidelines of SIE (Società Italiana di Ematologia) regarding platelet lowering treatment in adult ET patients [88]. Another similar risk classification has been proposed by Vannucchi and Barbui [89]: it considers three risk factors: age >60 years, history of thrombosis, cardiovascular risk factors (diabetes, hypertension, smoking, hypercholesterolemia).

Table 2. *V617F* and thrombosis in ET

association	No association
Campbell PJ et al 2005 [121] (venous events)	Antonioli E et al, 2005 [125]
Cheung B et al, 2006 [122]	Wolanskjy A et al, 2005 [126]
Kittur J et al, 2007 [123] (venous events)	Pemmaraju N et al, 2007 [127]
Finazzi G et al, 2007 [124]	Carobbio A et al, 2007 [85]
	Antonioli E et al, 2007 [128]

Authors	MPD	N. pts	JAK2 mutational burden
Vannucchi AM et al, 2007 [129]	ET	639	More thrombosis in homozygous
Vannucchi AM et al, 2007 [129]	PV	323	More thrombosis if > 75% mutated alleles
Antonioli E et al, 2008 [86]	ET	260	>25%: more arterial thrombosis (at diagnosis)
Kittur J et al, 2007 [123]	ET	176	More venous thrombosis (at follow-up)

Table 3. MRC Risk stratification of ET patients in PTI trial [87]

Low Risk	Intermediate Risk	High Risk
Patients <40y with all the following factors	Patients aged 40-60y with all the following factors	Patients either aged >60y or one of the following factors
No prior Thrombosis	No prior Thrombosis	Prior thrombosis or hemorrhage
No Hypertension or diabetes	No Hypertension or diabetes	Hypertension or Diabetes
Platelet count <1000-1500x10^9/l	Platelet count <1000-1500x10^9/l	Platelet count >1000x10^9/l; >1500x10^9/l if aged < 60y

Table 4. Class of risk and treatment of ET patients according to Vannucchi et al.

Category of risk	Age> 60 or history of thrombosis	Cardiovascular risk factors	Treatment
LOW	NO	NO	No treatment or LD aspirin
INTERMEDIATE	NO	YES	LD aspirin (no consensus)
HIGH	YES	N/A	LD aspirin and Myelosuppression (HU, α-IFN, anagrelide, others)

The treatment proposed can include antiplatelets agents in the lower classes, while in the highest risk patients cytoreduction must be included together with antiplatelets, in presence of increased platelet count. In case of a platelet count > 1000 x 10^3, before starting antiplatelets it is advisable to exclude an acquired von Willebrand disease. Antiplatelets are contraindicated in presence of hemorrhagic symptoms (Table 4).

Landolfi and Di Gennaro recently proposed a composed scoring system for the assessment of thrombotic risk and the treatment policy in ET and PV: the parameters have a different weight; history of thrombosis is the most relevant with age that has an increasing value [72] (Table 5).

According to the current SIE guidelines (Barbui 2004), the 1st line drug for antiaggregation is low-dose aspirin (75-100 mg/day). Clopidogrel at the dosage of 75 mg/day is the 2nd line for subjects intolerant to ASA. As cytoreductive therapy IFN and anagrelide are preferred in young subjects because they don't have mutagenic potential. HU has a not well established mutagenic potential, even though at the moment there aren't in literature cases of acute leukemia related to HU exposure. On the other hand HU could have adjunctive favorable effect for its action in reducing the interaction leukocyte-platelet and the expression of tissue factor by polymorphonucleated leukocytes [90]. Due to the fact that history of thrombosis is constantly considered a major risk for further events, interesting information about the efficacy of the therapy in the secondary prevention of the stroke can be drawn from a recent paper by De Stefano et al [73]. The Authors examined the recurrence of thrombosis in patients with PV and ET. They evaluated risk factors, the characteristics of the recurrence and the effect of treatment. Recurrence of thrombothic events is 5.6%/year; about 60% are in the arterial district. Patients aged less than 60 years are at lesser risk of recurrence both for all the events (HR > 60yrs *vs* < 60 yrs: 1.67, range 1.19 to 2.32; $p < 0.002$ in multivariate analysis), both for subjects with first cerebrovascular thromboembolism (HR > 60 yrs *vs* < 60 yrs: 2.09, range 1.12 to 3.86; $p < 0.01$ in multivariate analysis). Recurrences are more frequent in the same vascular district of the 1st event. Different rate of risk reduction are obtained in the different clinical settings of thrombosis: while for cardiovascular events cytoreductive drugs achieve a risk reduction of 70%, with no significant impact of the antiaggregating drugs, for cerebral ischemia the antiaggregation is the most effective prophylaxis with a risk reduction of 67%; in this case the cytoreduction does not give any significant protection. Hemorrhagic adverse events occurred in 0.9 patient/year in the whole group, and in 0.8 patient/year in those receiving antiaggregating agents.

The use of anti-platelet agents such as aspirin at low dose might reduce risk of cardiovascular events in young patients with microcirculatory symptoms and or cardiovascular risk factors, when platelet lowering or cytoreduction is contraindicated. Treatment is mandatory in young patients with previous thrombotic events, with more than one million of platelets or with splenomegaly.

Table 5. Thrombotic risk in ET and PV and their treatment according to Landolfi et al

Risk Factor	Score
Age <40	0
Age 40-55	1
Age 56-65	2.5
Age > 63	3.5
Hypertension	0.5
Dyslipidemia	0.5
Platelet count (>1000x 10^9/l)	1
Leukocyte count (>12x 10^9/l)	1
Smoking	1.5
Diabetes	1.5
Past History of thrombosis	3.5

Score	Risk	PV treatment	ET treatment	Absolute risk % patients/year
<1	Low	Phlebotomy Consider aspirin	Consider aspirin	<1.5
1-3	Moderate	Phlebotomy Aspirin	Aspirin Consider cytoreduction using IFN or HU	1.5-3
3.1-5.5	High	Aspirin HU	Aspirin HU	3.1-6
>5.5	Very high	Aspirin HU Consider more aggressive treatment	Aspirin HU Consider more aggressive treatment	>6

In young patients requiring cytoreduction and intolerant to anagrelide, interferon alpha is the drug of second choice. If interferon is not well tolerated, hydroxyurea might to be useful, in consideration of its low, but still not well established mutagenic potential.

Idiopathic Myelofibrosis and Chronic Myelogenous Leukemia

Stroke in young people with idiopathic myelofibrosis and chronic myelogenous leukemia is a rare event, probably linked to polymorphonucleated cell expression of tissue factor or to its activation, as demonstred by mixed aggregates leukocytes-platelets.

Thrombotic Thrombocytopenic Microangiopathies

Thrombotic thrombocytopenic microangiopathies clearly cause stroke. Effective treatment is now available for these disorders. They are a group of disorders characterized by thrombocytopenia, a microangiopathic hemolytic anemia evident by fragmented RBCs (schistocytes) and laboratory evidence of hemolysis (elevated serum levels of lactate dehydrogenase and indirect bilirubin, decreased haptoglobin and eventually increased reticulocyte count) not immune-mediated (Coomb's antiglobulin test negative), and microvascular thrombosis. These include thrombotic thrombocytopenic purpura (TTP) and hemolytic uremic syndrome (HUS), as well as syndromes complicating bone marrow transplantation, certain medications and infections, pregnancy, and vasculitis. The PT and aPTT are characteristically normal in TTP or HUS: this is a differential feature from Disseminated Intravascular Coagulation (DIC) where thrombocytopenia and microangiopathy are present together with a severe coagulopathy with consumption of clotting factors and fibrinogen resulting in a prolongation of prothrombin time (PT) and often activated partial thromboplastin time (aPTT). The two main clinical forms, TTP and HUS, were previously considered overlapping syndromes. In the past few years a better knowledge of the pathophysiology of inherited and idiopathic TTP has allowed us to differentiate TTP from HUS.

Thrombotic Thrombocytopenic Purpura (TTP)

TTP is still one of the most difficult diagnoses for the clinical hematologist to make, due to the rarity of the disease and the poor specificity of clinical and laboratory signs and symptoms. The classic pentad (thrombocytopenia, anemia, fever, neurologic and renal abnormalities), firstly described in 1924 by Eli Moschcowitz is fully present in only a minority of patients, nowadays probably due also to an earlier diagnosis and treatment. On the other hand consumptive thrombocytopenia and mechanical hemolytic anemia, may also be present in other thrombotic microangiopathies, so that the diagnosis of TTP requires their exclusion. vWF is normally secreted as ultra-large multimers, which are then cleaved by a metalloprotease, ADAMTS13. The pathogenesis of inherited TTP (Upshaw-Schulman syndrome) is related to a deficiency of ADAMTS13 (2% to 3% of patients). Idiopathic TTP is caused by antibodies to ADAMTS13, neutralizing the enzymatic activity and/or accelerating protease removal from the circulation. The persistence of ultra-large vWF molecules are thought to contribute to pathogenic platelet adhesion and aggregation. ADAMTS13 activity and antibody presence can now be detected by laboratory assays, even though, sensitivity and specificity can be improved. This defect of ADAMTS13 alone is not sufficient to cause TTP. In fact the subjects with congenital absence of ADAMTS13 develop TTP only episodically. Additional provocative factors are necessary, but they have not been completely defined. Idiopathic TTP appears to be more common in women than in men, and in patients with HIV infection and in pregnant women. In some cases the syndrome can be related to drugs: they can induce antibody formation, as ticlopidine and clopidogrel) or direct endothelial toxicity (cyclosporine, mitomycin C, tacrolimus, quinine).

TTP is a devastating disease if not diagnosed and treated promptly. The presence of microangiopathic hemolytic anemia and thrombocytopenia, in the absence of another known cause, is considered sufficient to establish the diagnosis and to justify prompt therapy with fresh frozen plasma (FFP) exchange. Simple FFP infusion could be used in patients with inherited disease. The introduction of treatment with plasma exchange markedly improved the prognosis in patients, with a decrease in mortality from 85–100% to 10–30%. It remains the mainstay of treatment of TTP. Idiopathic TTP (antibody mediated) appears to respond best to plasma exchange. It should be continued until the platelet count is normal and signs of hemolysis are resolved for at least 2 days. However, the hematologic findings are not specific for TTP, and other diagnoses must still be considered, even in the case of an apparently favorable response to treatment. Though never evaluated in clinical trial, the use of glucocorticoids seems a reasonable approach. They are currently used as an adjunct to plasma exchange [91]. Other immunomodulatory therapies, such as rituximab, vincristine, cyclophosphamide, and splenectomy, have been reported to be successful in refractory or relapsing TTP. The role of rituximab in the treatment of this disorder needs to be defined [92]. A significant relapse rate is noted: 25–45% within 30 days of initial "remission" and 12–40% with late relapses. Relapses may be more frequent in patients with severe ADAMTS13 deficiency at presentation.

Hemolytic Uremic Syndrome (HUS)

HUS is a syndrome characterized by acute renal failure, microangiopathic hemolytic anemia, and thrombocytopenia. It is seen predominantly in children and in most cases is preceded by an episode of diarrhea, often hemorrhagic in nature. *Escherichia coli* O157:H7 is the most frequent, although not only, etiologic serotype. HUS not associated with diarrhea (termed DHUS) is more heterogeneous in presentation and course [93]. Some children who develop DHUS have been found to have mutations in genes encoding Factor H, a soluble complement regulator, and membrane cofactor protein that is mainly expressed in the kidney. Treatment of HUS is primarily supportive. In D+HUS, many (~40%) children require at least some period of support with dialysis; however, the overall mortality is <5%. In D–HUS the mortality is higher, approximately 26%. Plasma infusion or plasma exchange has not been shown to alter the overall course. ADAMTS13 levels are generally reported to be normal in HUS, although occasionally they have been reported to be decreased. As ADAMTS13 assays improve, they may help in defining a subset that better fits a TTP diagnosis and may respond to plasma exchange [94].

Heparin Induced Thrombocytopenia (HIT)

Heparin induced thrombocytopenia is a serious side effect of a drug that is widely used in clinical practice. There are two clinical forms of HIT. HIT type I is benign and is characterized by reversible thrombocytopenia [95] while HIT type II is an immune-mediated disease with severe life-threatening complications [96]. Type I HIT, caused by the direct non-immune platelet-aggregating effect of heparin [95] usually starts 1–3 days after the start of heparin, with platelet counts rarely below 100,000 / ml. The thrombocytopenia resolves despite the continuation of heparin and does not present with any associated thrombosis. Type II HIT is an antibody-mediated thrombocytopenia, often associated with thrombosis, while bleeding and petechiae are generally absent. The pathogenesis of the syndrome is due to production of immunoglobulin G (IgG) antibodies against complexes of heparin and PF4, a small peptide stored within the alpha granules of platelets which binds to heparin and is released into the blood during treatment with heparin. In vitro, IgG–PF4–heparin complexes can activate platelets; this finding raises the possibility that platelet activation *in vivo*, together with endothelial cell immune-mediated injury, contributes to the thrombotic complications of HIT, originating the HITTS (Heparin Induced Thrombocytopenia Thrombotic Syndrome). Heparin specific antibodies, in the presence of PF4, trigger monocyte activation leading to expression of proinflammatory cytokine, interleukin-8, and of functional cell-surface tissue factor activity [97]. The frequency of HIT varies considerably and is probably related to different heparin preparations: bovine *vs* porcine heparin; unfractionated (1% - 3%) *vs* LMWH (0.1%). Some relevance has also the exposed patient population (more frequent after surgery than in medical patients and less frequent in pregnancy). Patients with HIT can have a dramatic presentation and often an unfortunate outcome. Each episode has the real potential to result in clinical catastrophe. Retrospective and prospective studies suggest that >90% of patients with clinical HIT have a platelet count fall >50% during their heparin treatment [98,99] between days 5 and 14 after the start of therapy, typically 4–5 days after the initiation of heparin therapy. Delayed recognition continues to contribute to the morbidity and mortality of these patients. Thus, platelet count should be monitored during those times when HIT usually occurs. The potential beneficial impact of therapy with direct thrombin inhibitors makes it more important to maintain awareness of and vigilance for this syndrome. In case of recent exposure to heparin the thrombocytopenia can begin also after few hours (median of 10.5 h). The median time for recovery of platelets to more than 150,000 is about 4 days, but sometimes thrombocytopenia can persist for weeks even after heparin administration is stopped [100]. Thrombosis occurs in approximately 33% of HIT patients and can produce devastating complications, including necrosis and thrombosis of the extremities, stroke, MI and pulmonary embolism, the last one occurring more frequently than all arterial thrombosis considered together. In fact venous thrombotic complications predominate in HIT [101]. The literature on neurologic complications in HITTS and, in particular, on brain infarcts, is limited. In an 11-year retrospective study of 120 patients with HIT [102], 11 (9.2%) had strokes: seven arterial ischemic events (the distribution described in only one case, a middle cerebral artery stroke), 3 dural venous sinus thromboses, and one transient confusional state. Another study of 960 patients with HIT disclosed 30 (3.2%) strokes [103]. The ischemic strokes appear to affect primarily the middle cerebral artery territory, but clinical details are sparse, and there have been no imaging reports. In the series of Pohl et al [102], two of the patients had a normal platelet count at the time of stroke onset. An extensive literature review of 29 case reports of HITTS and neurologic complications found 5 patients with MCA ischemic strokes, 3 with sagittal sinus thrombosis, and one with a parietal focal seizure. The clinical manifestations of the remaining patients were not reported [104].

The diagnosis must be clinically suspected based on the following criteria:

- decrease in platelet count by 50% from baseline or decrease in platelet count to less than $100–150x10^9$ / l, after heparin treatment for more than 5 days (in patients without recent exposure to heparin), in absence of other causes of thrombocytopenia
- development of new or extension of existing thrombosis while receiving heparin therapy

and confirmed by laboratory testing:

- functional assays, which detect heparin-dependent platelet activation in the presence of the patient's sera and UFH or LMWH.

They include heparin-induced platelet aggregation (HIPA) test and the serotonin release assay (SRA). Antigen assays (immunoassays such as ELISA), which measure IgG, IgM or IgA antibodies that bind PF4 to UFH. They are less specific for clinical HIT than is the SRA but offer higher sensitivity [105,106].

An additional diagnostic criterion is the return to normal platelet count when heparin is discontinued.

When HIT is clinically suspected heparin administration should be immediately suspended, and alternative anticoagulant agents such as lepirudin and argatroban can be used to rapidly control thrombin generation [107], without any delay, even if laboratory confirmation is not immediately available [108]; thrombocytopenia itself is not a contraindication to the treatment that should continue at least until the thrombosis is under control and the platelet counts reach a safe stable plateau. The administration of coumarin anticoagulants may promote an early, transient hypercoagulability by impairing production of fully functional proteins C and S, natural anticoagulant proteins whose synthesis is vitamin K-dependent. Therefore, in acute phase warfarin should be postponed until substantial platelet count recovery has been achieved. In this period also agents reducing thrombin generation (e.g. danaparoid, fondaparinux) can be administered as anticoagulant therapy. At the moment the reported use of Fondaparinux in HIT is not frequent. Danaparoid is preferred for parenteral anticoagulation of pregnant patients with HIT because it does not cross the placenta, but its effect is difficult to monitor, has a long duration and cannot be neutralized. LMWH is absolutely contraindicated in patients with acute HIT.

Acute Leukemias

Intracranial hemorrage and, more rarely, ischemic stroke are caused by acute leukemias, myeloid or lymphoid [109,110]. Acute promyelocytic leukemia frequently causes disseminated intravascular coagulation. This phenomenon is due to the release of a procoagulant, especially after chemotherapy-mediated cell lysis. the mortality rates, mainly due to hemorrhagic complications, is near 30% [111]. Diagnosis of disseminated intravascular coagulation is based on detection of schistocytes on the blood smear, elevated prothrombin time, decreased fibrinogen, increased plasma level of D-dimer. In patients with fulminant leukocytosis, particularly those with a leukocyte count over $200000x10^6/l$, leukostasis, or blast cell thrombi within small arterioles can occur, resulting in tissue ischemia and hyperviscosity syndrome [109,110]. The phenomenon can be observed in acute leukemias as well as in Chronic Granulocytic Leukemia. Its treatment is include leukopheresis and chemotherapy. Leukopheresis alone has no significant effect on early death and survival. Therefore chemotherapy should be started as soon as possible [112].

Hyperleukocytosis frequently produces vascular damage and massive hemorrhage through endothelial damage. Cerebral infarction is less common in oncohematologic patients than hemorrhage and is mainly related to sinovenous thrombosis. When lungs and brain are affected, patients complaint shortness of breath, headache, visual and/or auditory disturbances, dizziness, or lethargy, progressing to an acute confusional state, focal neurologic deficits, or seizures.

Acute lymphoid leukemia, acute myeloid leukemia, and acute promyelocytic leukemia have the highest incidence of leukostasis. Sinovenous thrombosis is frequently encountered in acute lymphoid leukemia and manifests clinically with headache, seizures, focal deficits, or altered consciousness. The pathogenic mechanisms contributing to venous occlusion are leukostasis, hypercoagulability (e.g., prothrombin G20210A mutation, factor V G1691A mutation), and use of certain chemotherapeutic agents, particularly L–asparaginase.

Another cause of stroke is vasculitis, frequently drug-induced (e.g., hydroxyurea, vincristine, cytarabine, methotrexate, alltrans retinoic acid) [109,110,113]. Finally, ischemic strokes may also occur as a result of radiation-induced vascular damage.

Plasma Cells Dyscrasias

Multiple myeloma is a possible, but infrequent malignant plasma-cell disease in young people. Most frequent symptoms are fatigue, bone pain, bleeding, infections, or renal impairment. The diagnosis is based on the presence of bone lesions, monoclonal immunoglobulin increase and plasma-cell infiltrate in the bone marrow [114]. The outcome is highly variable (survival ranging from a few months to more than 10 years). Classical prognostic factors as cytogenetic and molecular markers (e.g., hyperdiploidy, translocation at 14q32, chromosome 13 delection) are now overcome from the new therapies. Novel anti-multiple myeloma therapies include thalidomide and its more potent immunomodulatory derivative lenalidomide, the proteasome inhibitor bortezomib, and arsenic trioxide [115].

Waldenstrom's macroglobulinemia is an uncommon disease, very rare in young people. Median age of onset is 63 years (range 25–92). It accounts for approximately 2% of all hematologic malignancies [115]. Disease onset is insidious, and patients may present with weakness, weight loss, pallor, fever, purpura or hemorrhagic manifestations, splenomegaly, hepatomegaly, and polyneuropathy. Anemia is the most common laboratory finding, and raised erythrocyte sedimentation rate is almost constantly observed. High-resolution electrophoresis combined with immunofixation of serum and urine are recommended for identification and characterization of the IgM monoclonal protein [116]. Age, sex, hemoglobin level, serum albumin, IgM level, and b2M predict outcome [115]. Therapeutic regimens include glucocorticoids and cytotoxic agents, and more recently thalidomide and monoclonal antibodies [115,116].

The above-mentioned disorders, as well as the related POEMS syndrome (poly neuropathy, organomegaly, endocrinopathy, monoclonal gammopathy, skin changes), are associated with ischemic stroke and intracerebral hemorrhage [110,117]. Cerebrovascular complications generally result from hyperviscosity mostly due to hypergammaglobulinemia. The reasons for elevated viscosity are increased protein content and large molecular size, abnormal polymerization, and abnormal shape of immunoglobulin molecules. Other hematologic (elevated fibrinogen) and metabolic abnormalities (renal dysfunction) seen in patients with plasma cell dyscrasias also contribute to hyperviscosity. Hyperviscosity occurs when IgM concentration is higher than 3g/dl, IgG 4g/dl and IgA 6g/dl. Plasmapheresis can rapidly reduce hyperviscosity, but chemotherapy is necessary for the control of the disease.

Henoch–Schonlein Purpura (HSP)

Henoch–Schonlein purpura (HSP) is an immune complex-mediated generalized small-vessel vasculitis, characterized by vascular wall deposits of predominantly IgA, typically involving small vessels in the skin, gut, joints, and kidneys. HSP is associated with palpable cutaneous purpura, intestinal colic, arthralgia, and hematuria. The nervous system may be involved, but manifestations are usually mild and transient (e.g., headache, behavioral alterations, and reduction in the level of consciousness). Intracerebral and subarachnoid hemorrhage have been reported rarely as severe complications resulting from cerebral vasculitis. Plasmapheresis has been used in HSP cerebral vasculitis with intracerebral hemorrhage with anecdotally good success [118].

Neonatal alloimmune thrombocytopenia can occur when a mother is immunized against fetal platelet antigens inherited from the father. Five major human platelet antigen (HPA) systems are capable of causing this disorder (most frequently HPA-1a). Early diagnosis and appropriate platelet transfusion therapy are essential to prevent life-threatening intracranial hemorrhage in the thrombocytopenic fetus or neonate. Stroke has been rarely reported.

Intravascular Lymphoma

Intravascular lymphoma is an uncommon malignancy, defined pathologically by neoplastic proliferation of lymphoid cells within the lumens of capillaries, small veins, and arteries with little or no adjacent parenchymal involvement. It used to be called malignant angioendotheliosis but recent immunohistochemical studies have demonstrated that the tumours are neoplastic lymphoid cells more commonly of B-cell origin and therefore it is now referred to as intravascular lymphoma or angiotrophic large cell lymphoma. Most commonly symptoms are confined to the skin or CNS until later stages of the disease when systemic features may develop. A literature review of 114 patients found that 63% had neurological manifestations without abnormalities on bone marrow biopsy, chest and abdominal CT, or CSF examination. One neurological presentation is with recurrent stroke-like episodes. It may also present with a dementia with or without focal neurological signs, a spinal cord syndrome, and peripheral or cranial neuropathies. It may produce an identical clinical picture to primary angiitis of the CNS, including similar angiographic appearances, and distinction may only be possible on brain biopsy or postmortem. Similarly the peripheral nervous system findings may mimic systemic vasculitis and again only be differentiated on biopsy. Autoantibodies may occur which can make distinction from vasculitis even more difficult. Most of the cases of CNS involvement have been diagnosed at postmortem. In some cases an improvement has been made after corticosteroid therapy although this may only be partial or transient. Chemotherapy has resulted in remission in a few case reports.

Severe Iron Deficiency Anemia

Rarely, severe iron deficiency anemia has been recognized as a cause of ischemic stroke or cerebral venous thrombosis in adult or pediatric populations [119,120]. The main cause is intestinal blood loss, but inadequate dietary iron intake is rare in Western countries. Several potential pathophysiological mechanisms are hypothesized. Thrombocytosis occurring in iron-deficiency anemia is thought to be the major contributing factor of venous thrombosis. In ischemic stroke, rheological changes due to decreased blood viscosity may lead to turbulent flow, damage of endothelium, and platelet aggregation. Finally, microcytosis is associated with a reduction in the red cell deformability, which could facilitate small-vessel thrombosis [119,120].

Conclusion

Hematologic diseases sometimes can give origin to ischemic strokes. The absolute incidence among the general population is not high. However, because of their peculiar pathogenesis and clinical course, clinicians must have a high level of suspicion that a cerebral ischemic event might be due to an underlying hemopathy. In many cases, simple and routine laboratory tests can support the diagnostic suspect: thrombocytosis, erythocytosis, high number of blasts in the peripheral blood, microcytosis, alterations of RBC morphology, monoclonal gammopathy etc. can be relevant for the diagnosis and are easily and promptly available in any hospital. Making a timely diagnosis and starting early an appropriate treatment have a great prognostic relevance in these cases.

References

[1] Arboix A, Besses C. Cerebrovascular disease as the initial clinical presentation of haematological disorders. *Eur. Neurol.* 1997;37(4):207-11.

[2] Angastiniotis M, Modell B. Global epidemiology of haemoglobin disorders. *Ann. N. Y. Acad. Sci.* 1998;850:251–259.

[3] Higgs DR, Thein SL, Woods WG. The molecular pathology of the thalassaemias. In Weatherall DJ, Clegg B. The Thalassaemia Syndromes, 2001; 4th ed, pp. 133–191. Blackwell Science, Oxford, England.

[4] Lang F, Lang KS, Lang PA, Huber SM, Wieder T. Mechanisms and significance of eryptosis. *Antioxid. Redox. Signal.* 2006;8:1506-28.

[5] Shinar E, Rachmilewitz EA. Hemoglobinopathies and red cell membrane function. *Baill. Clin. Haematol.* 1993;6:357-369.

[6] Wood KC, Hsu LL, Gladwin MT. Sickle cell disease vasculopathy: A state of nitric oxide resistance. *Free Radical. Biol. Med.* 2008;44:1506–1528

[7] Eldor A, Rachmilewitz EA. The hypercoagulable state in thalassemia. *Blood* 2002;99: 36-43.

[8] Borgna-Pignatti C, Rugolotto S, De Stefano P, Zhao H, Cappellini MD, Del Vecchio GC, Romeo MA, Forni GL, Gamberini MR, Ghilardi R, Piga A, Cnaan A. Survival and complications in patients with thalassemia major treated with transfusion and deferoxamine. *Hematologica* 2004;89:1187-93

[9] Eldor A, Durst R, Hy-Am E, Goldfarb A, Gillis S, Rachmilewitz EA, Abramov A, MacLouf J, Godefray YC, De Raucourt E, Guillin MC. A chronic hypercoagulable state in patients with beta-thalassemia major is already present in childhood. *Br. J. Haematol.* 1999;107:739-746.

[10] Del Principe D, Menichelli A, Di Giulio S, De Matteis W, Cianciulli P, Papa G. PADGEM/GMP-140 expression on platelet membranes from homozygous beta thalassemic patients. *Br. J. Haematol.* 1993;84:111-117.

[11] Ruf A, Pick M, Deutsch V, Patscheke H, Goldfarb A, Rachmilewitz EA, Rund D, Rachmilewitz E. β Thalassemia. *N. Engl. J. Med.* 2005;353:1135-1146.

[12] Cappellini MD, Robbiolo L, Bottasso BM, Coppola R, Fiorelli G, Mannucci AP. Venous thromboembolism an hypercoagulability in splenectomized patients with thalassaemia intermedia. *Br. J. Haematol.* 2000;111:467-473.

[13] Setty BNY, Kulkarni S, Rao AK, Stuart MJ. Fetal haemoglobin in sickle cell disease: relationship to erythrocyte phosphatidylserine exposure and coagulation activation. *Blood* 2000;96:1119–1124.

[14] Kuypers FA, Yuan J, Lewis RA, Snyder LM, Kiefer CR, Bunyaratvej A, Fucharoen S, Ma L, Styles L, de Jong K, Schrier SL. Membrane phospholipid asymmetry in human thalassemia. *Blood* 1998;91:3044-3048.

[15] Ataga KI, Cappellini MD, Rachmilewitz EA. B-Thalassemia and siclke cell anemia as a paradigms of hypercoagulability. *Br. J. Haematol.* 2007;139:3-13.

[16] Borenstain-Ben Yashar V, Barenholz Y, Hy-Am E, Rachmilewitz EA, Eldor A. Phosphatidylserine in the outer leaflet of red blood cells from beta thalassemia patients may explain the chronic hypercoagulable state and thrombotic episodes. *Am. J. Hematol.* 1993;44:63-65.

[17] Helley D, Eldor A, Girot R, Ducrocq R, Guillin MC, Bezeaud A. Comparison of the procoagulant activity of red blood cells from patients with homozygous sickle cell disease and β-thalassemia. *Thromb Haemost.* 1996;76:322-327

[18] Shirahata A, Funahara Y, Opartkiattikul N, Fucharoen S, Laosombat V, Yamada K. Protein C and protein S deficiency in thalassemic patients. *South As. J. Trop. Med. Pub. Health* 1992;23:65-73.

[19] Musumeci S, Leonardi S, Di Dio R, Fischer A, Di Costa G. Protein C and antithrombin III in polytransfused thalassemic patients. *Acta Haematol.* 1997;77:30-33.

[20] Iolascon A, Giordano P, Storelli S, Li HH, Coppola B, Piga A, Fantola E, Forni G, Cianciulli P, Perrotta S, Magnano C, Maggio A, Mangiagli A. Thrombophilia in thalassaemia major patients: analysis of genetic predisposition factors. *Haematologica* 2004;86:1112–1113.

[21] Zalloua PA, Shbaklo H, Mourad YA, Koussa S, Taher A. Incidence of thromboembolic events in Lebanese thalassemia intermedia patients. *Thromb Haemost.* 2003;89:767–8.

[22] Tahar A, Isma'eel H, Mehio G, Bignamini D, Kattamis A, Rachmilewitz EA, Cappellini MD. Prevalence of thromboembolic events among 8, 860 patients with thalassaemia major and intermedia in the Mediterranean area and Iran. *Thromb Haemost.* 2006;96:488–491.

[23] Logothetis J, Constantoulakis M, Economidou J, Stefanis C, Hakas P, Augoustaki O, Sofroniadou K, Loewenson R, Bilek M. Thalassemia major (homozygous beta-thalassemia). A survey of 138 cases with emphasis on neurologic and muscular aspects. *Neurology* 1972;22:294–304.

[24] Borgna-Pignatti C, Carnelli V, Caruso V, Dore F, DeMattia D, Di Palma A, DiGregorio F, Romeo MA, Longhi R, Mangiagli A, Pizzarelli G, Musumeci S. Thromboembolic events in beta thalassaemia major: an Italian multicenter study. *Acta Haematol.* 1998; 99:76–79.

[25] Mandre L, Giarratano E, Maggio A, Banco A, Vaccaro G, Lagalla R. MR imaging of the brain: findings in asymptomatic patients with thalassaemia intermedia and sickle cell disease. *Am. J. Roentg.* 1999;173:1477–1480.

[26] Wun T, Paglieroni T, Rangaswami A, Franklin PH, Welborn J, Cheung A, Tablin F. Platelet activation in patients with sickle cell disease. *Br. J. Haematol.* 1998;100:741–749.

[27] Tomer A, Harker LA, Kasey S, Eckman JR. Thrombogenesis in sickle cell disease. *J. Lab. Clin. Med.* 2001;13:7398-407.

[28] Lee SP, Ataga KI, Orringer EP, Parise LV. Biologically active CD40 ligand is elevated in sickle cell disease: potential role for platelet-mediated inflammation. *Arterioscl. Thromb Vasc. Biol.* 2006;6:1626–1631.

[29] El Hazmi MAE, Warsy AS, Bahakim H. Blood protein C and S sickle cell disease. *Acta Haematol.* 1993;90:114-117.

[30] Karayaclin G, Lanzowsky P. Plasma protein C levels in children with sickle cell disease. *Am. J. Pediatr. Hematol. Oncol.* 1999;11:320-325

[31] Peters M, Plaat BE, ten Cate H, Wolters HJ, Weening RS, Brandjes DP. Enhanced thrombin generation in children with sickle cell disease. *Thromb Haemost.* 1994;71: 169-172

[32] Wright JG, Malia R, Cooper P, Thomas P, Preston FE, Serjeant GR. Protein C and S in homozygous sickle cell disease: does hepatic dysfunction contribute to low levels? *Br. J. Haematol.* 1997;98:627–631.

[33] Porter JB, Young L, Mackie IJ, Marshall L, Machin SJ. Sickle cell disorders and chronic intravascular haemolysis are associated with low plasma heparin cofactor II. *Br. J. Haematol.* 1993;83:459–465.

[34] O'Driscoll A, Mackie IJ, Porter JB, Machin SJ. Low plasma heparin cofactor II levels in thalassemia syndromes are corrected by chronic blood transfusion. *Br. J. Haematol.* 1995;90:65-70.

[35] Kinney TR, Sleeper LA, Wang WC, Zimmerman RA, Pegelow CH, Ohene-Frempong K, Wethers DL, Bello JA, Vichinsky EP, Moser FG, Gallagher DM, DeBaun MR, Platt OS, Miller ST. Silent cerebral infarcts in sickle cell anemia: a risk factor analysis. The Cooperative Study of Sickle Cell Disease. *Pediatrics* 1999;103:640-645.

[36] Bernaudin F, Verlhac S, Freard F, Roudot-Thoraval F, Benkerrou M, Thuret I, Mardini R, Vannier JP, Ploix E, Romero M, Cassé-Perrot C, Helly M, Gillard E, Sebag G, Kchouk H, Pracros JP, Finck B, Dacher JN, Ickowicz V, Raybaud C, Poncet M, Lesprit E, Reinert PH, Brugières P. Multicenter prospective study of children with sickle cell disease: radiographic and psychometric correlation. *J. Child Neurol.* 2000;15:333-343.

[37] Powars D, Wilson B, Imbus C, Pegelow C, Allen J. The natural history of stroke in sickle cell disease. *Am. J. Med.* 1978;65:461-471.

[38] Ohene-Frempong K, Weiner SJ, Sleeper LA, Miller ST, Embury S, Moohr JW, Wethers DL, Pegelow CH, Gill FM. Cerebrovascular accidents in sickle cell disease: rates and risk factors. *Blood* 1998;91:288–294.

[39] Wang WC. The pathophysiology, prevention, and treatment of stroke in sickle cell disease. *Curr. Opin. Hematol.* 2007;14:191–197.

[40] Adams RJ. Sickle cell disease and stroke. *J. Child Neurol.* 1995;10:75-76.

[41] Adams RJ, McKie VC, Hsu L, Pegelow C, Abboud M, Gallagher D, Kutlar A, Nichols FT, Bonds DR, Brambilla D. Prevention of a first stroke by transfusion in children with sickle cell anemia and abnormal results on transcranial Doppler ultrasonography. *N. Engl. J. Med.* 1998;339: 5-11.

[42] Adams RJ, Brambilla DJ, Granger S, Gallagher D, Vichinsky E, Abboud MR, Pegelow CH, Woods G, Rohde EM, Nichols FT, Jones A, Luden JP, Bowman L, Hagner S, Morales KH, Roach ES. STOP Study. Stroke and conversion to high risk in children screened with transcranial Doppler ultrasound during the STOP study. *Blood* 2004;103: 3689-3694.

[43] Vichinsky E, Onyekwere O, Porter J, Swerdlow P, Eckman J, Lane P, Files B, Hassell K, Kelly P, Wilson F, Bernaudin F, Forni GL, Okpala I, Ressayre-Djaffer C, Alberti D, Holland J, Marks P, Fung E, Fischer R, Mueller BU, Coates T, Deferasirox in Sickle Cell Investigators. A randomised comparison of deferasirox versus deferoxamine for the treatment of transfusional iron overload in sickle cell disease. *Br. J. Haematol.* 2007;136:501-8.

[44] Gladwin MT, Shelhamer JH, Ognibene FP, Pease-Fye ME, Nichols JS, Link B, Patel DB, Jankowski MA, Pannell LK, Schechter AN, Rodgers GP. Nitric oxide donor properties of hydroxyurea in patients with sickle cell disease. *Br. J. Haematol.* 2002; 116:436–444.

[45] Covas DT, Angulo I, Palma PVB, Zago MA. Effects of hydroxyurea on the membrane of erythrocytes and platelets in the sickle cell anaemia. *Haematologica* 2004;89:273–280.

[46] Chang Milbauer L, Wie P, Enenstein J, Jiang A, Hillery CA, Scott JP, Nelson SC, Bodempudi V, Topper JN, Yang RB, Hirsch B, Pan W, Hebbel RP. Genetic endothelial systems biology of sickle stroke risk. *Blood* 2008;111:3872-9.

[47] Hoppe C, Klitz W, D'Harlingue K, Cheng S, Grow M, Steiner L, Noble J, Adams R, Styles L, for the Stroke Prevention Trial in Sickle Cell Anemia (STOP) Investigators: Confirmation of an Association Between the TNF(-308) Promoter Polymorphism and Stroke Risk in Children With Sickle Cell Anemia. *Stroke* 2007;38:2241-2246

[48] Krishnan S, Siegel J, Pullen G Jr, Hevelow M, Dampier C, Stuart M. Increased von Willebrand factor antigen and high molecular weight multimers in sickle cell disease associated with nocturnal hypoxemia. *Thromb Res.* 2008;122:455-8.

[49] Tam DA. Protein C and S activity in sickle cell disease and stroke. *J. Child Neurol.* 1997;12:19–21.

[50] Hankinson TC, Bohman LE, Heyer G, Licursi M, Ghatan S, Feldstein NA, Anderson RC. Surgical treatment of moyamoya syndrome in patients with sickle cell anemia: outcome following encephaloduroarteriosynangiosis. *J. Neurosurg. Pediatrics* 2008;1: 211-216.

[51] Hulbert ML, Scothorn DJ, Panepinto JA, Scott JP, Buchanan GR, Sarnaik S, Fallon R, Chu JY, Wang W, Casella JF, Resar L, Berman B, Adamkiewicz T, Hsu LL, Smith-Whitley K, Mahoney D, Woods G, Watanabe M, DeBaun MR. Exchange blood transfusion compared with simple transfusion for first overt stroke is associated with a lower risk of subsequent stroke: a retrospective cohort study of 137 children with sickle cell anemia. *J. Pediatr* 2006;149:710-712.

[52] Socie G, Mary JY, de Gramont A, Rio B, Leporrier M, Rose C, Heudier P, Rochant H, Cahn JY, Gluckman E. Paroxysmal nocturnal haemoglobinuria: long-term follow-up and prognostic factors. French Society of Haematology. *Lancet* 1996;348:573–577

[53] Hall C, Richards S, Hillmen P. Primary prophylaxis with warfarin prevents thrombosis in paroxysmal nocturnal hemoglobinuria (PNH). *Blood* 2003;102:3587-3591.

[54] Rosse WF, Nishimura J. Clinical manifestations of paroxysmal nocturnal haemoglobinuria: present state and future problems. Int J Hematol 2003;77:113-120.

[55] Ziakas PD, Poulou LS, Rokas GI, Bartzoudis D, Voulgarelis M. Thrombosis in Paroxysmal Nocturnal Hemoglobinuria: sites, risks, outcome. An overview. *J. Thromb Haemost.* 2007;5:642–645.
[56] Hayag-Barin JE, Smith RE, Tucker FC. Hereditary spherocytosis, thrombocytosis, and chronic pulmonary emboli. A case report and review of the literature. *Am. J. Hematol.* 1998;57:82–4.
[57] Chou R, DeLoughery TG. Recurrent thromboembolic disease following splenectomy for pyruvate kinase deficiency. *Am. J. Hematol.* 2001;67:197–9.
[58] Pinkus M, Stark RA, O'Neill JH. Ischaemic stroke complicating pyruvate kinase deficiency. *Int. Med. J.* 2003;33:1-2.
[59] Vaquez H. Sur une forme spéciale de cyanose s'accompagnant d'hyperglobulie excessive et persistante. *CR Soc. Biol.* (Paris). 1892;44:384–388.
[60] Osler W. Chronic cyanosis with polycythaemia and enlarged spleen: a new clinical entity. *Am. J. Med. Sci.* 1903;126:187–201.
[61] James C, Ugo V, Le Couedic JP, Staerk J, Delhommeau F, Lacout C, Garçon L, Raslova H, Berger R, Bennaceur-Griscelli A, Villeval JL, Constantinescu SN, Casadevall N, Vainchenker W. A unique clonal JAK2 mutation leading to constitutive signalling causes polycythaemia vera. *Nature* 2005;434:1144–1148.
[62] Baxter EJ, Scott LM, Campbell PJ, East C, Fourouclas N, Swanton S, Vassiliou GS, Bench AJ, Boyd EM, Curtin N, Scott MA, Erber WN, Green AR; Cancer Genome Project. Acquired mutation of the tyrosine kinase JAK2 in human myeloproliferative disorders. *Lancet* 2005;365:1054–1061.
[63] Levine RL, Wadleigh M, Cools J, Ebert BL, Wernig G, Huntly BJ, Boggon TJ, Wlodarska I, Clark JJ, Moore S, Adelsperger J, Koo S, Lee JC, Gabriel S, Mercher T, D'Andrea A, Fröhling S, Döhner K, Marynen P, Vandenberghe P, Mesa RA, Tefferi A, Griffin JD, Eck MJ, Sellers WR, Meyerson M, Golub TR, Lee SJ, Gilliland DG. Activating mutation in the tyrosine kinase JAK2 in polycythemia vera, essential thrombocythemia, and myelofibrosis with myeloid metaplasia. *Cancer Cell* 2005;7: 387–397.
[64] Kralovics R, Passamonti F, Buser AS, Teo SS, Tiedt R, Passweg JR, Tichelli A, Cazzola M, Skoda RC. A gain-of-function mutation of JAK2 in myeloproliferative disorders. *N. Engl. J. Med.* 2005;352:1779–1790.
[65] Tefferi A, Vardiman JW. Classification and diagnosis of myeloproliferative neoplasms: the 2008 World Health Organization criteria and point-of-care diagnostic algorithms. *Leukemia* 2008;22:14-22.
[66] James C. The JAK2V617F Mutation in Polycythemia Vera and Other Myeloproliferative Disorders: One Mutation for Three Diseases? *Hematology Am. Soc. Hematol. Educ. Progr.* 2008:69-75.
[67] Chievitz E, Thiede T. Complications and causes of death in polycythaemia vera. *Acta Med. Scand.* 1962;172:513-523
[68] Najean Y, Mugnier P, Dresch C, Rain JD. Polycythaemia vera in young people: An analysis of 58 cases diagnosed before 40 years. *Br. J. Haematol.* 1987;67:285-291

[69] Harrison MJ. The hematocrit and cerebrovascular accidents. *Presse Med.* 1983;12(48): 3095-7.

[70] Landolfi R, Di Gennaro L, Barbui T, De Stefano V, Finazzi G, Marfisi R, Tognoni G, Marchioli R; European Collaboration on Low-Dose Aspirin in Polycythemia Vera (ECLAP).Leukocytosis as a major thrombotic risk factor in patients with polycythemia vera. *Blood* 2007; 109(6):2446-52.

[71] Landolfi R, Cipriani MC, Novarese L. Thrombosis and bleeding in polycythemia vera and essential thrombocytemia: pathogenetic mechanism and prevention. *Best Pract. Res. Clin. Haemat*. 2006;19:617-633.

[72] Landolfi R, Di Gennaro L. Prevention of thrombosis in polycythemia vera and essential thrombocythemia. *Haematologica* 2008;93(3):331-5

[73] De Stefano V, Za T, Rossi E, Vannucchi AM, Ruggeri M, Elli E, Micò C, Tieghi A, Cacciola RR, Santoro C, Gerli G, Vianelli N, Guglielmelli P, Pieri L, Scognamiglio F, Rodeghiero F, Pogliani EM, Finazzi G, Gugliotta L, Marchioli R, Leone G, Barbui T, for the GIMEMA CMD-Working Party. Recurrent thrombosis in patients with polycythemia vera and essential thrombocythemia: incidence, risk factors, and effect of treatments. *Haematologica* 2008;93(3):372-380.

[74] Prchal JT, Crist WM, Goldwasser E, Prchal JF: Autosomal dominant polycythemia. *Blood* 1985;66:1208-1214

[75] Perloff JK, Rosove MH, Child JS, Wright GB: Adults with cyanotic congenital heart disease: Hematologic management. *Ann. Intern. Med.* 1988;109:406-413

[76] Rosove MH, Hocking WG, Canobbio MM, Perloff JK, Child JS, Skorton DJ. Chronic hypoxaemia and decompensated erythrocytosis in cyanotic congenital heart disease. *Lancet* 1986;2:313-315

[77] Silverstein A, Gilbert H, Wasserman LR: Neurologic complications of polycythemia. *Ann. Intern. Med.* 1962;57:909-916

[78] Pearce JMS, Chandrasekera CP, Ladusans EJ: Lacunar infarcts in polycythemia with raised packed cell volumes. *Brit. Med. J.* 1983;287:935-937

[79] Burge PS, Johnson WS, Prankerd TAJ: Morbidity and mortality in pseudopolycythemia. *Lancet* 1975;1:1266-1269

[80] Doll DC, Greenberg BR: Cerebral thrombosis in smoker's polycythemia. *Ann. Intern. Med.* 1985;102:786-787

[81] Humphrey PRD, Michael J, Pearson TC: Management of relative polycythaemia: Studies of cerebral blood flow and viscosity. *Br. J. Haematol.* 1980;46:427-433

[82] Vannucchi, AM; Barbui, T. Thrombocitosis and thrombosis. *Hematology Am. Soc. Hematol. Educ. Progr*. 2008, 363-70.

[83] Tefferi A, Thiele J, Orazi A, Kvasnicka HM, Barbui T, Hanson CA, Barosi G, Verstovsek S, Birgegard G, Mesa R, Reilly JT, Gisslinger H, Vannucchi AM, Cervantes F, Finazzi G, Hoffman R, Gilliland DG, Bloomfield CD, Vardiman JW. Proposals and rationale for revision of the World Health Organization diagnostic criteria for polycythemia vera, essential thrombocythemia, and primary myelofibrosis: recommendations from an ad hoc international expert panel. *Blood* 2007;110:1092-1097.

[84] Passamonti F, Rumi E, Arcaini L, Boveri E, Elena C, Pietra D, Boggi S, Astori C, Bernasconi P, Varettoni M, Brusamolino E, Pascutto C, Lazzarino M. Prognostic factors for thrombosis, myelofibrosis, and leukemia in essential thrombocythemia: a study of 605 patients. *Haematologica* 2008 Nov;93(11):1645-51..

[85] Carobbio A, Finazzi G, Guerini V, Spinelli O, Delaini F, Marchioli R, Borrelli G, Rambaldi A, Barbui T. Leukocytosis is a risk factor for thrombosis in essential thrombocythemia: interaction with treatment, standard risk factors, and Jak2 mutation status. *Blood* 2007;109:2310-2313

[86] Antonioli E, G uglielmelli P, Poli G, Bogani C, Pancrazzi A, Longo G, Ponziani V, Tozzi L, Pieri L, Santini V, Bosi A, Vannucchi AM, for the Myeloproliferative Disorders Research Consortium (MPD-RC). Influence of *JAK2*V617F allele burden on phenotype in essential thrombocythemia. *Haematologica* 2008;93(1):41-8

[87] Harrison CN, Campbell PJ, Buck G, Wheatley K, East CL, Bareford D, Wilkins BS, van der Walt JD, Reilly JT, Grigg AP, Revell P, Woodcock BE, Green AR. United Kingdom Medical Research Council Primary Thrombocythemia 1 Study. Hydroxyurea compared with anagrelide in high-risk essential thrombocythemia. *N. Engl. J. Med.* 2005; 353(1):33-45.

[88] Barbui T, Barosi G, Grossi A, Gugliotta L, Liberato LN, Marchetti M, Mazzucconi MG, Rodeghiero F, Tura S. Practice guidelines for the therapy of essential thrombocythemia. A statement from the Italian Society of Hematology, the Italian Society of Experimental Hematology and the Italian Group for Bone Marrow Transplantation. *Haematologica* 2004;89:215-232

[89] Vannucchi, A.M; Barbui, T. Stratified management of essential thrombocythaemia and polycythaemia vera. Haematologica. Hematology Education (Education program for the 13th Congress of the European Hematology Association) 2008;2(1)201-208

[90] Maugeri N, Giordano G, Petrilli MP, Fraticelli V, de Gaetano G, Cerletti C, Storti S, Donati MB. Inhibition of tissue factor expression by hydroxyurea in polymorphonuclear leukocytes from patients with myeloproliferative disorders: a new effect for an old drug? *J. Thromb Haemost.* 2006;4(12):2593-8.

[91] Allford SL, Hunt BJ, Rose P, Machin SJ. Haemostasis nd Thrombosis Task Force, British Committee for Standards in Haematology. Guidelines on the diagnosis and management of the thrombotic microangiopathic haemolytic anemias. *Br. J. Haematol.* 2003;120:556-73

[92] Stein GY, Zeidman A, Fradin Z, Varon M, Cohen A, Mittelman M. Treatment of resistant thrombotic hrombocytopenic purpura with rituximab and cyclophosphamide. *Int. J. Haematol.* 2004;80:94–96

[93] Martin DL, MacDonald KL, White KE, Soler JT, Osterholm MT. The epidemiology and clinical aspects of the hemolytic uremic syndrome in Minnesota. *N. Engl. J. Med.* 1990;323:1161-1167.

[94] Garg AX, Suri RS, Barrowman N, Rehman F, Matsell D, Rosas-Arellano MP, Salvadori M, Haynes RB, Clark WF. Long-term renal prognosis of diarrhea-associated hemolytic uremic syndrome: a systematic review, meta-analysis, and meta-regression. *JAMA* 2003;290(10):1360-70

[95] Chong BH. Heparin-induced thrombocytopenia. *Br. J. Haematol.* 1995;89:431–9.

[96] Warkentin TE. Clinical presentation of heparin-induced thrombocytopenia. *Semin. Hematol.* 1998;5:9–16; discussion 35–6.

[97] Daneschvar HL, Daw H. Heparin-induced thrombocytopenia (an overview). *Int. J. Clin. Pract.* 2007;61(1):130-7

[98] Warkentin TE, Roberts RS, Hirsh J, Kelton JG. An improved definition of immune heparin-induced thrombocytopenia in postoperative orthopedic patients. *Arch Intern. Med.* 2003;163:2518–24.

[99] Warkentin TE. Heparin-induced thrombocytopenia: pathogenesis and management. *Br. J. Haematol.* 2003;121:535–55.

[100] Warkentin TE, Kelton JG. Temporal aspects of heparin-induced thrombocytopenia. *N. Engl. J. Med.* 2001;344:1286–92.

[101] Nand S, Wong W, Yuen B, Yetter A, Schmulbach E, Gross Fisher S. Heparin-induced thrombocytopenia with thrombosis: incidence, analysis of risk factors, and clinical outcomes in 108 consecutive patients treated at a single institution. *Am. J. Hematol.* 1997;56:12–6.

[102] Pohl C, Harbrecht U, Greinacher A, Theuerkauf I, Biniek R, Hanfland P, Klockgether T. Neurologic complications in immune-mediated heparin induced thrombocytopenia. *Neurology* 2000;54:1240–5.

[103] LaMonte MP, Browm PM, Hursting MJ. Stroke in cases with heparin-induced thrombocytopenia and the effects of argatroban therapy. *Crit. Care Med.* 2004;32:976–80.

[104] Becker PS, Miller VT. Heparin-induced thrombocytopenia. *Stroke* 1989;20:1449–59.

[105] Ganzer D, Gutezeit A, Mayer G, Greinacher A, Eichler P. Prevention of thromboembolism as a cause of thromboembolic complications. A study of the incidence of heparin-induced thrombocytopenia type II. *Z. Orthop. Ihre Grenzgeb.* 1997;135:543–9.

[106] Visentin GP, Ford SE, Scott JP, Aster RH. Antibodies from patients with heparin-induced thrombocytopenia thrombosis are specific for platelet factor 4 complexed with heparin or bound to endothelial cells. *J. Clin. Invest* 1994;93:81-8.

[107] Tardy-Poncet B, Tardy B, Reynaud J, Mahul P, Mismetti P, Mazet E, Guyotat D. Efficacy and safety of danaparoid sodium (ORG 10172) in critically ill patients with heparin-associated thrombocytopenia. *Chest* 1999;115:1616–20.

[108] Greinacher A, Eichler P, Lubenow N, Kwasny H, Luz M. Heparin-induced thrombocytopenia with thromboembolic complications: meta-analysis of 2 prospective trials to assess the value of parenteral treatment with lepirudin and its therapeutic aPTT range. *Blood* 2000;96:846–51.

[109] Demopoulos A, Deangelis LM . Neurologic complications of leukemia. *Curr. Opin. Neurol.* 2002;15:691–699.

[110] Recht L, Mrugala M. Neurologic complications of hematologic neoplasms. *Neurol. Clin.* 2003;21:87–105.

[111] Kwaan HC, Wang J, Boggio LN . Abnormalities in hemostasis in acute promyelocytic leukemia. *Hematol. Oncol.* 2002;20:33–41.

[112]Porcu P, Farag S, Marcucci G, Cataland SR, Kennedy MS, Bissell M. Leukocytoreduction for acute leukaemia. *Therapeutic Apheresis* 2002;6:15-23.

[113]Paydas S, Zorludemir S, Sahin B. Vasculitis and leukemia. *Leuk. Lymphoma* 2000; 40:105–112.

[114]Kyle RA, Rajkumar SV. Multiple myeloma. *N. Engl. J. Med.* 2004;351:1860–1873.

[115]Merlini G, Baldini L, Broglia C, Comelli M, Goldaniga M, Palladini G, Deliliers GL, Gobbi PG. Prognostic factors in symptomatic Waldenstrom's macroglobulinemia. *Semin. Oncol.* 2003;30:211–215.

[116]Gertz MA, Merlini G, Treon SP. Amyloidosis and Waldenstro¨m's macroglobulinemia. *Hematology Am. Soc. Hematol. Educ. Program* 2004;257–282.

[117]Drappatz J, Batchelor T. Neurologic complications of plasma cell disorders. *Clin. Lymphoma* 2004;5:163–171.

[118]Wen YK, Yang Y, Chang CC. Cerebral vasculitis and intracerebral hemorrhage in Henoch–Schonlein purpura treated with plasmapheresis. *Pediatr. Nephrol.* 2005;20: 223–225.

[119]Belman AL, Roque CT, Ancona R, Anand Ak, Davis RP. Cerebral venous thrombosis in a child with iron deficiency anemia and thrombocytosis. *Stroke* 1990;21:488–493.

[120]Akins PT, Glenn S, Nemeth PM, Derdeyn CP. Carotid artery thrombus associated with severe iron-deficiency anemia and thrombocytosis. *Stroke* 1996;27:1002–1005

[121]Campbell PJ, Scott LM, Buck G, Wheatley K, East CL, Marsden JT, Duffy A, Boyd EM, Bench AJ, Scott MA, Vassiliou GS, Milligan DW, Smith SR, Erber WN, Bareford D, Wilkins BS, Reilly JT, Harrison CN, Green AR; United Kingdom Myeloproliferative Disorders Study Group; Medical Research Council Adult Leukaemia Working Party; Australasian Leukaemia and Lymphoma Group. Definition of subtypes of essential thrombocythaemia and relation to polycythaemia vera based on JAK2 V617F mutation status: a prospective study. *Lancet* 2005;366(9501):1945-53.

[122]Cheung B, Radia D, Pantelidis P, Yadegarfar G, Harrison C. The presence of the JAK2 V617F mutation is associated with a higher haemoglobin and increased risk of thrombosis in essential thrombocythaemia. *Br. J. Haematol.* 2006;132(2):244-5.

[123]Kittiur J, Knudson RA, Lasho TL, Finke CM, Gangat N, Wolanskyj AP, Li CY, Wu W, Ketterling RP, Pardanani A, Tefferi A. Clinical correlates of JAK2V617F allele burden in essential thrombocythemia. *Cancer* 2007;109(11):2279-84

[124]Finazzi G, Rambaldi A, Guerini V, Carobbo A, Barbui T.Risk of thrombosis in patients with essential thrombocythemia and polycythemia vera according to JAK2 V617F mutation status. *Haematologica* 2007;92(1):135-6.

[125]Antonioli E, Guglielmelli P, Pancrazzi A, Bogani C, Verrucci M, Ponziani V, Longo G, Bosi A, Vannucchi AM. Clinical implications of the JAK2 V617F mutation in essential thrombocythemia. *Leukemia* 2005;19(10):1847-9.

[126]Wolanskyj AP, Lasho TL, Schwager SM, McClure RF, Wadleigh M, Lee SJ, Gilliland DG, Tefferi A. JAK2 mutation in essential thrombocythaemia: clinical associations and long-term prognostic relevance. *Br. J. Haematol.* 2005;131(2):208-13.

[127]Pemmaraju N, Moliterno AR, Williams DM, Rogers O, Spivak JL. The quantitative JAK2 V617F neutrophil allele burden does not correlate with thrombotic risk in essential thrombocytosis. *Leukemia* 2007;21(10):2210-2.

[128] Antonioli E, Guglielmelli P, Poli G, Santini V, Bosi A, Vannucchi AM. Polycythemia vera following autologous transplantation for AML: insights on the kinetics of JAK2V617F clonal dominance. *Blood* 2007;110(13):4620-1.

[129] Vannucchi AM, Antonioli E, Guglielmelli P, Rambaldi A, Barosi G, Marchioli R, Marfisi RM, Finazzi G, Guerini V, Fabris F, Randi ML, De Stefano V, Caberlon S, Tafuri A, Ruggeri M, Specchia G, Liso V, Rossi E, Pogliani E, Gugliotta L, Bosi A, Barbui T. Clinical profile of homozygous JAK2 617V>F mutation in patients with polycythemia vera or essential thrombocythemia. *Blood* 2007;110(3):840-6.

In: Cerebral Ischemia in Young Adults
Editors: A. Pezzini and A. Padovani
ISBN 978-1-60741-627-2

Chapter 18

Venous Infarcts in Young Adults

José M Ferro[3] and Patrícia Canhão
Department of Neurosciences, Serviço de Neurologia,
Hospital de Santa Maria, University of Lisboa, Lisboa, Portugal

Abstract

Thrombosis of the dural sinus and cerebral veins (CVT) are an uncommon cause of stroke in the young adult, accounting for less than 5% of the cases in most series. CVT predominantly affect young females and are associated with oral contraceptive use, pregnancy and puerperium, genetic and acquired prothrombotic conditions such as the antiphospholipid syndrome, and several other systemic conditions. The confirmation of the diagnosis of CVT and venous infarct is based on MRI, including T2*SE sequences combined with MR-venography. In half of the young adults with CVT a venous infarct is present in the admission CT or MRI. Venous infarcts are often multiple, and they can be combined with hemorrhagic lesions. They may undergo hemorrhagic transformation or disappear in subsequent scans. Venous infarcts are due to increased venous and capillary pressure with blood-brain barrier disruption, vasogenic oedema, venous hemorrhage and eventually decreased perfusion pressure with infarct. The most common clinical presentation in young patients with venous infarcts is a combination of headache with a focal syndrome (motor deficit, aphasia) with or without seizures. Mental status disturbances and decreased alertness are present in about ¼ of these patients. The prognosis of patients with venous infarcts is similar to that of CVT subjects without venous infarcts, with complete recovery in 87%, but with 7% mortality.

Treatment of venous infarcts includes treatment of the underlying condition, antithrombotic treatment (heparin followed by oral anticoagulants), treatment of intracranial hypertension and of infarcts producing impending herniation, and treatment and prevention of seizures.

3 Correspondence: José M. Ferro, Tel/fax:351 217957474, E-mail: jmferro@fm.ul.pt.

Introduction

Thrombosis of the dural sinus and cerebral veins (CVT) is less common than other types of stroke, has a more diverse clinical presentation [1,2] and is more difficult to diagnosis. CVT predominantly affect young adults, mostly females. CVT are a rare cause of stroke in the young adult, accounting for less than 5% of the cases in most series [3,4]. CVT are more frequent in particular clinical circumstances such as pregnancy and puerperium [5-7] or as a complication of a systemic diseases such as the antiphospholipid syndrome and other prothrombotic conditions, Behçet's disease or other vasculitis, malignancies in particular haematological ones and inflammatory diseases such as Chron´s disease.

CVT symptoms and signs at presentation can be grouped in three major syndromes: isolated headache with or without features of the intracranial hypertension syndrome (vomiting, papilloedema and visual symptoms), focal syndrome (focal deficits, seizures or both) and encephalopathy (multifocal signs, mental status changes, stupor or coma) [2]. Less common presentations include subarachnoid hemorrhage [8,9], TIAs, cranial nerve palsies and pulsatile tinnitus [10]. The symptoms and signs can develop acutely in a stroke like picture, but often had a subacute course or even a chronic presentation. CVT can also be an incidental finding in magnetic resonance imaging (MRI) performed for the investigation of unrelated complaints. Clinical symptoms and signs depend on: a) the interval from onset to presentation, chronic cases present mostly as isolated headache and intracranial hypertension syndrome[11]; b) the age of the patient [12,13], presentation as an isolated intracranial hypertension syndrome is more frequent in younger patients, while depressed consciousness and mental status changes are less frequent, when compared to elderly patients; c) the site and number of occluded sinus and veins, and d) the presence of parenchymal lesions.

We retrieved from the International Study on Cerebral Vein and Dural Sinus Thrombosis (ISCVT) [14] database information relative to venous infarcts in young adults (younger than 45 years). There were 415 young adults with CVT in the ISCVT cohort, 225 with brain lesions: 195 with infarcts, 149 with hemorrhages and 89 with both types of lesions. One hundred and six had only infarcts.

We will describe the characteristics of subgroup of the 106 patients with venous infarcts in more detail along the text.

Parenchymal Brain Lesions in CVT

In more than half of CVT young adult patients (54% in the ISCVT young adult venous infarct cohort) the initial neuroimaging of the brain, either CT or MRI, disclosed a parenchymal lesion: a venous infarct (47%), a hemorrhagic lesion (36%) or both (21%). These infarcts were quite often bilateral (40 patients; 37.7%) or multiple, and in 9 cases (8.4%) they were located in the posterior fossa. In 94 patients we had information on the nº and size of the infarct. Concerning lesions between 1-5 cm there 54 patients with single lesions and 25 with multiple lesions (15 with 2 lesions, 8 with 3 lesions, and 2 with 4 or more lesions). Nineteen patients had lesions > 5 cm: single infarcts in 17 patients, multiple in 2 (2 and 3 lesions respectively).

Hemorrhagic lesions include subarachnoid bleeding, subdural hematoma (suggestive of dural fistulae), intracerebral hematoma and hemorrhagic transformation of a venous infarct. Intracerebral hemorrhagic lesions can be single or multiple and are often associated with infarcts or oedema.

In acute severe cases or in patients who deteriorate, new infarcts or hemorrhages can develop in repeated CT or MRI.

Venous infarcts can be readily visible in CT but usually they are better depicted by MRI. MRI T1 and T2 WI may show a localised or diffuse brain swelling with normal or abnormal signal suggestive of oedema and/or infarct. Hyperintensities on T2 WI usually represent reversible oedema. In fact vasogenic oedema appears earlier in venous than in arterial stroke. Contrary to ischaemic stroke of arterial origin, in venous infarct the area of abnormal signal is larger in FLAIR than in DWI. Venous infarcts have several other distinctive features: they are often multiple, they do not follow an arterial vascular territory distribution and they may show marked mass effect, disproportionate to size of infarct and extending beyond the infarct zone [15]. Preferred locations include the parietal, frontal and posterior temporal lobes and the whole thalamus, often bilaterally, in cases with thrombosis of the deep cerebral venous system. Rarer locations include the basal ganglia and the splenium [16]. Often, there is no correlation between the extent and site of dural sinus thrombosis with the location and size of brain lesions [17]. In follow up imaging the ischemic lesions may undergo hemorrhagic transformation, they may enlarge in size but they may also decrease or even disappear (vanishing infarcts). About 2/3 of the ischemic parenchymal abnormalities can resolve completely even in the absence of complete recanalisation of the thrombosed sinus and veins [18]. Hemorrhagic transformation usually starts centrally and has a finger-like appearance on CT [15].

Pathophysiology

Few data on the pathophysiology of cerebral venous infarct is available compared with that of arterial ischemic infarct. This is partly due to the rarity of cerebral venous thrombosis, the high variability of venous system anatomy, and the comparative lack of experiments in adequate animal models of CVT [19]. Recently, advances in imaging modalities such as diffusion- and perfusion-weighted magnetic resonance have contributed to improve the understanding of some differences between venous and arterial occlusion and infarction [20-23].

At an early stage of venous occlusion, the collateral venous circulation allows for a significant compensation, and parenchymal lesions may not appear. The increase in venous and capillary pressure leads to dilatation of veins and capillaries, to blood-brain barrier disruption, causing vasogenic edema, with leakage of blood plasma into the interstitial space. As intravenous pressure increases, progression from mild parenchymal change to severe cerebral oedema and even to venous hemorrhage may occur due to venous or capillary rupture. The increase of intravenous pressure produces intracerebral venous congestion, increases intravascular pressure and lowers cerebral perfusion pressure. Cerebral blood flow may fall below penumbra or ischaemic thresholds, with failure of energetic metabolism, loss of the Na^{+}-K^{+}- ATPase pump activity and intracellular entry of water, with consequent cytotoxic oedema [23,24].

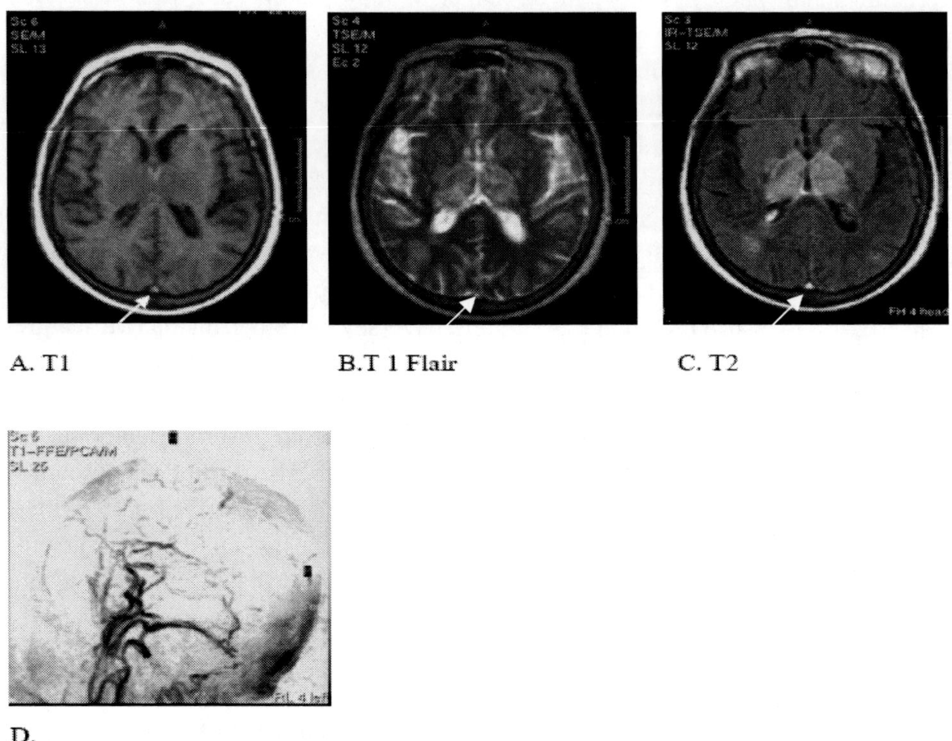

Figure 1. MRI of a patient presenting with 2 days of progressing mental status disturbances showed bithalamic lesions, not following an arterial vascular territory distribution (A. B. and C.). Thrombus is visible as a hyperintense signal in the superior sagittal sinus in all the sequences (arrows). D. MR venography confirmed the absence of flow in the superior saggital sinus, straight sinus and deep cerebral veins.

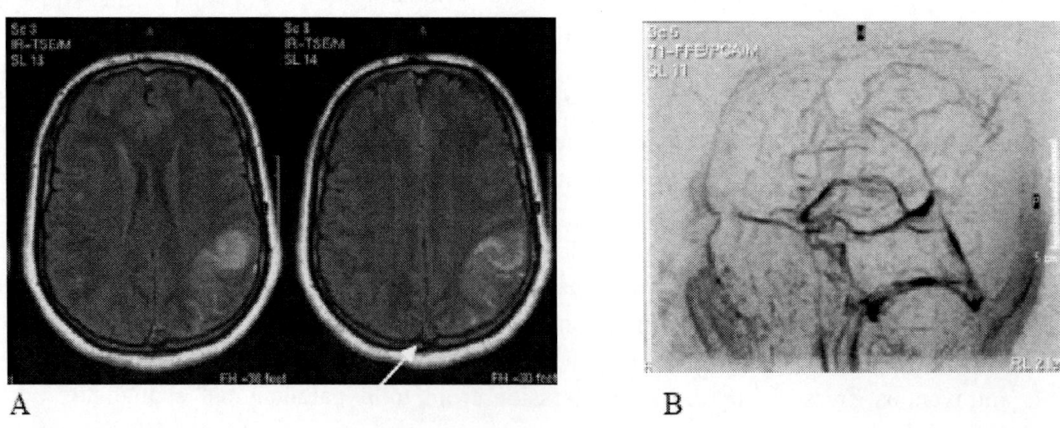

Figure 2. MRI (T1 flair) of a patient presenting with transient aphasia and paresthesias in the right hand showed a localised parietal hyperintensity suggestive of oedema and/or infarction. A thrombus is seen as isointense signal in the superior sagittal sinus (arrow) B. MR venography confirm the absence of flow in the superior sagittal sinus.

Magnetic resonance imaging has demonstrated the co-existence of both types of oedema, cytotoxic and vasogenic [20,22,25,26] in patients with CVT. Various patterns of DWI changes have been described [27-32]. The most frequent pattern is heterogeneous signal intensity with normal or increased ADC corresponding to vasogenic oedema [29,30]. A second pattern has areas of decreased ADC suggestive of cytotoxic oedema [31]. A third less frequent pattern is that of decreased diffusion with complete resolution and no lesion on follow up T2WI [32] which has been observed mostly in patients with seizures [2,32]. Overall DWI/ADC pattern is highly different from that of arterial infarcts, mostly suggestive of vasogenic oedema and far less frequently of cytotoxic oedema.

After venous occlusion, large areas of the brain may be functionally and metabolically disturbed, but not irreversibly. If collateral pathways drain the venous blood, adequate tissue perfusion may be possible, and swollen brain cells, although functionally impaired may be potentially recoverable [33]. This reversibility is very typical of venous infarcts, reflected both in favourable clinical recovery and vanishing lesions on neuroimaging.

Diagnosis of CVT

The confirmation of the diagnosis of CVT is based on demonstration of an occluded sinus/vein and of the thrombus, by MRI combined with MR venography (MRV), which is the most sensitive examination technique for the diagnosis CVT (Figures 1 and 2). Nevertheless, there are some diagnostic pitfalls with these techniques [34], namely concerning the diagnosis of cortical vein thrombosis [35]. Gradient echo (GRE) T_2* - weighted images with thrombus susceptibility effect (SE) improve the diagnosis of CVT enabling the identification of isolated cortical venous thrombosis as a hypointense area [36-38]. Multidetector CT venography (CTA) can also be as an alternative to MRV [39,40]. Intra-arterial digital venography is rarely performed today, except in doubtful cases and when it is necessary to confirm or exclude dural fistulae and to investigate its feeding and draining vessels.Clinical Aspects

In contrast to arterial stroke, only 43 patients (40.6%) with venous infarcts had an acute onset, with the full clinical picture becoming established in less than 4 days. The remaining patients had a subacute (4 - 30 days) (59 patients; 55.7%) or even chronic (> 30 days) (4 patients; 3.8%) mode of onset. The distribution of mode of onset was similar in CVT patients with and without venous infarcts ($p = 0.411$).

The most common symptoms and signs of young patients with venous infarcts (Figure 3) between onset of symptoms and diagnosis were headache (91 patients, 85.8%), focal deficits (aphasia – 15 patients, 14.2%; motor – 54 patients, 50.9%; sensory – 9 patients, 8.5%; other cortical deficits – 2 patients, 1.9%) and seizures (52; 49.1%), focal (26 patients, 24.5%) or with generalization (42 patients, 39.6%). Motor deficits were bilateral in 8 patients (7.5%). Mental status disturbance could be detected in 27 patients (25.5%), 22 (22%) had a Glasgow Coma Scale score (GCS) on admission below 14, but only 3 (3%) were comatose (GCS < 9). Only 28 (26.9%) subjects had papilloedema and 9 (8.6%) mentioned decreased visual acuity. Fourteen (13.2%) complained of diplopia or displayed an oculomotor palsy.

Overall, only 12 patients (11.3%) presented as a syndrome of isolated intracranial hypertension, while 83 (78.3%) featured a focal syndrome, with (52; 49.1%) or without (31; 29.2%) seizures.

When compared to the remaining young patients (n = 309), patients with venous infarcts (n = 106) had more often occlusion of the straight sinus (30/105, 28.6% vs. 52/309, 16.8%; p = 0.009), cortical vein (27/105, 25.7% vs. 46/309, 14.9%; p = 0.012), and deep venous system (23/105, 21.9% vs. 22/308, 7.1%; p < 0.001), motor deficits (54/106, 50.9% vs. 95/309, 30.7%; p < 0.001), bilateral motor deficits (8/106, 7.5% vs. 7/309, 2.3%; p = 0.012), and seizures (52/106, 49.1% vs. 113/309, 36.6%; p = 0.023). On the other hand they had less often left lateral sinus occlusion (33/105, 31.4% vs. 150/309, 48.5%; p = 0.002), headache (91/106, 85.8% vs. 290/308, 94.2%; p = 0.006), visual loss (9/105, 8.6% vs. 52/307, 16.9%; p = 0.037) and presentation as intracranial hypertension syndrome (12/106, 11.3% vs. 97/309, 31.4%; p < 0.001).

Symptoms and signs clustered differently according to the localization of the venous occlusion. In the 15 patients with isolated superior sagittal sinus thrombosis the clinical picture was dominated by headache, motor deficits and seizures. Bilateral motor deficits, decreased alertness and papilloedema were present in 13% of these subjects. In contrast,patients with isolated right (8 patients) or left (7 patients) lateral sinus thrombosis presentedmainly with headache, combined with seizures in about 1/3-1/2 and aphasia in 1/3 of the occlusions on the left side. In cases with thrombosis of the straight sinus and/or deep venous system the predominant features were headache, mental disturbance, decreased alertness and motor deficits, quite often bilateral.

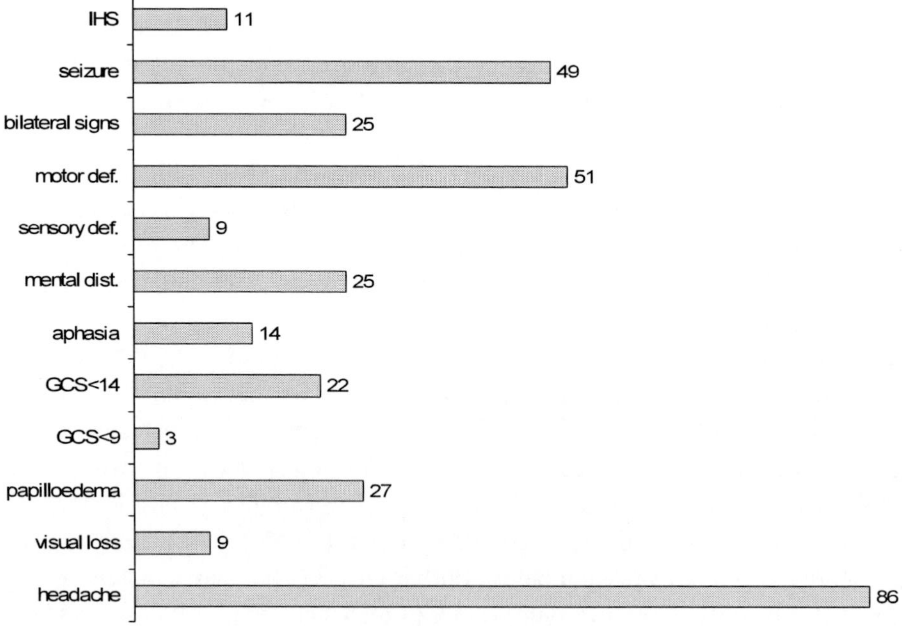

Figure 3. Presenting symptoms and signs.

Associated Conditions

The table (Table 1) listing the conditions associated with CVT in the ISCVT young infarct series illustrates that there are many potential causes for CVT and that about ½ of the cases have multiples causes, namely the combination of a prothrombotic latent condition (Table 2) with a precipitant (e.g. oral contraceptives [41,42], puerperium, sinusitis or other infection).

The most frequent associated conditions were oral contraceptive intake, pregnancy/ puerperium, acquired and genetic prothrombotic conditions, infections and non-malignant hematological diseases, in particular severe anemia [43,44]. Pregnancy/puerperal (30/106, 28.3% vs. 47/309, 15.2%; $p = 0.003$), CNS infections (6/106, 5.7% vs. 4/309, 1.3%; $p = 0.031$ with continuity correction), other (non-malignancies) hematological conditions (19/105, 17.9% vs. 29/309, 9.4%; $p = 0.018$) were more often present in patients with than in patients without venous infarct.

Table 1. Conditions associated with venous infarcts in young adults – ISCVT cohort

	Males n=17		Females n=89		Total n=106	
Associated condition	n	%	n	%	n	%
None	4	23.5	4	4.5	8	7.5
Multiple	7	41.2	47	52.8	54	50.9
Oral contraceptives	-	-	42	47.2	42	39.6
Pregnancy/puerperium	-	-	30	33.7	30	28.3
Prothrombotic conditions	3	17.6	28	31.5	31	29.2
Genetic	3	13.6	19	21.3	22	20.8
Acquired	0	0	10	11.2	10	9.4
Infections	7	41.2	9	10.1	16	15.1
CNS	3	17.6	3	3.4	6	5.7
ENT	2	11.8	6	6.7	8	7.5
Malignancies	3	17.6	4	4.5	7	6.6
Hematological	2	11.8	1	1.1	3	2.8
Other hematological diseases	4	23.5	15	16.9	19	17.9
Vasculitis	0	0	4	4.5	4	3.8
Other systemic diseases	0	0	5	5.6	5	4.7
Dehydration	1	5.9	1	1.1	2	1.9
Mechanical precipitants	3	17.6	1	1.1	4	3.8
Prothrombotic medications	1	5.9	5	5.6	6	5.7

Table 2. Recommended workup for prothrombotic screening in CVT patients

Protein C, protein S, anti-thrombin III
Factor V Leiden and prothrombin mutation
Factor VIII
Homocysteine
Lupus anticoagulant, antiphospholipid and anti-cardiolipin antibodies

Prognosis

In 28 patients (26.4%) the neurological condition worsened after admission: depressed consciousness in 14 (13.2%), altered mental status in 7 (6.6%), worsening of previous focal deficit in 6 (5.7%), new focal deficit in 5 (4.7%), new seizure in 9 (8.5%) and visual loss in 2 (1.9%).

Fifty patients had a repeated CT/MRI in the acute phase, which disclosed new infarcts in 6 (12%) patients and new hemorrhages in 6 (12%) cases.

At discharge, 6 months and last follow up (median 503 days) the modified Rankin Scale (mRS) distribution was as described in Table 3.

Table 3. Outcome of young adult patients with venous infarcts - ISCVT cohort

mRS	discharge	6 months	last follow up
0	23 (21.7%)	56 (53.3%)	66 (62.3%)
1	44 (41.5%)	35 (33.3%)	26 (24.5%)
2	23 (21.7%)	5 (4.8%)	4 (3.8%)
3	11 (10.4%)	1 (1%)	1 (0.9%)
4	0	2 (1.9%)	2 (1.9%)
5	1 (0.9%)	0	0
6	4 (3.8%)*	6 (5.7%)	7 (6.6%)
0-1	67 (63.2%)	91 (86.7%)	92 (86.8%)
3-6	16 (15.1%)	9 (8.6%)	10 (9.4%)

* All 4 cases died within 30 days from onset

The outcome at discharge was similar to that of the remaining patients ($p = 1.00$ for the 0-6 mRS distribution; $p = 0.51$ for complete recovery; $p = 0.63$ for death or dependency), as well as at 6 months ($p = 0.57$ for the 0-6 mRS distribution; $p = 0.37$ for complete recovery; $p = 0.63$ for death or dependency) or at the end of follow up ($p = 0.43$ for the 0-6 mRS distribution; $p = 0.42$ for complete recovery; $p = 0.75$ for death or dependency)

Predictors of poor long term prognosis in CVT are CNS infection, malignancy, deep cerebral venous system thrombosis, hemorrhage on CT/MRI, GCS score on admission <9, mental status disorder, age > 37 years and male gender [14]. In this subgroup of young patients with venous infarct the only significant predictor of death or dependency at the end of follow up was coma (GCS < 9) with a unadjusted OR of 4.17 (95% CI, 1.06 to 16.7) and a OR adjusted for age, mental status disturbance and deep cerebral venous system thrombosis of 4.20 (95% CI, 1.04 to 16.9). The main cause of death is transtentorial herniation secondary to a large lesion [45], other causes are herniation due to multiple lesions or to diffuse brain oedema, status epilepticus, medical complications and pulmonary embolism [46].

Long term complications in these young adults with venous infarct included seizures (7, 6.6%), severe headaches (12, 11.4%), visual loss (4, 3.8%), recurrent venous thrombosis of the brain (1, 0.9%), extremities or pelvis (1, 0.9%). Recurrent CVT is difficult to document, in particular if a previous follow up MRI/MRV is not available. Arterio-venous fistulae is another possible remote complication that needs intra-arterial angiography for confirmation.

Treatment

The treatment of CVT and associated venous infarct includes:

1. Treatment of the underlying condition
2. Antithrombotic treatment
3. Symptomatic treatment
4. Prevention/treatment of complications

Antithrombotic Treatment

The evidence supporting the use of heparin in acute CVT comes from three clinical trials [47-49] and a meta-analysis of two of these trials, which showed a relative risk of 0.46 (95% CI, 0.16 to 1.31) of death or dependency after anticoagulant therapy as compared to placebo [50]. In our series 82% of the patients (87) were anticoagulated with IV heparin or subcutaneous low molecular weight heparin (LMWH). Only 1 patient was treated with local thrombolysis. This data indicates that there is a large consensus on the use of either IV heparin or SC LMWH in acute CVT to prevent thrombus propagation and pulmonary embolism and to increase the chances of recanalisation. Heparin is safe and can be used in acute CVT patients with hemorrhagic lesions.

Subcutaneous LMWHs are preferable to IV heparin because they have longer half-life, more predictable clinical response and less interaction with platelets compared with standard heparin and are less labour-intensive.

Endovascular thrombolysis aims to dissolve the venous clot by delivering a thrombolytic substance (urokinase or rtPA) within the occluded sinus through an intravenous catheter. It is used as an alternative to heparin in severe cases or in patients who fail to improve on anticoagulation. No randomised trials of endovascular treatment for sinus thrombosis have been performed. A systematic review including 169 patients with CVT treated with local thrombolysis, suggested a possible benefit for severe CVT cases, indicating that thrombolytics may reduce case fatality in critically ill patients. Intracranial hemorrhage after thrombolysis was reported in 17 percent of cases, and was associated with clinical worsening in 5 percent [51]. However the possibility of publication bias must be kept in mind. In a Dutch series of 20 patients treated with IV local thrombolysis 12 recovered to independent living while 6 died [52]. Local thrombolysis was not useful in patients with large infarcts and impending herniation. A randomised trial to compare endovascular treatment vs. heparin in acute CVT is needed, before this treatment option can be routinely recommended.

Prevention of Recurrent Venous Thrombosis

After the acute phase of CVT, anticoagulation with warfarin is mandatory to prevent further thrombotic events. Optimal duration of anticoagulation is unknown, but it is usually maintained for 3 to 12 months after acute CVT, aiming at an international normalized ratio (INR) of 2 to 3. Chronic oral anticoagulation is reserved for patients with inherited or acquired prothrombotic conditions, including those with the antiphospholipid syndrome. If CVT was related to a transient risk factor (e.g. pregnancy, infection) current recommendation suggest anticoagulants for 3 months. In patients with idiopathic CVT or CVT associated with "mild" thrombophilia, the period of anticoagulation must be extended for 6 to 12 months. In patients with "severe thrombophilia (e.g. 2 or more prothrombotic abnormalities; antiphospholipid syndrome) anticoagulants should be given for life [53].

Symptomatic Treatment

Treatment of Intracranial Hypertension

In patients with severe headache and papilloedema, intracranial hypertension can be reduced and symptoms relieved by elevating the head of the bed and through a therapeutic lumbar puncture (5 patients in our series), if there is no contraindication such as a large infarct.

In more severe cases, diuretics such as furosemide (2 patients) or mannitol (15 patients; 14%) may be needed. Comatose patients need intensive care unit admission with sedation, hyperventilation to a target PaCO2 of 30 to 35 mmHg, and ICP monitoring.

Corticosteroids do not improve outcome in the acute phase of CVT [54] and should be avoided, unless they are needed to treat an underlying condition. They were prescribed in 32 (31%) of the patients of the ISCVT young adult venous infarct cohort.

Despite lack of randomised trials, acetazolamide is often (11 patients, 11%) used to relief symptoms of increased intracranial hypertension.

Hemicraniectomy may be life-saving when performed in CVT patients aged less than 60 years (1 patient) with parenchymal lesions producing impending herniation [55,56].

A lumboperitoneal shunt may be indicated in patients (2 patients) with persistent symptoms of increased intracranial hypertension and /or visual loss who do not improve with repeated lumbar punctures.

Treatment and Prevention of Seizures: Antiepileptics

Early Seizures

Acute seizures and supratentorial lesion are the risk factors for subsequent early seizures. Patients with both risk factors should be prescribed antiepileptic drugs. Prophylactic antiepileptics can also be considered in patients with one of the risk factors and should be avoided in patients with none of the two risk factors [57].

Prevention of Remote Seizures and Epilepsy

The long term risk of seizures is approximately 11% [14, 58]. The risk factors for seizures and post-CVT epilepsy are acute seizures, supratentorial hemorrhagic lesions and motor deficits. Antiepileptics are recommended for patients with seizures in the acute phase and for those who experience a seizure after the acute phase. Antiepileptics can also be considered for patients without seizures but with either supratentorial hemorrhagic lesions or motor deficits.

Contraception and Future Pregnancies

Oral contraception and hormonal replacement therapy should be stopped. Emergency contraception is also contraindicated [59]. Alternative methods of contraception can be used. Women on fertile age should not become pregnant while on oral anticoagulants, because of their teratogenic effects.

CVT and pregnancy or puerperium-related CVT are not a contraindication for future pregnancy. Although pregnancy and the puerperium are risk factors for CVT, the risk of complications during subsequent pregnancy among women who have a history of CVT is low [14,58,60,61,62].

Conclusion

Although CVT are a rare cause of stroke in the young adult, the possibility of a venous infarct should always be sought in cases with a) multiple infarcts, infarcts with hemorrhagic transformation, or infarcts combined with intracerebral hemorrhage and in b) young females using oral contraception or during pregnancy and puerperium or in c) subjects with history or clinical evidence of genetic or acquired prothrombotic conditions or infections. The management of venous infarct is similar to that of CVT in general, but special attention is required concerning the treatment of intracranial hypertension and seizures.

Our understanding of the pathogenesis of venous infarcts is incomplete and requires further investigation in animal models of CVT or in studies using serial MRI examinations.

References

[1] Stam J. Thrombosis of the cerebral veins and sinuses. *N. Engl. J. Med.* 2005;352:1791-1798.

[2] Bousser MG, Ferro JM. Cerebral venous thrombosis: an update. *Lancet Neurol.* 2007; 6:162-170.

[3] Otero Palleiro MM, Barbagelata López C. Etiologic subtypes of ischemic stroke in young adults aged 18 to 45 years: a study of a series of 93 patients. *Rev. Clin. Esp.* 2007;207:158-65.

[4] Woitmant F. Ischemic stroke in young adults. *Presse Med.* 2007;36:1s59-64.

[5] Sharshar T, Lamy C, Mas JL. Incidence and causes of strokes associated with pregnancy and puerperium. A study in public hospitals of Ile de France. Stroke in Pregnancy Study Group. *Stroke* 1995;26:930-936.

[6] Lanska DJ, Kryscio RJ. Risk factors for peripartum and postpartum stroke and intracranial venous thrombosis. *Stroke* 2000;31:1274-1282.

[7] Skidmore FM, Williams LS Fradkin, KD, Alonso RJ, Biller J. Presentation, etiology, and outcome of stroke in pregnancy and puerperium. *J. Stroke Cerebrovasc. Dis.* 2001; 10:1-10.

[8] Oppenheim C, Domigo V, Gauvrit JY, Lamy C, Mackowiak-Cordoliani, MA, Pruvo JP, Méder JF. Subarachnoid hemorrhage as the initial presentation of dural sinus thrombosis. *AJNR Am. J. Neuroradiol.* 2005;26:614-617.

[9] Shukla R, Vinod P, Prakash S, Phadke RV, Gupta RK. Subarachnoid haemorrhage as a presentation of cerebral venous sinus thrombosis. *J. Assoc. Physicians India* 2006;54: 42-44.

[10] Sigari F, Blair E, Redleaf M. Headache with unilateral pulsatile tinnitus in woman can signal dural sinus thrombosis. *Ann. Otol. Rhinol. Laryngol.* 2006;115:686-689.

[11] Ferro JM, Lopes MG, Rosas MJ, Fontes J, VENOPORT Investigators. Delay in hospital admission of patients with cerebral vein and dural sinus thrombosis. *Cerebrovasc. Dis.* 2005;19:152-156.

[12] deVeber G, Andrew M, Adams C, Bjornson B, Booth F, Buckley DJ, Camfield CS, David M, Humphreys P, Langevin P, MacDonald EA, Gillett J, Meaney B, Shevell M, Sinclair DB, Yager J and the Canadian Pediatric Ischemic Stroke Study Group: Cerebral sinovenous thrombosis in children. *N. Engl. J. Med.* 2001;345:417-423.

[13] Ferro JM, Canhão P, Bousser MG, Stam J, Barinagarrementeria F, ISCVT Investigators: Cerebral vein and dural sinus thrombosis in elderly patients. *Stroke* 2005; 36:1927-1932.

[14] Ferro JM, Canhão P, Stam J, Bousser MG, Barinagarrementeria F, ISCVT Investigators: Prognosis of cerebral vein and dural sinus thrombosis: results of the International Study on Cerebral Vein and Dural Sinus Thrombosis (ISCVT). *Stroke* 2004;35:664-670.

[15] Bakaç G, Wardlaw JM. Problems in the diagnosis of intracranial venous infarction. *Neuroradiology* 1997;39:566-570.

[16] Lai W, Katirji B. Splenium infarct due to cerebral venous thrombosis. *Arch Neurol.* 2007;64:1540.

[17] Bergui M, Bradac GB, Daniele D. Brain lesions due to cerebral venous thrombosis do not correlate with sinus involvement. *Neuroradiology* 1999;41:419-224.

[18] Röttger C, Trittmacher S, Gerriets T, Blaes F, Kaps M, Stolz E. Reversible MR imaging abnormalities following cerebral venous thrombosis. *AJNR Am. J. Neuroradiol.* 2005;26:607-613.

[19] Schaller B, Graf R. Cerebral venous infarction: the pathophysiological concept. *Cerebrovasc. Dis.* 2004;18:179-188.

[20] Corvol JC, Oppenheim C, Manai R, Logak M, Dormont D, Samson Y, Marsault C, Rancurel G. Diffusion-weighted magnetic resonance imaging in a case of cerebral venous thrombosis. *Stroke* 1998;29:2649-2652.

[21] Lövblad KO, Bassetti C, Schneider J, Guzman R, El-Koussy M, Remonda L, Schroth G. Diffusion-weighted MR in cerebral venous thrombosis. *Cerebrovasc. Dis.* 2001;11: 169-176.

[22] Yoshikawa T, Abe O, Tsuchiya K, Okubo T, Tobe K, Masumoto T, Hayashi N, Mori H, Yamada H, Aoki S, Ohtomo K. Diffusion-weighted magnetic resonance imaging of dural sinus thrombosis. *Neuroradiology* 2002;44:481-488.

[23] Makkat S, Stadnik T, Peeters E, Osteaux M. Pathogenesis of venous stroke: Evaluation with diffusion- and perfusion- weighted MRI. *J. Stroke. Cerebrovascular. Dis.* 2003; 12:132-136.

[24] Gotoh M, Ohmoto T, Kuyama H. Experimental study of venous circulatory disturbance by dural sinus occlusion. *Acta Neurochir* (Wien) 1993;124:120-126.

[25] Rother J, Waggie K, van Bruggen N, de Crespigny AJ, Moseley ME. Experimental cerebral venous thrombosis: Evaluation using magnetic resonance imaging. *J. Cereb. Blood Flow Metab.* 1996;16:1353-1361.

[26] Chu K, Kang DW, Yoon BW, Roh JK. Diffusion-weighted magnetic resonance in cerebral venous thrombosis. *Arch Neurol.* 2001;58:1569-1576.

[27] Keller E, Flacke S, Urbach H, Schild HH. Diffusion- and Perfusion-Weighted Magnetic Resonance Imaging in Deep Cerebral Venous Thrombosis. *Stroke* 1999;30:1144-1146.

[28] Manzione J, Newman GC, Shapiro A, Santo-Ocampo R. Diffusion- and perfusion-weighted MR imaging of dural sinus thrombosis. *AJNR Am. J. Neuroradiol.* 2000; 21:68-73.

[29] Ducreux D, Oppenheim C, Vandamme X, Dormont D, Samson Y, Rancurel G, Cosnard G, Marsault C. Diffusion-weighted imaging patterns of brain damage associated with cerebral venous thrombosis. *AJNR Am. J. Neuroradiol.* 2001;22:261-268.

[30] Doege CA, Tavakolian R, Kerskens CM, Romero BI, Lehmann R, Einhäupl KM, Villringer A. Perfusion and diffusion magnetic resonance imaging in human cerebral venous thrombosis. *J. Neurol.* 2001;248:564-571.

[31] Forbes KP, Pipe JG, Heiserman JE. Evidence for cytotoxic edema in the pathogenesis of cerebral venous infarction. *AJNR Am. J. Neuroradiol.* 2001;22:450-455.

[32] Mullins ME, Grant PE, Wang B, Gonzalez RG, Schaefer PW. Parenchymal abnormalities associated with cerebral venous sinus thrombosis: assessment with diffusion-weighted MR imaging. *AJNR Am. J. Neuroradiol.* 2004;25:1666-1675.

[33] Frerichs KU, Deckert M, Kempski O, Schurer L, Einhäupl K, Baethmann A. Cerebral sinus and venous thrombosis in rats induces long-term deficits in brain function and

morphology – Evidence for a cytotoxic genesis. *J. Cereb. Blood Flow Metab.* 1994;14: 289-300.

[34] Leach JL, Fortuna RB, Jones BV, Gaskill-Shipley MF. Imaging of cerebral venous thrombosis: current techniques, spectrum of findings and diagnostic pitfalls. *RadioGraphs* 2006;26:S19-S43.

[35] Ferro JM, Morgado C, Sousa R, Canhão P. Interobserver agreement in the magnetic resonance location of cerebral vein and dural sinus thrombosis. *Eur. J. Neurol.* 2007; 14:353-356.

[36] Fellner FA, Fellner C, Aichner FT, Mölzer G. Importance of T2*- weighted gradient-echo MRI for diagnosis of cortical vein thrombosis. *Eur. J. Neurol.* 2005;56:235-239.

[37] Idbaih A, Boukobza M, Crassard I, Porcher R; Bousser MG, Chabriat H. MRI of clot in cerebral venous thrombosis: high diagnostic value of susceptibility- weighted images. *Stroke* 2006;37:991-995.

[38] Leach JL, Strub WM, Gaskill-Shipley MF. Cerebral venous thrombus signal intensity and susceptibility effect on gradient recalled-echo MR imaging. *AJNR Am. J. Neuroradiol.* 2007;28:940-945.

[39] Rodallec MH, Krainik A, Feydy A, Hélias A, Colombani J-M, Jullès M-C, Marteau V, Zins M. Cerebral venous thrombosis and multidetector CT angiography: tips and tricks. *RadioGraphics* 2006;26:S5-S18.

[40] Linn J, Erti-Wagner B, Seelos KC, Strupp M, Reiser M, Brückmann H, Bruning R. Diagnostic value of multidetector-row CT angiography in the evaluation of thrombosis in the cerebral venous sinuses. *AJNR Am. J. Neuroradiol.* 2007;28:946-152.

[41] Dentali F, Crowther M, Ageno W. Thrombophilic abnormalities, oral contraceptives, and risk of cerebral vein thrombosis: a meta-analysis. *Blood* 2006;107:2776-2773.

[42] Mohllajee AP, Curtis KM, Martins SL, Peterson HB. Does use of hormonal contraceptives among women with thrombogenic mutations increase their risk of venous thromboembolism? A systematic review. *Contraception* 2006;73:166-178.

[43] Balci K, Utku U, Asil T, Büyükkoyuncu N. Deep cerebral vein thrombosis associated with iron deficiency anaemia in adults. *J. Clin. Neurosci.* 2007;14:181-184.

[44] Cantu C, Alonso E, Jara A, Martinez L, Rios C, Fernandez Mde L, Garcia I, Barinagarrementeria F. Hyperhomocysteinemia, low folate and vitamin B12 concentrations, and metylene tetrahydrofolate reductase mutation in cerebral venous thrombosis. *Stroke* 2004;35:1790-179.

[45] Canhão P, Ferro JM, Lindgren AG, Bousser MG, Stam J, Barinagarrementeria F, ISCVT Investigators. Causes and predictors of death in cerebral venous thrombosis. *Stroke* 2005:36:1720-1725.

[46] Del Sette M, Dinia L, Gandolfo C. Brain-to-brain paradoxical embolism through patent foramen ovale after cerebral vein thrombosis. *Eur. Neurol.* 2007,57:176-177.

[47] Einhäupl KM, Villringer A, Meister W, Mehraein S, Garner C, Pellkofer M, Haberl RL, Pfister HW, Schmiedek P. Heparin treatment in sinus venous thrombosis. *Lancet* 1991;338:597-600.

[48] de Bruijn SF, Stam J, CVST study group: Randomized, placebo-controlled trial of anticoagulant treatment with low-molecular-weight heparin for cerebral sinus thrombosis. *Stroke* 1999;30:484-488.

[49] Nagaraja D, Rao B, Taly AB, Subhash MN. Randomized controlled trial of heparin in puerperal cerebral venous/sinus thrombosis. *Nimhans Journal* 1995;13:111-115.

[50] Stam J, de Bruijn SF, deVeber G. Anticoagulation for cerebral sinus thrombosis. *Cochrane Database Syst. Rev*. 2002, CD002005.

[51] Canhão P, Falcão F, Ferro JM. Thrombolytics for cerebral sinus thrombosis: a systematic review. *Cerebrovasc. Dis*. 2003;15:159-166.

[52] Stam J, Majoie BLM, van Delden OM, van Lienden KP, Reekers JA. Endovascular thrombectomy and thrombolysis for severe cerebral sinus thrombosis. *Stroke* 2008;39: 1487-1490.

[53] Einhäupl K, Bousser MG, de Bruijn SF, Ferro JM, Martinelli I, Masuhr F, Stam J. EFNS guideline on the treatment of cerebral venous and sinus thrombosis. *Eur. J. Neurol*. 2006,13:553-559.

[54] Canhão P, Cortesão A, Cabral M, Ferro JM, Stam J, Bousser M-G, Barinagarrementeria F, for the ISCVT investigators: Are steroids useful to treat cerebral venous thrombosis? *Stroke* 2008;39:105-110.

[55] Stefini R, Latronico N, Cornali C, Rasulo F, Bollati A. Emergent decompressive craniectomy in patients with fixed dilated pupils due to cerebral venous and dural sinus thrombosis: report of three cases. *Neurosurgery* 1999;45:626-629.

[56] Keller E, Pangalu A, Fandino J, Könü D, Yonekawa Y. Decompressive craniectomy in severe cerebral venous and dural sinus thrombosis. *Acta Neurochir* 2005;94(supp):177-183.

[57] Ferro JM, Canhão P, Bousser MG, Stam J, Barinagarrementeria F, ISCVT Investigators. Early seizures in cerebral vein and dural sinus thrombosis. Risk factors, and role of antiepileptics. *Stroke* 2008;39:1152-1158.

[58] Ferro JM, Lopes MG, Rosas MJ, Ferro MA, Fontes J, Cerebral Venous Thrombosis Portugese Collaborative Study Group. Long-term prognosis of cerebral vein and dural sinus thrombosis. Results of the VENOPORT study. *Cerebrovasc. Dis*. 2002;13:272-278.

[59] Horga A, Santamaria E, Quinlez A, de Francisco J, Garcia-Martinez R, Alvarez-Sabin J. Cerebral venous thrombosis associated with repeated use of emergency contraception. *Eur. J. Neurol*. 2007;14:e-5.

[60] Srinivasan K. Cerebral venous and arterial thrombosis in pregnancy and puerperium: a study of 135 patients. *Angiology* 1983;34:731-746.

[61] Lamy C, Hamon JB, Coste J, Mas JL. Ischemic stroke in young women: risk of recurrence during subsequent pregnancies: French Study Group on Stroke in Pregnancy. *Neurology* 2000;55:269-274.

[62] Mehraein S, Ortwein H, Busch M, Weih M, Einhäupl K, Masuhr F. Risk of recurrence of cerebral venous and sinus thrombosis during subsequent pregnancy and puerperium. *J. Neurol. Neurosurg. Psychiatry* 2003;74:814-816.

In: Cerebral Ischemia in Young Adults
Editors: A. Pezzini and A. Padovani

ISBN 978-1-60741-627-2

Chapter 19

Cerebral Autosomal Dominant Arteriopathy with Subcortical Infarcts and Leucoencephalopathy (CADASIL): Clinical and Pathogenetic Aspects of a Form of Genetic Vascular Dementia

Antonio Federico*[*]*, Silvia Bianchi and Maria Teresa Dotti
Department of Neurological, Neurosurgical and Behavioural Sciences,
Medical School, University of Siena, Siena, Italy

Abstract

Cerebral Autosomal Dominant Arteriopathy with Subcortical Infarcts and Leucoencephalopathy (CADASIL) is a clinical disorder due to Notch3 mutation, involving endothelial cells. The main symptoms are migraine, stroke, and leucoencephalopathy. We here report on clinical findings and their pathogenetic aspects.

Introduction

In 1977, Sourander and Walinder described an inherited condition clinically characterized by recurrent strokes and dementia, further defined as multi-infarct dementia [1]. In the same time, Stevens described a second similar family in England [2]. Other families were described, in particular French families in which recurrent strokes were associated with migraine as first symptom: the condition was called CADASIL, whose acronym was for

* Correspondence: Antonio Federico, Viale Bracci, 2, 53100 Siena, Italy. Tel 39.0577.585763-60, fax 39.577.40327. e-mail federico@unisi.it.

Cerebral Autosomal Dominant Arteriopathy with Subcortical Infarcts and Leucoencephalopathy [3]; the gene was linked to *NOTCH3* mutation [4]. Further studies described the mutation pattern in 50 French CADASIL patients, reporting that all mutations were located within the EGF repeats in the extracellular domain of the *NOTCH3* gene, with a strong clustering of the mutations observed within exons 3 and 4 [5]. However, de novo mutations have also been reported [6].

Actually, CADASIL seems to be more frequent than previously considered, with a wide spectrum of clinical presentations and present in all countries.

Clinical Presentation

Hemelsoet *et al.* hypothesized that Friedrich Nietzsche's disease (consisting in migraine, psychiatric disturbances, cognitive decline with dementia and stroke) despite the prevalent opinion that the cause of this illness was neurosyphylis, lacking of support for this diagnosis, was CADASIL [7].

Dichgans *et al.* reported the clinical spectrum of CADASIL from more than 100 cases [8]. The main clinical signs are reported in Table 1. However the clinical presentation is very heterogeneous, with a marked intra-familial variability.

Migraine

Among other neurological symptoms, migraine with aura (MA) is reported in 20% to 40% of CADASIL patients. In 2004 Vahedi *et al.* described the migraine characteristic in a population of 41 CADASIL patients: 18 (44%) of them reported attacks with typical aura [9]. The frequency of attacks and the triggering factors, when reported, were similar to those of migraine in the general population. However, some differences with usual migraine were observed, including the late age at onset (the third decade), the low frequency of migraine without aura present in less than one fourth of the patients, and the high number of patients experiencing atypical aura (56%).

Table I. Clinical presentation of CADASIL

- TIA or stroke in 71 % of cases
- Cognitive deficit in 48% of cases
- Dementia (28%) accompanied by gait disturbances (90%), urinary incontinence (86%) and pseudobulbar palsy (52%)
- History of migraine (38%)(mean age at onset 26 years) classified as migraine with aura in 87%
- Psychiatric disturbances (30%)
- Epileptic seizures (10%)
- 55% of the patients older than age 60 were unable to walk without assistance
- 14% in this age group exhibited no disability at all
- Medial survival times of 64 years (males) and 69 years (females).
- Marked intrafamilial variation

Psychiatric Symptoms

Psychiatric changes as starting symptom in CADASIL have firstly reported by Kumar and Mahr in 1998, as bipolar disorder, and by Lagas and Juvonen in 2002 as schizophrenia [10,11]. Behavioural abnormalities (present in 10-20% of patients) are frequently associated with various degree of cognitive impairment. They have been recently reviewed by Chabriat and Bousser and correlate with ischemic lesions within the basal ganglia or the frontal white matter [12]. More recently, our group found, in a large series of families with exon 10 mutation, the presence of mood disorders as one of the most important clinical findings (personal data).

In a review of the literature, the prevalence of psychiatric disorders in CADASIL patients is reported to range from 20% to 41%. The psychiatric disturbances reported with the highest frequency are mood disturbances (9-41%). Pooling together the studies and considering a total of 454 CADASIL patients reported in the literature, 106 of these were affected by mood disturbances (24%). The majority of the studies however did not use any defined criteria to assess the presence of psychiatric disorders and diagnoses were mainly based on history or review of clinical records [13].

Ocular Abnormalities

Rufa *et al.* described acute unilateral visual loss as the first symptom of CADASIL [14]. This finding has been reported also by other Authors [15], and has been related to haemodynamic changes in the optic nerve [16], related to the presence of arterial vessels with thickened walls, granular osmiophilic material (GOMs) and PAS positive material in tunica media, and positivity with anti-amyloid antibodies, evident at neuropathologic examination [17].

Other Atypical Presentations

They consist in reversible coma with raised intracranial pressure [18] and acute vestibular syndrome [19].

Neuromuscular involvement has been described in several cases, mainly with mitochondrial abnormalities: Finnila *et al.* and De La Pena *et al.* described deficiency of complex I activity, COX negative fibers, and ragged red fibres in muscle of CADASIL patients discussing them as an epiphenomenon or OXPHOS defect linked to the pathophysiology of the disease [20,21]. Malandrini A *et al.* showed paracrystalline mitochoncrial inclusions, asymptomatic cores without mtDNA and RYR1 gene mutations in a large family [22]. Finally, fatigue, thyroid dysfunction, morphological mitochondrial changes in muscle biopsy associated with classical CADASIL symptoms have been described by Dotti *et al.* associated to a frameship deletion: 5 bp deletion from aminoacid 127 to 158, with premature termination of translation (stop codon at aminoacid 159) of Notch3 gene [23].

We also have described peripheral nerve abnormalities investigated by neurophysiological and histopathological techniques, confirming a generalized defect, not only involving brain vessels but also peripheral nerve vessels [24].

Neuroimaging

It is widely accepted that magnetic resonance imaging (MRI) is the most relevant tool for diagnosis and monitoring the cerebral pathology of CADASIL. MRI reveals white matter microangiopathy and signal abnormalities suggestive of ischemic infarts, lacunes, microbleeding, diffuse leucoencephalopathy in the periventricular white matter, the basal ganglia, the thalamus, the internal capsule and the pons.

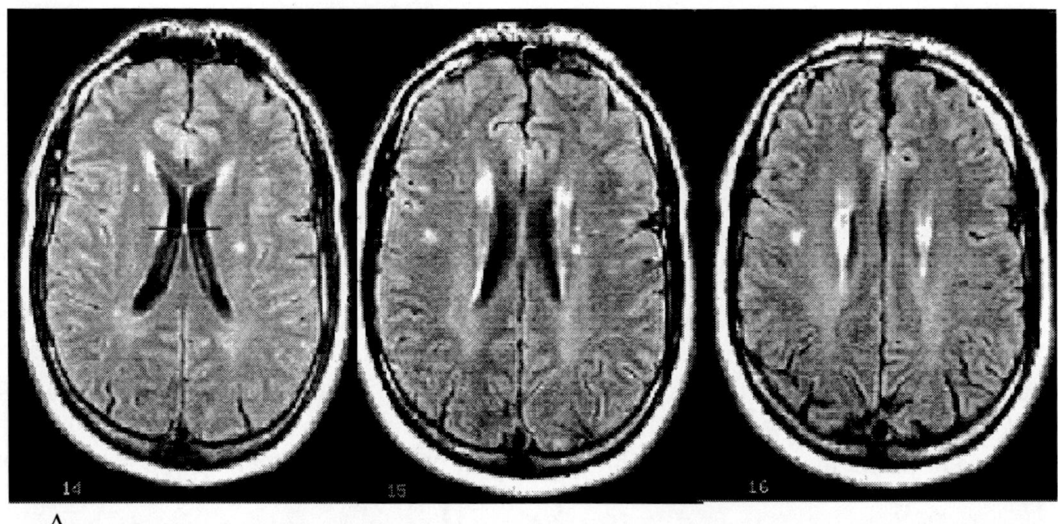

A.

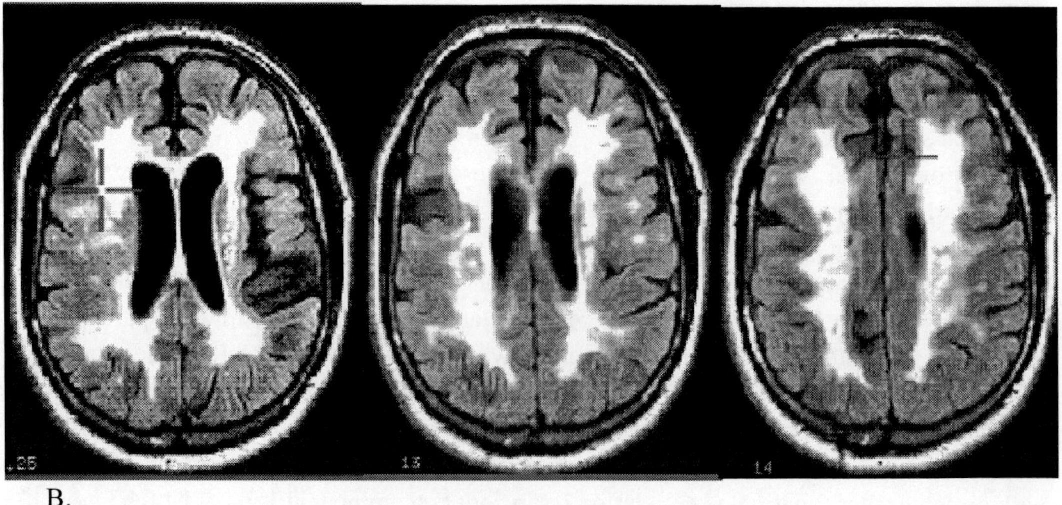

B.

Figure 1. RM of two CADASIL patients, the first at onset (A) and the second in an advanced stage (B).

White matters lesions are most easily detected with FLAIR sequences and abnormalities in the temporal pole appear the most characteristic [25]. Dichgans *et al.* have shown a correlation between MRI lesion volume with clinical characteristics and disability [26]. More recently three-dimensional MRI segmentation has been utilized to investigate the lacunar infarctions volume and its correlation with age, vascular risk factors measuring the individual lacunar volume (ILV) in a large CADASIL cohort, showing that the ILV is not related to the associated lesions or to vascular risk factors, but that and individual predisposition may explain predominating small or predominating large lacunes [27].

Besides white matter changes, important morphological alterations of cortical sulci occur in association with clinical worsening, extension of subcortical tissue damage and progression of global cerebral atrophy [28]. Structural and metabolic brain abnormalities have been shown by Stromillo *et al.* also in preclinical stages, demonstrating that the pathological process occurring in CADASIL leads to damage of white matter and neuocortex before the evidence of clinical symptoms [29]. In an early phase, pathological changes at MRI and MR-spectroscopy seem to be more evident in the frontal brain region (Figure 1).

Cerebral Blood Flow

By dynamic contrast-enhanced MRI, single photon emission computed tomography (SPECT) or positron emission tomography (PET) cerebral blood flow in CADASIL has been evaluated and correlated with cognition and lesion observed from MRI [30-32], confirming reduced CBF in CADASIL, that correlated with disability and cognitive impairment. Transcranial Doppler sonography and proton MR spectroscopy have shown reduced cerebrovascular CO2 reactivity as well as reduced glucose consumption, reduced N-acetylaspartate, choline, creatine compared to control [33,34].

Vascular Risk Factors

Abnormalities in classical vascular risk factors such as hyperglycemia, hypercholesterolemia, trombophilic factors are absent in CADASIL. Hyperomocysteinemia has been reported, but its correlation with the severity of clinical manifestations is not proven. Increased homocysteine levels or abnormalities in homocysteine metabolism may have a role in the pathogenesis of CADASIL [35].

A lower nocturnal blood pressure fall may be partly associated with incidence and/or worsening of deep white matter lesions in CADASIL [36]. This findings was further confirmed by our group [37], showing that BP profile correlated with cognitive decline but not with MRI lesions and that abnormalities in BP profile could be related to impaired central or peripheral mechanism controlling BP variations. This observation prompted us to further investigate for autonomic nervous system dysfunction in CADASIL patients.

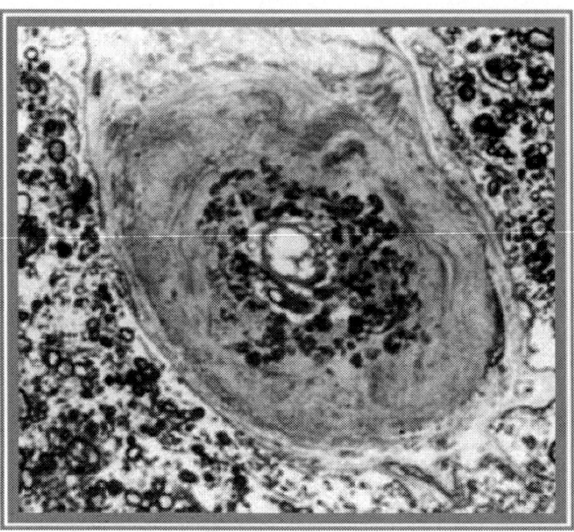

Figure 2. A cerebral artery with the presence of GOMs.

Cardiac autonomic nervous system and risk of arrhythmias was investigated in a cohort of CADASIL patients [38], founding a statistically significant reduction in all frequency domain parameters of heart rate variability associated with a higher low frequency/high frequency ratio for CADASIL patients with respect to normal subjects. These data are consistent with autonomic derangement and suggests that CADASIL patients may be at risk for life-threatening arrhythmias. This could at least in part explain the higher recurrence of sudden unexpected death and should be taken into account in planning therapy. In fact Opherk *et al.* in a study on long term prognosis and cause of death of CADASIL patients, reported that 25% of them have a sudden unexpected death [39]. More recently, increase QT variability has been described, with the hypothesis that this abnormality may explain sudden death occurring in these patients [40].

Angeli *et al.* reported a very high prevalence of right-to-left shunt on transcranial Doppler in an Italian family with CADASIL [41]. Zicari *et al.* investigated this abnormality in 23 patients founding right-lo-left shunt in 47% of patients, with no significant clinical or MRI differences between patients with or without shunt [42]. This may not be a coincidence, but it can be rather related to the role of the Notch receptor family in the development of cardiovascular system.

Vasoreactivity induced by L-arginine, which is the substrate for endothelial nitric oxide synthase, is a parameter of endothelial function and has been shown to be altered in patients with cerebrovascular disease. L-arginine-induced vasoreactivity was significantly increased in patients compared to controls, indicating a pathogenic role of impaired cerebral hemodynamics and endothelial dysfunction in CADASIL. Increase levels of plasma dimethylarginine have been described by Rufa *et al.* [43].

All these data are consistent with the morphological evidence that cerebral vessels are narrowed by intimal thickening and expansion of the extracellular matrix in CADASIL. This is accompanied by disruption and degeneration of smooth muscle cells in vessel wall and the deposition of the GOM. Both intracranial and extracranial arterial vessels may acquire 1-2 μm size extracellular GOM, which still remain to be characterized (Figure 2). In addition to

GOM, the ectodomain of the Notch3 receptors accumulates within the cerebral vasculature, using an antibody against the amino-terminal region of the Notch3 receptor [44].

Molecular Genetic of Notch 3

CADASIL is caused by mutations in the *NOTCH3* gene [4]. Notch3 is one of four mammalian homologous of Drosophila Notch [45]. *NOTCH* genes code for large transmembrane receptors involved into cell fate decision during embryonic development. Unlike other members of the mammalian *NOTCH* gene family such as *NOTCH1* that is ubiquitously expressed in several cell types, *NOTCH3* was found to be predominantly expressed in the vascular smooth muscle cells suggesting the importance of specific Notch3 signalling in these cells [46]. The Notch 3 receptor is proteolytically processed in the trans-Golgi network as it traffics from the endoplasmatic reticulum to the plasma membrane [47]. Proteolytic cleavage results in a large extracellular fragment and a small intracellular fragment that contains the tramsmembrane region (Figure 3A). Interaction of Notch receptor with its ligand leads to cleavage of the transmembrane receptor which migrates into the nucleus and, associated with a transcription factor, activates transcription of primary target genes (Figure 3B) [48].

Current evidence suggests Notch first undergoes constitutive cleavage at a site designed S1 by a furin like convertase to form heterodimeric receptor, which is presented at cell surface [49]. Receptor ligands such as Jagged (jag) and Delta (D) which are also type I transmembrane receptors, expressed on juxtaposed cells, interact with Notch [47]. The interaction results in a second and third cleavage of the receptors S2 and S3 sited by a disintegrin-metalloprotease and a presenilin-dependent gamma-secretase, resulting in the generation of an intracellular demain [48].

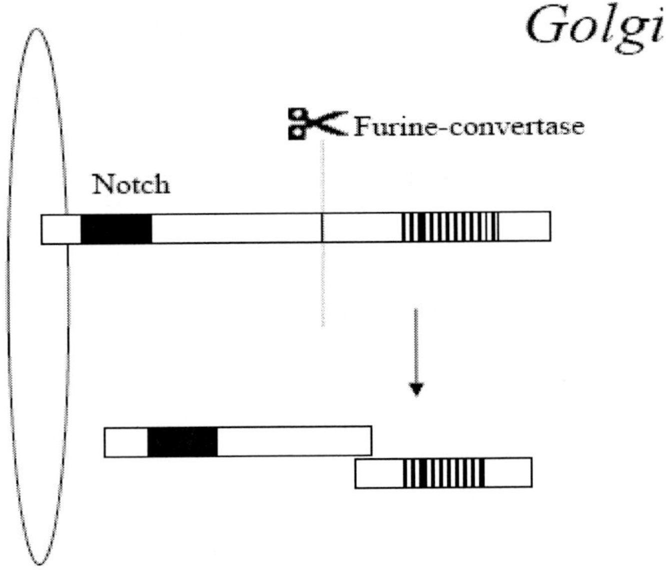

Figure 3A. Maturation of the Notch3 receptor.

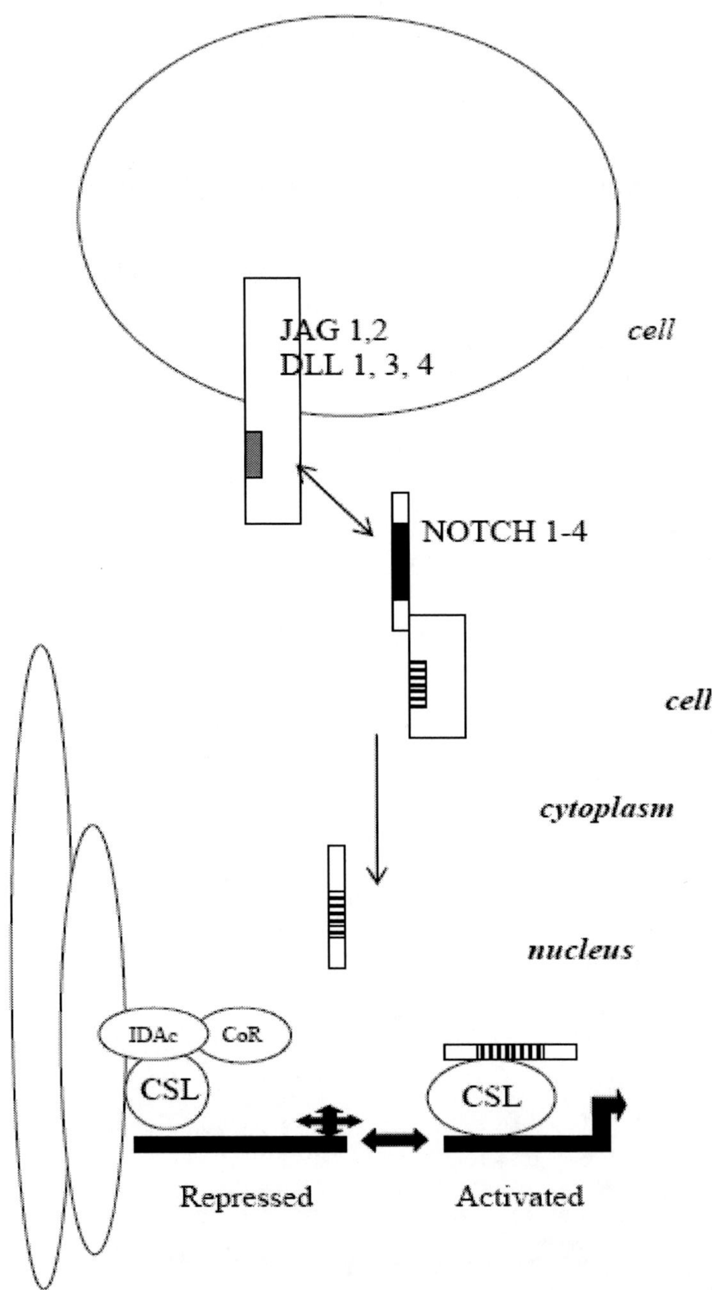

Figure 3B. Simplified overview of Notch signalling in mammals.

Like all Notch receptors, Notch 3 contains a large number of tandemly arranged epidermal growth factor-like (EGF-like) repeat domains, which account for most of the extracellular part of protein. The gene consists of 34 exons, all of them virtually may have pathogenetic mutations (Figure 4).

Numerous mutations have been in the recent years described in this gene, giving to the disease a large genetic heterogeneity (for a list of sequence variants, see *http://chromium.*

liacs.nl/LOVD2/variants.php?select_db=NOTCH3&action=view_unique). Until now, no genotype-phenotype relationship has been described.

All CADASIL-related mutations occur in exons that encodes one of the 34 EGF-repeat domains [5]. To date, about 150 different mutations in Notch3 gene have been reported in CADASIL patients, the 95% being missense point mutations (Figure 5). The remaining consists of six little deletions (five in frame and one frame shift) and two splice site mutation. Many polymorphisms have also been identified in the *NOTCH3* coding sequence. All mutations (except some missense mutations) result in an odd number of cysteine residues, suggesting the occurence of abnormal disulfide bridging and protein misfolding. These would cause changes in receptor activation and abnormal signal transduction. Having said that though, the mechanism by which CADASIL mutations become pathogenic are actually unknown.

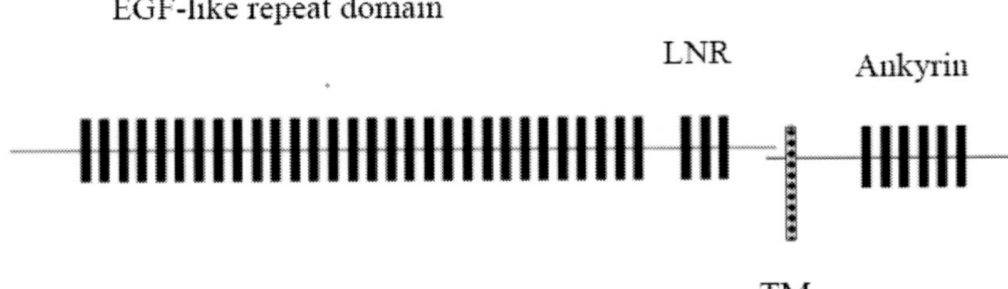

EGF-like repeat domains: extracellular domain containing 34 tandemly arranged EGF-like repeats.
LNR: 3 cysteine-rich Notch/Lin-12 repeats.
TM: transmembrane region.
Ankyrin: intracellular domain containing 6 ankyrin repeats.

Figure 4. Notch3 predicted protein structure.

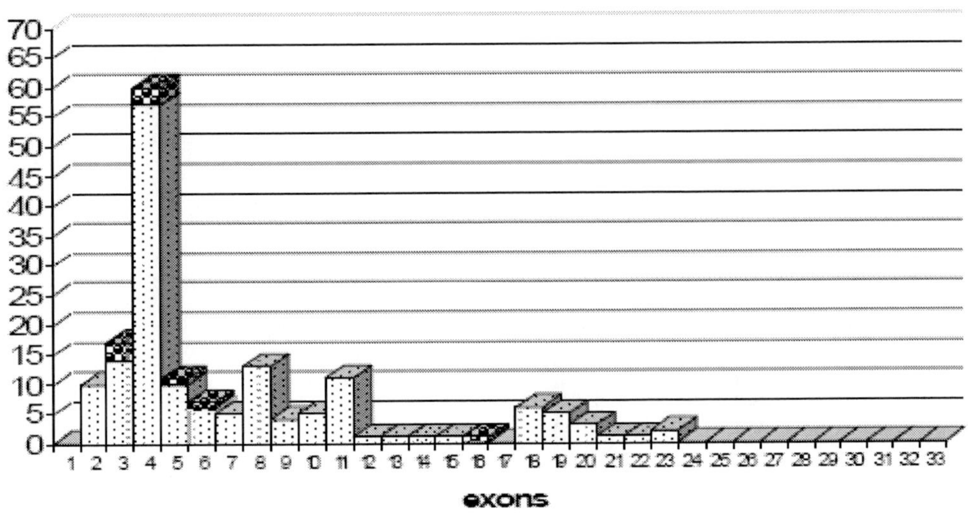

missense mutations;

deletion, splice site mutation.

Figure 5. Mutations identified in the different exons of the Notch3 gene.

Spectrum of Mutations in CADASIL

The low sensitivity of skin biopsy for diagnosis of CADASIL, reported by Markus *et al* [50] and also in our experience give to the molecular genetic approach the diagnostic key of this disorder. However, the length of the gene (34 exons) is one of limitation for a complete gene sequencing for its time and money cost. Since the article of Joutel *et al.* [5] and more recently of Markus *et al.* [50] it has been reported that most mutations were located in exon 4, followed by exon 3, 5 and 6, and 8, 18 and 22, based on experience on 48 index patients. Lesnik Oberstein reported his experience in Dutch families, confirming the high exon 4 mutation frequency, but the second highest frequency of mutations has been found in exon 11, and then exons 5, 6 and 19, suggesting a variation in mutational spectrum between CADASIL populations [51]. Similar geographic variations have been described also in Italy, with an higher frequency of exon 3 and 4 mutations in the north, of exons 4 and 11 in the centre and of 8 in the south (Figure 6) [52].

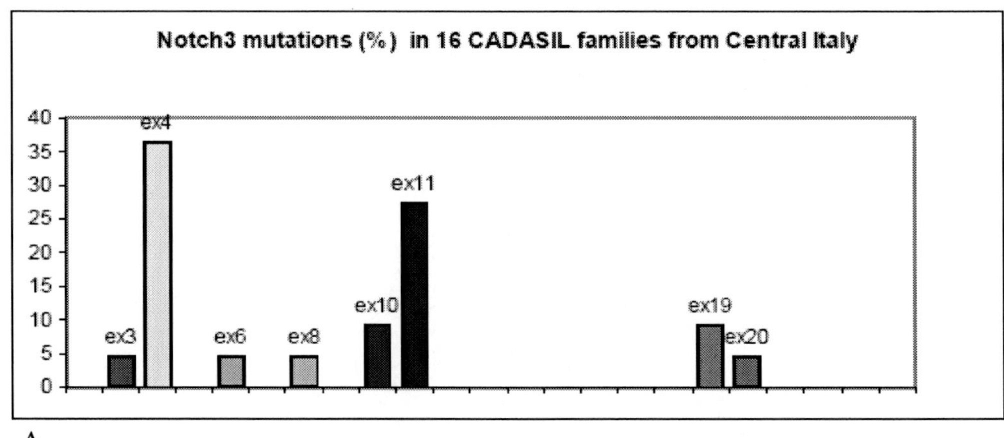

A.

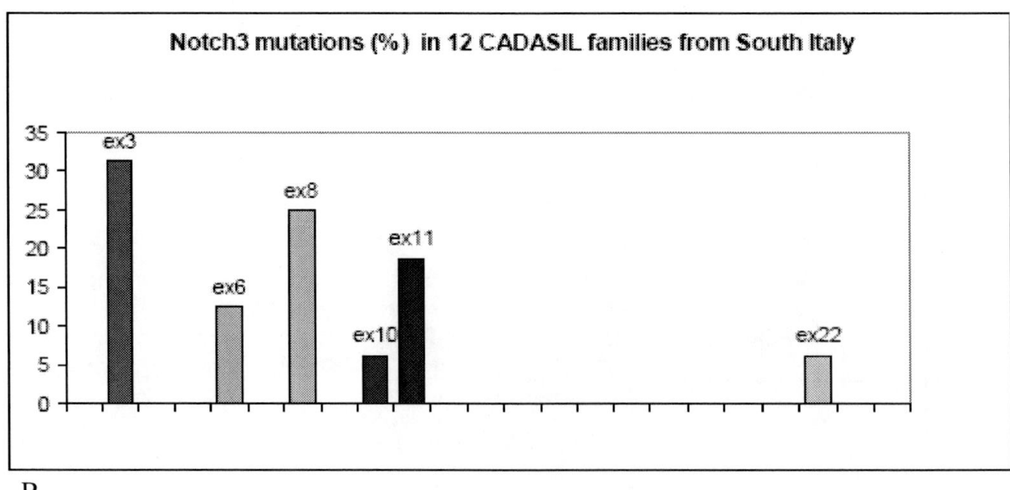

B.

Figure 6. Different mutation in families deriving from Centre (A) and South Italy (B).

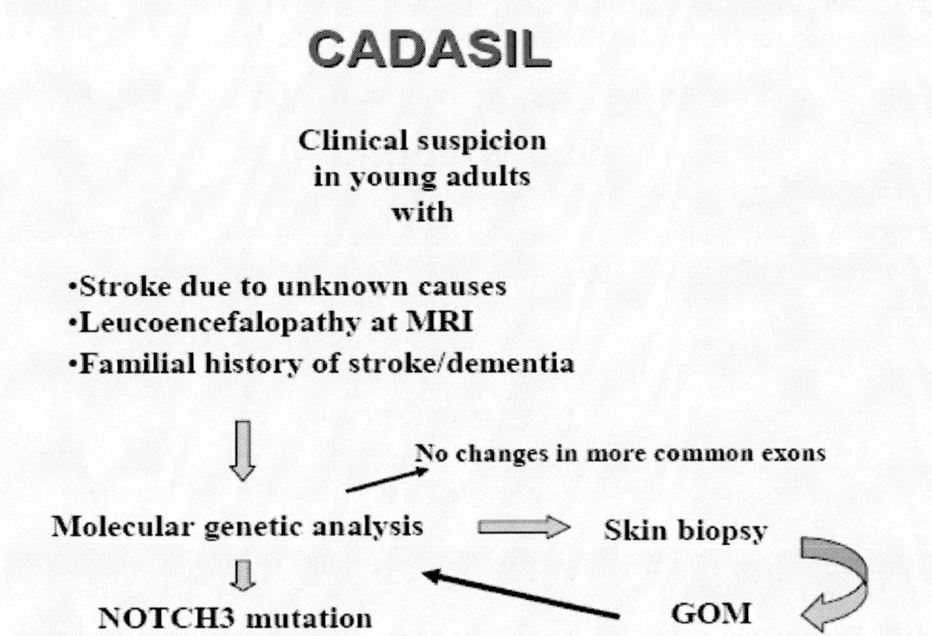

Figure 7. Algorithm for CADASIL diagnosis.

CADASIL Diagnosis

Clinical diagnosis of CADASIL is based on the familiarity, symptoms and neuroimaging aspect of leucoencephalopathy. The diagnosis is confirmed by the evidence in skin, muscle or other biopsies of GOMs and by molecular genetic analysis of *NOTCH3* gene.

A diagnostic flow chart is reported in Figure 7. Diagnostic value of GOMs for CADASIL diagnosis has been recently analyzed in an article [53], discussing the specificity and the sensitivity of the analysis. We have also detected regional differences in the mutational analysis in relationship to the area of origin of the family (Figure 6) [52]. This finding is of great help in the economy and strategy of the planning of molecular analysis of a large gene as *NOTCH3* gene.

Treatment

Recent efforts have been dedicated to investigate the effects of cholinesterase inhibitors drugs in CADASIL. Dichgans *et al.* in a collaborative study in 168 patients reported that Donepezil had no effect on the primary endpoint, the V-ADAS-cog score in CADASIL patients with cognitive impairment [54]. Improvements were noted on several measures of executive function, but the clinical relevance of these findings is not clear.

Short term treatment with atorvastatin resulted in no significant improvement of hemodynamic parameters [55].

The recent data on L-arginine [56,43] and on the role of the glycosilation in the normal functioning of the Notch patway [57] suggest new therapeutical approachs.

Acknowledgments

Research in part supported by a grant from Regione Toscana to AF, Fondazione Monte dei Paschi di Siena to AF e MTD e from Ministery of Research and University (PRIN) to MTD.

References

[1] Sourander P and Walinder J. Hereditary multi-infarct dementia. *Acta Neuropathol.* 1977; 39: 247-54
[2] Stevens DL, Hewlett RH, Browel B. Chronic familial vascular encephalopathy. *Lancet* 1977; 1: 1364-5
[3] Chabriat H, Vahedi K, Iba-Zizen MT, Joutel A, Nibbio A, Nagy TG, et al. Clinical spectrum of Cadasil: a study of seven families. *Lancet* 1995; 346: 934-49
[4] Joutel A, Corpechot C, Ducros A, Vahedi K, Chabriat H, Mouton P et al. Notch 3 mutations in CADASIL, a hereditary adult onset condition causing stroke and dementia. *Nature* 1996; 383: 707-710
[5] Joutel A, Vahedi K, Corpechot C, Troesch A, Chabriat H, Vayssiere C et al. Strong clustering and stereotyped nature of Notch 3 mutations in CADASIL patients. *Lancet* 1997; 350: 1511-5
[6] Joutel A, Dodick DD, Parisi JE, Cecillon M, Tournier-Lasserve E, Bousser MG. De novo mutation in the Notch 3 gene causing CADASIL. Ann Neurol. 2000; 3: 388-91
[7] Hemelsoet D, Hemelsoet K, Devreese D. The neurological illness of Friedrich Nietzsche. *Acta Neurol. Belg.* 2008; 108: 9-16
[8] Dichgans M, Mayer M, Uttner I, Brüning R, Müller-Höcker J, Rungger G, Ebke M, Klockgether T, Gasser T. The phenotypic spectrum of CADASIL: clinical findings in 102 cases. *Ann. Neurol.* 1998;44:731-9
[9] Vahedi K, Chabriat H, Levy C, Joutel A, Tournier-Lasserve E, Bousser MG. Migraine with aura and brain magnetic resonance imaging abnormalities in patients with CADASIL. *Arch Neurol.* 2004;61:1237-40
[10] Kumar SK and Mahr G. CADASIL presenting as bipolar disorder. *Psychosomatics* 1997; 38:393-8
[11] Lagas PA and Juvonen V. Schizophrenia in a patient with cerebral autosomal dominant arteriopathy with subcortical infarcts and leucoencephalopathy (CADASIL). *Nord. J. Psychiat.* 2001, 55: 41-42
[12] Chabriat H and Bousser MG. Neuropsychiatric manifestations in CADASIL. *Dialogues Clin. Neurosci.* 2007; 9: 199-208

[13] Valenti R, Poggesi A, Pescini F, Inzitari D, Pantoni L. Psychiatric disturbances in CADASIL: a brief review. *Acta Neurol. Scand.* 2008;118:291-5

[14] Rufa A, De Stefano N, Dotti MT, Bianchi S, Sicurelli F, Stromillo ML, D'Aniello B, Federico A. Acute unilateral visual loss as the first symptom of cerebral autosomal dominant arteriopathy with subcortical infarcts and leukoencephalopathy. *Arch Neurol.* 2004; 61:577-80

[15] Parisi V, Pierelli F, Fattapposta F, Bianco F, Parisi L, Restuccia R, Malandrini A, Ferrari M, Carrera P. Early visual function impairment in CADASIL. *Neurology* 2003; 60:2008-10

[16] Rufa A, Dotti MT, Frezzotti P, De Stefano N, Caporossi A, Federico A. Hemodynamic evaluation of the optic nerve head in cerebral autosomal dominant arteriopathy with subcortical infarcts and leukoencephalopathy. *Arch Neurol.* 2004;61:1230-3

[17] Rufa A, Malandrini A, Dotti MT, Berti G, Salvadori C, Federico A. Typical pathological changes of CADASIL in the optic nerve. *Neurol. Sci.* 2005;26:271-4

[18] Feuerhake F, Volk B, Ostertag CB, Jungling FD, Kassubek J, Orszagh M, Dichgans M. Reversible coma with raised intracranial pressure: an unusual clinical manifestation of CADASIL. *Acta Neuropathol.* 2002;103:188-92

[19] Rufa A, Cerase A, Monti L, Battisti C, Forte F, Federico A, Dotti MT. Acute vestibular syndrome in a patient with cerebral autosomal dominant leukoencephalopathy with subcortical infarcts and leukoencephalopathy (CADASIL). *J. Neurol. Sci.* 2008;271: 211-3

[20] Finnilä S, Tuisku S, Herva R, Majamaa K. A novel mitochondrial DNA mutation and a mutation in the Notch3 gene in a patient with myopathy and CADASIL. *J. Mol. Med.* 2001;79:641-7

[21] de la Peña P, Bornstein B, del Hoyo P, Fernández-Moreno MA, Martín MA, Campos Y, Gómez-Escalonilla C, Molina JA, Cabello A, Arenas J, Garesse R. Mitochondrial dysfunction associated with a mutation in the Notch3 gene in a CADASIL family. *Neurology* 2001;57:1235-8

[22] Malandrini A, Albani F, Palmeri S, Fattapposta F, Gambelli S, Berti G, Bracco A, Tammaro A, Calzavara S, Villanova M, Ferrari M, Rossi A, Carrera P. Asymptomatic cores and paracrystalline mitochondrial inclusions in CADASIL. *Neurology* 2002;59: 617-20

[23] Dotti MT, De Stefano N, Bianchi S, Malandrini A, Battisti C, Cardaioli E, Federico A. A novel NOTCH3 frameshift deletion and mitochondrial abnormalities in a patient with CADASIL. *Neurol.* 2004;61:942-5

[24] Sicurelli F, Dotti MT, De Stefano N, Malandrini A, Mondelli M, Bianchi S, Federico A. Peripheral neuropathy in CADASIL. *J. Neurol.* 2005;252:1206-9

[25] O'Sullivan M, Jarosz JM, Martin RJ, Deasy N, Powel JF, Markus HS. MRI hyperintensities of the temporal lobe and external capsule in patients with CADASIL. *Neurology* 56: 628-34, 2001

[26] Dichgans M, Filippi M, Brüning R, Iannucci G, Berchtenbreiter C, Minicucci L, Uttner I, Crispin A, Ludwig H, Gasser T, Yousry TA. Quantitative MRI in CADASIL correlation with disability and cognitive performances. *Neurology* 1999; 52: 1361-7

[27] Hervè D, Godin O, Dufouil C, Viswanathan A, Jouvent E, Pachai C, Guichard JP, Bousser MG, Dichgans M, Chabriat H. Three dimensional MRI analysis of individual volume of lacunae in CADASIL. *Stroke* 2008 (Epub ahead of print)

[28] Jouvent E, Mangin JF, Porcher R, Viswanathan A, O'Sullivan M, Guichard JP, Dichgans M, Bousser MG, Chabriat H. Cortical changes in cerebral small vessel diseases: a 3D MRI study of cortical morphology in CADASIL. *Brain* 2008; 131: 2201-08

[29] Stromillo ML, Dotti MT, Battaglini M, Mortilla M, Bianchi S, Plewnia K, Pantoni L, Inzitari D, Federico A, De Stefano N. Structural and metabolic brain abnormalities in preclinical CADASIL. *J. Neurol. Neurosurg. Psychiat.* 2008 (Epub ahead of print)

[30] Iannucci G, Dichgans M, Rovaris M, Brüning R, Gasser T, Giacomotti L, Yousry TA, Filippi M. Correlations between clinical findings and magnetization transfer imaging metrics of tissue damage in individuals with cerebral autosomal dominant arteriopathy with subcortical infarcts and leukoencephalopathy. *Stroke* 2001;32:643-8

[31] Bruening R, Dichgans M, Berchtenbreiter C, Yousry T, Seelos KC, Wu RH, Mayer M, Brix G, Reiser M. Cerebral autosomal dominant arteriopathy with subcortical infarcts and leukoencephalopathy: decrease in regional cerebral blood volume in hyperintense subcortical lesions inversely correlates with disability and cognitive performance. AJNR *Am. J. Neuroradiol.* 2001;22:1268-74

[32] Mellies JK, Bäumer T, Müller JA, Tournier-Lasserve E, Chabriat H, Knobloch O, Hackelöer HJ, Goebel HH, Wetzig L, Haller P. SPECT study of a German CADASIL family: a phenotype with migraine and progressive dementia only. *Neurology* 1998;50: 1715-21

[33] Pfefferkorm T, Struckrad-Barre SV, Herzog J, Gasser T, Hamann GF, Dichgans M. Reduced cerebrovascular CO2 reactivity in CADASIL. A transcranial Doppler sonography study. *Stroke* 2001: 32: 17-21

[34] Auer DP, Schirmer T, Heidenreich JO, Herzog J, Putz B, Dichgans M. Altered white and grey matter metabolism in CADASIL. A proton MR spectroscopy and 1H-MRSI study. *Neurology* 2001; 56: 635-42

[35] Flemming KD, Nguyen TT, Abu-Lebdeh HS, Parisi JE, Wiebers DO, Sicks JD, O'Fallon WM, Petty GW. Hyperhomocysteinemia in patients with cerebral autosomal dominant arteriopathy with subcortical infarcts and leukoencephalopathy (CADASIL). *Mayo Clin. Proc.* 2001;76:1213-8

[36] Manabe Y, Murakami T, Iwatsuki K, Narai H, Warita H, Hayashi T, Shoji M, Imai Y, Abe K. Nocturnal blood pressure dip in CADASIL. *J. Neurol. Sci.* 2001 Dec 15;193(1): 13-6

[37] Rufa A, Dotti MT, Franchi M, Stromillo ML, Cevenini G, Bianchi S, De Stefano N, Federico A. Systemic blood pressure profile in cerebral autosomal dominant arteriopathy with subcortical infarcts and leukoencephalopathy. *Stroke* 2005;36:2554-8

[38] Rufa A, Guideri F, Acampa M, Cevenini G, Bianchi S, De Stefano N, Stromillo ML, Federico A, Dotti MT Cardiac autonomic nervous system and risk of arrhythmias in cerebral autosomal dominant arteriopathy with subcortical infarcts and leukoencephalopathy (CADASIL). *Stroke* 2007;38:276-80

[39] Opherk C, Peters N, Herzog J, Luedtke R, Dichgans M. Long-term prognosis and causes of death in CADASIL: a retrospective study in 411 patients. *Brain* 2004;127: 2533-9

[40] Piccirillo G, Magrì D, Mitra M, Rufa A, Zicari E, Stromillo ML, De Stefano N, Dotti MT. Increased QT variability in cerebral autosomal dominant arteriopathy with subcorticinfarcts and leukoencephalopathy. *Eur. J. Neurol.* 2008;15:1216-21

[41] Angeli S, Carrera P, Del Sette M, Assini A, Grandis M, Biancolini D, Ferrari M, Gandolfo C. Very high prevalence of right-to-left shunt on transcranial Doppler in an Italian family with cerebral autosomal dominant angiopathy with subcortical infarcts and leukoencephalopathy. *Eur. Neurol.* 2001;46:198-201

[42] Zicari E, Tassi R, Stromillo ML, Pellegrini M, Bianchi S, Cevenini G, Gistri M, De Stefano N, Federico A, Dotti MT. Right-to-left shunt in CADASIL patients: prevalence and correlation with clinical and MRI findings. *Stroke* 2008;39:2155-7

[43] Rufa A, Blardi P, De Lalla A, Cevenini G, De Stefano N, Zicari E, Auteri A, Federico A, Dotti MT. Plasma Levels of Asymmetric Dimethylarginine in Cerebral Autosomal Dominant Arteriopathy with Subcortical Infarct and Leukoencephalopathy. *Cerebrovasc. Dis.* 2008;26:636-640

[44] Joutel A, Andreux F, Gaulis S, Domenga V, Cecillon M, Battail N, et al. The ectodomain of the Notch3 receptor accumulates within the cerebrovasculature of CADASIL patients. *J. Clin. Invest.* 2000; 105: 597-605

[45] Artavanis-Tsakonas S, Rand MD, Lake RJ. Notch signaling: cell fate control and signal integration in development. *Science* 1999;284:770-6

[46] Domenga V, Fardoux P, Lacombe P, Monet M, Maciazek J, Krebs LT, Klonjkowski B, Berrou E, Mericskay M, Li Z, Tournier-Lasserve E, Gridley T, Joutel A. Notch3 is required for arterial identity and maturation of vascular smooth muscle cells. *Genes. Dev.* 2004;18:2730-5

[47] Weinmaster G. The ins and outs of notch signaling. *Mol. Cell Neurosci.* 1997;9:91-102

[48] Kopan R. Notch: a membrane-bound transcription factor. *J. Cell Sci.* 2002;115:1095-7

[49] Logeat F, Bessia C, Brou C, LeBail O, Jarriault S, Seidah NG, Israël A. The Notch1 receptor is cleaved constitutively by a furin-like convertase. *Proc. Natl. Acad. Sci. USA* 1998;95:8108-12

[50] Markus HS, Martin RJ, Simpson MA, Dong YB, Ali N, Crosby AH, Powell JF . Diagnostic strategies in CADASIL. *Neurology* 2002;59:1134-8

[51] Lesnik Oberstein SAJ. Diagnostic strategies in CADASIL. *Neurology* 2003;60:2019

[52] Dotti MT, Federico A, Mazzei R, Bianchi S, Scali O, Conforti FL, Sprovieri T, Guidetti D, Aguglia U, Consoli D, Pantoni L, Sarti C, Inzitari D, Quattrone A. The spectrum of Notch3 mutations in 28 Italian CADASIL families. *J. Neurol. Neurosurg. Psychiatry* 2005; 76:736-8

[53] Malandrini A, Gaudiano C, Gambelli S, Berti G, Serni G, Bianchi S, Federico A, Dotti MT. Diagnostic value of ultrastructural skin biopsy studies in CADASIL. *Neurology* 2007; 68:1430-2

[54] Dichgans M, Markus HS, Salloway S, Verkkoniemi A, Moline M, Wang Q, Posner H, Chabriat HS. Donepezil in patients with subcortical vascular cognitive impairment: a randomised double-blind trial in CADASIL. *Lancet Neurol.* 2008;7:310-8

[55] Peters N, Freilinger T, Opherk C, Pfefferkorn T, Dichgans M. Effects of short term atorvastatin treatment on cerebral hemodynamics in CADASIL. *J. Neurol. Sci.* 2007; 260:100-5

[56] Peters N, Freilinger T, Opherk C, Pfefferkorn T, Dichgans M. Enhanced L-arginine-induced vasoreactivity suggests endothelial dysfunction in CADASIL. *J. Neurol.* 2008 Jun 13. [Epub ahead of print]

[57] Rampal R, Luther KB, Haltiwanger RS. Notch signaling in normal and disease states: possible therapies related to glycosylation. *Curr. Mol. Med.* 2007;7:427-45

In: Cerebral Ischemia in Young Adults
Editors: A. Pezzini and A. Padovani
ISBN 978-1-60741-627-2

Chapter 20

Fabry Disease and Stroke

Christoph Lichy* and Pilar Peredo**
*Department of Neurology, University of Heidelberg, Heidelberg, Germany
**Laboratory of Genetics and Inborn Errors of Metabolism, Institute of Nutrition and Food Technology, Universidad de Chile, Santiago de Chile, Chile

Abstract

Fabry disease is a X-chromosomal inherited storage disease. It affects male and female individuals and finally results into multiorganic failure. A lack of activity of the enzyme alpha-galactosidase A causes widespread lysosomal accumulation of sphingolipids, especially of globotriaosylceramid (Gb3). Beside a high morbidity and mortality due to renal and cardiac failure, classical Fabry disease is characterized by harmless but pathognomonic skin (angiokeratoma) and cornea lesions (cornea verticillata). In the peripheral nervous system, a small fiber neuropathy with typical painful acroparesthesias and hypohydrosis predominates.

Central nervous system involvement in Fabry disease has been recognized for a long time. Cerebrovascular events in Fabry patients commonly occur before the age of 50 and a premature cerebral white matter disease is found in a majority of affected male and female adults. Ischemic events involve mainly the vertebrobasilar territory suggesting an important role of dolichoectatic basilar vessels found in many Fabry patients. Additionally, Fabry patients may suffer from stroke due to secondary mechanisms like cardiac embolism following heart failure or premature atherosclerosis induced by renal hypertension. Magnetic resonance imaging (MRI) depicting premature white matter disease, vertebrobasilar dolichoectasia, and/or pulvinar T1 hyperintensities may lead to the suspicion of an underlying Fabry disease in younger stroke patients.

Recognizing oligosymptomatic Fabry patients in a juvenile stroke population is relevant not only for appropriate genetic counselling. With enzyme replacement therapy (ERT), a specific treatment option for Fabry disease is available. However, it is unclear

* Correspondence: Christoph Lichy, Im Neuenheimer Feld 400, D-69120 Heidelberg, Germany. e-mail: christoph_lichy@med.uni-heidelberg.de.

whether this expensive treatment is able to reverse late stage tissue damage to a clinically meaningful degree. Oral chaperon therapy may become an alternative for some affected subjects in the near future.

Up to date, the true prevalence of Fabry disease in juvenile stroke populations is largely unknown. In 2005, a multicentric observational study reported on an unexpectedly high frequency of Fabry defining gene mutations in patients younger than 55 years with cryptogenic stroke (4.9% of men and 2.4% of females). Remarkably, quiet few of those patients had clinical stigmata typical for Fabry disease. A large-scale Pan-European study currently is underway to investigate the disease's prevalence in stroke of any etiology at age < 55 years.

Introduction

Among the large group of hereditary lysosomal storage disorders, traditionally only the X-linked Fabry disease has been recognized to bear a considerable cerebrovascular morbidity [1,2]. This either is attributable to a cerebral white matter disease found in most Fabry patients or to territorial infarcts predominantly involving the vertebrobasilar system. In Fabry patients, stroke usually occurs within the third to fifth decade of life. Therefore, it should be considered in the differential diagnosis of juvenile stroke, especially but not exclusively in male patients.

In the past, however, the enthusiasm to take Fabry disease into account as a potential etiology was rather low, as was the awareness of the disease's clinical characteristics. This probably reflected the conception of the disease as an extremely rare one. More recent data, mainly derived from one large observational study in juvenile cryptogenic strokes, suggested a much higher prevalence of Fabry disease in this population than would have been expected. Remarkably, none of these patients (including a considerable number of females) with a mean age of almost 40 years was known to have Fabry disease before [3]. Together with specific treatment options now being available [4-6], this finding raises the question if in the future an increased awareness or even standard testing for Fabry disease is needed in the diagnostic work up of juvenile stroke.

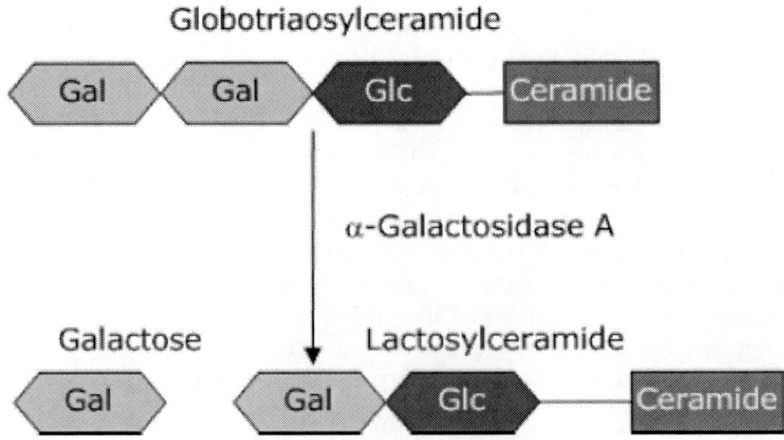

Figure 1. Metabolic pathway of degradation of globotriasylceramide by alpha-galactosidase A.

General Pathophysiology, Epidemiology and Clinical Characteristics of Fabry Disease

Fabry disease is an X-linked hereditary error of glycosphingolipid catabolism resulting from deficiency of a lysosomal hydroxylase, alpha-galactosidase A (AGLA) [7]. Up to now, over 350 mostly private mutations of the AGLA gene located on Xq21.1 have been described, thus making genetic testing quiet a challenge in Fabry disease [8-11]. The predominantly lysosomal storage of the glycosphingolipid substrates, globotriaosylceramide (Gb3) and ceramide dihexoside, occurs in almost all human tissues (Figure 1).

Despite being an X-linked disorder, it is well established that also about 70% of females develop clinically relevant symptoms, even in the presence of low-normal AGLA serum levels. This phenomenon classically is explained by the "Lyon-hypothesis", i.e. arbitrary inactivation of one of both female X chromosomes in different tissues.

The prevalence of Fabry disease in Caucasian populations has been estimated to be about 2 in 100.000 males [12]. However, more recently much higher prevalence rates have been reported. By neonate screening, Spada and collegues in 2006 described a deficiency of AGLA and corresponding gene mutations in 12 (0.03%) out or approximately 37.000 Italian male babies [13]. Further, in certain patient populations, Fabry patients may be a relevant subgroup. For example, in male Japanese patients with final stage renal disease, 2% were found to suffer from Fabry disease [14].

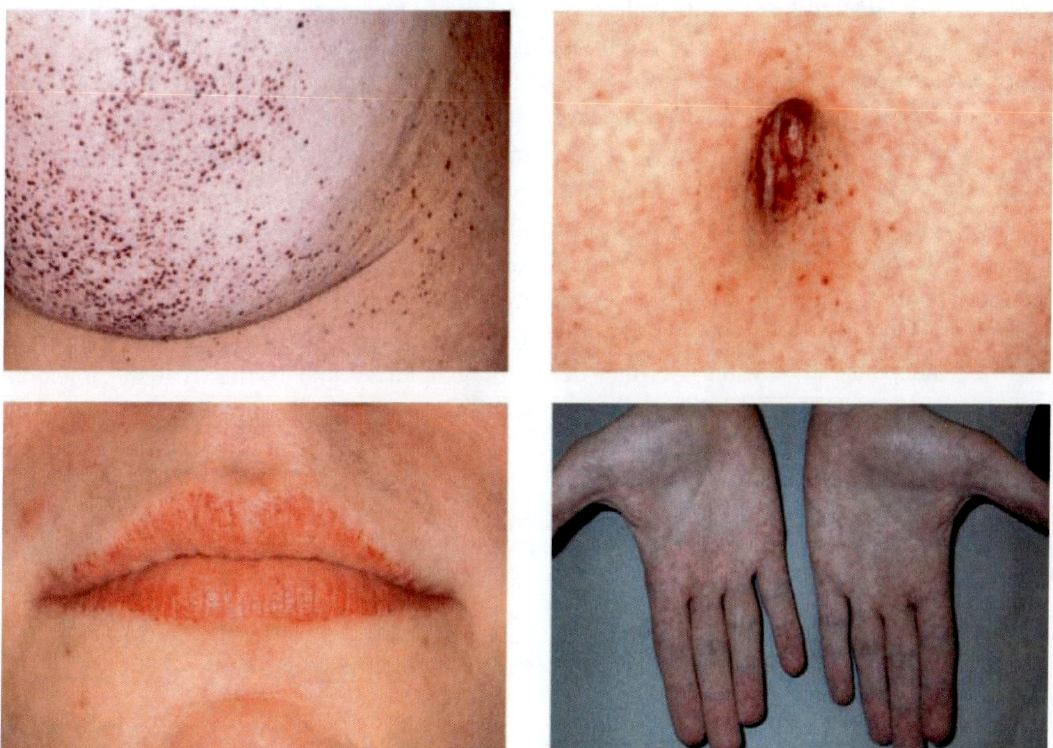

Figure 2. Angioceratoma in Fabry disease.

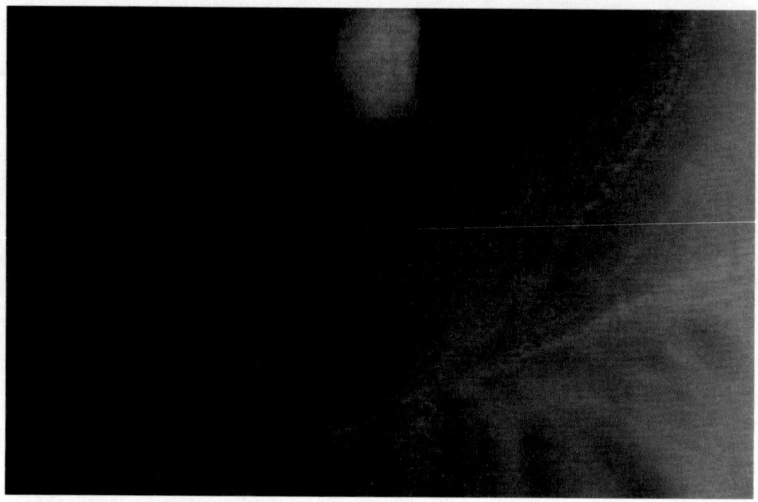

Figure 3. Cornea verticillata in Fabry disease.

The accumulation of Gb3 results in multiple organ involvement and accordingly in a broad variety of clinical manifestations [7,15]. Heterozygous females may either be asymptomatic or exhibit fewer signs and symptoms of disease, although there is an increasing number of reports describing females with symptoms similar to those of affected males [16]. Individuals suffering from classical Fabry disease usually become symptomatic during the second life decade and have a modestly decreased life expectancy, mainly attributable to the complications of renal failure, cardiomyopathy, and major cerebrovascular events. Renal failure evolves over about three to four life decades from asymptomatic proteinuria to final renal insufficiency [17]. It is the leading cause of death in patients with Fabry disease [18]. A peripheral neuropathy predominantly affects small unmyelinated fibers and leads to severe acrodistal pain crises which severely affect the quality of patients' life [19-21]. They go along with a high psychiatric comorbidity including suicide and opiate addiction [22,23]. Vegetative manifestations as hypohidrosis are another common finding [24]. Other clinical signs and symptoms rarely cause relevant impairment but still are very important for recognizing Fabry patients. These include the typical angioceratoma of the skin first described independently by the German dermatologist Fabry and by his British colleague Anderson in 1898. These small lilac skin lesions often are not very prominent and may easily be overlooked due to their predominantly periumbilical and perigenital localization (Figure 2) [25-27]. The so-called cornea verticillata is a further pathognomonic and early detectable finding on ophthalmologic slit lamp examination. It rarely affects vision to a relevant degree (Figure 3)[28,29].

Stroke in Fabry Disease

The incidence of ischemic stroke has been described to be about 40% in hemizygous males [1]. Of the approximately 1300 Fabry patients registered within one of two web based registries ("Fabry Outcome Survey"; www.fos-tkt5s.com), 12% were reported to have had a stroke (14% of males and 10 % of females). By contrast, reports on cerebral hemorrhage are scarce in Fabry patients. The cerebrovascular manifestations include vertebrobasilar large-vessel ectasia, large vessel occlusive disease, and small vessel disease. Even in individuals free from vascular clinical events, inevitably some degree of white matter disease is seen during later adulthood on MRI. Overall, the cerebral vasculopathy of Fabry disease could be classified into large and small vessel pathologies. Additionally, cardioembolic mechanisms as a consequence of the often present cardiomyopathy need to be considered [30-33].

Pathophysiology

PET investigations suggest a chronic alteration of the nitric oxide pathway in Fabry disease [34]. On the other hand, an increased endothelium-mediated vascular reactivity, has been described. An increased vessel response to acetylcholine with and without N^G-monomethyl-L-arginine (L-NNMA) suggests altered functionality of non-NO endothelium-dependent pathways for vasodilatation. Vessel wall alterations with narrowing of cerebral resistance vessels are likely to comprise cerebral blood flow (CBF) and to contribute to the early and increased incidence of stroke.

There are also clear data of abnormalities of cerebrovascular autoregulation and vasoreactivity [35]. Moore and co-workers investigated, in the course of a randomized double-blind placebo-controlled 6-month ERT trial, the functional blood flow response of the brain, the cerebral vasoactivity and PET in Fabry patients. They demonstrated that Fabry patients had a significantly greater increase in rCBF and that the time for recovery of the cerebral vasculature following acetazolamide was prolonged in Fabry patients as well. ERT was able to reverse the exaggerated cerebrovascular response [34]. Similarly, Hilz and colleagues speculate that both, reduced rCBF and impaired cerebral autoregulation are likely to be involved in the increased risk of stroke in Fabry patients [35].

An increased endothelium-dependent vascular reactivity to acetylcholine in the forearm vascular bed has been described [36]. Interestingly, this seems to be still present after infusion of a competitive inhibitor of arginine which indicates changing of function of the non-nitric oxide pathways. Also based on the high incidence of vertebrobasilar dolichoectasia these data might argue that the vascular dysfunction in Fabry disease is due to increased release of reactive oxygen species what induces increased oxidative stress and peroxynitrite formation potentially resulting in persistent vasodilation [34].

Stroke Subtypes and Typical Manifestations

Strokes and transient ischemic events in Fabry disease seem to have a predominant distribution in the vertebrobasilar circulation. Accordingly, signs and symptoms rising from dysfunction of brain stem and cerebellum like vertigo or dizziness, diplopia, nystagmus, dysarthria, and ataxia are common findings in Fabry stroke patients [3]. There is an increased likelihood for arterial dolichoectasia or elongation and dilation [37]. This most commonly involves the basilar artery but the carotid artery may also be affected [3,38]. Such arterial dilation may induce flow stagnation resulting in an increased risk of artery-to-artery embolization or thrombosis with consecutive cerebrovascular events. The reason for the predilection of the vertebrobasilar system is not clear, as it seems reasonable to presume that the endothelial changes in the scope of Fabry disease should affect the cerebral arteries in a uniform manner. Mitsias and Levine reported in their careful neuropathologic analysis of cerebrovascular complications in 12 hemizygotic and 3 heterozygotic Fabry patients a prevalence of thickened vessels of the circle of Willis with narrowing of the lumina in about one third of the cases, moderate atheroma of the major cerebral vessels or intracellular deposits in arteries and arterioles in about 15%. A massive dilatation of the basilar was seen in 1 case. There are a many reports of Fabry patients demonstrating the marked thickening of the medium- and small-sized arteries as well as the dolichoectasia in the posterior circulation [37,39]. In non-Fabry cases the incidence of dolichoectasia varies between 0.06% and 5.8%. (Figure 4)

Several studies have reported an increased number of lacunar, predominantly periventricular, infarctions, as well as small cortical infarcts [40]. As Fellgiebel and co-workers have demonstrated Fabry patients present more commonly with radiological finding consistent with small-vessel disease either as a cause of symptomatic stroke or as clinically silent lesions [31]. The swollen vascular endothelial cells, often accompanied by endothelial cell proliferation, encroach upon the lumen of involved vessels and might lead to focal increase of intraluminal pressure, dilatation and angiectasis of small cerebral arteries. Grewal described eight Fabry patients with CVE which involved in all cases the deep or penetrating arteries similar to those arteries which cause lacunar strokes [38]. This is in accordance with the study from Rolfs and co-workers as well as Schiffman and Riess where nearly 50% of the Fabry patients with stroke demonstrate periventricular white-matter hyperintensities [3,41].

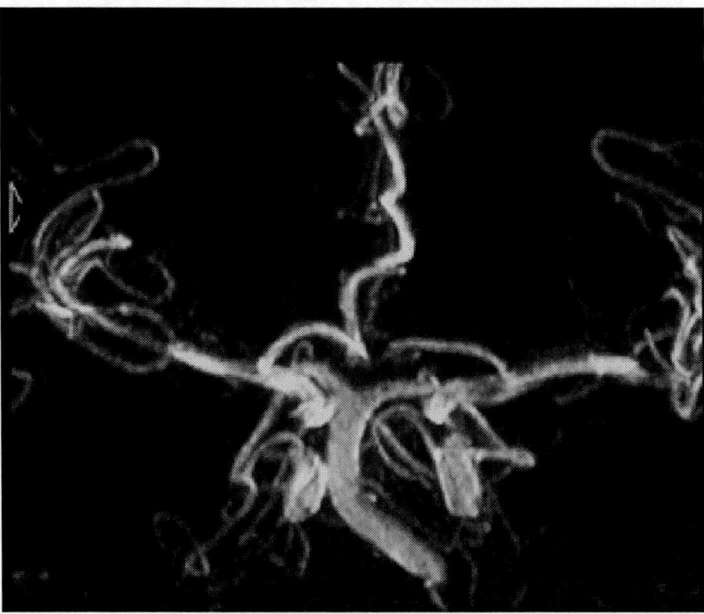

Figure 4. MR angiographic appearance of a dolichoectatic basilar artery in a Fabry patient presenting with cerebellar infarction.

Epidemiology of Stroke in Fabry Patients

In 2005, Rolfs and co-workers reported on a cohort of 721 (432 males and 289 females) unrelated patients 18 to 55 years of age who had had an unexplained acute cerebrovascular event classified as cryptogenic stroke after appropriate work up [3]. Biologically significant mutations within the AGLA gene were found in 28 patients (21 males, 7 females). The mean age of onset of symptomatic cerebrovascular disease was 38.4 ± 13.0 years in the group of the male stroke patients and 40.3 ± 13.1 years in the female group compared to the non-Fabry cohort with a mean age of 47.9 years. The most important result of this study is the unexpected high frequency of Fabry disease in a cohort of stroke patients with cryptogenic stroke aged between 18 and 55 years: the number of newly diagnosed Fabry patients corresponds to 4.9% and 2.4% of the male and female groups of stroke patients, respectively. Remarkably, only a minority of the patients having Fabry defining mutations appeared to have other typical stigmata of the disease as are renal impairment, pain crises, or recognized typical skin lesions. This partly might be an effect of the non-systematic evaluation by physicians who were not familiar with Fabry disease. By contrast to the findings by Rolfs and colleagues, the monocentric Middelheim Fabry Study from Belgium published in 2007 failed to identify Fabry patients in a consecutive series of 103 cryptogenic strokes aged 16 to 60 years [42]. Still, the findings by Rolfs raise the question whether there is a significant number of oligosymptomatic patients who relatively late present with a stroke.

Diagnostics

At present, general genetic testing for Fabry disease even in a juvenile population of stroke patients cannot be recommended without clinical studies. It is important to stress that the presence of some established stroke etiology, as e.g. cardiac embolism with atrial fibrillation (which might be a consequence of a Fabry disease caused cardiomyopathy), does NOT exclude Fabry disease as a relevant differential diagnosis.

Family History

A positive family history (also taking into account female relatives!) for early ischemic events, but also for neuropathic pain crisis, unexplained renal disease or cardiopathy may indicate a monogenetic stroke etiology, including Fabry disease.

Imaging

MRI-imaging might reveal findings suspicious of Fabry disease.

This includes otherwise unexplained, unspecific periventricular white matter disease. Further, the finding of dolichoectatic arteriopathy, predominantly in the vertebrobasilar arteries, is an unspecific but typical finding in Fabry patients.

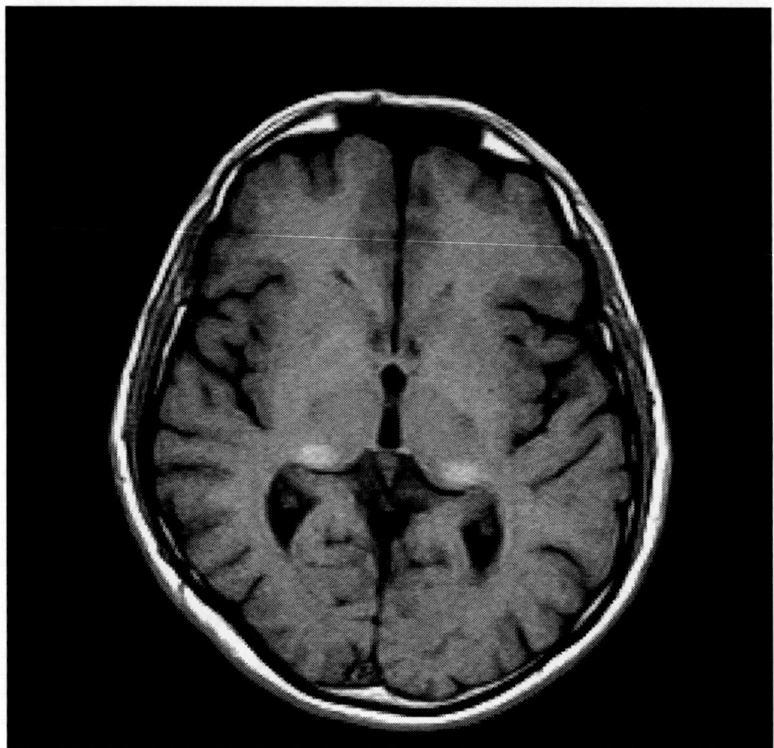

Figure 5. Bilateral pulvinar T1-hyperintensitiy typically seen on cranial MRI in Fabry patients.

A typical bilateral hyperintensity in the pulvinar on T1-weighted MRI seems to be an important but also nonpathognomonic finding in Fabry disease. It is likely to reflect the presence of calcification rather than being of vascular origin [43]. Cerebral hyper-perfusion is also associated with calcifications in the cerebral white matter and in the pulvinar or posterior thalamic regions. In the study from Takanashi and co-workers bilateral T1 shortening in the lateral pulvinar was recognized in at least seven out of 10 patients, all over the age of 30 years, who also had small areas of T2 prolongation in the white matter [44]. In the study from Moore and co-workers overall, 22 patients (about 23%) demonstrated pulvinar hyperintensity on T1-weighted images; the frequency increased with age to over 30% by age 50 years [43]. The group from Burlina and co-workers has analysed 36 patients (16 males, 20 females) and was able to demonstrate the pulvinar sign only in 5 male patients. Seven patients had had at least one stroke (territorial or lacunar). There was no correlation between stroke and the pulvinar sign [45]. Thus, the absence of a pulvinar T1-hyperintensity evidently does not exclude Fabry disease by any means (Figure 5)

Urine Analysis

Increased urine protein seems to be an early and sensitive marker for renal impairment in Fabry patients. This cheap test might be helpful for screening [46].

Clinical Examination

Inspection of the patient's skin including the genital and periumbilical area should not be missed. The Fabry-typical angiokeratoma predominate in these body areas and therefore are easily overlooked. In unclear cases, the diagnosis easily can be made by the dermatologist. It also might be advisable to perform an ophthalmologic investigation in younger stroke patients. Whilst also evaluating other relevant features like e.g. presence of a fundus hypertonicus, an experienced (!) ophthalmologist would not miss the pathognomonic cornea verticillata found in most Fabry patients.

Laboratory Testing

If Fabry disease is considered in a stroke victim, genetic and / or biochemical blood tests can confirm the diagnosis. Testing, as for any hereditary disease, should only be performed after appropriate counselling of patients with respect to the meaning of a potentially positive finding, also for other family members.

In male patients, serum levels of Gb3 can be measured easily and at low cost. In patients found to have abnormal or borderline high levels, genetic testing should follow to identify the specific responsible mutation. In females, however, the much more elaborate sequencing of the alpha-galactosidase A gene a priori is necessary [47].

Treatment

General Treatment of Stroke in Fabry Patients

No evidence based data exist suggesting the most appropriate general therapeutic approach. However, it is common sense to give platelet inhibitors after a first ischemic event for secondary prevention. In the presence of a cardiac source of embolism, oral anticoagulation is recommended as in non-Fabry stroke patients. No reports on a relevantly increased bleeding risk exist.

Specific Treatment of Fabry Disease

The management of Fabry disease warrants a multidisciplinary approach involving neurologists with expertise in stroke medicine and in pain therapy, cardiologists and nephrologists, opthalmologists, experts in genetic counselling, and others. Regular follow-up including echocardiography and tests of renal function is essential for the management of Fabry disease. Inclusion of newly diagnosed Fabry patients into one of the existing observational Fabry data benches is recommended (www.fabryregistry.com; www.fos-tkt5s.com).

Recently, enzyme replacement therapy (ERT) with recombinant alpha-galactosidase A has become available for specific treatment of Fabry disease [48-52]. Positive effects of ERT on renal function and on pain relief have been demonstrated by small randomized controlled trials. At least partly, reversibility of Gb3 tissue accumulation could be demonstrated, too. However, data from placebo-controlled trials on long-term outcome under ERT are lacking. The influence of ERT on primary or secondary cerebrovascular risk also is largely unknown. ERT causes high costs of approximately 200.000 Euro per year and patient. Despite a low rate of relevant side-effects, the need of biweekly intravenous application considerably affects patients' quality of life and requires appropriate logistics.

In the future, oral medication with individual chaperon drugs may become an alternative or additional option. Chaperons enhance the residual functionality of an abnormally folded enzyme. However, this approach is suitable only for a subset of the more than 350 different ALGA gene mutations known to cause Fabry disease [53].

Stroke in Other Storage Disorders

Despite less well known than for Fabry patients, also for patients with Pompe disease an increased cerebrovascular morbidity has been described. Pompe disease is an autosomal recessive disorder caused by a deficiency in the lysosomal acid alpha-glucosidase activity. The clinical manifestation in children is mainly restricted to the muscles due to accumulation of lysosomal glycogen. However, several reports of strokes related to intracranial aneurysms or dilatative arteriopathy in late-onset patients suggest that cerebrovascular events are an underrecognized complication of this disease. As for Fabry disease, ERT is available for Pompe disease.

Perspective

The real role of Fabry disease in the context of juvenile ischemic stroke is likely to be elucidated by the results of the ongoing European SIFAP ("Stroke In young FAbry Patients"; www.sifap.de) trial expected in 2010. SIFAP investigates the prevalence of Fabry disease in a cohort of 5000 well characterised patients aged 18 to 55 years with stroke or TIA of any etiology. Fabry patients identified within this cohort will receive follow up and individual treatment including ERT within the SIFAP II protocol. This hopefully will elucidate the best medical treatment helpful for this disease. In the meanwhile, however, increased awareness of signs and symptoms suggesting Fabry disease in stroke victims is needed. Some findings of a thorough clinical work up as discussed in this article may lead to the diagnosis of an underlying Fabry disease in individual patients with important consequences for both, individual and family health counselling and management.

References

[1] Fellgiebel A, Muller MJ, Ginsberg L. Cns manifestations of fabry's disease. *Lancet Neurol.* 2006;5:791-795

[2] Mehta A, Ginsberg L. Natural history of the cerebrovascular complications of fabry disease. *Acta Paediatr. Suppl.* 2005;94:24-27; discussion 29-10

[3] Rolfs A, Bottcher T, Zschiesche M, Morris P, Winchester B, Bauer P, Walter U, Mix E, Lohr M, Harzer K, Strauss U, Pahnke J, Grossmann A, Benecke R. Prevalence of fabry disease in patients with cryptogenic stroke: A prospective study. *Lancet* 2005; 366:1794-1796

[4] Brady RO, Murray GJ, Moore DF, Schiffmann R. Enzyme replacement therapy in fabry disease. *J. Inherit. Metab. Dis.* 2001;24 Suppl 2:18-24; discussion 11-12

[5] Wanner C. Fabry disease: Clinical outcomes of agalsidase enzyme replacement therapies. *Int. J. Clin. Pract.* 2007;61:1234-1235; author reply 1235

[6] Bodary PF, Shayman JA, Eitzman DT. Alpha-galactosidase a in vascular disease. *Trends Cardiovasc. Med.* 2007;17:129-133

[7] Clarke JT. Narrative review: Fabry disease. *Ann. Intern. Med.* 2007;146:425-433

[8] Eng CM, Resnick-Silverman LA, Niehaus DJ, Astrin KH, Desnick RJ. Nature and frequency of mutations in the alpha-galactosidase a gene that cause fabry disease. *Am. J. Hum. Genet.* 1993;53:1186-1197

[9] Ashley GA, Shabbeer J, Yasuda M, Eng CM, Desnick RJ. Fabry disease: Twenty novel alpha-galactosidase a mutations causing the classical phenotype. *J. Hum. Genet.* 2001; 46:192-196

[10] Ashton-Prolla P, Tong B, Shabbeer J, Astrin KH, Eng CM, Desnick RJ. Fabry disease: Twenty-two novel mutations in the alpha-galactosidase a gene and genotype/phenotype correlations in severely and mildly affected hemizygotes and heterozygotes. *J. Investig. Med.* 2000;48:227-235

[11] Askari H, Kaneski CR, Semino-Mora C, Desai P, Ang A, Kleiner DE, Perlee LT, Quezado M, Spollen LE, Wustman BA, Schiffmann R. Cellular and tissue localization of globotriaosylceramide in fabry disease. *Virchows Arch.* 2007;451:823-834

[12] Masson C, Cisse I, Simon V, Insalaco P, Audran M. Fabry disease: A review. *Joint Bone Spine.* 2004;71:381-383

[13] Spada M, Pagliardini S, Yasuda M, Tukel T, Thiagarajan G, Sakuraba H, Ponzone A, Desnick RJ. High incidence of later-onset fabry disease revealed by newborn screening. *Am. J. Hum. Genet.* 2006;79:31-40

[14] Ichinose M, Nakayama M, Ohashi T, Utsunomiya Y, Kobayashi M, Eto Y. Significance of screening for fabry disease among male dialysis patients. *Clin. Exp. Nephrol.* 2005;9:228-232

[15] Eng CM, Germain DP, Banikazemi M, Warnock DG, Wanner C, Hopkin RJ, Bultas J, Lee P, Sims K, Brodie SE, Pastores GM, Strotmann JM, Wilcox WR. Fabry disease: Guidelines for the evaluation and management of multi-organ system involvement. *Genet. Med.* 2006;8:539-548

[16] Maier EM, Osterrieder S, Whybra C, Ries M, Gal A, Beck M, Roscher AA, Muntau AC. Disease manifestations and x inactivation in heterozygous females with fabry disease. *Acta Paediatr. Suppl.* 2006;95:30-38

[17] Warnock DG, West ML. Diagnosis and management of kidney involvement in fabry disease. *Adv. Chronic. Kidney Dis.* 2006;13:138-147

[18] Raas-Rothschild A, Friedlaender MM, Pizov G, Backenroth R. The kidney in fabry disease. *J. Pediatr.* 2005;146:148

[19] Schiffmann R, Scott LJ. Pathophysiology and assessment of neuropathic pain in fabry disease. *Acta Paediatr. Suppl.* 2002;91:48-52

[20] MacDermot J, MacDermot KD. Neuropathic pain in anderson-fabry disease: Pathology and therapeutic options. *Eur. J. Pharmacol.* 2001;429:121-125

[21] Dutsch M, Marthol H, Stemper B, Brys M, Haendl T, Hilz MJ. Small fiber dysfunction predominates in fabry neuropathy. *J. Clin. Neurophysiol.* 2002;19:575-586

[22] Gold KF, Pastores GM, Botteman MF, Yeh JM, Sweeney S, Aliski W, Pashos CL. Quality of life of patients with fabry disease. *Qual. Life Res.* 2002;11:317-327

[23] Cole AL, Lee PJ, Hughes DA, Deegan PB, Waldek S, Lachmann RH. Depression in adults with fabry disease: A common and under-diagnosed problem. *J. Inherit. Metab. Dis.* 2007;30:943-951

[24] Lidove O, Ramaswami U, Jaussaud R, Barbey F, Maisonobe T, Caillaud C, Beck M, Sunder-Plassmann G, Linhart A, Mehta A. Hyperhidrosis: A new and often early symptom in fabry disease. International experience and data from the fabry outcome survey. *Int. J. Clin. Pract.* 2006;60:1053-1059

[25] Karen JK, Hale EK, Ma L. Angiokeratoma corporis diffusum (fabry disease). *Dermatol. Online J.* 2005;11:8

[26] Mohrenschlager M, Braun-Falco M, Ring J, Abeck D. Fabry disease: Recognition and management of cutaneous manifestations. *Am. J. Clin. Dermatol.* 2003;4:189-196

[27] Orteu CH, Jansen T, Lidove O, Jaussaud R, Hughes DA, Pintos-Morell G, Ramaswami U, Parini R, Sunder-Plassman G, Beck M, Mehta AB. Fabry disease and the skin: Data from fos, the fabry outcome survey. *Br. J. Dermatol.* 2007;157:331-337

[28] Franceschetti AT. Fabry disease: Ocular manifestations. *Birth Defects Orig. Artic. Ser.* 1976;12:195-208

[29] Hauser AC, Lorenz M, Voigtlander T, Fodinger M, Sunder-Plassmann G. Results of an ophthalmologic screening programme for identification of cases with anderson-fabry disease. *Ophthalmologica* 2004;218:207-209

[30] Moore DF, Kaneski CR, Askari H, Schiffmann R. The cerebral vasculopathy of fabry disease. *J. Neurol. Sci.* 2007;257:258-263

[31] Fellgiebel A. Stroke and brain structural alterations in fabry disease. *Clin. Ther.* 2007; 29 Suppl A:S9-10

[32] Fellgiebel A, Muller MJ, Mazanek M, Baron K, Beck M, Stoeter P. White matter lesion severity in male and female patients with fabry disease. *Neurology* 2005;65:600-602

[33] Kampmann C, Wiethoff CM, Perrot A, Beck M, Dietz R, Osterziel KJ. The heart in anderson fabry disease. *Z. Kardiol.* 2002;91:786-795

[34] Moore DF, Scott LT, Gladwin MT, Altarescu G, Kaneski C, Suzuki K, Pease-Fye M, Ferri R, Brady RO, Herscovitch P, Schiffmann R. Regional cerebral hyperperfusion

and nitric oxide pathway dysregulation in fabry disease: Reversal by enzyme replacement therapy. *Circulation* 2001;104:1506-1512

[35] Hilz MJ, Kolodny EH, Brys M, Stemper B, Haendl T, Marthol H. Reduced cerebral blood flow velocity and impaired cerebral autoregulation in patients with fabry disease. *J. Neurol.* 2004;251:564-570

[36] Altarescu G, Moore DF, Pursley R, Campia U, Goldstein S, Bryant M, Panza JA, Schiffmann R. Enhanced endothelium-dependent vasodilation in fabry disease. *Stroke* 2001;32:1559-1562

[37] Maisey DN, Cosh JA. Basilar artery aneurysm and anderson-fabry disease. *J. Neurol. Neurosurg. Psychiatry* 1980;43:85-87

[38] Grewal RP. Stroke in fabry's disease. *J. Neurol.* 1994;241:153-156

[39] Gavazzi C, Borsini W, Guerrini L, Della Nave R, Rocca MA, Tessa C, Buchner S, Belli G, Filippi M, Villari N, Mascalchi M. Subcortical damage and cortical functional changes in men and women with fabry disease: A multifaceted mr study. *Radiology* 2006;241:492-500

[40] Crutchfield KE, Patronas NJ, Dambrosia JM, Frei KP, Banerjee TK, Barton NW, Schiffmann R. Quantitative analysis of cerebral vasculopathy in patients with fabry disease. *Neurology* 1998;50:1746-1749

[41] Schiffmann R, Ries M. Fabry's disease--an important risk factor for stroke. *Lancet* 2005;366:1754-1756

[42] Brouns R, Sheorajpanday R, Braxel E, Eyskens F, Baker R, Hughes D, Mehta A, Timmerman T, Vincent MF, De Deyn PP. Middelheim fabry study (mifas): A retrospective belgian study on the prevalence of fabry disease in young patients with cryptogenic stroke. *Clin. Neurol. Neurosurg.* 2007;109:479-484

[43] Moore DF, Altarescu G, Barker WC, Patronas NJ, Herscovitch P, Schiffmann R. White matter lesions in fabry disease occur in 'prior' selectively hypometabolic and hyperperfused brain regions. *Brain Res. Bull.* 2003;62:231-240

[44] Takanashi J, Barkovich AJ, Dillon WP, Sherr EH, Hart KA, Packman S. T1 hyperintensity in the pulvinar: Key imaging feature for diagnosis of fabry disease. *AJNR Am. J. Neuroradiol.* 2003;24:916-921

[45] Burlina AP, Manara R, Caillaud C, Laissy JP, Severino M, Klein I, Burlina A, Lidove O. The pulvinar sign: Frequency and clinical correlations in fabry disease. *J. Neurol.* 2008;255:738-744

[46] Fervenza FC, Torra R, Lager DJ. Fabry disease: An underrecognized cause of proteinuria. *Kidney Int.* 2008;73:1193-1199

[47] Ashton-Prolla P, Ashley GA, Giugliani R, Pires RF, Desnick RJ, Eng CM. Fabry disease: Comparison of enzymatic, linkage, and mutation analysis for carrier detection in a family with a novel mutation (30delg). *Am. J. Med. Genet.* 1999;84:420-424

[48] Clarke JT, Iwanochko RM. Enzyme replacement therapy of fabry disease. *Mol. Neurobiol.* 2005;32:43-50

[49] Beck M, Ricci R, Widmer U, Dehout F, de Lorenzo AG, Kampmann C, Linhart A, Sunder-Plassmann G, Houge G, Ramaswami U, Gal A, Mehta A. Fabry disease: Overall effects of agalsidase alfa treatment. *Eur. J. Clin. Invest.* 2004;34:838-844

[50] Pastores GM, Thadhani R. Advances in the management of anderson-fabry disease: Enzyme replacement therapy. *Expert Opin. Biol. Ther*. 2002;2:325-333

[51] Schiffmann R, Kopp JB, Austin HA, 3rd, Sabnis S, Moore DF, Weibel T, Balow JE, Brady RO. Enzyme replacement therapy in fabry disease: A randomized controlled trial. *JAMA* 2001;285:2743-2749

[52] Eng CM, Banikazemi M, Gordon RE, Goldman M, Phelps R, Kim L, Gass A, Winston J, Dikman S, Fallon JT, Brodie S, Stacy CB, Mehta D, Parsons R, Norton K, O'Callaghan M, Desnick RJ. A phase 1/2 clinical trial of enzyme replacement in fabry disease: Pharmacokinetic, substrate clearance, and safety studies. *Am. J. Hum. Genet.* 2001;68:711-722

[53] Fan JQ, Ishii S. Active-site-specific chaperone therapy for fabry disease. Yin and yang of enzyme inhibitors. *FEBS J.* 2007;274:4962-4971

In: Cerebral Ischemia in Young Adults
Editors: A. Pezzini and A. Padovani

ISBN 978-1-60741-627-2

Chapter 21

Other Monogenic Causes of Ischemic Stroke

Alessandro Pezzini[1*], Elisabetta Del Zotto[1,2], Alessia Giossi[1], Irene Volonghi[1], Paolo Costa[1] and Alessandro Padovani[1]

1. Dipartimento di Scienze Mediche e Chirurgiche, Clinica Neurologica, Università degli Studi di Brescia, Brescia, Italia
2. Dipartimento di Scienze Biomediche e Biotecnologie, Università degli Studi di Brescia, Brescia, Italia

Abstract

Mendelian conditions are an important cause of stroke, especially in young patients without known risk factors. In some disorders stroke is the prevailing manifestation, whereas in others it is part of a wider phenotypic spectrum. Most single-gene disorders are associated with specific stroke subtypes, which together with the accompanying systemic features can lead to diagnosis. Within recent years considerable progress has been made in defining the underlying genetic basis of many Mendelian and mitochondrial diseases which can cause ischemic stroke and most of the major genes loci have been mapped. Many of these genes have been cloned thus allowing a direct diagnosis in the index patient and its relatives. Furthermore, cloning of the genes has provided new insights into the molecular mechanisms underlying these disorders. However, although monogenic stroke disorders represent a useful model for understanding the molecular basis of cerebral ischemia, they account for only a minority of cases of stroke, even in young adults.

This chapter summarizes present data regarding clinical and genetic aspects of some rare monogenic conditions associated with ischemic stroke. Other specific single-gene diseases which are especially relevant in clinical practice because of their frequency in young adults (i.e, CADASIL, Fabry disease, MELAS, Moya-Moya disease, sickle cell

---

* Correspondence: Alessandro Pezzini, P.le Spedali Civili, 1, 25100 Brescia, Italia. Tel: +39.030.399 5631 – 5632, Fax: +39.030.399 5027. e-mail: ale_pezzini@hotmail.com.

disease, and prothrombotic disorders) are discussed in more detail in separate chapters of this book.

Introduction

Although the monogenic disorders are an important recognized cause of ischemic stroke, they comprise less than 1 per cent of all cases. To what extent these specific heritable disorders contribute to the population of patients with cerebral ischemia at young age is currently unknown. However, indirect data indicate that the frequency of such single-gene conditions in this age category is probably higher because they often remain undiagnosed, reflecting the substantial variability in their phenotypic expression. In order to recognize Mendelian stroke syndromes it is essential to perform a systematic family inquiry and to search for neurological and non-neurological signs and symptoms in index cases and relatives. Family history also may be negative because the disease can be caused by a new mutation. The diagnosis may have implications both for therapeutic decisions and genetic counseling.

Table 1. Monogenic disorders causing ischemic stroke

Disorders with stroke as a principal manifestation
Small Vessel
Cerebral autosomal dominant arteriopathy with subcortical
infarcts and leukoencephalopathy (CADASIL)
Cerebral autosomal recessive arteriopathy with subcortical
infarcts and leukoencephalopathy (CARASIL)
Hereditary endotheliopathy with retinopathy, nephropathy and stroke (HERNS)
Large Vessel
Moya-Moya disease
Disorders with stroke as a recognised manifestation
Large vessel
Ehlers-Danlos syndrome Type IV
Marfan syndrome
Pseudoxanthoma elasticum
Neurofibromatosis Type I
Small and large vessel
Sickle cell disease
Fabry disease
Homocystinuria
Thrombo-embolic disease
Hereditary haemorrhagic telangiectasia types 1 and 2
Inherited cardiomyopathies
Familial atrial myxomas and cardiac arrhythmias
Mitochondrial disorders
Prothrombotic disorders
Familial hemiplegic migraine

At present, there is no uniform classification for Mendelian stroke syndromes. Criteria that may be useful include underlying mechanisms (Table 1), mode of inheritance, and the presence or absence of associated symptoms.

Single-gene Disorders with Ischemic Stroke as a Principal Manifestation

Cerebral Autosomal Dominant Arteriopathy with Subcortical Infarcts and Leukoencephalopathy (CADASIL)

Clinical, genetic and pathophysiological aspects of CADASIL are discussed in Chapter 19.

Hereditary Endotheliopathy, Retinopathy, Nephropathy and Strokes (HERNS), Cerebroretinal Vasculopathy (CRV), and Hereditary Vascular Retinopathy (HVR)

Jen and colleagues first described a Chinese American family in 1997, with eleven affected members over three generations [1]. The cardinal features were a hereditary syndrome consisting of retinopathy, nephropathy, and stroke. Presentation was usually either with visual or renal symptoms. Retinal changes included macular oedema with capillary dropout and perifoveal microangiopathic telangiectases. Renal dysfunction was accompanied by proteinuria and haematuria. Neurological symptoms appeared in the third to fourth decade and included migraine-like headaches, psychiatric disturbances, dysarthria, hemiparesis and apraxia.

A distinctive feature of this disorder was the presence of progressive subcortical contrast-enhancing lesions with surrounding oedema (pseudotumours) typically located within the fronto-parietal white matter. Retinopathy was characterised by micro-angiopathy of the retina, with micro-aneurysms and telangiectatic capillaries, preferentially around the posterior lobe, which may be seen even in asymptomatic individuals on fluorescein angiography. Advanced stages were characterized by occlusion of branches of large retinal arteries and avascular areas in the retinal periphery. Pathological studies showed a vasculopathy with distinctive multi-laminated vascular basement membranes in the brain and other organs including the kidney, stomach, omentum, intestine and skin. In particular, small intracerebral vessels exhibited amorphous thickening of their walls with adventitial fibrosis. Based on these findings, the Authors suspected a primary endothelial injury and coined the acronym HERNS (hereditary endotheliopathy retinopathy, nephropathy and stroke).

Microangiopathy of the brain in combination with a vascular retinopathy are also the leading features of cerebroretinal vasculopathy (CRV) [2].

A group from the University of Leiden, the Netherlands, later evaluated a large Dutch family with hereditary vascular retinopathy (HVR) associated with migraine and Raynaud's phenomenon [3]. Of the 289 pedigree members (151 males, 138 females) 198 were interviewed. Retinopathy was found in 20 (6.9 %), migraine in 65 (22.5%) and Raynaud's phenomenon in 50 (17.3 %). A combination of all three symptoms was found in 11 individuals. Although white matter T2-hypersignals where observed in some patients, yet stroke does not appear to be part of the syndrome.

A genome-wide search was subsequently performed using a high throughput capillary sequencer. This showed significant evidence of linkage to chromosome 3p21.1-p21.3 (maximum pairwise LOD score 5.25, with D3S1578) [4].Testing of two additional families that had a similar phenotype, cerebroretinal vasculopathy, and hereditary endotheliopathy with retinopathy, nephropathy, and stroke, revealed linkage to the same chromosomal region (combined maximum LOD score 6.30, with D3S1588). Haplotype analysis of all three families defined a 3-cM candidate region between D3S1578 and D3S3564. The group therefore demonstrated that the aforementioned three autosomal dominant vasculopathy syndromes with cerebro-retinal features mapped to the same 3-cM interval on 3p21.

In summary, CRV, HERNS, and HRV represent allelic disorders. The three conditions are transmitted in an autosomal dominant manner with high penetrance and are considered exceptionally rare. From the reported pedigrees the major clinical features include progressive visual loss secondary to retinopathy, headaches of migrainous nature, renal dysfunction and focal neurological deficits and progressive cognitive worsening with psychiatric illness. Raynaud's phenomenon has been reported in only one of these families.

The differential diagnosis of CRV, HERNS and HRV includes diabetic retinopathy, hypertensive small vessel disease, and Susac syndrome [5]. Corticosteroids have been advocated for the treatment of oedema in the acute stage of CRV/HERNS. Surgical resection of the pseudotumour has not been beneficial for those who underwent this procedure. Thus, management consists of symptom control, counselling and support.

Moya-Moya Disease

Clinical, genetic, pathophysiological, and therapeutic aspects of Moya-Moya disease are discussed in Chapter 12.

Single-gene Disorders with Stroke as a Recognised Feature

Sickle Cell Disease

Clinical, genetic, pathophysiological, and therapeutic aspects of Sickle cell disease are discussed in Chapter 17.

Fabry Disease

Clinical, genetic, pathophysiological, and therapeutic aspects of Fabry disease are discussed in Chapter 20.

Single-gene Disorders Occasionally Associated with Stroke

Ehlers-Danlos Syndrome Type IV (EDS type IV)

EDS type IV is an autosomal dominant condition that results from mutations in the COL3A1 gene (located on chromosome 2q31 and encoding collagen type III). The clinical diagnosis is made on the basis of at least two of the following criteria: easy bruising, translucent skin with visible veins, characteristic facial features, and rupture of arteries, uterus, or intestines [6]. Patients often have ecchymoses in well-protected areas. Smaller joints are often hypermobile, but skin hyper-extensibility and large joint hypermobility are rare. The diagnosis is confirmed by mutational screening or biochemical studies (cultured fibroblasts synthesize abnormal type III procollagen). The mutational spectrum is wide with more than 200 different mutations reported thus far (http://www.le.ac.uk/genetics/collagen/col3a1.html), all leading to synthesis of an abnormal type III procollagen protein. New mutations are common. Actually, about 50% of affected individuals have *de novo* mutations and therefore no apparent family history for the disorder. Neurological complications include intracranial aneurysms, arterial dissection (see also Chapter 10) and spontaneous rupture of large- and medium-sized arteries [7]. Aneurysmal rupture can also lead to spontaneous carotid-cavernous sinus fistulae. Fistulae involving the carotid artery and cavernous sinus are the most common complication (2.4%) followed by aneurysms (1.2%) and rupture (0.5%) according to the analysis of a large series of index cases reported by Pepin et al [6].

Death is most often due to arterial dissection or rupture of abdominal or thoracic aorta. Other causes include organ rupture (uterus, liver, spleen, heart) and gastrointestinal rupture. Rupture of any artery into a free space, such as pleural cavity, require immediate intervention, even though the tissues are friable and repair may be difficult. In contrary, rupture into a confined space may be sealed by tamponade, and, in such cases, surgery may be deleterious. Arteriography carries special risks and should be avoided if possible. Whether incidental aneurysms should be treated is still unclear. Prompt surgical intervention is crucial in the treatment of bowel rupture. Women with EDS type IV who become pregnant have to be considered at high risk for uterine and vessel rupture and should therefore be followed at specialized centres.

Marfan Syndrome (MFS)

This autosomal dominant condition is caused by mutations in the epidermal growth factor-like regions of the fibrillin-1 (FBN1) gene on chromosome 15q21.1 (65 exons). More than 90% of families have private mutations in a very large gene, which renders mutational screening very laborious [8]. Thus, the diagnosis is usually established on clinical grounds (the Ghent criteria, Table 2) [9], whereas the role of genetic testing is limited. Fibrillin 1 shares homology with TGFβ binding proteins and there is increasing evidence for a key role of TGFβ signalling in Marfan syndrome [10,11]. It is expressed in many tissues, including the heart and elastic arteries (it is found in abundance in the suspensory ligament of the lens and elastin-rich tissues such as the aorta). Features include tall stature, arm span greater than height, arachnodactyly, high arched palate, ectopia lentis, scoliosis, pectus excavatum or carinatum, and varying degrees of joint hypermobility. Cardiac abnormalities include mitral valve prolapse, aortic incompetence and aortic dissection.

Contrary to popular belief, the prevalence of intracranial aneurysms is not higher in Marfan syndrome than in the general population [12,13]. Cerebrovascular complications themselves are not common and in one retrospective 8-year study occurred in only 3.5% of patients [14]. In this retrospective series on 513 patients, neurovascular manifestations were associated with cardiac sources of embolism, in particular prosthetic heart valves, mitral valve prolapse, and atrial fibrillation, whereas there was no association with aortic disease or cerebral artery dissection. However, other studies have observed an association with aortic and cerebral artery dissection [15,7]. Important risk factors for neurovascular events included older age, valvular heart disease, prosthetic heart valves, atrial fibrillation and anticoagulation. The presence of aortic disease was not different in patients with or without neurovascular complications. Interestingly, no significant association with dissection was demonstrated. With regard to pregnancy in Marfan syndrome, a Dutch study of 78 pregnancies beyond 24 weeks gestation demonstrated two strokes. Pre-conception aortic diameter of 40 mm or more, progressive dilatation and impaired cardiac function conferred additional risk [16]. Patients with artificial valves or significant mitral valve prolapse require life-long anticoagulation to reduce stroke risk.

Pseudoxanthoma Elasticum (PXE)

Dominant and recessive forms of PXE are both due to mutations on the ATP-binding cassette ABCC6 gene on chromosome 16p13 [17]. These result in abnormal deposition of calcium on elastic fibres of skin, blood vessels and eyes. However, the mechanisms by which these mutations become pathogenic are still unknown. The prevalence is estimated to be about 1 in 100,000.

Flexural areas of skin (such as neck, inguinal area, axillae) are especially involved. Numerous yellow papules coalesce to form large plaques resembling a plucked chicken. In long-standing disease, redundant folds of skin hang down from affected areas. Calcium deposition in the elastic lamina of Bruch's membrane in the eye results in angioid streaks visualised on ophtalmoscopic examination. Cardiovascular complications are common due to calcification of the internal elastic lamina of mostly medium-sized arteries. Patients with PXE are at an increased risk of developing ischemic infarction. Focal cerebral ischemia in PXE may be caused by large artery disease, or, less frequently, small vessel disease. Hypertension, also common in PXE, acts as an accelerating factor. A network of abnormal vessels between the external carotid and internal carotid system (*rete mirabile*) associated with carotid hypoplasia has repeatedly been reported in patients with PXE [7]. There are several case reports on a co-occurrence of PXE with intracranial aneurysms or spontaneous cervical artery dissection. However, these observations are likely to be fortuitous [18]. Platelet inhibitors, high systemic blood pressure, and contact sports should be avoided because of an increased risk of bleeding. Nutritional restrictions (calcium) are controversial.

Neurofibromatosis Type 1 (NF1)

NF1 is one of the most common autosomal dominant disorders with a prevalence of about 1 in 3500 live births and with high (virtually complete) penetrance by adulthood. NF1 is a systemic disease affecting mesodermal and ectodermal structures. The rate of *de novo* mutations is high [19] with about one half of index cases having no family history. The NF1 gene is located on chromosome 17q11.2 and codes for neurofibromin, a large (12 kB transcript) tumor suppressor protein [20,21]. Hundreds of different NF1 mutations have been reported thus far (http://archive.uwcm.ac.uk/uwcm/mg/hgmd0.html), the majority of them leading to a truncated protein and can be detected at the protein level. Diagnosis is based on clinical criteria [20].

Clinical manifestations include peripheral neurofibromas, café-au-lait lesions, skeletal anomalies and iris hamartomas (Lisch nodules). Hypertension is a major cerebrovascular risk (children – renal artery stenosis, adults – phaeochromocytoma). Neurological manifestations of NF1 include headache, epilepsy, hydrocephalus, optic nerve tumours, gliomas, meningiomas, peripheral nerve malignant tumours and polyneuropathy [20]. The incidence of intracranial aneurysms has not been found to be higher in NF1 compared with the general population [22]. Although cerebrovascular symptoms are rare, NF1 predisposes to a Moya-Moya-like phenomenon with collateral vessels of the intracranial vasculature leading to both ischemic and haemorrhagic stroke. Stenosis, and eventually occlusion of the supraclinoid internal carotid artery is the most commonly reported abnormality.

The vascular pathology in NF1 includes concentric growth of the intima, disruption of the elastica, and nodular aggregates of proliferating smooth muscle cells. These findings are in agreement with studies that have demonstrated a vascular expression of NF1 within smooth muscle cells and vascular endothelium [23]. The impact of NF1 mutations on the vascular pathology is further corroborated by a mouse model of mutations in p120-rasGAP and NF1 genes [24]. Like p120-rasGAP, neurofibromin has been shown to act as a GTPase activating protein (GAP) on Ras. Disruption of p120-rasGAP in mice affects the ability of endothelial cells to organize into vascularised networks, and mutations in GAP and NF1 genes have a synergistic effect on the observed phenotype which includes thinning and rupture of large- and medium-sized arteries during embryonic development.

There is no specific therapy for cerebrovascular complications in NF1. Thus, management is mainly supportive.

Hereditary Haemorrhagic Teleangiectasia (HHT)

HHT (Osler-Weber-Rendu disease) is an autosomal dominant condition inherited with high penetrance and variable expressivity. The prevalence is estimated at 1 in 50,000. There are 2 recognised entities, HHT1 (endoglin gene on chromosome 9q33) and HHT2 (activator receptor-like kinase 1 gene - ALK1 gene – on chromosome 12q13).

Table 2. Summary of the major and minor suggested Ghent criteria used to establish the diagnosis of Marfan syndrome

Skeletal

Major (at least four of the following constitutes a major criterion):
- Pectus carinatum
- Pectus excavatum requiring surgery
- Reduced upper to lower segment ratio OR arm span to height ratio >1.05
- Wrist and thumb signs
- Scoliosis of >20° or spondylolisthesis
- Reduced extension at the elbows (<170°)
- Medial displacement of the medial malleolus causing pes planus
- Protrusio acetabuli of any degree

Minor
- Pectus excavatum
- Joint hypermobility
- Highly arched palate with crowding of teeth
- Facial appearance: dolichocephaly (long narrow skull)
  - Malar hypoplasia (flattening)
  - Enophthalmos (sunken eyes)
  - Retrognathia (recessed lower mandible)
  - Down-slanting palpebral fissures

For involvement of the skeletal system, at least two features contributing to major criteria, or one major and two minor criteria must be present.

Ocular

Major
- Ectopia lentis

Minor
- Flat cornea
- Increased axial length of globe (<23.5 mm)
- Hypoplastic iris OR hypoplastic ciliary muscle causing decreased miosis

For involvement of the ocular system, at least two of the minor criteria must be present.

Cardiovascular

Major (either of the following constitutes a major criterion)
- Dilatation of the ascending aorta with or without aortic regurgitation and involving at least the sinuses of Valsalva
- Dissection of the ascending aorta

Minor
- Mitral valve prolapse with or without mitral valve regurgitation
- Dilatation of the main pulmonary artery, in the absence of valvular or peripheral pulmonic stenosis below the age of 40 years
- Calcification of the mitral annulus below the age of 40 years
- Dilatation or dissection of the descending thoracic or abdominal aorta below the age of 50 years

For involvement of the cardiovascular system, only one of the minor criteria must be present.

Pulmonary System

Major
- None

Minor
- Spontaneous pneumothorax
- Apical blebs

For involvement of the pulmonary system, only one of the minor criteria must be present.

Skin and Integument

Major
- None

Minor
- Striae atrophicae (stretch marks) not related to marked weight gain, pregnancy, or repetitive stress
- Recurrent or incisional herniae

For involvement of the skin and integument, only one of the minor criteria must be present.

Dura

Major
- Lumbosacral dural ectasia by CT or MRI

Minor
- None

Family/Genetic History

Major (one of the following constitutes a major criterion)
- First-degree relative who independently meets the diagnostic criterion
- Presence of mutation in FBN1
- Presence of a haplotype around FBN1 inherited by descent and unequivocally associated with diagnosed Marfan syndrome in the family

Minor
- None

Endoglin is a homodimeric transmembrane receptor which is highly expressed on endothelial cells. Endoglin binds transforming growth factor-beta (TGFβ) isoforms 1 and 3 in combination with the signalling complex of TGFβ receptors type I and II. Its expression increases during angiogenesis, wound healing, and inflammation, all of which are associated with TGFβ signaling and alteration in vascular structure. Mouse embryos lacking both copies of the endoglin gene die due to defects in vessel and heart development [25,26].

HHT2 is, like endoglin, a cell-surface receptor for the TGFβ superfamily of ligands that is heavily expressed in endothelial and vascular smooth muscle cells [27]. Mice deficient in ALK1 show severe vascular abnormalities characterized by fusion of capillary plexes into cavernous vessels [28]. Thus, both HHT1 and HHT2 highlight the role of receptors for TGFβ family members in the regulation of vascular differentiation.

Vascular malformations are found in skin, lung, liver, kidney and brain. Clinical features include mucocutaneous telangiectasias (especially peri-oral), recurrent epistaxis, gastrointestinal bleeds and dyspnoea and haemoptysis secondary to lung arteriovenous malformations (AVMs) (20 %). In a large systematic study the frequency of classic AVMs was found to be 11 per cent [29]. Teleangiectasias tend to enlarge and multiply over time. Cerebral embolism from a pulmonary AVM is the most common neurological manifestation (usually paradoxical from venous system, occasionally from thrombus within AVM itself). TIAs during haemoptysis may be caused by air embolism from a bleeding pulmonary arteriovenous fistula.

One-third of patients with HHT have pulmonary AVMs. Approximately 5% of those with pulmonary AVMs develop a brain abscess. Intra-cranial AVMs (10%) are multiple, mostly low grade (Spetzler-Martin grade I or II), either supra-tentorial or infra-tentorial and may lead to both intracerebral and subarachnoid haemorrhage though actual risk of bleeding is relatively low (1.4–2% per year) [30]. In a series of 321 cases with HHT the frequency of intracranial hemorrhage (ICH) was found to be 2.1 per cent with a mean age of onset for ICH of 25.4 years [31].

Cavernous and venous malformations and indeterminate malformations are also found.

Treatment is restricted to management of bleeding malformations. Recurrent bleeds necessitate iron replacement and periodic transfusions. Surgical resection and occlusion of pulmonary and cerebral AVMs may be recommended in some cases.

Cardiac Disorders Possibly Associated with Stroke

Inherited cardiac disorders of myocardium and rhythm may be associated with cardio-embolic stroke. The cardiomyopathies include dilated cardiomyopathies (DCM, chromosomes 15q14, 14q12, 1q21.2), hypertrophic cardiomyopathies (HC, chromosomes 20q13.3, 15q14, 14q12, 14q12), restrictive cardiomyopathies (RCM, chromosome 19q13.4) and arrhythmogenic right ventricular cardiomyopathy (ARVC, chromosomes 14q23-q24, 2q32.1-q32.3, 1q42-q43, 10p14-p12, 3p23, 14q12-q22, 6p24)[32]. Inheritance is usually autosomal dominant. HCM is common (about 1 in 500 young adults) and has been identified as an important cause of sudden unexpected death. DCM (prevalence, about 1 in 20,000) and ARVC are less frequent.

Of the above, stroke is most common in dilated cardiomyopathy and is secondary to a cardio-embolic event, either due to mural thrombi or atrial fibrillation (more often). Associated congestive cardiac failure is also a risk factor for ischemic stroke. Of 900 patients followed over a mean of 7 ± 7 years, 44 (4.9%) developed an ischemic stroke [33]. Of these, 89 per cent (n = 39) had AF. Twenty per cent (n = 10) died as a direct consequence of their event.

Inherited arrhythmias, such as those involving supraventricular structures (e.g, familial atrial fibrillation) may also predispose to stroke. It is also plausible that ventricular arrhythmias occurring in the Romano-Ward syndrome (long QT syndrome linked to chromosome 11p15 and encoding for potassium channels, others linked to 4q25, 3p21, 21q22) and in the Brugada syndrome (right bundle branch block and ST elevation syndrome linked to chromosome 3p21 and encoding for sodium channels) may on occasion lead to cardio-embolic stroke [34]. However, there are no systematic studies addressing the frequency of cerebrovascular events in this group of disorders.

Therapeutic options include anticoagulation, pacing and implantable defibrillators. In patients with long QT intervals, precautions with diet, electrolytes and pharmacotherapy must be exercised.

Familial Hemiplegic Migraine (FHM)

Clinical and genetic aspects of FHM are discussed in Chapter 3.

Mitochondrial Encephalopathy, Lactic Acidosis and Stroke-like Episodes (MELAS)

Clinical, genetic, pathophysiological, and therapeutic aspects of MELAS are discussed in Chapter 23.

Familial Dyslipidaemias

Disorders of lipoprotein metabolism predispose to premature vascular disease. Most such disorders are polygenic. Monogenic disorders include autosomal dominant familial hypercholesterolaemia, which can be caused by mutations in the low density lipoprotein receptor gene [35] or ligand-defective apolipoprotein-B 100 [36], and autosomal recessive hypercholesterolaemia [37,38]. There is strong family history of early cardiovascular disease and premature death. Clinical features occasionally detected include corneal arcus and xanthomas. It is still not established if familial hypercholesterolaemia predisposes to stroke or not [39-41].

Homocystinuria

Homocystinuria encompasses a group of mostly autosomal recessive enzyme deficiencies, which cause high (>100 μmol/L) plasma concentrations of homocysteine and homocystinuria. Homocystinuria must be distinguished from milder (15–100 μmol/L) hyperhomocysteinaemia, which is a risk factor for stroke in the general population and is associated with deficient dietary B6, B12, or folate. The most common cause of homocystinuria is a deficiency of cystathionine betasynthase (CBS), a key enzyme in the degradation of homocysteine, in which the conversion of homocysteine to cystathionine is impaired. The estimated incidence of CBS deficiency varies from 1 in 50,000 to 1 in 400,000. Over 90 different mutations have been described, with most being quite rare [42] (http://www.uchsc.edu/sm/cbs). More rarely, homocystinuria results from disturbances in the conversion of homocysteine to methionine by a pathway that requires the formation of methylated derivatives of folate and B12.

The disease should be considered in any child with stroke [43], mental retardation, atraumatic (mostly downward) dislocation of the ocular lenses, or Marfan-like skeletal abnormalities [44]. About 50% of untreated patients with CBS deficiency have a thromboembolic event by the age of 30 years and about a third of these events involve the cerebrovascular system [43]. Homocystinuria can cause stroke not only through atherosclerosis and thromboembolism but also through small-vessel disease and arterial dissection [45,46]. Homocysteine has been shown to injure endothelial cells and increase smooth-muscle-cell proliferation *in vitro* [46]. Putative factors by which homocysteine might induce vascular injury further include extracellular matrix modification, lipoprotein oxidation, and effects on platelets and coagulation [47]. Patients with concurrent homocystinuria and factor V Leiden have an increased risk of thrombosis [48]. Around a half of the patients with CBS deficiency respond to B6. Those who respond tend to have a later onset, a milder phenotype, and a better prognosis than non-responders [49]. The mutational spectrum of CBS deficiency is broad [42]. There are many private mutations (ie, unique to one family) but some mutations, in particular Ile278Thr and Gly307Ser, are relatively common [42,50]. An important observation regarding genotype–phenotype correlations has been that some mutations, including Ala114Val and Ile278Thr, are associated with B6 responsiveness whereas others, in particular Gly307Ser, are associated with B6 resistance. Early diagnosis of homocystinuria is essential as complications can be reduced by early treatment. Diagnosis is established upon the basis of urine amino acid analysis (homocysteine in the urine) and elevated plasma methionine (in CBS deficiency, in the range of 500 – 2000 μM). Management consists of a methionine-restricted diet and initiation of pyridoxine (vitamin B6). Based on observations that some patients with CBS deficiency may respond to pyridoxine therapy, two major subgroups have been traditionally defined: pyridoxine responsive homocystinuria and pyridoxine non-responsive homocystinuria. Those who are responsive tend to have a later onset, a milder phenotype and a better prognosis.

Betaine, a methyl donor that recycles homocysteine to methionine, may be beneficial in both those responding or not to dietary measures and pyridoxine [51,52]. Folate therapy is also recommended as secondary deficiency often occurs. Prophylactic antiplatelet therapy may potentially prevent thromboembolic complications and stroke. Patients with homocystinuria are at increased risk for surgery and need special perioperative care [53].

References

[1] Jen J, Cohen AH,Yue Q, Stout JT, Vinters HV,Nelson S, Baloh RW. Hereditary *endotheliopathy with retinopathy, nephropathy, and stroke (HERNS).* Neurology 1997; 49:1322–1330

[2] Grand MG, Kaine J, Fulling K, Atkinson J, Dowton SB, Farber M, Craver J, Rice K. Cerebroretinal vasculopathy. A new hereditary syndrome. *Ophthalmology* 1988;95: 649-59

[3] Terwindt GM, Haan J, Ophoff RA, Groenen SM, Storimans CW, Lanser JB, Roos RA, Bleeker-Wagemakers EM, Frants RR, Ferrari MD (1998) Clinical and genetic analysis of a large Dutch family with autosomal dominant vascular retinopathy, migraine and Raynaud's phenomenon. *Brain* 1998;121(Pt 2):303–316

[4] Ophoff RA, DeYoung J, Service SK, Joosse M, Caffo NA, Sandkuijl LA, Terwindt GM, Haan J, van den Maagdenberg AM, Jen J, Baloh RW, Barilla-La Barca ML, Saccone NL, Atkinson JP, Ferrari MD, Freimer NB, Frants RR (2001) Hereditary vascular retinopathy, cerebroretinal vasculopathy, and hereditary endotheliopathy with retinopathy, nephropathy, and stroke map to a single locus on chromosome 3p21.1-p21.3. *Am. J. Hum. Genet.* 2001;69:447–453

[5] Papo T, Biousse V, Lehoang P, Fardeau C, N'Guyen N, Huong DL, Aumaitre O, Bousser MG, Godeau P, Piette JC. Susac syndrome. *Medicine* (Baltimore) 1998;77:3-11

[6] Pepin M, Schwarze U, Superti-Furga A, Byers PH. Clinical and genetic features of Ehlers-Danlos syndrome type IV, the vascular type. *N. Engl. J. Med.* 2000;342:673–680

[7] Schievink WI, Michels VV, Piepgras DG. Neurovascular manifestations of heritable connective tissue disorders. A review. *Stroke* 1994;25:889-903

[8] Nollen GJ, Mulder BJ. What is new in the Marfan syndrome? *Int. J. Cardiol.* 2004; 97(suppl 1):103–08.

[9] De Paepe A, Devereux RB, Dietz HC, Hennekam RC, Pyeritz RE. Revised diagnostic criteria for the Marfan syndrome. *Am. J. Med. Genet.* 1996;62:417–26.

[10] Judge DP, Dietz HC. Marfan's syndrome. *Lancet* 2005;366:1965–76.

[11] Neptune ER, Frischmeyer PA, Arking DE, Myers L, Bunton TE, Gayraud B, Ramirez F, Sakai LY, Dietz HC. Dysregulation of TGF-beta activation contributes to pathogenesis in Marfan syndrome. *Nat. Genet.* 2003;33:407–11.

[12] Conway JE, Hutchins GM, Tamargo RJ. Marfan syndrome is not associated with intracranial aneurysms. *Stroke* 1999;30:1632–1636

[13] Schievink WI, Parisi JE, Piepgras DG, Michels VV. Intracranial aneurysms in Marfan's syndrome: an autopsy study. *Neurosurgery* 1997;41:866–870

[14] Wityk RJ, Zanferrari C, Oppenheimer S. Neurovascular complications of Marfan syndrome: a retrospective, hospital-based study. *Stroke* 2002;33:680–684

[15] Spittell PC, Spittell JA, Joyce JW, Tajik AJ, Edwards WD, Schaff HV, Stanson AW. Clinical features and differential diagnosis of aortic dissection: experience with 236 cases (1980 through 1990). *Mayo Clin. Proc.* 1993;68:642–51.

[16] Lind J, Wallenburg HC. The Marfan syndrome and pregnancy: a retrospective study in a Dutch population. *Eur. J. Obstet. Gynecol. Reprod. Biol.* 2001;98:28–35

[17] Ringpfeil F, Lebwohl MG, Christiano AM, Uitto J. Pseudoxanthoma elasticum: mutations in the MRP6 gene encoding a transmembrane ATP-binding cassette (ABC) transporter. *Proc. Nat. Acad. Sci. USA* 2000;97:6001-6

[18] van den Berg JS,Hennekam RC, Cruysberg JR, Steijlen PM, Swart J, Tijmes N, Limburg M. Prevalence of symptomatic intracranial aneurysm and ischaemic stroke in pseudoxanthoma elasticum. *Cerebrovasc. Dis.* 2000;10:315–319

[19] Riccardi VM. Neurofibromatosis: past, present, and future. *N. Eng. J. Med.* 1991;324; 1283-1285

[20] Gutmann DH, Collins FS. The neurofibromatosis type 1 gene and its protein product, neurofibromin. *Neuron* 1993;10:335-43

[21] Sezinger BR. NF1: a prevalent cause of tumorigenesis in human cancers? *Nat. Genet.* 1993;3:97-9

[22] Conway JE, Hutchins GM, Tamargo RJ. Lack of evidence for an association between neurofibromatosis type I and intracranial aneurysms: autopsy study and review of the literature. *Stroke* 2001;32:2481–2485

[23] Norton KK, Xu J, Gutmann DH. Expression of the neurofibromatosis type 1 gene product, neurofibromin, in blood vessel endothelial cells and smooth muscle. *Neurobiol. Dis.* 1995;2:13-21

[24] Henkemeyer M, Rossi DJ, Holmyard DP, Puri MC, Mbamalu G, Harpal K, Shih TS, Jacks T, Pawson T. Vascular system defects and neuronal apoptosis in mice lacking ras GTPase-activating protein. *Nature* 1995;377:695-701

[25] Bordeau A, Dumont DJ, Letarte M. A murine model of hereditary hemorrhagic teleangiectasia. *J. Clin. Invest* 1999;104:1343-51

[26] Arthur HM, Ure J, Smith AJ, Renforth G, Wilson DI, Torsney E, Charlton R, Parums DV, Jowett T, Marchuk DA, Burn J, Diamond AG. Endoglin, an ancillary TGFbeta receptor, is required for extraembryonic angiogenesis and plays a key role in heart development. *Devlop. Biol.* 2000;217;42-53

[27] Johnson DW, Berg JN, Baldwin MA, Gallione CJ, Marondel I, Yoon SJ, Stenzel TT, Speer M, Pericak-Vance MA, Diamond A, Guttmacher AE, Jackson CE, Attisano L, Kucherlapati R, Porteous ME, Marchuk DA. Mutations in the activin receptor-like kinase 1 gene in hereditary haemorrhagic teleangiectasia type 2. *Nat. Genet.* 1996; 13: 189-95

[28] Urness LD, Sorensen LK, Li DY. Arteriovenous malformations in mice lacking activin receptor-like kinase-1. *Nat. Genet.* 2000;26:328-31

[29] Willemse RB, Mager JJ, Westermann CJ, Overtoom TT, Mauser H, Wolbers JG. Bleeding risk of cerebrovascular malformations in hereditary hemorrhagic teleangiectasia. *J. Neurosurg.* 2000;92:779-84

[30] Easey AJ,Wallace GM,Hughes JM, Jackson JE, Taylor WJ, Shovlin CL (2003) Should asymptomatic patients with hereditary haemorrhagic telangectasia (HHT) be screened for cerebral vascular malformations? Data from 22.061 years of HHT patient life. *J. Neurol. Neurosurg. Psychiatry* 74:743–748

[31] Maher CO, Piepgras DG, Brown RD, Friedman JA, Pollock BE. Cerebrovascular manifestations in 321 cases of hereditary hemorrhagic teleangiectasia. *Stroke* 2001;32: 877-82

[32] Franz WM, Muller OJ, Katus HA. cardiomyopathies: from genetics to the prospect of treatment. *Lancet* 2001;358:1627-37

[33] Maron BJ, Olivotto I, Bellone P, Conte MR, Cecchi F, Flygenring BP, Casey SA, Gohman TE, Bongioanni S, Spirito P. Clinical profile of stroke in 900 patients with hypertrophic cardiomyopathy. *J. Am. Coll. Cardiol.* 2002;39:301-7

[34] Roberts R, Brugada R. Genetic aspects of arrhythmias. *Am. J. Med. Genet.* 2000;97: 310-318

[35] Lindgren V, Luskey KL, Russell DW, Francke U. Human genes involved in cholesterol metabolism: chromosomal mapping of the loci for the low density lipoprotein receptor and 3-hydroxy-3-methylglutarylcoenzyme A reductase with cDNA probes. *Proc. Natl. Acad. Sci. USA* 1985;82: 8567–8571

[36] Corsini A, Fantappie S,Granata A, Bernini F, Catapano AL, Fumagalli R, Romano L, Romano C. Bindingdefective low-density lipoprotein in family with hypercholesterolaemia. *Lancet* 1989;1:623

[37] Garcia CK,Wilund K, Arca M, Zuliani G, Fellin R,Maioli M, Calandra S, Bertolini S, Cossu F, Grishin N, Barnes R, Cohen JC, Hobbs HH. Autosomal recessive hypercholesterolemia caused by mutations in a putative LDL receptor adaptor protein. *Science* 2001;292:1394–1398

[38] Zuliani G, Vigna GB, Corsini A, Maioli M, Romagnoni F, Fellin R. Severe hypercholesterolaemia: unusual inheritance in an Italian pedigree. *Eur. J. Clin. Invest* 1995;25:322–331

[39] Hutter CM, Austin MA, Humphries SE. Familial hypercholesterolemia, peripheral arterial disease, and stroke: a HuGE minireview. *Am. J. Epidemiol.* 2004;160:430–435

[40] Kaste M, Koivisto P. Risk of brain infarction in familial hypercholesterolemia. *Stroke* 1988;19:1097–1100

[41] Mabuchi H, Miyamoto S, Ueda K, Oota M, Takegoshi T,Wakasugi T, Takeda R. Causes of death in patients with familial hypercholesterolemia. *Atherosclerosis* 1986; 61:1–6

[42] Kraus JP, Janosik M, Kozich V, Mandell R, Shih V, Sperandeo MP, Sebastio G, de Franchis R, Andria G, Kluijtmans LA, Blom H, Boers GH, Gordon RB, Kamoun P, Tsai MY, Kruger WD, Koch HG, Ohura T, Gaustadnes M. Cystathionine beta-synthase mutations in homocystinuria. *Hum. Mutat.* 1999;13:362-75

[43] Mudd SH, Skovby F, Levy HL, Pettigrew KD, Wilcken B, Pyeritz RE, Andria G, Boers GH, Bromberg IL, Cerone R. The natural history of homocystinuria due to cystathionine betasynthase deficiency. *Am. J. Hum. Genet.* 1985;37:1–31

[44] Brenton DP. Skeletal abnormalities in homocystinuria. *Postgrad. Med. J.* 1977;53:488–496

[45] Kelly PJ, Furie KL, Kistler JP, Barron M, Picard EH, Mandell R, Shih VE. Stroke in young patients with hyperhomocysteinemia due to cystathionine beta-synthase deficiency. *Neurology* 2003;60:275–79.

[46] Hassan A, Hunt BJ, O'Sullivan M, Bell R, D'Souza R, Jeffery S, Bamford JM, Markus HS. Homocysteine is a risk factor for cerebral small vessel disease, acting via endothelial dysfunction. *Brain* 2004;127:212–19.

[47] Bellamy MF, McDowell IF. Putative mechanisms for vascular damage by homocysteine. *J. Inherit. Metab.* Dis. 1997;20:307–15.

[48] Mandel H, Brenner B, Berant M, Rosenberg N, Lanir N, Jakobs C, Fowler B, Seligsohn U. Coexistence of hereditary homocystinuria and factor V Leiden: eff ect on thrombosis. *N. Engl. J. Med.* 1996;334:763–68.

[49] Yap S, Boers GH, Wilcken B, Wilcken DE, Brenton DP, Lee PJ, Walter JH, Howard PM, Naughten ER. Vascular outcome in patients with homocystinuria due to cystathionine beta-synthase defi ciency treated chronically: a multicenter observational study. Arterioscler *Thromb Vasc. Biol.* 2001;21:2080–85.

[50] Sebastio G, Sperandeo MP, Panico M, de Franchis R, Kraus JP, Andria G. The molecular basis of homocystinuria due to cystathionine beta-synthase defi ciency in Italian families, and report of four novel mutations. *Am. J. Hum. Genet.* 1995; **56:** 1324–33.

[51] Wilcken DE, Dudman NP, Tyrrell PA. Homocystinuria due to cystathionine beta-synthase deficiency – the effects of betaine treatment in pyridoxine-responsive patients. *Metabolism* 1985;34:1115–1121

[52] Wilcken DE, Wilcken B, Dudman NP, Tyrrell PA. Homocystinuria – the effects of betaine in the treatment of patients not responsive to pyridoxine. *N. Engl. J. Med.* 1983; 309: 448–453

[53] Weksler BB. Hematologic disorders and ischemic stroke. *Curr. Opin. Neurol.* 1995;8: 38-44

In: Cerebral Ischemia in Young Adults
Editors: A. Pezzini and A. Padovani

ISBN 978-1-60741-627-2

Chapter 22

Polygenic Ischemic Stroke

Anna Bersano* [*]

Dipartimento di Scienze Neurologiche, Ospedale Maggiore Policlinico, Mangiagalli e Regina Elena, Università degli Studi di Milano, Milano, Italy

Abstract

Many ischemic strokes in young patients are considered cryptogenic and remain of undetermined aetiology, despite extensive investigations. However, epidemiological and familial studies provided evidences that genetic factors have a role in stroke occurrence. In particular, it has been suggested that genetic factors are more important in individuals presenting with stroke at a young age. Single gene disorders explain only a minority of juvenile strokes. Stroke represents a complex trait, which is usually assumed to be polygenic. The role of a several of candidate genes has been investigated in juvenile stroke, mostly through association studies, with controversial results. Therefore, it is difficult for the clinician to establish the validity and the level of clinical applicability of the previously reported associations between genetic factors and stroke. This chapter is an update and an extensive analysis of the more recent association studies conducted in stroke patients younger than 50 years. We evaluated a number of studies on several candidate genes providing a final panel of genes and molecular variants, which we categorized in relation to the degree of association with juvenile stroke, supported by the results of case-control studies and, when available, by meta-analyses.

Introduction

The prevalence of ischemic stroke affecting young adults between the ages of 15 and 45 years has been reported ranging from 3 to 5%-12.3% [1, 2]. Many ischemic strokes in young patients are considered cryptogenic [1] and remain of undetermined aetiology despite

[*] Correspondence: Anna Bersano, IRCCS, Via F. Sforza, 35, Milano, Italy. Ph.: +39 02 55033830 - 02 50320433, Fax: +39 02 50320430. E-mail: anna.bersano@unimi.it.

extensive investigation [2]. Studies in twins, families and animal models [3-5] provided substantial evidence that genetic factors are important. In particular, it has been suggested that genetic factors are more important in individuals presenting with stroke at a young age and in certain stroke subtypes [6-7]. Thus, genetic factors seem to be more important in large and small vessels stroke than in cryptogenetic stroke [7].

Although monogenic disorders are an important recognized cause of juvenile stroke, they comprise less than 1% of all cases. Stroke is thought to be a complex multifactorial and polygenic disorder for which classic patterns of inheritance cannot be shown. However the extent of the genetic predisposition is unclear and difficult to understand for variable gene penetrance and presence of confounding effect of coexisting risk factors. As a consequence the relation between genotype and phenotype in sporadic stroke is complicated. Therefore to study the influence of genetic factors on stroke it is helpful to consider at what level in the stroke pathway genetic factors could act to increase stroke risk [6]. It is believed that stroke arises from a wide number of gene-gene and gene-environment interactions [7,8]. Genetic factors could act by predisposing to conventional cerebrovascular risk factors, by modulating the effects of such risk factors on the end organs or in alternative by a direct independent effect on stroke risk and on infarct evolution in acute phase and outcome [7-10]. Thus, mechanisms that trigger cerebrovascular disease in young, in whom atherosclerosis is minimal, may lead to insights into the initiation of endothelial damage in general. As for adult stroke, genes controlling intermediate risk factors, such as arterial stenosis, hypertension, and hyperhomocysteinemia, may be important.

However studies on stroke genetics present some methodological difficulties. The late onset, difficulty in collecting genealogic tree, phenotypic heterogeneity and coexistence of confounding risk factors made it difficult to apply a direct approach analysis such as linkage-based method [6,8].

Therefore, the major line of multifactorial stroke investigation is the candidate-gene approach that consists in identifying molecular variants within a functional relevant gene and establishing its function in stroke risk by association case-control or cohort studies. Following some reports of positive association in venous thrombosis and ischemic heart disease, a wide number of candidate genes has been investigated in stroke even if, so far, only few polymorphisms have been consistently associated with stroke occurrence [6,11]. Most of these studies have been criticized for some bias related to small sample size, lack of classification by stroke phenotype or subtype, use of ethnically different populations and unmatched controls [12-13].

An important issue is that stroke is a phenotypically heterogeneous disorder. Stroke is not a single disease but a syndrome caused by a number of different pathologies with different underlying disease mechanisms. The development of neuroimaging made easier to appropriately classify stroke in most cases. For example, a quarter of ischaemic stroke is caused by large artery atherosclerosis, a quarter by small artery disease, 25-30% by cardioembolic sources, and the rest by an assorted variety of different pathologies. Previous family history studies demonstrated that the genetic components for the different stroke subtypes vary. Therefore, to identify with more success genetic factors, it is essential that patients are well phenotyped or subtyped to detect gene associations with particular types of stroke. This has not happened in many studies to date. Moreover despite family history studies demonstrated that genetic factors are much more important in younger individuals, most studies conducted so far have included patients of all ages.

The differences in patients' characteristics together with the heterogeneity in study design could explain much of the inconsistence between studies [14]. Although association studies are considered a powerful instrument to identify risk factors, both implementation of methodologically appropriated studies and replication of results, in independent cohorts, are necessary to demonstrate a causal relationship between a genetic marker and stroke. Therefore the results of existing studies identified a list of possible candidate genes associated with stroke whose clinical utility and validity has still to be assessed [11]. Hassan and Markus in 2000 (6) provided an extensive review of studies, in which the role of a large number of candidate genes was explored in stroke. They included some studies conducted on young stroke patients. In 2004 Casas et al. [15] published a detailed meta-analysis and a quality evaluation study on some association studies between stroke and some candidate genes in white patients older than 18 y.o. We previously published a complete review on polymorphisms associated with stroke in patients of all ages [16]. However no reviews are, so far, available evaluating the association between molecular variants and stroke in youngs. In this chapter we performed an updated literature review about the role of several candidate gene in juvenile stroke. For this purpose we considered only papers evaluating stroke patients younger than 50 years. As previous reviews [15-16], we analyzed only studies in which genotype frequency was reported. In our literature revision we focused on ischemic stroke, excluding association analyses on hemorrhagic stroke patients. Since genetic factors seem to have more influence in young age, we retain important to evaluate separately the possible influence of molecular variants of some candidate genes in stroke occurrence in young subjects.

Finally this comprehensive review will give a panel of possible genes associated with juvenile ischemic stroke risk that could be useful either for planning future meta-analyses either for deciding new research strategies for stroke genetics studies.

Search Strategy

Articles were searched until November 2008 using electronic databases (MEDLINE, EMBASE and HuGE Published Literature Database). We used also the MEDLINE option 'related articles' for all the relevant papers, and additionally, we consulted the references of all evaluated articles. We considered only published English language papers including abstracts, letters, articles, case control studies, prospective cohort studies, reviews and meta-analyses on stroke genes. The search key words used were: stroke, juvenile stroke, cerebrovascular disease, brain infarction combined with genetics, candidate gene name,polymorphism and mutation names. We included only studies evaluating stroke patients aged from 0 to 50 y.o. The statistically significant or not-significant results of association and linkage studies (case control studies and meta-analysis) were reported as odds ratio (OR) and 95% confidence intervals (95% CI) as calculated by the authors. No further statistical or quality analysis was performed in our paper. We judged the association between genetic variants and juvenile stroke 'possible' when supported at least by one meta-analysis and at least one case-control study with statistical significant results, 'uncertain' when there were not enough data to conclude about the relationship and 'not demonstrated' when the association did not seem reliable. We did not consider studies specifically conducted on cerebral haemorrhages, but we reported association studies between candidate genes and specific stroke subtypes. The OMIM accession numbers, the HUGO-approved gene symbols, the GenBank accession numbers and the mutation nomenclature system suggested by Dunnen and Antonakis were used to indicate, respectively, genes and molecular variants, when available from papers included [17].

Association Studies

We found 47 case control studies and two meta-analyses evaluating the association between molecular variants and juvenile stroke.

Haemostasis

Coagulation System

Factor V Leiden

Factor V Leiden (FV) is a large single-chain glycoprotein, encoded by a 25 exons gene mapped on chromosome 1q23 (F5), involved in the coagulation process and regulated by activated protein C [18]. Coagulation factor V (FV) acts as cofactor of FXa and plays an important role in regulation of coagulation process. It is a large, single-chain glycoprotein of about 330 kDa, which circulates in plasma at a concentration of 20 nmol/l (4–14 mg/l) as inactive profactor. FV can be activated by a limited proteolysis of several peptide bonds by thrombin and FXa [19]. In prothrombinase complex, FVa enhances the rate of prothrombin activation by FXa by several orders of magnitude. FV is also found in the α-granules of platelets. The regulation of the procoagulant activity of FVa is mediated by the proteolysis of FVa at positions Arg306, Arg506, and Arg679 by activated protein C [18]. Resistance to activated protein C was first described by Dahlback et al. in 1993 [20]. In most cases it has been related to the F5 gene single point mutation c.1691G>A leading to a p.Arg506Gln aminoacid exchange (rs6025), which is the most studied single nucleotide polymorphism (SNP) (MIM#227400; NM_000130.4). This SNP occurs in about 5% of the Caucasian population and has been considered one of the most important risk factor for inherited thrombophilia. Even if the association between F5 c.1691G>A polymorphism and venous thrombosis is well established, Sykes et al. [21] and Endler et al. [22], in their reviews, reported some doubts on the contribution of FV Leiden to cerebral ischemia.

We found one meta-analysis and 23 case-control studies on young stroke, represented in Table 1a [23-45]. Of these the meta-analysis and most papers, which demonstrated a positive association between ischemic stroke and F5 c.1691G>A, were on children stroke patients. This positive association was confirmed by the meta-analysis of Haywood et al 2005 [46] conducted on children with neuroradiological diagnosis of ischemic stroke, which concluded that F5 c.1691G>A is significantly more common in children with first ischemic stroke than controls. The other studies describing a positive association between F5 c.1691G>A and stroke were conducted on specific phenotypes [32, 41,43] or on small series [37]. Some other studies attempted to demonstrate an association between F5 c.1691G>A and stroke in PFO [39, 44]. Both the case control studies of Pezzini et al 2003 [39] and Botto et al 2007 [44] did not report an association between this molecular variant and ischemic stroke in patients with patent foramen ovale (PFO). This lack of relationship was confirmed by Belvis et al 2007, that did not find any association between prothrombotic markers and stroke in PFO patients belonging to a consecutive series of young strokes.

In conclusion, the c.1691G>A variant would seem to predispose to a higher stroke risk in children. The role of this SNP in young adults has still to be clearly assessed. Thus, it could be useful to implement new studies confirming this association in young strokes.

Otherwise. the role of another polymorphism of F5 gene, the c.4070 A>G variant in exon 13, leading to p.His1299Arg, has still to be assessed in young stroke patients, after the report of Akar et al., 2000 of an association of this variant with cerebral infarction in children [34].

Prothrombin

The proenzyme of thrombin, or prothrombin, is a vitamin K-dependent glycoprotein that converts fibrinogen into fibrin. The gene coding for prothrombin, F2, (MIM#176930; NM_000506.2) is located on chromosome 11p11-q12 and consists of 14 exons, 13 introns and a 5' and 3' untranslated region (UTR). Poort et al.1996 [47] identified a single nucleotide G>A transition, at position 20210 (c.20210G>A) in the 3' UTR of prothrombin gene. The prevalence of this molecular variant is between 1 to 5% in general European population but it is rare in Asians or Africans [21]. This molecular defect represents a gain-of-function mutation that causes enhanced cleavage site recognition, increased 3'-end processing and increased mRNA accumulation and protein synthesis [48-49]. As a consequence, carriers of the G20210A mutation have higher plasma prothrombin levels than non-carriers. For this reason, this variant has been previously correlated to an increased risk of venous thrombosis [21-22, 50].

The nineteen case-control studies we identified on young stroke patients [25, 27, 29-32, 35, 37, 40, 42-45) (Table 1a) were not able singularly to strongly demonstrate the same association. Some positive, but not significant, associations, were found in specific subgroups such as Aznar et al 2004 [40] who reported that c.20210G>A increases cryptogenetic strokerisk, Pezzini et al. [45] who detected an higher frequency c.20210G>A variant in women < 45 y.o with acute ischemic stroke and Botto et al [44], who found an increased risk of cerebral ischemia in PFO patients, carriers of this polymorphism. However the association between c.20210G>A and PFO is controversial. In fact a previous work of Pezzini et al in 2003 [39] did not find the same association. In conclusion, we believe that the role of c.20210G>A variant in stroke risk could be reliable and worthy of further investigations both in ischemic stroke and in specific patients' subgroups.

Table 1a. Coagulation system polymorphisms

Reference	Type of study	Polymorphism	Subtype of population	Case/ controls	Results OR	95%CI
		F5 (Factor V Leiden)				
Juul et al 2002	Meta analysis	c.1691G>A	Ischemic stroke (childhood)	453/1180	4.79	3.26-7.03
Landi et al 1996	Case-control	c.1691G>A	Focal cerebral ischemia (<45 y.o)	95/190	n.s	
Bentolila et al 1997	Case-control	c.1691G>A	Non transient cerebral ischemia (18-49 y.o)	125/134	n.s	
Iniesta et al 1997	Case-control	c.1691G>A	Cerebrovascular diseases <45 y.o	125/102	n.s	
Longstreth et al 1998	Case-control	c.1691G>A	Stroke (54 haemorrages) (women 18-44 y.o)	106/391	n.s	
Nabavi et al 1998	Case control	c.1691G>A	TIA or ischemic stroke (<45 y.o)	225/200	n.s 3	1.3-6.6[1]
De Stefano et al 1998	Case control	c.1691G>A	Ischemic stroke (<50 y.o)	72/196	n.s	
Margaglione et al 1999	Case-control	c.1691G>A	Ischemic stroke (<50 y.o)	202/1036	2.56	1.28-5.14[2]
Heller et al. 1999	Case-control	c.1691G>A	Arterial cerebral infarction (<16 y.o)	26/150	3.7	1-13.7
Nowak-Göttl et al 1999	Case-control	c.1691G>A	Spontaneous Ischemic Stroke (0..5-16 y.o)	148/296	6.00	2.97-12.1
Kenet et al 2000	Case-control	c.1691G>A	Ischemic stroke (Children)	65/145	4.82	1.4-16.5
Voetsch et al 2000	Case-control	c.1691G>A	Ischemic stroke (15-45 y.o) (124 Caucasian/ 43 Africans)	167/225	n.s	
Lopaciuk et al 2001	Case-control	c.1691G>A	Ischemic stroke not cardioembolic (<45 y.o)	100/238	n.s	
Grossmann et al 2002	Case-control	c.1691G>A	TIA/ Ischemic stroke (15-50 y.o)	93/186	3.19	1.38-7.39
Madonna et al 2002	Case-control	c.1691G>A	Ischemic stroke (<51 y.o)	132/262	n.s	
Pezzini et al 2003	Case-control	c.1691G>A	Ischemic stroke in PFO (<46 y.o)	125/149	n.s	
Aznar et al 2004	Case-control	c.1691G>A	Juvenile ischemic stroke (<50 y.o)	49/294	n.s	
Pezzini et al 2005	Case-control	c.1691G>A	Ischemic stroke (<45 y.o)	163/158	n.s	
Slooter et al 2005	Case-control	c.1691G>A	Ischemic stroke (women 18-49 y.o)	193/767	1.8	0.9-3.6
De Paula Sabino et al 2006	Case-control	c.1691G>A	Arterial Thrombosis <50 y.o (33 Ischemic stroke)	53/275	7.11	1.55-32.73[3]
Komitopoulou et al 2006	Case-control	c.1691G>A	Ischemic stroke children (2-5400 days)	90/103	4.2	1.5-12.1
Botto et al 2007	Case-control	c.1691G>A	Ischemic stroke in PFO	97/160	n.s	

Reference	Type of study	Polymorphism	Subtype of population	Case/ controls	Results OR	95%CI
			(<55 y.o)			
Pezzini et al 2007	Case-control	c.1691G>A	Acute ischemic stroke (women<45 y.o)	108/216	n.s	
Akar et al. 2000	Case-control	c.4070A>G	Ischemic childhood stroke (<18y.o)	43/113	2.4	.90-6.8
			F2 (Prothrombin)			
Bentolila et al 1997	Case-control	c.20210G>A	Non transient cerebral ischemia (18-49 y.o)	125/134	n.s	
De Stefano et al 1998	Case control	c.20210G>A	Ischemic stroke (<50 y.o)	72/196	3.8	1.1-13.1 4
Longstreth et al 1998	Case-control	c.20210G>A	Stroke (54 haemorrages) (women 18-44 y.o)	106/391	n.s	
Heller et al. 1999	Case-control	c.20210G>A	Arterial cerebral infarction (<16 y.o)	26/150	n.s	
Margaglione et al 1999	Case-control	c.20210G>A	Ischemic stroke (<50 y.o)	202/1036	n.s	
Nowak-Göttl et al 1999	Case control	c.20210G>A	Spontaneous Ischemic Stroke (0,5-16 y.o)	148/296	4.7	1.4-15.6
Kenet et al 2000	Case-control	c.20210G>A	Ischemic stroke (Children)	65/145	n.s	
Voetsch et al 2000	Case-control	c.20210G>A	Ischemic stroke 15-45 y.o (124 Caucasian/ 43 Africans)	167/225	n.s	
Lopaciuk et al 2001	Case-control	c.20210G>A	Ischemic stroke not cardioembolic (<45 y.o)	100/238	n.s	
Gomez Garcia et al 2002	Case-control	c.20210G>A	Ischemic stroke not cardioembolic or ATS (<45 y.o)	49/87	2.3	0.6-8.3
Madonna et al 2002	Case-control	c.20210G>A	Ischemic stroke (<51 y.o)	132/262	n.s	
Pezzini et al 2003	Case-control	c.20210G>A	Ischemic stroke in PFO (<46 y.o)	125/149	n.s	
Aznar et al 2004	Case-control	c.20210G>A	Juvenile ischemic stroke (<50 y.o)	49/294	3.75	1.05-13.34
Pezzini et al 2005	Case control	c.20210G>A	Ischemic stroke (<45 y.o)	163/158	n.s	

Table 1.a. (Continued).

Slooter et al 2005	Case-control	c.20210G>A	Ischemic stroke (women 18-49 y.o)	193/767	n.s	
Komitopoulou et al 2006	Case-control	c.20210G>A	Ischemic stroke children (2-5400 d)	90/103	n.s	
De Paula Sabino et al 2006	Case-control	c.20210G>A	Arterial Thrombosis (33 Ischemic stroke)	53/275	n.s	
Botto et al 2007	Case-control	c.20210G>A	Ischemic stroke in PFO (<55 y.o)	97/160	4.7	1.2-18.2
Pezzini et al 2007	Case-control	c.20210G>A	Acute ischemic stroke (women <45 y.o)	108/216	6.52	1.73-24.6[4]

[1] cryptogenetic stroke
[2] afetr correction
[3] All positive patients for FV R506Q had stroke as clinical manifestation of arterial thrombosis;
[4] A variant

Fibrinogen

Fibrinogen is a glycoprotein composed of three polypeptidic chains named α, ß, γ encoded by different genes FGA (MIM# 134820; NM_000508.3), FGB (MIM#134830; NM_005141.2), FGG (MIM#134850; NM_021870.2), clustered on the long arm of chromosome 4q28. This glycoprotein was considered from a long time an independent risk factor for myocardial infarction, peripheral vascular disease and stroke [51]. Several mechanisms, including increased fibrin formation, blood viscosity, platelet aggregation and vascular endothelial and smooth muscle cell proliferation, might explain the association between increased fibrinogen and arterial thrombotic disease. In addition, high fibrinogen concentrations lead to a fibrin clot formation with thin and tightly packed fibers that has high thrombogenicity, possibly because the small pore size restricts access of fibrinolytic enzymes [52]. However, fibrinogen levels are also strongly correlated with traditional vascular risk factors, including age, physical inactivity, hypertension, smoking and features of the insulin resistance syndrome. Genetic factors are estimated to contribute to about 50% of total variability in fibrinogen levels. Several polymorphisms have been identified in the genes encoding the 3 pairs of fibrinogen polypeptide chains, α, ß, and γ; however, because the synthesis of the ß-chain is rate-limiting in vitro, most studies have focused on this gene.

The most studied ß chain variants are *Bcl*I (detected by the *Bcl*I restriction enzyme) and the G to A transition at nucleotide position -455 within promoter of FGB gene, which is in complete linkage disequilibrium with the C to T substitution at position -148 (also called HindIII beta-148 polymorphism) in promoter region of FGB gene. The *-455AA* genotype is present in about 10% to 20% of population and is correlated with fibrinogen levels that are reported 10% higher than in individuals with the *GG* genotype. Although a certain association evidence between high plasma fibrinogen levels and arterial thrombosis and between some fibrinogen polymorphisms and high fibrinogen levels, the relation between the c.455G>A polymorphism and thrombotic disease is still unclear.

Another described SNP is c.4266A>G transition of FGA gene which results in the substitution p.Thr312Ala in α chain within its carboxy-terminal end, which is a region important for factor XIII–dependent processes, including α-α chain cross-linking. Clots generated in vitro in the presence of the Ala312 fibrinogen isoform have more extensive α-chain crosslinking and in consequence, thicker fibers.

Initial studies, included in Hassan and Markus' review [6], demonstrated an association between the c.455 G>A and c.148 C>T polymorphisms and atherosclerotic stroke in elderly [53-54]

We found only one case-control study focusing on young strokes [43] (Table 1b), which did not report any significant association between c.455 G>A variant and stroke. In conclusion, according to studies conducted on all age strokes, it does not seem to exist a link between these SNPs and stroke. It has still to be also assessed the role of the polymorphism c.4266A>G of FGA gene, p.Thr312Ala, in acute stroke, after the report of Carter et al. 1999 [55] of an association with post stroke mortality in cardioembolic stroke [56].

Factor VII

Factor VII (FVII) is a vitamin K-dependent coagulation factor, which is converted into activated factor VII by thrombin and factor Xa, owing to its role in initiation of coagulation. It is encoded by a gene located on chromosome 13q34 in which five polymorphisms have been identified. (MIM#227500; NM_019616.2). Similar to fibrinogen, various environmental factors influence plasma FVII levels, including age, body mass index and plasma triglycerides. In fact, correlation between plasma triglyceride levels and FVII coagulant activity has been suggested to explain in part the close association between hypertriglyceridemia and arterial thrombotic disease. Seven polymorphisms in the FVII gene have been described, which account for about 30% of variation in FVII plasma levels [57].
The molecular variants include a decanucleotide insertion, the c.323_324 insCCTATATCCT from ATG-translation initiation codon, in the promoter region of F7 gene, a single substitution in exon 8 c.10976G>A (rs6046), the SNP p.Arg353Gln, two additionalpromoter polymorphisms c.401G>T and c.402G>A and a polymorphism within the hypervariable region 4 of intron 7 which determines three different alleles termed H5, H6, H7 [21, 22, 58]. Whether these polymorphisms, which are well known determinants of circulating FVII concentrations, are associated with arterial thrombosis is still unclear. A large Netherland case control study [59] did not find any correlation between myocardial infarction and high FVII level. Previous studies, just reported by the Hassan and Markus 2000 review [6], failed in finding any link between stroke and F7 polymorphisms [60] in adults. Some other studies on stroke [61, 62] and the meta-analysis of Casas et al. 2004 [15] concluded for lack of association between F7 gene variants and stroke. We found only one prospective case-control study on juvenile stroke from Yeh et al. 2004 [63] (Table 1b) that evaluated the c.10976G>A variant in a population of young stroke patients. This study failed in confirming a relationship

between this molecular variant and ischemic stroke. In conclusion, despite there is only one case-control study on young stroke, the lack of association between F7 gene variants with stroke both in adults and youngs, makes it poor reliable that F7 gene SNPs have a role in juvenile stroke.

Factor XIII

Coagulation factor XIII (FXIII) is a transglutaminase involved in the final step of coagulation cascade. At this stage, thrombin cleavage of factor XIIIA results in formation of activated factor XIII, a transglutaminase that cross-links adjacent fibrin molecules to increase clot stability and resistance to fibrinolysis. Factor XIII also participates in extracellular matrix remodeling, cell adhesion and migration and tissue repair. In a rat model of experimental cerebral aneurysm formation, exogenous administration of factor XIII abrogated the defective intimal proliferative response to arterial wall injury. The plasma FXIII heterotetramer consists of two A-subunits (active site) and two B-subunits (carrier molecule), encoded respectively by genes located on chromosome 6p25-p24 and 1q31-q32.1.

A deficiency of factor XIII has been associated with severe bleeding, illustrating that its main function is the formation of stable cross-linked fibrin.

Several polymorphisms of A subunit have been described in F13A1 gene on chromosome 6 (MIM#134570; NM_000129.3). Of these the most studied is c.143G>T in the exon 2 of the F13A1 gene, leading Valine (Val) to Leucine (Leu) substitution at aminoacid position 34. Located only 3 amino acid residues from the thrombin cleavage site, residue 34 plays a critical role in interaction between FXIII and thrombin. The less common 34Leu isoform is activated more rapidly, with a 2.5-fold higher catalytic efficiency and shortened clot-formation time when compared with its 34Val counterpart [64]. More rapid activation influences fibrin formation and molecular structure of fibrin clot. Fibrin cross-linked in presence of 34Leu isoform does not aggregate laterally, generating clots that consist of thinner fibers, smaller pores, and ultimately, a finer meshwork with altered permeation characteristics.

Thus, it was thought that c.143G>T variant determines FXIII inactivation and contributes to pathogenesis of thrombotic disorders. Two other less described variants of F13A1 are p.Ty204Phe which lowers both FXIII plasma levels and FXIII activity and p.Pro564Leu which also lowers FXIII plasma levels but increases FXII activity [65]. However, contradictory results have been reported about role of c.143G>T polymorphism in myocardial infarction, in which some authors did not find a correlation underlining, instead, a protective role of Leu34 allele [66, 67]. The association between F13A1 p.Val34Leu polymorphism and ischemic stroke is still under discussion. The paper of Catto et al. [68] did not find any significant difference in frequencyof p.Val34Leu between adult cases with brain infarction and controls, reporting that this mutation, on the contrary, seems to predispose for intracerebral haemorrhage. This result is confirmed also by a study on Spanish stroke patients showing that the incidence of severe hemorrhagic transformation after thrombolytic therapy was higher among the L34 variant carriers [69]. The meta-analysis of Casas et al. 2004 [15] and the most recent studies on adults did not find a significant association between F13A1 variants and stroke [70-72]. We found only five studies on young stroke patients [43, 34, 73-75] (Table 1b). Of these only Reiner et al in 2001 and 2002 [73-74] (on the same series) and

Pruissen et al in 2008 demonstrated an association between this candidate gene and stroke occurrence in young women. In particular Pruissen et al identified a strong association between pTyr204Phe while His905 Arg was only slightly associated with ischemic stroke. The heterozygous and homozygous genotypes increasingly affected stroke risk indicating a gene-dose effect compatible with an additive model of inheritance. In this study Val34Leu and Pro564Leu did not increase ischemic stroke risk. In conclusion not enough and convincible studies were conducted on young stroke patients to establish the role of these gene variants in stroke occurrence.

Table 1b. Coagulation system polymorphisms

Reference	Type of study	Polymorphism	Subtype of population	Case/ controls	Results OR	95% CI
FGA/FGB (Fibrinogen)						
Komitopoulou et al 2006	Case-control	FGB c.455 G>A	Ischemic stroke children (2-5400 d)	90/103	n.s	
F7 (Factor VII)						
Yeh et al 2004	Case-control	c.10976 G>A	Acute ischemic stroke (25-49 y.o)	231/200	.97	.31-3[1]
F13A1(Factor XIII)						
Reiner et al 2001	Population Based Case-control	c. 143G>T p.Tyr204Phe p. Pro564Leu	Non-fatal ischemic stroke (women<45y.o)	36/345	3.88 n.s n.s	1.33-11.34[2]
Reiner et al 2002	Population Based Case-control	c. 143G>T p. Pro564Leu	Non-fatal ischemic stroke (women <45y.o)	42/345	3.59 1.95	.25-10.28 [2] .63-6.05 [3]
Komitopoulou et al 2006	Case-control	c. 143G>T	Ischemic stroke children (2-5400 d)	90/103	n.s	
Akar et al 2007	Case-control	c. 143G>T	Cerebral Infarct (Turkey) (10m-18y.o)	116/100	n.s	
Pruissen et al 2008	Case-control	c. 143G>T p.Tyr204Phe p. Pro564Leu p.His95Arg	First Ischemic stroke (women 18-50 y.o)	190/767	.77 9.1 .89 1.7	.53-1.11 5.5-15 .61-1.29 1.1-2.7

[1] at multivariate analysis after correction for risk factors.
[2] Leu34/Leu34 .
[3] Tyr204/Phe204

Von Willebrand Factor (vWF)

Synthesized exclusively by endothelial cells and megakaryocytes, Von Willebrand factor (vWF) is a high-molecular weight multimerized glycoprotein that promotes platelet adhesion and aggregation at a high shear rate, and also acts as a carrier of coagulation factor VIII and as a stabiliser of FVIII in the circulation. The stabilization is achieved by the formation of a non-covalently bound vWF–FVIII complex, which protects FVIII from degradation by activated protein C (APC) and localizes it to sites of platelet plug and clot formation [76]. Reduced levels of vWF are frequently accompanied by reduced levels of circulating FVIII.

Raised levels of vWf have been reported in a number of vascular disorders including deep venous thrombosis. Some studies revealed that vWf levels remain high 3 months after a stroke, and they suggested that raised vWf levels might reflect the repair to endothelial damage after ischemic stroke [77].

Persistently high vWf levels for a few months after stroke may play an important role in the enlargement of the infarct area or the incidence of recurrent strokes because vWf is an important factor in platelet aggregation and adhesion to the subendothelium of an injured vessel wall [77] However, the timecourse or significance of persistently high vWf levels is not fully explained. VWf also increases in response to an acute insult and, therefore, reflects an acute inflammatory event, partly in response to tissue ischemia or necrosis.

The gene encoding for vWF contains 52 exons and is localized on chromosome 12p13.3. Several variants have been identified in vWF gene (MIM#193400; NM_000552.3): c.1051G>A and c.1793 C>G in the promoter of gene, c.1234C>T, c.1185A>G and c.1423C>T in exon 12, the *Sma* I located in intron 2 and the p.Thr789Ala substitution in the coding region of the gene. The two SNP c.1051G>A and c.1793C>G and the aminoacid change p.Thr789Ala have been associated with an increased risk of ischemic heart disease, probably mediated by high vWF levels [78]. Of the few studies conducted on adults only Dai et al. described an association between a Sma I polymorphism and ischemic stroke [79]. We did not find any study on young stroke patients.

Factor XII

Factor XII (FXII) is a plasma protein and a member of the serin protease family involved in intrinsic pathway of coagulation, fibrinolysis and kinin formation. The N terminal portion binds to negatively charged surfaces, while the carboxy terminal portion contains the enzymatic active site. In vivo Factor XII is activated by negatively charged surfaces (contact activation) leading to further proteolytic cleavage of FXII molecule and activation to FXII, which induces factor XI activation. FXII also participates to the conversion of plasminogen to plasmin. While in vitro FXII plays a central role in the initiation of coagulation and fibrinolysis, the role of FXII in vivo is still under discussion. Usually no increased bleeding tendency was observed in patients with severe deficiency of FXII. In contrast severe as well as mild factor XII deficiency has been associated with increased risk for venous and arterial thromboembolism [80-81].

The gene for FXII (F12), composed by 14 exons, is located on chromosome 5q33-qter (MIM#610619; NM_000505.3). A common polymorphism within the F12 gene is the substitution from C to T at nucleotide 46, in the 5'untransletd region of exon 1, [82] probably responsible for decreased FXII plasma levels. The role of the c.46C>T F12 variant in venous thrombosis and coronary heart diseases is still under discussion [84-85]. The few case-control studies on elderly stroke did not show any convincing association between F12 polymorphisms and ischemic stroke [86-87]. No studies are available in literature considering F12 gene variants in stroke patients younger than 50 years.

Fibrinolitic System

Plasminogen Activator Inhibitor-1 (PAI-1)

Plasminogen activator inhibitor 1 (PAI-1) is a fast acting inhibitor of tissue plasminogen (t-PA), thereby attenuates fibrinolysis. PAI-1 levels show circadian variation and are highly dependent on other factors that are involved in cardiovascular risk such as lipids, insulin, sex hormones and inflammatory response [88-89]. High levels of PAI-1 have been detected in the atheromasic plaque [90] and related to the development of myocardial infarction [91]. The human gene for PAI-1 (SERPINE 1) is located on the long arm of chromosome 7(7q21.3-q22) (MIM#173360; NM_000602.1). Several polymorphic loci have been described, including the single nucleotide insertion deletion, c.675_676delinsG from the ATG-translation initiation codon in the SERPINE 1 promoter region, resulting in 4G or 5G alleles, a 3' *Hind*III site and a CA (n) dinucleotide repeat in intron 3 [21, 58, 92]. Despite a wide number of publications, including a recent meta-analysis of nine studies [93], attempted to associate 4G allele with myocardial infarction, other authors did not find this association [94-95]. The evidence for SERPINE 1 role in stroke is less clear. Most of studies [62, 96-101], which considered the association between SERPINE 1 and stroke, excluded an association between SERPINE-1 variants and stroke in adults. Only Bang et al. [102], in a small series of 60 patients with atherosclerotic stroke, Casas et al. in their meta-analysis [15], even if on small data set, and Wiklund et al. [103], studying two independent cohorts, concluded that carriers of 4G/5G genotype are more likely to develop stroke. Roest et al. 2000 [104] and Boncoraglio et al. 2006 [105] reported a protective role of the 5G/5G and 4G/4G homozygosity for cerebrovascular mortality. The lack of a role of SERPINE 1 variants in old stroke patients was confirmed by a population based prospective study on 2995 participants aged 70-79 y.o (101 patients developing stroke), in which the stroke risk was not associated with SERPINE-1 polymorphisms [106]. We found 5 case-control studies on c.675_676delinsG in juvenile stroke [43, 63,107-109]. These studies were not able to demonstrate a significant association between this molecular variant and stroke in youngs. Reiner et al (2001) in genotyping a population of young stroke women (<45 y.o) for FXIII subunit A SNPs found that women who carried either Leu 564/leu 564 genotype or Phe 204 allele in combination with tPAI-1 5G/5G genotype had a nearly 20-fold increased risk of heamorragic stroke (OR 18.9, 95% CI 3.8 to 95.1). In conclusion c.675_676delinsG does not seem to be a risk factor for ischemic stroke occurrence in youngs. The role of this variant in determining heamorragic stroke alone or in combination with other coagulation factor molecular variants has still to be assessed.

Table 2. Fibrinolitic system polymorphisms

Reference	Type of study	Polymorphism	Subtype of population	Case/ controls	Results OR	95% CI
SERPINE 1 (Plasminogen Activator Inibithor-I)						
Akar et al 2001	Case control	c.675_676delinsG	Ischemic childhood stroke (<18y.o)	43/113	n.s	
Nowak-Gottl et al 2001	Case control	c.675_676delinsG	Stroke children (6m-16 y.o)(Germany)	198/951	n.s	
Hindorff et al 2002	Case control	c.675_676delinsG	Ischemic stroke (women 18-44 y.o)	42/386	n.s	
Yeh et al 2004	Case control	c.675_676delinsG	Acute ischemic stroke (25-49 y.o)	231/200	1.04	.49-2.21[1]
Komitopoulou et al 2006	Case-control	c.675_676delinsG	Ischemic stroke children (2-5400 d)	90/103	n.s	

[1] at multivariate analysis after correction for risk factors.

Platelet Receptors

Platelet Glycoprotein IIb-IIIa Complex (GpIIb-IIIa Complex)

Surface membrane glycoproteins (GPs) are essential for adhesion of platelets to exposed subendothelial extracellular matrix components and for platelet-platelet interactions. Platelet glycoprotein receptors mediate the effect of platelets in thrombosis and thus they were considered good candidate genes for ischemic stroke.

GpIIb–IIIa complex is a receptor belonging to the integrin family playing a role in platelet activation, aggregation and clot formation. GPIIb/IIIa is the primary platelet surface receptor for fibrinogen. It also binds von Willebrand factor (vWF) and several other adhesion ligands.

The genes encoding for GpIIb–IIIa complex, named ITGB3 and ITGA2B, are both located on chromosome 17q21.32. The ITGB3 gene (MIM#173470; NM_000212.2), which encodes for glycoprotein IIIa, consists of 7 alleles and the two most common isoforms are PLA1 (HPA-1a) and PLA2 (HPA-1b) [92]. The heritable PLA1/PLA2 polymorphism is due to the nucleotide T to C substitution in nucleotide 1565 within exon 2 (rs5918), resulting in the amino acid substitution of proline (Pro) to leucine (Leu) at position 33 that determines a conformational change in the N-terminal disulfide loop of the receptor [21, 58, 92, 110]. Other ITGB3 gene dimorphisms are c.526G>A (p.Arg143Gln) and c.1564G>A inducing the aminoacid change p.Arg489Gln. The relationship between PLA2 allele and coronary artery disease is still unclear [111-113]. The meta-analyses and case-control studies on stroke patients, without age subgroup analyses, including the two meta-analyses of Wu et al. [114] and more recently of Casas et al., failed in confirming the relationship between ITGB3 gene variants and stroke [15, 57, 62, 101, 114-119]. We found 6 case-control studies on children and youngs, including the subgroup analysis of young patients of the study of Carter et al 1998 [43, 120-125] (Table 2). Of these four studies, conducted, in some cases on small series, found an association between PLA2 and juvenile ischemic stroke. However, since the small sample size of these studies, the role of ITGB3 gene SNPs in the occurrence of ischemic stroke in youngs has to be furtherly investigated.

The most common polymorphism of ITGA2B, which encodes for Glycoprotein IIb (GPIIb) (MIM#607759; NM_000419.3) gene is a substitution of isoleucine/serine at position 843 (p.Ile843Ser) (HPA-3a/3b). We collected only one case-control studies about GPIIb variants and stroke in young people [122] (Table 2). The study reported an association only with the women subgroups with diabetes, hypertension and high plasma homocysteine levels. In conclusion there are not enough data to conclude if carriers of ITGA2B variants have an increased risk of ischemic stroke.

Platelet Glycoprotein Ia-IIa Complex (GPIa-IIa Complex)

Platelet Glycoprotein Ia-IIa Complex is the major platelet/collagen receptor responsible for platelet adhesion to exposed vascular subendothelium. Via GPIa-IIa, platelets adhere to collagen exposed in subendothelial structures and subsequently become activated leading to thrombus formation. The N-terminal extracellular portion of the glycoprotein Ia $\alpha 2$ integrin) subunit contains an insert domain or I-domain (aminoacides 140-349), that shares sequence homology with the wWF A domain and provides the metal ion-dependent binding site for collagen. Congenital or acquired deficiencies of Glycoprotein Ia/IIa have been described in patients with clinical bleeding diathesis and defective in vitro platelet response to collagen. Moreover the $\alpha 2$-$\beta 1$ integrin receptor, other than on platelets, is present on fibroblasts, activated T lymphocytes, epithelial cells and endothelial cells. On epithelial and endothelial cells the receptor binds both collagen and laminin, and it is involved in extracellular matrix remodelling.

Two SNPs in the gene for GPIa subunit, the ITGA2 gene, on chromosome 5q23-31 (MIM#192974; NM_002203.3), have been described at position c.807C>T and c.873 G>A. Another SNP c.1648 G>A, which produces the amino acid substitution p.Glu505Lys, is responsible for the HPA-5 platelet antigen system. This polymorphism is always present together with the c.807C>T variant providing three different haplotypes (Allele A1 807C/Glu505; AlleleA2 807T/Glu 505; Allele A3 807C/Lys 505). A number of case-control studies found a link between GPIa-IIa complex variants and myocardial infarction [126-128], but other authors did not confirm these results [129]. We found 4 case-control studies on young stroke patients. We found one meta-analysis and four further case-control studies [122,125, 130-131] (Table 3). Of these Carlsson et al [130] observed a 2-3 fold increased stroke risk in carriers of 807T allele only in patients <50 y.o. and Reiner et al [122] reported an increased, although not significant, risk of stroke in women <45 y.o carriers of c.807C>T polymorphism. These preliminary results, although on a small number of studies, did not find a strong relation between c.807C>T and ischemic stroke. Therefore, the role of ITGA2 gene variants has to be furtherly studied in juvenile stroke.

Platelet Glycoprotein Ib/IX/V Complex (GPIb /IX/V Complex)

The Platelet Glycoprotein Ib/IX/V (GPIb/IX/V) complex, which combines four glycoprotein chains GP1bα, Gp1bβ, GpIX and GpV, is the major platelet receptor for von Willebrand factor. It is present at a density of about 25.000 copies per platelet. Binding platelet to subendothelial vWF trough glycoprotein Ib/IX/V is important for the initial stage of platelet adhesion to injured blood vessel wall. The Platelet Glycoprotein Ib/IX/V receptor also contains a high affinity binding site for thrombin and contributes to thrombin-mediated platelet activation and procoagulant activity. Moreover this receptor is also a counter receptor for endothelial P-selectin and mediates platelet rolling on inflamed endothelium. Glycioprotein Ib is composed of two disulfide-linked polypeptides, glycoprotein 1bα and 1bβ which are encoded by two distinct genes on chromosome 17 and 22.

Table 3. Platelet receptor polymorphisms

Reference	Type of study	Polymorphism	Subtype of population	Case/ controls	Results OR	95% CI
ITGB3 (GpIIb –IIIa complex)						
Carter et al 1998	Case-control	GPIIIa PLA2	Ischemic stroke	37/74	1.68	1-2.82
Wagner et al 1998	Population Case-control	GPIIIa PLA2	Cerebral infarction (15-44 y.o)	65/122	1.1	.6-2.3
Reiner et al 2000	Population Case-control	GPIIIa PLA2	Non fatal stroke (women <45 y.o)	78/346	1.01	.48-2.13[1]
Van Goor et al 2003	Case-control	GPIIIa PLA2	Ischemic stroke/TIA (45 y.o)	45/60	.8	.3-1.9
Chen et al 2004	Case-control	GPIIIa PLA2	Ischemic stroke (Taiwan) (15-45 y.o)	157/157	n.s	
Komitopoulou et al. 2006	Case-control	GPIIIa PLA2	Ischemic stroke children (2-5400 d)	90/103	n.s	
Reiner et al 2000	Case-control	GPIIb p.Ile843Ser	Non fatal stroke (women <45 y. o)	78/346	1.20	.59-2.45
ITGA2 (GpIa-IIa complex)						
Carlsson et al 1999	Case-control	GPIa c.807C>T GPIa c.873G>A	Stroke patients (<50 y.o)	45/41	3.02	1.2-7.6
Reiner et al 2000	Case-control	GPIa c.807C>T	Non fatal stroke (women <45 y.o)	78/346	2.24	.99-5.06
Akar et al 2001	Case-control	GPIa c.807C>T	Cerebral infarct (Turkish) (10m-18y.o)	44/99	n.s	
Chen et al 2004	Case-control	GPIa c.807C>T	Ischemic stroke (Taiwan) (15-45 y.o)	157/157	n.s	
GP1BA (GpIb/IX/V complex)						
Reiner et al 2000	Case-control	GPIb HPA-2	Non fatal stroke (women <45 y. o)	78/346	10.36	1.43-79.34 [2]
Frank et al 2001	Case-control	GPIb (-5)T/C Kozak	Non fatal stroke (women 18-44 y.o)	106/384	n.s	
Chen et al 2004	Case-control	GPIb HPA-2	Ischemic stroke (15-45 y.o)	157/157	n.s	

Several polymorphisms have been characterised in the four genes encoding for the complex, mostly in the gene encoding for GPIbα subunit (GP1BA), which is located on chromosome 17pter-p12 (MIM#606672; NM_000173.4). The rs41439349 polymorphism, characterized by variable numbers of tandem repeats (VNTR), was identified within the GP1BA gene causing a replication of a 13 aminoacid sequence (from Serine 399 to Threonine 411) and consequently four different size variants D, C, B, A, (in order of the increasing number of repeats from 1 to 4 times) [130]. A second polymorphism identified in the GP1BAgene is c.3550C>T resulting in a p.Thr145Met substitution linked to HPA-2

(Human Platelet Antigen 2) alloantigen system [126, 132]. HPA-2 and VNTR polymorphism are in strong linkage disequilibrium each other. More recently, a third polymorphism, the Kozack sequence, occurring in the region of translation start site at position 5' from the initiator ATG codon (where either T or C is present) of GP1BA gene was identified [133-134].

We found three case-control studies focused on juvenile stroke as shown in Table 3 [122,125,135]. Of these only Reiner et al 2000 [122] found an association between GPIb HPA-2 and stroke in young women but the results are not convincing since the small series. Thus, despite some data on adults support a role of GP1BA gene variants in stroke [15, 136-137], the specific role of these molecular changes and in young stroke has been assessed in large series.

Renin Angiotensin Aldosterone System

The renin–angiotensin–aldosterone system (RAAS) influences blood pressure, vasoconstriction, thrombosis, and vessel wall damage. Renin, released from the kidney, cleaves angiotensinogen (AGT) to angiotensin I, which then is modified by angiotensin-converting enzyme (ACE) to angiotensin II (ATII). ATII is an extremely potent vasoconstrictor that acts within seconds. ATII also stimulates aldosterone secretion, which absorbs sodium and increases intravascular volume. In addition, ATII and aldosterone promote coagulation by increasing plasminogen-activator inhibitor and activating platelets at sites of injury. Several studies have suggested that RAAS contributes to brain infarction. Two major antihypertensive drug classes can directly interact with the RAS, that is, ACE inhibitors and b-blockers. ACE inhibitors inhibit the conversion from angiotensin I to angiotensin II, resulting in a reduction of the peripheral vascular resistance.

1) Angiotensin-Converting Enzyme (ACE)

Angiotensin-converting enzyme (ACE) is a membrane-bound dipeptidil-carboxypeptidase ectoenzyme that has an important role within the renin angiotensin aldosterone system.

Its most important substrates are angiotensin I, which it converts to angiotensin II, which plays a major role in vasoconstriction and bradykinin, which it inactivates. It also cleaves ekephalins and substance P even though the significance of this action is unclear. ACE is located on the luminal surface of vascular endothelial cells. Despite there are not indications that plasma ACE levels are directly related to blood pressure levels, the study of molecular variants of this gene has developed during years, since hypertension is one of the most important risk factor for stroke. Plasma ACE activity shows considerable interindividual variation, although intraindividual variations are small.

The ACE gene is located on chromosome 17q23 and consists of 26 exons and 25 introns (MIM#107180; NM_152830.1). An insertion (I)/deletion (D) polymorphism situated in intron 16 of the ACE gene of 287-bp (g.11417_11704del287), the so-called ACE I/D polymorphism, has been described. This polymorphism result in three genotypes homozygous DD, heterozygous ID, homozygous II [138-139]. This variant, in particular DD genotypes, was found associated with high ACE plasma and tissue levels [140]. ACE gene polymorphisms have been widely studied in stroke, after the report of increased risk of myocardial infarction in DD genotype carriers [141]. Two meta-analyses and some case-control studies conducted on stroke patients of all ages [15, 142-148] concluded for an association between the 16 bp i/d variant and stroke both in European and non-European subjects. We found only one case–control study evaluating the association between 16 bp i/d variant and stroke [149] (Table 4). This study was on a small series and did not report a relationship between this variant and juvenile stroke. Doi et al demonstrated a significant association between the ACE gene polymorphism and thrombotic brain infarction in patients age 60 years or younger in a Japanese population [150]. This molecular variant has been studied also in subgroup of patients with the same range of age both with carotid atherosclerosis (< 60 y.o) [151] and IMT (50-64 y.o) [152] with controversial results.

In conclusion, since 16 bp i/d variant seems strongly associated with stroke in patients of all ages, it could be interesting better investigating in youngs and through different ethnic groups, the role of ACE variants in stroke.

2) Angiotensinogen

Angiotensinogen is a glycoprotein secreted by the liver, which represents the substrate for renin action. It is believed that angiotensinogen levels, which are influenced by estrogens, glucocorticoids and thyroid hormones, contribute to hypertension [153]. The gene encoding for angiotensinogen (AGT) is located on chromosome 1q41-qter (MIM#106150; NM_000029.2). The most common SNPs reported are the substitution of Threonine for Methionine at amino acid position 235 (p.Met235Thr) and the aminoacid change Methionine for Threonine at 174. Two other polymorphisms, in the promoter region at position c.6G>A (6 bp upstream from the site of transcription initiation), which is in very tight linkage disequilibrium with Thr235 and c.20A>C, have been described and seem to alter the gene transcriptional activity. We did not find any study evaluating the link between AGT variants and juvenile stroke. The studies considering stroke, without any age differentiation [62, 101, 142, 143, 154-156] did not find a link between stroke and angiotensinogen polymorphisms. Recently van Rijn et al [157] found an association between angiotensinogen p.Met235Thr and increased blood pressure, carotid plaques and white matters lesions suggesting that AGT gene variants could act at intermediate phenotype level. It could be probably interesting to assess the role of AGT SNPs in these intermediate phenotypes in young people.

Table 4. Renin-angiotensin-aldosterone system polymorphisms

Reference	Type of study	Polymorphism	Subtype of population	Case/ controls	Results OR	95% CI
ACE (Agiotensin-converting enzyme)						
Varda et al 2005	Case-control	g.11417_11704del287	Cerebrovascular disease (8-34 y.o)	58/58	n.s	

Endothelial Nitric Oxid Synthase (e-NOS)

Nitric Oxide Synthase (NOS) catalyzes the formation of soluble nitric oxide (NO) from L-arginine. Endothelial NO has several functions, including maintaining basal cerebral flow, cerebral vasodilatation and autoregulation. Nitric oxide (NO) synthesized from L-arginine by endothelial constitutive NO synthase (ecNOS) is permanently released from arterial and arteriolar endothelium. NO plays a key role in the relaxation of vascular smooth muscle cells (VSMCs); it reduces VSMC proliferation, adhesion of platelets and leukocytes, endothelial permeability, and extracellular matrix collagen synthesis. Conversely, an excess of NO may be harmful because of its oxidative role. In animal models, ecNOS inhibition accelerates atherosclerosis whereas its administration prevents it. In humans with atherosclerosis, abnormalities in endothelial NO pathway have been shown.

A lack of endothelium-derived NO would be expected to lead to cerebral hypoperfusion, impaired cerebral autoregulation, endothelial damage with breakdown of the blood-brain barrier and vessel remodelling. Several key genes are concerned with the endothelial system, including endothelial nitric oxide synthase (eNOS), the enzyme catalyzing formation of soluble nitric oxide (NO) from L-arginine.

There are three isoforms of NOS, named in relation to the tissue, which they were first cloned from [158]: neuronal (NOS1), immunologic (NOS2) endothelial (eNOS or NOS3). NOS1 and NOS3 are involved in cerebral ischemia. The NOS3 gene, composed of 26 exons, is located on chromosome 7q36 (MIM#163729; NM_000603.3). Several variable tandem repeats and dinucleotide repeats (CA^n) have been reported. In particular, a promoter polymorphism c.786 T>C, a 27-bp tandem repeat in intron 4 closer to the 5-prime end of the NOS3 gene, the g.3726_3834insGAAGTCTAGACCTGCTGCGGGGGTGAG, and the c.894G>T SNP in exon 7, resulting in p.Glu298Asp, have been described to impair the enzymatic activity. Hassan and Markus 2000 [6], reviewing papers until 1999, conclude that there is not a relation between NOS3 gene polymorphisms and stroke. The meta-analysis and the case-controls studies on stroke [15, 62, 101, 144, 158-161], without age distinction did not demonstrate a convincing association between c.894G>T variant and stroke. On youngs we identified only two case control studies [162-163] (Table 5). The first one, although on a small series, did not report any relationship between NOS3 variant and stroke, the second one on women aged 15 to 44 years reported an association between c. 922 G>A and c.786 T>C and stroke in blacks.

In conclusion, wider series of patients have to be studied to clarify the association between NOS3 variants and juvenile stroke.

Homocysteine (Hcy) Metabolism

Homocysteine (Hcy) is a sulphidryl-containing amino-acid derived from the metabolism (demethylation) of dietary methionin [164]. The homocystein metabolism occurs through two remethylation pathways to methionine that are catalysed by *methionine synthase* and *betaine-homocysteine-methyltransferase* and one pathway of trans-sulfuration to cysteine cathalized by *cystathionine-ß-synthase* (CßS). In the first pathway cobalamine acts as cofactor and methyl group derivates from 5-methyl-tetrahydrofolate that is a product of the reduction of

5,10-methylenetetrahydrofolate by methylenetetrahydrofolate reductase (MTHFR) (164). When remetylation pathways is saturated the homocysteine is converted to cystathionine (and then to cysteine) by cystathionine ß-synthase that uses as cofactor a derivate of vitamine B6 (pyridoxal-5'-phosphate) [164-165].

Plasma levels of homocysteine (Hcy), which is a sulphidryl-containing amino acid derived from the metabolism of dietary methionin [164] are well known to increase with age, vitamin B12, B6 and folate deficiency, renal dysfunction and other less, well established, determinants such as smoke, arterial hypertension, hypercholesterolemia, coffee and alcohol consumption. It is possible to distinguish between severe and mild to moderate concentration levels of homocysteine [165]. Severe hyperhomocysteinemia (Hcy>100 μmol/l), more frequently caused by homozygous deficit of CßS and in only 5-10 percent of cases by homozygous deficit of methylenetetrahydrofolate reductase (MTHFR), is responsible for theclinical feature of homocystinuria, ectopic lens, skeletal abnormalities, premature vascular disease such as thromboembolism, mental retardation, seizures and peripheral neuropathy.

Mild to moderate hyperhomocysteinemia (Hcy15-100 μmol/l) occurs in phenotypically normal subjects with genetic defects (heterozygosity of MTHFR or CßS), acquired conditions or an association of both. At least 60 mutations have been recognised on the CßS gene (MIM#236200; NM_000071.1), located on chromosome 21q22.3, of which the most frequently detected are the nucleotide changing c.833C>T resulting in p.Ile278Thr, the c.919G>A substitution resulting in p.Gly307Ser both in exon 8 and the splice alteration c.844 ins68. However, the most common gene variant associated with moderate hyperomo cysteinemia is the substitution c.677C>T of the gene encoding for MTHFR (MIM#607093; NM_005957.3), mapped on chromosome 1p36.3, resulting in a p.Ala222Val substitution. This molecular variant is responsible for the reduction of 50 percent of enzymatic activity, indicating that it is possible that other factors contribute to determine the different phenotypic expressions. Other common MTHFR variants are the substitution c.1298 A>C in the C terminal region that converts glutamate to alanine (p.Glu429Ala) and c.983 A>G transition, resulting in a p.Asn324Ser. A strong positive and dose-related association between homocystein serum concentration and risk of stroke has been widely demonstrated by case controls and cohort studies [166-167]. However, although the studies [62, 119, 168-171] in adults showed a trend toward the association between c.677C>T and stroke, the results are controversial.

We collected one meta-analysis and fifteen case-control studies on young stroke patients (Table 5) [29, 30,35, 36, 37, 38, 39, 41, 42, 43, 45 46, 173-174]. Of these, other than the meta-analysis of Haywood [46], only 4 studies [30, 41, 45, 173, 176] demonstrated a positive association between MTHFR 677 TT genotype a stroke. Particularly this association was observed in women since the studies of Slooter et al 2005, Pezzini et al in 2005 and 2007 (which is the same series of the study of 2006) [41, 45, 173, 176] were all conducted on populations of young women with ischemic stroke. Two other studies [101,177] conducted on stroke patients younger than 60 years also did not demonstrated this relationship.

In conclusion, the association between c.677C>T and juvenile stroke is still doubt and the only reliable association seems to be between TT genotype and stroke in women. Thus, it has still to be defined in further studies whether this association in youngs as well in adults, is causal or related, to several confounding concausal factors [178].

Table 5. Endothelial nitric oxide and homocysteine methabolism polymorphisms

Reference	Type of study	Polymorphism	Subtype of population	Case/ controls	Results OR	95% CI
NOS3 (eNOS)						
Akar et al 2000	Case-control	c.894G>T	Ischemic stroke (10 m-18 y.o)	43/82	n.s	
Howard et al 2005	Case-control	c.922G>A c.786T>C c.1468T>A c.894G>T	Ischemic stroke (women 15-44 y.o)	110/206	3 2.9 n.s n.s	1.3-6.8[1] 1.3-6.4[1]
MTHFR-CBS-MTR (Homocysteine)						
Haywood et al 2004	Meta-analysis	MTHFR c.677C>T	Acute ischemic stroke Children (2 d-18 y.o)	3235/9019	1.7	1.23- 2.34
De Stefano et al 1998	Case-control	MTHFR c.677C>T	Ischemic stroke (<50 y.o)	72/198	n.s	
Kristensen et al 1999	Case-control	MTHFR c.677C>T	Ischemic stroke (18-44 y.o)	80/41	n.s	
Margaglione et al 1999	Case-control	MTHFR c.677C>T	Ischemic stroke (3-50 y.o)	202/1036	1.6	1-2.54[2]
Voetsch et al 2000	Case-control	MTHFR c.677C>T	First ischemic stroke (15-45 y.o)	153/225	n.s	
Lopaciuk et al 2001	Case-control	MTHFR c.677C>T	Ischemic stroke without a cardiac source (<45 y.o)	100/238	n.s	
Madonna et al 2002	Case-control	MTHFR c.677C>T	Ischemic stroke (6m-50 y.o)	132/262	n.s	
Grossmann et al 2002	Case-control	MTHFR c.677C>T CBS c.844ins68	Ischemic stroke/TIA (<50 y.o)	93/186	n.s	
Pezzini et al 2003	Case-control	MTHFR c.677C>T	Ischemic stroke with or without PFO (<45 y.o)	125/149	n.s	
Slooter et al 2005	Case-control	MTHFR c.677C>T	Ischemic stroke (women 20-49 y.o)	193/767	1.5 5.4	0.9-2.6 2.4-12[3]
Pezzini et al 2005	Case-control	MTHFR c.677C>T	First ischemic stroke (45 y.o)	163/158	1.93	1-3.71[2]
Sirachainan et al 2006	Case-control	MTHFR c.677 C>T MTHFR c.1298 A>C	Ischemic stroke children (Thailand) (<18 y.o)	27/99	n.s	
Sanchez-Marin et al 2006	Case-control	MTHFR c.677 C>T	Ischemic stroke (<50 y.o)	99/90	n.s	
Komitopoulou et al 2006	Case-control	MTHFR c.677C>T MTHFR c.1298A>C	Ischemic stroke children (2-5400 d)	90/103	n.s	
De Paula Sabino et al 2006	Case-control	MTHFR c.677C>T	Arterial Thrombosis (<50 y.o) (33 Ischemic stroke)	53/275	n.s	
Pezzini et al 2007	Case-control	MTHFR c.677C>T	Acute ischemic stroke (women <45 y.o)	108/216	3.36	1.60-7.05[2]

[1] Black population.
[2] TT compared to CC genotype.
[3] using oral contraceptives.

Lipoprotein Metabolism

Apolipoprotein E (ApoE)

Apolipoprotein E (ApoE) is a plasma glycoprotein involved in lipids transport and in growth and regeneration of peripheral and central nervous system tissues [179]. The three common human isoforms, which differ by single amino acid interchanges, are apo E2, E3, E4, encoded by three alleles (ε2, ε3, ε4) of the apo E gene located on chromosome 19q13.2 (MIM#107741; NM_000041.2). Apolipoprotein E (APOE) is very important in cholesterol transport and other physiologic processes, including supplying lipids to neurites to aid regeneration after injury. APOE gene molecular variants have been associated with atherosclerosis and Alzheimer's disease (AD).

Their distribution in Caucasian population is respectively 60 percent for E3/E3, 22 percent for E3/E4, 12 percent for E2/E3, 3 percent for E4/E4, 2 percent for E2/E4, 1 percent for E2/E2.

The role of APOE and ischemic stroke is controversial. The case controls identified on adults and the results of meta-analysis reported very heterogenous results [15, 62, 101, 142, 181-187]. Only one study focused on juvenile stroke [173] (Table 6). Pezzini et al 2005 [173], on the same population of the study of 2004 (188) reported an increased risk of stroke in allele ε4 carriers. The study of Jin et al 2004 confirmed the relationship between apo ε4 and cerebral infarction in a study on 226 Chinese stroke patients aged 40 to 60 years old [189]. Sturgeon et al 2005 [190] did not confirm an association between this variant and incident stroke in a cohort study involving 15792 subjects aged 45 to 65 years.

We conclude that the role of apoE ε4 allele as risk factor for stroke in young patients has still to be verify in further wider studies.

Apolipoproteins (APO) AI –B

Apolipoproteins (APO) represent the proteic component of lipoproteins, involved in lipid transportation. Two major types of APOs have been recognized, APO A1 and APO B. APO A1, encoded by a gene located on chromosome 11q23-q24 (MIM#107680; NM_000039.1) is the major component of high-density lipoprotein (HDL) and mediates the efflux of cholesterol from the peripheral cell membranes [191]. APO B, whose gene is located on chromosome 2p24-p23 (MIM#107730; NM_000384.2), is a component of very low-density lipoproteins (VLDL) and low-density lipoproteins (LDL) and plays a role in cholesterol delivery to tissues. The descriptions of a relation between APOs and lipid levels suggested that APOs could be a cardiovascular risk factor. Despite APO A-I and APO B have been described as cardiovascular risk factors [192-193], the relation between these two lipoproteins and stroke is still uncertain. Cristopher et al (1996) [194] and Qureshi et al. 2002 [191] did not find an association between apolipoptoteins A-I and B levels and stroke. However in a recent study Walldius et al. [195] described a link between APOA-I/B ratio and the risk of fatal stroke. Some molecular variants of APOA1, such as c.75G>A and c.83C>T, have been described to determine variations in serum lipids whereas two SNPs in APO B p.Arg3500Gly and c.10800C>T, causing p.Arg353Cys, have been related to Familial hypercholesterolemia phenotype [196]. However the relation between these molecular variants and stroke has never been studied. Thus, it has still to be assessed if APO A1 and APO B variants have a role in pathogenesis of juvenile stroke.

Lipoprotein Lipase (LPL)

Lipoprotein Lipase (LPL) plays a key role in lipid metabolism hydrolyzing triglycerides from chylomicrons and very low-density lipoproteins (VLDL) and removing chylomicron remnants and VLDLs from the circulation (197-198). The LPL gene (MIM#609708; NM_000237.2) is located on chromosome 8p22 and contains 10 exons. A number of studies investigated the relationship between lipid levels and two variants in the human LPL gene, each changing the amino-acid sequence of the LPL protein. Several polymorphisms of theLPL gene such as *Hind* III in intron 8, which identifies a two-allele polymorphism with restriction fragments of 6 kb (Hl) and 11 kb (H2) and *Pvu* II in intron 6 have been associated to high triglycerid levels and coronary artery disease [198-200].

The three LPL polymorphisms most commonly associated with cerebrovascular disease are the stop mutation Ser447Ter in exon 9 (S447X), which results in the generation of a premature stop codon, truncating the last 2 amino acids of the mature LPL protein, c.1127A>G in exon 6 resulting in p.Asn291Ser and p.Asp9Asn. The first, a point mutation (A → G) at nucleotide 1127 in exon 6, results in the N291S variant, and the second is a C → G transversion at nucleotide 1595 in exon 9 that results in the premature truncation of theLPL enzyme by deleting two amino acids (S447X). The S291 allele has been associated with elevated plasma triglycerides and reduced high-density lipoprotein (HDL) cholesterol levels, while the X447 allele has been associated with reduced plasma triglycerides and increased HDL cholesterol levels.

From the analysis of literature, we found only studies including stroke patients, without age subgroup analysis [62, 101, 202-205], which did not give concordant results, probably because of different sample sizes and heterogeneity of phenotypes studied. We did not identify any study specifically conducted on young subjects. A positive association between S447X variant and stroke has been reported only in the prospective cohort study of Morrison et al. 2002 [206] described, evaluating a population of 15792 individuals aged 45-64 years, a positive association between men carriers of S447X and asymptomatic stroke lesions.

In conclusion, there are not enough data to establish if LPL variants increase the risk of ischemic stroke both in young and elderly patients.

Paraoxonase

The paraoxonase (PON) gene family contains at least three related genes, including PON1, PON2 and PON3, which are located on chromosome 7q21.3–22 and share 60–65% similarity at the amino acid level.

The PON1 gene product, the paraoxonase 1 (PON1) is a calcium dependent serum enzyme located on high-density lipoprotein (HDL), which was recently considered to have a role in atherosclerosis and cardiovascular disease. It is associated with apolipoprotein (Apo) A1 in high-density lipoprotein (HDL). PON1 is capable of preventing low-density lipoprotein (LDL) oxidation by hydrolyzing lipid peroxides in the lipoprotein. Therefore, it can reduce the risk of atherosclerosis development. The gene encoding for PON1 is mapped on chromosome 7q21.3 (MIM#168820; NM_000446.3). Two common polymorphisms in the coding region of the PON1 gene are the substitution of glutamine (A allele) to arginine (B allele) at position 192 (p.Glu192Arg) and of Methionine (M allele) to Leucine (L allele) at position 55 (p.Met55Leu). The two polymorphisms are in linkage disequilibrium. More recently five new polymorphic sites of PON1 were detected in the promoter region of PON1 gene: c.107C>T, c.126G>C, c.160G>A, c.824G>A and c.907G>C, variably associated to enzyme serum concentration. Schmidt et al., 1998 [207], as reported by Hassan and Markus 2000 [6], recognized paraoxonase LL genotype as a possible risk factor for carotid atherosclerosis. The studies on strokes [62, 186, 208-215] did not find any conclusive result on the relationship between PON1 variants and stroke. We identified only two case control studies by Voetsch et al., 2002 and 2004 on young stroke patients (Table 6). These authors reported a positive association between the p.Gln192Arg [216] and c.107C>T mutations [217] and stroke in the same population of young strokes, evaluated in two studies respectively.

Table 6. Lipoprotein metabolism polymorphisms

Reference	Type of study	Polymorphism	Subtype of population	Case/ controls	Results OR	95%CI
APO E (ApolipoproteinE)						
Pezzini et al 2005	Case-control	APO ε2/ε3/ε4	First ischemic stroke (45 y.o)	163/158	2.01	1.13-3.571
PON 1 (Paraoxonasi 1)						
Voetsch et al 2002	Case-control	p.Gln192Arg p.Leu55Met	Ischemic stroke (<45 y.o)	118/118	4.1	1.14-14.73
Voetsch et al 2004	Case-control	c.107C>T c. 824G>T	Ischemic stroke (<45y.o)	118/118	2.69	1.06-6.78 2

[1] ε4allele.
[2] R allele.

Genome Wide Studies: Linkage Approach

Phosphodiesterase-4D (PDE4D)

In last years, the DeCode group identified a new locus associated with stroke in the Icelandic stroke population, using a genome-wide linkage analysis through an extensive computerised genealogical database. This locus, mapped on chromosome 5q12 (STRK1), contains the 5' end of the gene PDE4D. The gene PDE4D, composed of 24 exons, encodes for eight isoforms, of the enzyme phosphodiesterase 4D, which is involved in regulation of second messenger cAMP levels (MIM#600129; NM_006203.3), through differential promoter and alternative splicing in gene expression. Low cAMP levels induce cell proliferation and vascular smooth muscle cells migration, while high levels of cAMP, in animal models, prevent neointimal lesions and smooth muscle cell proliferation after vessel injury [218]. Variants or mutations within this gene, according to authors' opinion, could be responsible for stroke susceptibility. In particular, PDE4D genotype has been associated with cardioembolic and atherosclerotic stroke [219-220]. The two most significant variants identified as contributing to an increased stroke risk were the microsatellite AC 008818-1 and the SNP 45 [220-221]. The results of Gretarsdottir et al 2002 and 2003 [219-220] have been criticized not only for the lack of accurate phenotyping but also because the finding was based on a relatively genetically isolated population, possibly having a strong founder effect [218,222].

In the following years, some authors tried to replicate these findings in other cohorts of every age stroke patients of different ethnicity reporting controversial results [218,221,223-231]. A positive association between PDE4D SNPs and stroke has been reported in some cohorts in different non-European countries such as USA, Pakistan, Japan, Australia [221,226, 228-229,231] but these results have not been strongly replicated in Europe where only the study of van Rijn et al. [224] reported a positive association in a small Netherland population. In addiction the heterogeneity of phenotypes associated with PDE4D variants in replication studies has not brought clarification [232]. No studies are available in literature evaluating PDE4D SNPs in young stroke patients except for Song et al 2006 [233] that studying a population of 224 ischemic stroke women aged 15-49 years demonstrated that SNP rs 91852 was significantly associated with all stroke subtypes (OR 1.38, 95%CI 0.99 to 1.9) except for cardioembolic stroke. This association was similar across African Americans and Caucasians.

A recent meta-analysis by Bevan et al 2008 [234] concluded that no genetic variant in PDE4D showed a robust and reproducible association with ischemic stroke and that any reported association is likely to be weak and restricted to specific population. In consideration of the lack of data on juvenile stroke and of the results of this recent paper it could be interesting to assess the role of PDE4D SNPs in the subgroup of young stroke patients.

5-Lipoxygenase-Activating-Protein

Another susceptibility locus predisposing to myocardial infarction and stroke has been identified, from the DeCode group, in Icelandic population on chromosome 13q12, through linkage studies [235]. The candidate gene was the ALOX5AP that encodes for 5-lipoxygenase-activating protein (FLAP), which converts unesterified arachidonic acid to leukotriens [236] (MIM#603700; NM_001629.2). It is well known that leukotriens promote leukocytes adhesion to vascular endothelium and chemotaxis (LTB4) and induce capillary permeability and vasoconstriction (LTC4, LTD4, LTE4). Leukotriens have been implicated in critical stages of atherosclerosis, both in animal models [237] and in human studies [238]. An haplotype of ALOX5AP (Hap A), defined by four SNPs (SG13S25, SG13S114-rs 10507391, SG13S89-rs4769874, SG13S32) in the first four exons, has been recognized as the most strongly associated with stroke and myocardial infarction. From the first description of Helgadottir et al. 2004 [235], who reported a 1.67 fold increase risk of stroke in Icelandics HapA carriers, further linkage and association studies evaluating this relationship in every age stroke patients were published [221, 225, 228, 239, 240]. Of these only Helgadottir et al. 2005 [239] replicated the association between HAP A and stroke in a Scottish population from Aberdeenshire and more recently Kaushal et al. 2007 [240] reported an association between two SNPs (SG13S106-rs9579646; SG13S89-rs4769874) and white stroke patients. No studies were conducted specifically on young stroke patients.

In conclusion studies specifically conducted on youngs and in populations belonging to different countries are necessary to assess the validity of this association in young stroke patient and to exclude the possible founder effect of some ethnic groups.

Conclusions

In this chapter we explored, in patients younger than 50 years, the role in stroke occurrence of a wide number of candidate genes and for each of them several polymorphisms. We found a total of 9 polymorphisms of 7 candidate genes possibly associated with an increased risk of stroke in youngs and worthy of deeper evaluation in further studies. Out of the other SNPs associated with stroke in literature, in 24 cases we did not find any studies evaluating the association with juvenile stroke and in 19 cases the association was not demonstrated by consistent data or was uncertain. These results are reported in Table 7.

The complexity of this reviewing work is related both to the lack of data on young subjects and to wide heterogeneity between data published due to the different populations studied, inadequate sample sizes and unselected phenotypes. Similar difficulties on reviewing studies on genetics of stroke were described by other authors [12, 232]. On this topic, Dichgans et al. [13] provided some guidelines to implement detailed and properly conducted large-scale association studies. Some other authors underlined the difficulty in assigning a causality role to polymorphisms for the multifactorial nature of the stroke pathogenesis, where many genetic variants could contribute together with environmental and other genes interactions [8,14]. Moreover some genetic factors such as the ones involved in lipoproteins metabolism or renin-angiotensin-aldosterone system could act indirectly through the influence of the common cerebrovascular risk factors.

However, although a consistent association with stroke, and even less for juvenile stroke, has been provided by studies conducted so far only for few candidate genes, some of them, particularly the ones related to trombophilia, are currently considered among the stroke non-modifiable risk factors [241], mostly in childhood and youngs. This fact is probably consequence of the difficulty in finding stroke aetiology in youngs despite extensive investigations and is supported by the evidences that genetic factors have more influence in young age. However, clinicians should careful evaluate which genetic test to administer to patients and above all which is the clinical implication of the results of genetic screening in terms of stroke management and treatment, since it is not supported by clear scientific evidence.

Despite we performed a comprehensive review on molecular variants associated with juvenile stroke, we decided to not combine the results into a meta-analysis, for which further work should be developed.

Otherwise, our analysis of literature could be relevant in addressing future association studies towards the candidate-genes SNPs, which seem more likely related to stroke in youngs. Advanced research approaches suggest the need of confirmation of associations

Table 7. Final panel of genetic factors with different degree of association with stroke

Type of Factor	Factor	Gene	Polymorphisms	Association
Coagulation system	*Factor V Leiden*	*F5*	c.1691G>A	Possible
			c.4070A>G	Not demonstrated
	Phrothrombin	F2	c.20210G>A	Possible
	Fibrinogen	FGA	c.4266A>G	No studies
		FGB	c.148C>T	No studies
			c.455G>A	Not demonstrated
	Factor VII	F7	A1/A2	No studies
			c.10976G>A	Not demonstrated
			c.323_324insCCTATATCT	No studies
			c. 402G>A	No studies
			c. 401G>T	No studies
	Factor XIII	F13A1	c. 143G>T	Uncertain
			p. Pro564Leu	Uncertain
	Von Willebrand factor	vWF	Sma I	Uncertain
			c.1423C>T	No studies
			c.1793C>G	Not demonstrated
	Factor XII	F12	c.46C>T	Uncertain
Fibrinolitic system	Plasminogen activator inhibitor 1	SERPINE-1	c.675_676delinsG	Uncertain
			c.1053 G>T	No studies
Platelet receptor	GpIIb–IIIa complex	ITGB3	GPIIIa PLA2	Possible
			GPIIIa c.1691G>A	No studies
		ITGA2B	GPIIb HPA-3	No studies
			GPIIb p.Ile843Ser	Not demonstrated
	Gp Ia-IIa Complex	ITGA2	GPIa c.807C>T	Not demonstrated
			GPIa c. 873 G>A	Not demonstrated
	GpIb/IX/V Complex	GP1BA	HPA2 c. 3550 C>T	Possible
			VNTR	No studies
			GPIb (-5) T/C Kozak	Not demonstrated
Renin-angiotensin-aldosterone system	ACE	ACE	g.11417_11704del287	Not demonstrated
	Angiotensinogen	AGT	p.Met174Thr	No studies
			p.Met235Thr	No studies
Homocysteine & eNOS methabolism	eNOS	NOS3	g.3726_3834insGAAGTCTAGACC TGCTGCGGGGGTGAG	Uncertain
			c.894G>T	Not demonstrated
			c.786T>C	Uncertain
	Hcy	MTHFR	MTHFR c.677C>T	Possible
			MTHFR c.1298A>C	Not demonstrated
		CBS	CBS c.844ins68	Not demonstrated
			CBS c.833T>C	No studies
		MTR	MTR c.2756 A>G	No studies
Lypoprotein metabolism	APOE	APO ε2/ε3/ε4	□□□□□□	Possible
			p. Cys112Arg	No studies
			p. Arg158Cys	No studies
	LPL	LPL	S447X	No studies
			p.Asp9Asn	No studies
			c.1127A>G	No studies
			c. 93 C>T	No studies
	PON1	PON1	p.Gln192Arg	Possible
			p. Leu55Met	Possible
			c.107 C>T	Possible
Linkage-association studies	PDE4D	PDE4D	SNP 39-44-56-83-87-89	No studies
	5-LIPOXYGENASE-ACTIVATING-PROTEIN	ALOX5AP	HAP A	No studies
			SG13S106- SG13S89	No studies

between molecular variants and stroke, performing replication studies on independent cohorts [14]. However, since multiple genetic factors could be involved in pathogenesis of stroke, new prospective could derive from the development of high-throughput genomic technologies such as genome-wide assays (GWA), which allows to identify contemporarily multiple SNPs across genome acting together in the genesis of stroke [242-243]. This approach has been recently validated by a big GWA association study, exploring some epidemiologically important complex diseases in British population, which provided also methodological insights relevant to the pursuit of new GWA studies [244].

References

[1] Hart RG, Miller VT. Cerebral infarction in young adults: A practical approach. *Stroke* 1983; 14: 110-114.

[2] Bogousslavsky J, Pierre P. Ischemic stroke in patients under age 45. *Neurol. Clin.* 1992; 10: 113-124.

[3] Bak S, Gaist D, Sindrup SH, Skytthe A, Christensen K.Genetic liability in stroke: a long-term follow-up study of Danish twins.*Stroke* 2002;33:769-774.

[4] Liao D, Myers R, Hunt S, Shahar E, Paton C, Burke G, Province M, Heiss G. Familial history of stroke and stroke risk. The Family Heart Study. *Stroke* 1997 ;28:1908-1912.

[5] Jeffs B, Clark JS, Anderson NH, Gratton J, Brosnan MJ, Gauguier D, Reid JL, Macrae IM, Dominiczak AF.Sensitivity to cerebral ischaemic insult in a rat model of stroke is determined by a single genetic locus. *Nat. Genet.* 1997;16:364-367.

[6] Markus H. Stroke Genetics.Oxford University Press, 2003

[7] Hassan A, Markus HS. Genetics and ischaemic stroke. *Brain* 2000; 123:1784-1812.

[8] Jerrard-Dunne P, Cloud G, Hassan A, Markus HS. Evaluating the genetic component of ischemic stroke subtypes: a family history study. *Stroke* 2003 ;34:1364-1369.

[9] Rubattu S, Giliberti R, Volpe M. Etiology and pathophysiology of stroke as a complex trait. *Am. J. Hypertens*. 2000; 13:1139-1148.

[10] Markus H. Genes for stroke. *J. Neurol. Neurosurg. Psychiatry* 2004; 75:1229-1231.

[11] Meschia JF, Brott TG, Brown RD Genetics of cerebrovascular Disorders. *Mayo Clin. Proc.* 2005; 80:122-132

[12] Flossmann E, Schulz UG, Rothwell PM. Systematic review of methods and results of studies of the genetic epidemiology of ischemic stroke. *Stroke* 2004; 35:212-227

[13] Dichgans M, Markus HS. Genetic association studies in stroke: methodological issues and proposed standard criteria. *Stroke* 2005; 36: 2027-2031

[14] Dichgans M. Genetics of ischaemic stroke. *Lancet Neurol.* 2007;6:149-161.

[15] Casas JP, Hingorami AD, Bautista LE, Sharma P. Meta-analysis of Genetic Studies in Ischemic stroke. *Arch Neurol.* 2004; 61:1652-1662.

[16] Bersano A, Ballabio E, Bresolin N, Candelise L.Genetic polymorphisms for the study of multifactorial stroke. *Hum. Mutat.* 2008, Apr 17.

[17] Johan T. den Dunnen Stylianos E. Antonarakis Mutation Nomenclature Extensions and Suggestion to Describe Complex Mutations: A Discussion. *Human. Mutation* 2000; 15: 7-12

[18] Kalafatis M, Rand MD, Mann Kg. The mechanism of inactivation of human factor V and human factor Va by activated protein C. *J. Biol. Chem*. 1994; 269: 31869-31880.

[19] Monkovic DD, Tracy PB. Activation of human factor V by factor Xa and thrombin. *Biochemistry* 1990;29:1118– 1128.

[20] Dahlback B, Carlsson M, Svensson PJ. Familial thrombophilia due to a previously unrecognized mechanism characterized by poor anticoagulant response to activated protein C: prediction of a cofactor to activated protein C. *Proc. Natl. Acad. Sci. USA* 1993;90:1004–1008.

[21] Sykes TCF, Fegan C, Mosquera D. Thrombophilia, polymorphisms, and vascular disease. *Mol. Pathol*. 2000; 53:300-306.

[22] Endler G, Mannhalter C. Polymorphisms in coagulation factors genes and thier impact on arterial and venous thombosis. *Clinica Chimica Acta* 2003; 330: 31-55.

[23] Juul K, Tybjærg-Hansen A, Steffensen R, Kofoed S, Jensen G, Nordestgaard BG. Factor V Leiden: the Copenaghen City Heart Study and 2 meta-analyses. *Blood* 2002; 100: 3-10.

[24] Landi G, Cella E, Martinelli I, Tagliabue L, Mannucci PM, Zerbi D. Arg506Gln factor V mutation and cerebral ischemia in the young. *Stroke* 1996;27:1697-1698.

[25] Bentolila S, Ripoll L, Drouet L, Mazoyer E, Woimant F.Thrombophilia due to 20210 G-->A prothrombin polymorphism and cerebral ischemia in the young. *Stroke* 1997;28:1846-1847.

[26] Iniesta JA, Corral J, Fernández-Pardo J, González-Conejero R, Vicente V. Factor-V (Arg506 --> Gln) mutation in ischemic cerebrovascular disease. *Haemostasis* 1997; 27:105-111.

[27] Longstreth WT Jr, Rosendaal FR, Siscovick DS, Vos HL, Schwartz SM, Psaty BM, Raghunathan TE, Koepsell TD, Reitsma PH.Risk of stroke in young women and two prothrombotic mutations: factor V Leiden and prothrombin gene variant (G20210A). *Stroke* 1998;29:577-580.

[28] Nabavi DG, Junker R, Wolff E, Lüdemann P, Doherty C, Evers S, Droste DW, Kessler C, Assmann G, Ringelstein EB. Prevalence of factor V Leiden mutation in young adults with cerebral ischaemia: a case-control study on 225 patients. *J. Neurol.* 1998; 245:653-658.

[29] De Stefano V, Chiusolo P, Paciaroni K, Casorelli I, Rossi E, Molinari M, Servidei S, Tonali PA, Leone G. Prothrombin G20210A mutant genotype is a risk factor for cerebrovascular ischemic disease in young patients. *Blood* 1998 ;91:3562-3565.

[30] Margaglione M, D'Andrea G, Giuliani N, Brancaccio V, De Lucia D, Grandone E, De Stefano V, Tonali PA, Di Minno G.Inherited prothrombotic conditions and premature ischemic stroke: sex difference in the association with factor V Leiden. *Arterioscler. Thromb Vasc. Biol.* 1999 ;19:1751-1756.

[31] Heller C, Becker S, Scharrer I, Kreuz W. Prothrombotic risk factors in childhood stroke and venous thrombosis. *Eur. J. Pediatr.* 1999;158 Suppl 3:S117-121.

[32] Nowak-Göttl U, Sträter R, Heinecke A, Junker R, Koch HG, Schuierer G, von Eckardstein A. Lipoprotein (a) and genetic polymorphisms of clotting factor V, prothrombin, and methylenetetrahydrofolate reductase are risk factors of spontaneous ischemic stroke in childhood. *Blood* 1999;94:3678-82.

[33] Kenet G, Sadetzki S, Murad H, Martinowitz U, Rosenberg N, Gitel S, Rechavi G, Inbal A. Factor V Leiden and antiphospholipid antibodies are significant risk factors for ischemic stroke in children. *Stroke* 2000;31:1283-1288.

[34] Akar N, Akar E, Yilmaz E. Coexistence of factor V 1691 G-A and factor V 4070 A-G mutation in turkish thromboembolic patients. *Am. J. Hematol.* 2000; 65:88.

[35] Voetsch B, Damasceno BP, Camargo EC, Massaro A, Bacheschi LA, Scaff M, Annichino-Bizzacchi JM, Arruda VR.Inherited thrombophilia as a risk factor for the development of ischemic stroke in young adults. *Thromb Haemost.* 2000;83:229-233.

[36] Lopaciuk S, Bykowska K, Kwiecinski H, Mickielewicz A, Czlonkowska A, Mendel T, Kuczynska-Zardzewialy A, Szelagowska D, Windyga J, Schröder W, Herrmann FH, Jedrzejowska H. Factor V Leiden, prothrombin gene G20210A variant, and methylenetetrahydrofolate reductase C677T genotype in young adults with ischemic stroke. *Clin. Appl. Thromb Hemost.* 2001;7:346-350.

[37] Grossmann R, Geisen U, Merati G, Műllges W, Schambeck CM, Walter U, Schwender S. Genetic risk factors in young adults with ‚cryptogenic' ischemic cerebrovascular disease. *Blood Coagulation and Fibrinolysis* 2002; 13: 583-590.

[38] Madonna P, de Stefano V, Coppola A, Cirillo F, Cerbone AM, Orefice G, Di Minno G. Hyperhomocysteinemia and other inherited prothrombotic conditions in young adults with a history of ischemic stroke. *Stroke* 2002 ;33:51-56.

[39] Pezzini A, Del Zotto E, Magoni M, Costa A, Archetti S, Grassi M, Akkawi NM, Albertini A, Assanelli D, Vignolo LA, Padovani A. Inherited thrombophilic disorders in young adults with ischemic stroke and patent foramen ovale. *Stroke* 2003;34:28-33.

[40] Aznar J, Mira Y, Vaya A, Corella D, Ferrando F, Villa P, Estelles A. Factor V Leiden and prothrombin G20210A mutations in young adults with cryptogenetic ischemic stroke. *Thromb Haemost.* 2004; 91:1031-1034.

[41] Slooter AJ, Rosendaal FR, Tanis BC, Kemmeren JM, van der Graaf Y, Algra . Prothrombotic conditions, oral contraceptives, and the risk of ischemic stroke. *J. Thromb Haemost.* 2005;3:1213-1217.

[42] de Paula Sabino A, Ribeiro DD, Carvalho MG, Cardoso J, Dusse LM, Fernandes AP. Factor V Leiden and increased risk for arterial thrombotic disease in young Brazilian patients.*Blood Coagul. Fibrinolysis* 2006 ;17:271-275.

[43] Komitopoulou A, Platokouki H, Kapsimali Z, Pergantou H, Adamtziki E, Aronis S. Mutations and polymorphisms in genes affecting hemostasis proteins and homocysteine metabolism in children with arterial ischemic stroke. *Cerebrovasc. Dis.* 2006; 22:13-20.

[44] Botto N, Spadoni I, Giusti S, Ait-Ali L, Sicari R, Andreassi MG.Prothrombotic mutations as risk factors for cryptogenic ischemic cerebrovascular events in young subjects with patent foramen ovale. *Stroke* 2007 Jul;38:2070-2073.

[45] Pezzini A, Grassi M, Iacoviello L, Del Zotto E, Archetti S, Giossi A, Padovani A. Inherited thrombophilia and stratification of ischaemic stroke risk among users of oral contraceptives. *J. Neurol. Neurosurg. Psychiatry* 2007; 78: 271-276.

[46] Haywood S, Liesner R, Pindora S, Ganesan V.Thrombophilia and first arterial ischaemic stroke: a systematic review. *Arch Dis. Child* 2005;90:402-425.

[47] Poort SR, Rosendaal FR, Reitsma PH, Bertina RM. A common genetic variation in the 3'untraslated region of the prothrombin gene is associated to an elevated plasma prothrombin level and an increase in venous thrombosis. *Blood* 1996; 88:3698-3703.
[48] Gehring NH, Frede U, Neu-Yilik G, et al. Increased efficiency of mRNA 30 end formation: a new genetic mechanism contributing to hereditary thrombophilia. *Nat. Genet.* 2001;28:389–392
[49] Soria JM, Almasy L, Souto JC, et al. Linkage analysis demonstrates that the prothrombin G20210A mutation jointly influences plasma prothrombin levels and risk of thrombosis. *Blood* 2000;95:2780–2785
[50] Girolami A, Simioni P, Scarano L, Carraro G. Prothrombin and the prothrombin 20210 G to A polymorphism: thei relationship with hypercoagulability and thrombosis. *Blood Reviews* 1999; 13: 205-210.
[51] Wilhelmsen L, Svardsudd K, Korsan-Bengtsen K, Larsson B, Welin L, Tibblin G. Fibrinogen as a risk factor for stroke and myocardial infarction. *N. Engl. J. Med.* 1984; 31: 501-505.
[52] Collet JP, Soria J, Mirshahi M, Hirsch M, Dagonnet FB, Caen J, Soria C. Dusart syndrome: a new concept of the relationship between fibrin clot architecture and fibrin clot degradability: hypofibrinolysis related to an abnormal clot structure. *Blood* 1993;82:2462–2469.
[53] Kessler C, Spitzer C, Stauske D, Mende S, Stadlmuller J, Walther R, Rettig R. The apolipoprotein E and beta-fibrinogen G/A-455 gene polymorphisms are associated with ischemic stroke involving large-vessel disease. *Arterioscler. Thromb Vasc. Biol.* 1997; 17: 2880-2884.
[54] Schmidt H, Schmidt R, Niederkorn K, Gradert A, Schumacher M, Watzinger N, et al. Paraoxonase PON1 polymorphism leu-Met54 is associated with carotid atherosclerosis: results of the Austrian Stroke Prevention Study. *Stroke* 1998; 29:2043-2048.
[55] Carter AM, Catto AJ, Grant PJ. Association of the alpha –fibrinogen Thr312Ala polymorphism with poststroke mortality in subject with atrial fibrillation. *Circulation* 1999; 99: 2423-2426.
[56] Rubattu S, Di Angelantonio E, Nitsch D, Gigante B, Zanda B, Stanzione R, Evangelista A, Pirisi A, Rosati G, Volpe M. Polymorphism in prothrombotic genes and their impact on ischemic stroke in a Sardinian population. *Thromb Haemost.* 2005; 93:1095-1100.
[57] Voetsch B, Loscalzo J. Genetic determinants of arterial thrombosis. *Arterioscler. Thromb Vasc. Biol.* 2004;24:216-229
[58] Lane DA., Grant PJ. Role of hemostatic gene polymorphisms in venous and arterial thrombotic disease. *Blood* 2000; 95: 1517-1532.
[59] Doggen CJ, Manger Cats V, Bertina RM, Reitsma PH, Vandenbroucke JP, Rosendaal FR. A genetic propensity to higher factor VII is not associated with the risk of myocardial infarction in men. *Thromb Haemost.* 1998; 80: 281-285.
[60] Heywood DM, Carter AM, Catto Aj, Bamford JM, Grant PJ. Polymorphisms of the factor VII gene and circulating FVII: C levels in relation to acute cerebrovascular disease and poststrokemortality. *Stroke* 1997: 28: 816-821.

[61] Petrovic D, Milanez T, Kobal J, Bregar D, Potisk KP, Peterlin B. Prothrombotic gene polymorphisms and atherothrombotic cerebral infarction. *Acta Neurol. Scand.* 2003; 108: 109-113

[62] Berger K, Stogbauer F, Stoll M, Wellmann J, Huge A, Cheng S, Kessler C, John U, Assmann G, Ringelstein EB, Funke H. The glu298asp polymorphism in the nitric oxide synthase 3 gene is associated with the risk of ischemic stroke in two large independent case-control studies. *Hum. Genet.* 2007; 121:169-178.

[63] Yeh PS, Lin HJ, Li YH, Lin KC, Cheng TJ, Chang CY, Ke DS. Prognosis of young ischemic stroke in Taiwan: impact of prothrombotic genetic polymorphism. *Thromb Haemost.* 2004; 92: 583-589.

[64] Ariens RA, Lai TS, Weisel JW, Greenberg CS, Grant PJ. Role of factor XIII in fibrin clot formation and effects of genetic polymorphisms. *Blood* 2002;100:743–754

[65] Anwar R, Gallivan L, Edmonds SD, Markham AF.Genotype/phenotype correlations for coagulation factor XIII: specific normal polymorphisms are associated with high or low factor XIII specific activity. *Blood* 1999; 93:897-905.

[66] Franco RF, Pazin-Filho A, Tavella MH, Simoes MV, Marin-Neto JA, Zago MA Factor XIII val34leu and the risk of myocardial infarction. *Haematologica* 2000; 85: 67-71.

[67] Kohler HP, Ariens RA, Whitaker P, Grant PJ. A common coding polymorphism in the FXIII A-subunit gene (FXIIIVal34Leu) affects cross-linking activity. *Thromb Haemost.* 1998; 80: 704.

[68] Catto AJ, Kohler HP, Bannan S, Stickland M, Carter A, Grant PJ. Factor XIII Val 34 Leu: a novel association with primary intracerebral hemorrhage. *Stroke* 1998; 29: 813–816.

[69] Gonzalez-Conejero R, Fernandez-Cadenas I, Iniesta JA, Marti-Fabregas J, Obach V, Alvarez-Sabin J, Vicente V, Corral J, Montaner J; Proyecto Ictus Research Group. Role of fibrinogen levels and factor XIII V34L polymorphism in thrombolytic therapy in stroke patients. *Stroke* 2006; 37: 2288-2293.

[70] Corral J, Gonzaàlez-Conejero R, Iniesta JA, Rivera J, Martinez C, Vincente V. The FXIII Val34Leu polymorphism in venous and arterial thromboembolism. *Haematologica* 2000; 85: 293-297.

[71] Elbaz A, Poirier O, Canple S, Chédru F, Cambien F, Amarenco P on behalf of the GENIC investigators. The association between the Val34Leu polymorphism in the factor XIII gene and brain infarction. *Blood* 2000; 95: 586-591.

[72] Slowik A, Dziedzic T,Pera J, Figlewicz DA, Szezudlik A. Coagulation factor XIII VaI34Leu polymorphism in patients with small vessel disease or primary intracerebral hemorrhage.*Cerebrovasc. Dis*. 2005;19:165-170.

[73] Reiner AP, Schwartz SM, Frank MB, Longstreth WT Jr, Hindorff LA, Teramura G, Rosendaal FR, Gaur LK, Psaty BM, Siscovick DS.Polymorphisms of coagulation factor XIII subunit A and risk of nonfatal hemorrhagic stroke in young white women. *Stroke* 2001 ;32:2580-2586.

[74] Reiner AP, Frank MB, Schwartz SM, Linenberger ML, Longstreth WT, Teramura G, Rosendaal FR, Psaty BM, Siscovick DS. Coagulation factor XIII polymorphisms and the risk of myocardial infarction and ischaemic stroke in young women. *Br. J. Haematol.* 2002; 116: 376-382.

[75] Pruissen DM, Slooter AJ, Rosendaal FR, van der Graaf Y, Algra A. Coagulation factor XIII gene variation, oral contraceptives, and risk of ischemic stroke. *Blood* 2008;111:1282-1286.

[76] Koppelman SJ, van Hoeij M, Vink T. Lankhof H, Schiphorst ME, Damas C, et al. Requirements of von Willebrand factor to protect factor VIII from inactivation by activated protein C. *Blood* 1996;87:2292–2300.

[77] Blann AD, McCollum CN.von Willebrand factor and soluble thrombomodulin as predictors of adverse events among subjects with peripheral or coronary atherosclerosis. *Blood Coagul. Fibrinolysis* 1999;10:375-380.

[78] Lacquemant C, Gaucher C, Delorme C, Chatellier G, Galois Y, Rodier M, Passa P, Balkau B, Mazurier C, Marre M, Froguel P. Association between high von willebrand factors levels and the Thr789Ala vWF gene polymorphism but not with nephropathy in type I diabetes. The GENEDIAB Study Group and the DESIR Study Group. *Kidney Int.* 2000; 57:1437-1443.

[79] Dai K, Gao W, Ruan C.The Sma I polymorphism in the von Willebrand factor gene associated with acute ischemic stroke. *Thromb Res.* 2001;104:389-395.

[80] Halbmayer WM, Mannhalter C, Feichtinger C, Rubi K, Fischer M. The prevalence of factor XII deficiency in 103 orally anticoagulated outpatients suffering from recurrent venous and/or arterial thromboembolism. *Thromb Haemost.* 1992;68:285–290.

[81] Halbmayer WM, Mannhalter C, Feichtinger C, Rubi K,Fischer M. Factor XII (Hageman factor) deficiency: a risk factor for development of thromboembolism. Incidence offactor XII deficiency in patients after recurrent venous orarterial thromboembolism and myocardial infarction. *Wien Med. Wochenschr* 1993;143:43–50.

[82] Kanaji T, Okamura T, Osaki K, Kuroiwa M, Shimoda K, Hamasaki N, Niho Y. A common gene polymorphism (46 C to T substitution) in the 5' untraslated region of the coagulation factor XII gene is associated with low translation efficacy and decrease in plasma factor XII level. *Blood* 1998; 91:2010-2014.

[83] Kanaji T, Okamura T, Osaki K, Kuroiwa M, Shimoda K, Hamasaki N, Niho Y. A common gene polymorphism (46 C to T substitution) in the 5' untraslated region of the coagulation factor XII gene is associated with low translation efficacy and decrease in plasma factor XII level. *Blood* 1998; 91:2010-2014.

[84] Zeerleder S, Schloesser M, Redondo M, Wuillemin WA, Engel W, Furlan M. Reevaluation of The Incidence of Throembolic Complications in Congenital factor XII Deficiency-A study on 73 Subjects from 14 Swiss Families.*Thromb Haemost.* 1999; 82: 1240-1246

[85] Zito F, Lowe GD, Rumley A, McMahon AD, Humphries SE; WOSCOPS Study Group West of Scotland Coronary Prevention Study.Association of the factor XII 46C>T polymorphism with risk of coronary heart disease (CHD) in the WOSCOPS study. *Atherosclerosis* 2002; 165: 153-158.

[86] Oguchi S, Ito D, Murata M, Yoshida T, Tananashi N, Fukuuchi Y, Ikeda Y, Watanabe K. Genotype Distribution of the 46C/T Polymorphism of Coagulation Factor XII in the Japanese Population: Absence of Its Association with Ischemic Cerebrovascular Disease. *Thromb Haemost.* 2000; 83:178-179.

[87] Santamaria A, Mateo J, Tirado I, Oliver A, Belvis R, Marti-Fabregas J, Felices R, Soria JM, Souto JC, Fontcuberta J. Homozygosity of the T allele of the 46 C->T polymorphism in the F12 gene is a risk factor for ischemic stroke in the Spanish population. *Stroke* 2004; 35:1795-1799.

[88] Vague P, Juhan-Vague I, Aillaud MF, Badier C, Viard R, Alessi MC, Collen D.Correlation between blood fibrinolytic activity, plasminogen activator inhibitor level, plasma insulin level, and relative body weight in normal and obese subjects. *Metabolism* 1986;35:250-253.

[89] Ridker PM, Vaughan DE, Stampfer MJ, Manson JE, Hennekens CH. Endogenous tissue-type plasminogen activator and risk of myocardial infarction. *Lancet* 1993;341:1165-1168.

[90] Schneiderman J, Sawdey MS, Keeton MR, Bordin GM, Bernstein EF, Dilley RB, Loskutoff DJ. Increased type I plasminogen activator inhibitor gene expression in atherosclerotic human arteries. *Proc. Natl. Acad. Sci.* 1992; 89: 6998-7002.

[91] Thogersen AM, Jansson JH, Boman K, Nilsson TK, Weinehall L, Huhtasaari F, Hallmans G. High plasminogen activator inhibitor and tissue plasminogen activator levels in plasma precede a first acute myocardial infarction in both men and women: evidence for the fibrinolytic system as an independent primary risk factor. *Circulation* 1998; 98:2241-2247.

[92] Reiner AP, Siscovick DS, Rosendaal FR. Hemostatic risk factors and arterial thrombotic disease. *Thromb Haemost*. 2001; 85: 584-595.

[93] Boekholdt SM, Bijsterveld NR, Moons AH, Levi M, Buller HR, Peters RJ. Genetic variation in coagulation and fibrinolytic proteins and their relation with acute myocardial infarction: a systematic review. *Circulation* 2001; 104:3063-3068.

[94] Doggen CJ, Bertina RM, Cats VM, Reitsma PH, Rosendaal FR. The 4G/5G polymorphism in the plasminogen activator inhibitor-1 gene is not associated with myocardial infarction. *Thromb Haemost*. 1999; 82:115-120.

[95] Ye S, Green FR, Scarabin PY, Nicaud V, Bara L, Dawson SJ, Humphries SE, Evans A, Luc G, Cambou JP, et al The 4G/5G genetic polymorphism in the promoter of the plasminogen activator inhibitor-1 (PAI-1) gene is associated with differences in plasma PAI-1 activity but not with risk of myocardial infarction in the ECTIM study. Etude CasTemoins de l'Infarctus du Myocarde. *Thromb Haemost*. 1995. 74: 837-841

[96] Catto AJ, Carter AM, Stickland M, Bamford JM, Davies JA, Grant PJ. Plasminogen activator inhibitor-1 (PAI-1) 4G/5G promoter polymorphism and levels in subjects with cerebrovascular disease. *Thromb Haemost*. 1997; 77:730-734

[97] Akar N, Akar E, Yilmaz E, Deda G. Plasminogen activator inhibitor -1 4G/5G polymorphism in Turkish children with cerebral infarct and effect on factor V 1691 A mutation. *J. Chil. Neurol*. 2001; 16: 294-295.

[98] Cheng CH, Eng HL, Chang CJ, Tsai TT, Lai ML, Chen HY, Liu Cj, Lin TM. 4G/5G promoter polymorphism of plasminogen activator inhibitor -1, lipid profiles, and ischemic stroke. *J. Lab. Clin. Med*. 2003; 142:100-105.

[99] van Goor MPJ, Gomez-Garcia EB, Leebek FWG, Brouwers GJ, Koudstaal PJ, Dippel DWJ. The -148 C/T fibrinogen gene polymorphism and fibrinogen levels in ischaemic stroke: a case- control study. *J. Neurol. Neurosurg. Psychiatry* 2005; 76:121-123.

[100]Jood K, Ladenvall P, Tjarnlund-Wolf A, Ladenvall C, Andersson M, Nilsson S, Blomstrand C, Jern C. Fibrinolytic gene polymorphism and ischemic stroke. *Stroke* 2005 ;36:2077-2081.

[101]Lalouschek W, Endler G, Schillinger M, Hsieh K, Lang W, Cheng S, Bauer P, Wagner O, Mannhalter C. Candidate Genetic Risk Factors of Stroke: Results of a Multilocus Genotyping Assay. *Clin. Chem.* 2007 ;53(4):600-605.

[102]Bang CO, Park HK, Ahn MY, Shin HK, Hwang KY, Homg SY. 4G/5G polymorphism of the plasminogen activator inhibitor -1 gene and insertion/deletion polymorphism of the tissue type plasminogen activator gene in atherothrombotic stroke. *Cerebrov Dis.* 2001; 11: 294-299.

[103]Wiklund PG, Nilsson L, Ardnor SN, Eriksson P, Johansson L, Stegmayr B, Hamsten A, Holmberg D, Asplund K. Plasminogen activator inhibitor-1 4G/5G polymorphism and risk of stroke: replicated findings in two nested case-control studies based on independent cohorts.*Stroke* 2005; 36:1661-1665.

[104]Roest M, van der Schouw YT, Banga jD, Tempelman MJ, de Groot PG, Sixma JJ, Grobbeee DE. Plasminogen Activator Inhibitor 4G Polymorphism Is Associated With Decreased Risk of Cerebrovascular Mortality in Older Women. *Circulation* 2000; 101: 67-70.

[105]Boncoraglio GB, Bodini A, Brambilla C, Carriero MR, Ciusani E, Parati EA. An effect of the PAI-1 4G/5G polymorphism on cholesterol levels may explain conflicting associations with myocardial infarction and stroke. *Cerebrovasc. Dis.* 2006; 22:191-195.

[106]Ding J, Nicklas BJ, Fallin MD, de Rekeneire N, Kritchevsky SB, Pahor M, Rodondi N, Li R, Zmuda JM, Harris TB. Plasminogen activator inhibitor type 1 gene polymorphisms and haplotypes are associated with plasma plasminogen activator inhibitor type 1 levels but not with myocardial infarction or stroke. *Am. Heart J.* 2006;152:1109-1115.

[107]Akar N, Akar E, Yilmaz E, Deda G.Plasminogen activator inhibitor-1 4G/5G polymorphism in Turkish children with cerebral infarct and effect on factor V 1691 A mutation. *J. Child Neurol.* 2001;16:294-295.

[108]Nowak-Gottl U, Strater R, Kosch A, von Eckadstein A, Schobess R, Luigs P, Nabel P, Vielhaber H, Kurnik K, Junker R. The plasminogen activator inhibitor (PAI)-1 promoter 4G/4G genotype is not associated with ischemic stroke in a population of German children. Childhood Stroke Study Group. *Eur. J. Haematol.* 2001; 66:57-62

[109]Hindorff LA, Schwartz SM, Siscovick DS, Psaty BM, Longstreth WT Jr, Reiner AP. The association of PAI-1 promoter 4G/5G insertion/deletion polymorphism with myocardial infarction and stroke in young women. *J. Cardiovasc. Risk* 2002; 9:131-137.

[110]Honda S, Honda Y, Bauer B, Ruan C, Kunicki TJ. The impact of three dimensional structure on the expression of PlA alloantigen oh human integrin beta 3. *Blood* 1995; 86: 234-242.

[111]Di Castelnuovo A, de Gaetano G, Benedetti Donati M, Iacoviello L. Platelet Glycoprotein Receptor IIIa Polymorphism PlA2/Pl A2 and Coronary Risk: a Meta-Analysis. *Thromb Haemost*. 2001; 85: 626-633.

[112]Ridker PM, Hennekens CH, Schmitz C, Stampfer MJ, Lindpaintner. PIA1/A2 polymorphism of platelet glycoprotein IIIa and risks of myocardial infarction, stroke, and venous thrombosis. *Lancet* 1997; 349: 385-388.
[113]Yee DL, Bray PF. Clinical and Funcional Consequences of Platelet Membrane Glycoprotein Polymorphisms. *Seminars in Thrombosis and Hemostasis* 2004; 30: 591-600.
[114]Wu AH, Tsongalis GJ. Correlation of polymorphism to coagulation and biochemical risk factors for cardiovascular diseases. *Am. J. Cardiol.* 2001; 87:1361-1366
[115]Meiklejohn DJ, Vickers MA, Morrison ER, Dijkhuisen R, Moore I, Urbaniak SJ, Greaves M. In vivo platelet activation in atherothrombotic stroke is not determined by polymorphisms of human platelet glycoprotein IIIa or Ib. *Br. J. Haematol.* 2001; 112: 621-31
[116]Slowik A, Dziedzic T, Turaj W, Pera J, Glodzik-Sobanska L, Szermer P, Malecki MT, Figlewicz DA, Szezudlik A. A2 Allele of GpIIIa Gene Is a Risk Factor for stroke Caused by large –Vessel Disease in Males. *Stroke* 2004; 35:1589-1593.
[117]Lanni F, Santulli G, Izzo R, Rubattu S, Zanda B, Volpe M, Iaccarino G, Trimarco B.The Pl(A1/A2) polymorphism of glycoprotein IIIa and cerebrovascular events in hypertension:increased risk of ischemic stroke in high-risk patients. *J. Hypertens.* 2007 25:551-556.
[118]Zhang Y, Wang Y, Cui C, Hiang P, Li X, Liu S, Lendon C, Guo N. Platelet glycoprotein polymorphisms: risk, in vivo expression and severity of atherothrombotic stroke in Chinese. *Clin. Chim. Acta* 2007;378: 99-104.
[119]Berge E, Haug KB, Charlotte Sandset E, Kristine Haugbro K, Turkovic M, Sandset PM. The factor V leiden, prothrombin gene 20210GA, methylenetetrahydrofolate reductase 677CT and platelet glycoprotein IIIa 1565TC mutations in patients with acute ischemic stroke and atrial fibrillation. *Stroke* 2007;38:1069-1071.
[120]Carter AM, Catto AJ, Bamford JM, Grant PJ. Platelet GP IIIa PlA and GP Ib variable number tandem repeat polymorphisms and markers of platelet activation in acute stroke. *Arterioscler. Thromb Vasc. Biol.* 1998 ;18:1124-1131.
[121]Wagner KR, Giles WH, Johnson CJ, Ou CY, Bray PF, Goldschmidt-Clermont PJ, Croft JB, Brown VK, Stern BJ, Feeser BR, Buchholz DW, Earley CJ, Macko RF, McCarter RJ, Sloan MA, Stolley PD, Wityk RJ, Wozniak MA, Price TR, Kittner SJ.Platelet glycoprotein receptor IIIa polymorphism P1A2 and ischemic stroke risk: the Stroke Prevention in Young Women Study. *Stroke* 1998;29:581-585.
[122]Reiner AP, Kumar PN, Schwartz SM, Longstreth WT Jr, Pearce RM, Rosendaal FR, Psaty BM, Siscovick DS. Genetic variants of platelet glycoprotein receptors and risk of stroke in young women. *Stroke* 2000; 31: 1628-1633.
[123]van Goor ML, Gómez García E, Brouwers GJ, Leebeek FW, Koudstaal PJ, Dippel DW.
[124]PLA1/A2 polymorphism of the platelet glycoprotein receptor IIb/IIIa in young patients with cryptogenic TIA or ischemic stroke. *Thromb Res*. 2002;108:63-65.
[125]Chen CH, LO YK, Ke D, Liu CK, Liou CW, Wu HL, Lai ML for the Southern Taiwan Young Stroke study Group. Platelet glycoprotein I a C807T, Ib C3550T, and IIa Pl A2/A1 polymorphisms and ischemic stroke in young Taiwanese. *J. Neurol. Sci.* 2004; 227: 1-5.

[126]Reiner AP, Siscovick DS, Rosendaal FR. Platelet glycoprotein gene polymorphisms and risk of thrombosis: facts and fancies. *Rev. Clin. Exp. Hematol.* 2001; 5:262-287

[127]Moshfegh K, Wuillemin WA, Redondo M, Lämmle B, Beer JH, Liechti-Gallati S, Meyer BJ Association of two silent polymorphisms of platelet glycoprotein Ia/IIa receptor with risk of myocardial infarction:A case-control study. *Lancet* 1999; 353: 351-354.

[128]Santoso S, Kunicki TJ, Kroll H, Haberbosch W, Gardemann A. Association of the platelet glycoprotein Ia C807T gene polymorphism with nonfatal myocardial infarction in younger patients. *Blood* 1999; 93:2449-2453

[129]Croft SA, Hampton KK, Sorrell JA, Steeds RP, Channer KS, Samani NJ, Daly ME. The GPIa C807T dimosphism associated with platelet collagen receptor density is not a isk factor for myocardial infarction. *Br. J. Haematol.* 1999; 106: 771-776.

[130]Carlsson LE, Santoso S, Spitzer C, Kessler C, Greinacher A. The alpha2 gene coding sequence T807/A873 of the platelet collagen receptor integrin alpha2beta1 might be a genetic risk factor for the development of stroke in younger patients. *Blood* 1999; 93: 3583-3586.

[131]Akar N, Duman T, Akar E, Deda G, Sipahi T.The alpha2 Gene alleles of the platelet collagen receptor integrin alpha2 beta1 in Turkish children with cerebral infarct. *Thromb Res.* 2001;102:121-123.

[132]Kuijpers R, Faber NM, Cuypers H, Ouwehand WH, von dem Borne AE. NH2-terminal globular domain of human platelet glycoprotein Ib alpha has a methionine 145/threonine 145 amino acid polymorphism which is associated with the HPA-2 (Ko)alloantigens. *J. Clin. Invest* 1992; 89: 381-384.

[133]Afshar-Kharghan V, Li C, Khoshnevis –Asl M, Lopez JA. Kozak sequence polymorphism in the glycoproetin (GP) Ib alpha gene is a major determinant of the plasma membrane levels of the platelet GPIb-IX-V complex. *Blood* 1999; 94:186-191.

[134]Kunicki TJ. The role of platelet collagen receptor (glycoprotein Ia/IIa; integrin alpha2 beta1) polymorphisms in atherombotic disease. *Curr. Opinion. Haematol.* 2001; 8: 277-285.

[135]Frank MB, Reiner AP, Schwartz SM, Kumar PN, Pearce RM, Arbogast PG, Longstreth WT Jr, Rosendaal FR, Psaty BM, Siscovick DS.The Kozak sequence polymorphism of platelet glycoprotein Ibalpha and risk of nonfatal myocardial infarction and nonfatal stroke in young women. *Blood* 2001;97:875-879.

[136]Sonoda A, Murata M, Ito D, Tanahashi N, Ohta A, Tada Y, Takeshita E, Yoshida T, Saito I, Yamamoto M, Ikeda Y, Fukuuchi Y, Watanabe K. Association between platelet glycoprotein Ibalpha genotype and ischemic cerebrovascular disease. *Stroke* 2000; 31: 493-497.

[137]Sonoda A, Murata M, Ikeda Y et al. Stroke and platelet glycoprotein Iba polymorphisms. *Thromb Haemost*. 2001; 85: 573-574.

[138]Agerholm-Larsen B, Tybjaerg-Hansen A, Frikke-Schmidt R, Gronholdt MLM, Jensen G and Nordestgaard BG. ACE gene polymorphism as a risk factor for ischemic cerebrovascular disease. *Ann. Int. Med.* 1997; 127: 346-355.

[139]Pfohl M, Fetter M, Koch M, Barth CM, Rudiger W, Häring HU. Association between angiotensin I-converting enzyme genotypes, extracranial artery stenosis, and stroke. *Atherosclerosis* 1998; 140:161-166.

[140]Rigat B, Hubert C, Alhenc–Gelas F, Cambien F, Corvol P, Soubrier F. An insertion/deletion polymorphism in angiotensin I converting enzyme gene accounting for half of the variance of the serum enzyme levels. *J. Clin. Invest* 1990; 86:1434-1436.

[141]Cambien F, Poirier O, Lecerf L, Evans A, Cambou JP, Arveiler D, Luc G, Bard JM, Bara L, Ricard S, Tiret L, Amouyel P, Alhenc-Gelas F, Soubrier F. Deletion polymorphism in the gene for angiotensin-converting enzyme is a potent risk factor for myocardial infarction. *Nature* 1992; 359: 641-644.

[142]Ariyaratnam R, Casas JP, Whittaker J, Smeeth L, Hingorani AD, Sharma P. Genetics of Ischaemic Stroke among Persons of Non-European Descent: A Meta-Analysis of Eight Genes Involving approximately 32,500 Individuals. *PLoS Med.* 2007; 4:e131

[143]Brenner D, Labreuche J, Poirier O, Cambien F, Amarenco P; GENIC Investigators. Renin-angiotensin-aldosterone system in brain infarction and vascular death. *Ann. Neurol.* 2005; 58:131-138.

[144]Szolnoki Z, Havasi V, Bene J, Komlosi K, Szöke D, Somogyvari F, Kondacs A, Szabo M, Fodor L, Gati I, Wittman I, Melegh B. Endothelial nitric oxide synthase gene interactions and the risk of ischaemic stroke. *Acta Neurol. Scand.* 2005; 111:29-33.

[145]Dikmen M, Gunes HV, Degirmenci I, Ozdemir G, Basaran A. Are the angiotensin-converting enzyme gene and activity risk factors for stroke? *Arq. Neuropsiquiatr.* 2006; 64:211-216

[146]Tuncer N, Tuglular S, Kilic G, Sazci A, Us O, Kara I. Evaluation of the angiotensin-converting enzyme insertion/deletion polymorphism and the risk of ischaemic stroke. *J. Clin. Neurosci.* 2006 ;13:224-227.

[147]Pera J, Slowik A, Dziedzic T, Wloch D, Szczudlik A. ACE I/D polymorphism in different etiologies of ischemic stroke. *Acta Neurol. Scand.* 2006;114: 320-322

[148]Gormley K, Bevan S, Markus HS. Polymorphisms in genes of the renin-angiotensin system and cerebral small vessel disease. *Cerebrovasc. Dis.* 2007; 23:148-155

[149]Varda NM, Peterlin B, Bradac SU, Gregari A. Carotid artery intima-media thickness and angiotensin-converting enzyme gene polymorphism in the offspring of parents with premature stroke. *Acta Paediatrica* 2005; 94:33-37.

[150]Doi Y, Yoshinari M, Yoshizumi H, Ibayashi S, Wakisaka M, Fujishima M.Polymorphism of the angiotensin-converting enzyme (ACE) gene in patients with thrombotic brain infarction. *Atherosclerosis* 1997 ;132:145-50.

[151]Aalto-Setälä K, Palomäki H, Miettinen H, Vuorio A, Kuusi T, Raininko R, Salonen O, Kaste M, Kontula K.Genetic risk factors and ischaemic cerebrovascular disease: role of common variation of the genes encoding apolipoproteins and angiotensin-converting enzyme. *Ann. Med.* 1998 ;30:224-233.

[152]Castellano M, Muiesan ML, Rizzoni D, Beschi M, Pasini G, Cinelli A, Salvetti M, Porteri E, Bettoni G, Kreutz R, et al.Angiotensin-converting enzyme I/D polymorphism and arterial wall thickness in a general population. The Vobarno Study. *Circulation* 1995; 91:2721-2724.

[153] Reid IA. The renin-angiotensin system: physiology, pathophysiology, and pharmacology. *Adv. Physiol. Educ.* 1998; 275: 236-245.

[154] Sethi AA, Tybjaerg-Hansen A, Gronholdt MLM, Steffensen R, Schnohr P, Nordestgaard BG. Angiotensinogen mutations and risk for ischemic heart disease, myocardial infarction, and ischemic cerebrovascular disease. Six case-control studies from the Copenhagen City Heart Study. *Ann. Intern. Med.* 2001; 134: 941-954

[155] Bis JC, Smith NL, Psaty BM, Heckbert SR, Edwards KL, Lemaitre RN, Lumley T, Rosendaal FR. Angiotensinogen Met235Thr polymorphism, angiotensin-converting enzyme inhibitor therapy, and the risk of nonfatal stroke or myocardial infarction in hypertensive patients. *American Journal of Hypertension* 2003; 16:1011-1017.

[156] Zhang JH, Kohara K, Yamamoto Y, Nakura J, Tabara Y, Fujisawa M, Katagi R, Miki T. Genetic predisposition to neurological symptoms in lacunar infarction. *Cerebrovasc. Dis.* 2004; 17: 273-279.

[157] van Rijn MJ, Bos MJ, Isaacs A, Yazdanpanah M, Arias-Vásquez A, Stricker BH, Klungel OH, Oostra BA, Koudstaal PJ, Witteman JC, Hofman A, Breteler MM, van Duijn CM.Polymorphisms of the renin-angiotensin system are associated with blood pressure, atherosclerosis and cerebral white matter pathology. *J. Neurol. Neurosurg. Psychiatry* 2007;78:1083-1087.

[158] MacLeod MJ, Dahiyat MT, Cumming A, Meiklejohn D, Shaw D, St Clair D. No association between Glu/Asp polymorphism of NOS3 gene and ischemic stroke. *Neurology* 1999; 53: 418-420.

[159] Elbaz A, Poirier O, Moulin T, Chédru F, Cambien F, Amarenco P on behalf of the GENIC investigators. Association between the Glu298Asp polymorphism in the endothelial constitutive Nitric Oxide Synthase gene and brain infarction. *Stroke* 2000; 31:1631-1639.

[160] Hou L, Osei –Hyiaman D, Yu H, Ren Z, Zhang Z, Wang B, Harada S. Association of a 27-bp repeat polymorphism in ecNOS gene with ischemic stroke in Chinese patients. *Neurology* 2001; 56: 490-496.

[161] Hassan A, Gormley K, O'Sullivan M, Knight j, Sham P, Vallance P, Bamford J, Markus H. Endothelial Nitric Oxide Gene Haplotypes and Risk of Cerebral Small-Vessel Disease. *Stroke* 2004; 35: 654-659.

[162] Akar N, Akar E, Deda G, Sipahi T. No association between Glu/Asp polymorphism of NOS3 gene and ischemic stroke. *Neurology* 2000; 55: 460-461.

[163] Howard TD, Giles WH, Xu J, Wozniak MA, Malarcher AM, Lange LA, Macko RF, Basehore MJ, Meyers DA, Cole JW, Kittner SJ.Promoter polymorphisms in the nitric oxide synthase 3 gene are associated with ischemic stroke susceptibility in young black women. *Stroke* 2005;36:1848-1851

[164] Hankey GJ, Eikelboom JW. Homocysteine and stroke. *Curr. Opin. Neurol.* 2001; 14: 95-102.

[165] Cattaneo M. Hyperhomocysteinemia, atherosclerosis and thrombosis. *Thromb Haemost.* 1999;81:165-176.

[166] The Homocysteine Studies Collaboration. Homocysteine and Risk of Ischemic Heart Disease and Stroke. *JAMA* 2002; 288: 2015-2022.

[167] Wald DS, Law M, Morris JK. Homocysteine and cardiovascular disease: evidence on causality from a meta-analysis. *BMJ* 2002; 325: 1-7.

[168] Szolnoki Z, Somogyvari F, Kondacs A, Szabo M, Fodor L, Bene J, Melegh B. Evaluation of the modifying effects of unfavourable genotypes on classical clinical risk factors for ischaemic stroke. *J. Neurol. Neurosurg. Psychiatry* 2003; 74: 1615-1620.

[169] Sazci A, Ergul E, Tuncer N, Akpinar G, Kara I. Methylenetetrahydrofolate reductase gene polymorphisms are associated with ischemic and hemorrhagic stroke: Dual effect of MTHFR polymorphisms C677T and A1298C. *Brain Res. Bull.* 2006 ;71:45-50.

[170] Hankey GJ, Eikelboom JW. Homocysteine and stroke. *Lancet* 2005;36:194-196.

[171] Dikmen M, Ozbabalik D, Gunes HV, Degirmenci I, Bal C, Ozdemir G, Basaran A. Acute stroke in relation to homocysteine and methylenetetrahydrofolate reductase gene polymorphisms.*Acta Neurol. Scand.* 2006;113:307-314

[172] Bosco P, Gueant-Rodriguez RM, Anello G, Spada R, Romano A, Fajardo A, Caraci F, Ferri R, Gueant JL. Association of homocysteine (but not of MTHFR 677 C>T, MTR 2756 A>G, MTRR 66 A>G and TCN2 776 C>G) with ischaemic cerebrovascular disease in Sicily. *Thromb Haemost.* 2006; 96:154-159.

[173] Kristensen B, Malm J, Nilsson TK, Hultdin J, Carlberg B, Dahlén G, Olsson T. Hyperhomocysteinemia and hypofibrinolysis in young adults with ischemic stroke. *Stroke* 1999 ;30:974-980.

[174] Pezzini A, Grassi M, Del Zotto E, Archetti S, Spezi R, Vergani V, Assanelli D, Caimi L, Padovani A.Cumulative effect of predisposing genotypes and their interaction with modifiable factors on the risk of ischemic stroke in young adults. *Stroke* 2005;36:533-539.

[175] Sirachainan N, Tapanapruksakul P, Visudtibhan A, Chuansumrit A, Cheeramakara C, Atamasirikul K, Chotsuppakarn S, Areekul S. Homocysteine, MTHFR C677 T, vitamin B12, and folate levels in Thai children with ischemic stroke: a case-control study. *J. Pediatr Hematol. Oncol.* 2006;28:803-808

[176] Sánchez-Marín B, Grasa JM. Methylenetetrahydrofolate reductase (MTHFR) C677T polymorphism in ischemic vascular disease *Rev. Neurol.* 2006;43:630-636.

[177] Pezzini A, Grassi M, Del Zotto E, Assanelli D, Archetti S, Negrini R, Caimi L, Padovani A. Interaction of homocysteine and conventional predisposing factors on risk of ischaemic stroke in young people: consistency in phenotype-disease analysis and genotype-disease analysis. *J. Neurol. Neurosurg. Psychiatry* 2006;77:1150-1156.

[178] Linnebank M, Montenarh M, Kölsch H, Linnebank A, Schnez K, Schweichel D, Pohl C, Urbach H, Heun R, Harbrecht U, Klockgether T, Wüllner U. Common genetic variants of homocysteine metabolism in ischemic stroke: a case-control study. *European Journal of Neurology* 2005; 12: 614- 618.

[179] Hankey GJ, Eikelboom JW. Homocysteine and stroke. *Lancet* 2005;365:194-196.

[180] Mahley RW, Rall SC. Apolipoptrotein E: Far More Than a Lipid Transport Protein. *Annu. Rev. Genomics Hum. Genet.* 2000; 1: 507-537.

[181] Mc Carron M. Delong D, Alberts M. APOE genotype as a risk factor for ischemic cerebrovascular disease: A meta-analysis. *Neurology* 1999; 53:1308-1311.

[182] Sudlow C, Martinez Gonzalez NA, Kim J, Clark C. Does apolipoprotein E genotype influence the risk of ischemic stroke, intracerebral hemorrhage, or subarachnoid

hemorrhage? Systematic review and meta-analyses of 31 studies among 5961 cases and 17,965 controls. *Stroke* 2006 ;37: 364-370.

[183]Banerjee I, Gupta V, Ganesh S. Association of gene polymorphism with genetic susceptibility to stroke in Asian populations: a meta-analysis. *J. Hum. Genet.* 2007; 52:205-219.

[184]Chowdhury AH, Yokoyama T, Kokubo Y, Zaman MM, Haque A, Tanaka H. Apolipoprotein E genetic polymorphism and stroke subtypes in a Bangladeshi hospital-based study. *J. Epidemiol.* 2001; 11:131-138.

[185]Szolnoki Z, Somogyvari F, Kondacs A, Szabo M, Fodor L. Evaluation of the interactions of common genetic mutations in stroke subtypes. *J. Neurol.* 2002; 249:1391-1397.

[186]Souza DRS, Campos BF, Arruda EF, Yamamoto LJ, Trindade DM, Tognola WA. Influenece of the polymorphism of apolipoprotein E in cerebral vascular disease. *Arq. Neuropsiquiatr.* 2003; 61: 7-13.

[187]Kolovou GD, Daskalova DCh, Hatzivassiliou M, Yiannakouris N, Pilatis ND, Elisaf M, Mikhailidis DP, Cariolou MA, Cokkinos DV. The epsilon 2 and 4 alleles of apolipoprotein E and ischemic vascular events in the Greek population--implications for the interpretation of similar studies. *Angiology* 2003; 54: 51-58.

[188]Baum L, Ng HK, Wong KS, Tomlinson B, Rainer TH, Chen X, Cheung WS, Tang J, Tam WW, Goggins W, Tong CS, Chan DK, Thomas GN, Chook P, Woo KS. Associations of apolipoprotein E exon 4 and lipoprotein lipase S447X polymorphisms with acute ischemic stroke and myocardial infarction. *Clin. Chem. Lab. Med.* 2006; 44:274-281.

[189]Pezzini A, Grassi M, Del Zotto E, Bazzoli E, Archetti S, Assanelli D, Akkawi NM, Albertini A, Padovani A. Synergistic Effect of Apolipoprotein E Polymorphisms and Sigarette Smoking on Risk of Ischemic Stroke in Young Adults. *Stroke* 2004; 35: 438-442.

[190]Jin ZQ, Fan YS, Ding J, Chen M, Fan W, Zhang GJ, Zhang BH, Yu SJ, Zhang YS, Ji WF, Zhang JG. Association of apolipoprotein E 4 polymorphism with cerebral infarction in Chinese Han population. *Acta Pharmacol. Sin.* 2004;25:352-356.

[191]Sturgeon JD, Folsom AR, Bray MS, Boerwinkle E, Ballantyne CM for the Atherosclerosis Risk in Communities Study Investigators. Apolipoprotein E genotype and incident ischemic stroke: the Atherosclerosis Risk in Communities Study. *Stroke* 2005; 36: 2484-2486.

[192]Qureshi AI, Giles WH, Croft JB, Guterman LR, Hopkins LN. Apolipoproteins A-1 and B and the likelihood of non-fatal stroke and myocardial infarction-data from The Third National Health and Nutrition Examination Survey. *Med. Sci. Monit.* 2002; 8: CR311-316.

[193]Lamarche B, Moorjani S, Lupien PJ, Cantin B, Bernard PM, Dagenais GR, Despres JP. Apolipoprotein A-I and B levels and the risk of ischemic heart disease during a five-year follow-up of men in the Quebec cardiovascular study. *Circulation* 1996; 94: 273-278.

[194]Florvall G, Basu S, Larsson A. Apolipoprotein A1 is a stronger prognostic marker than are HDL and LDL cholesterol for cardiovascular disease and mortality in elderly men. *J. Gerontol. A Biol. Sci. Med. Sci.* 2006;61:1262-1266

[195]Christopher R, Kailasanatha KM, Nagaraja D, Tripathi M.Case-control study of serum lipoprotein(a) and apolipoproteins A-I and B in stroke in the young. *Acta Neurol. Scand.* 1996 ;94:127-130.

[196]Walldius G, Aastveit AH, Jungner I.Stroke mortality and the apoB/apoA-I ratio: results of the AMORIS prospective study. *J. Intern. Med.* 2006;259:259-266.

[197]Hutter CM, Austin A, Humpries SE. Familial Hypercholesterolemia, Peripheral Arterial Disease, and Stroke: A HuGE Minireview. *American Journal of Epidemiology* 2004; 160: 430-435.

[198]Beisiegel U, Weber W, Bengtsson-Olivecrona G. Lipoprotein lipase enhances the binding of chylomicrons to low density lipoprotein receptor-related protein. *Proc. Natl. Acad. Sci. USA* 1991; 88: 8342-8346.

[199]Eckel RH.Lipoprotein lipase. A multifunctional enzyme relevant to common metabolic diseases. *N. Engl. J. Med.* 1989

[200]Mattu RK, Needham EWA, Morgan R, Rees A, Hackshaw AK, Stocks J, Elwood PC, Galton DJ. DNA Variants at the LPL Gene Locus Associate With Angiographically Defined Severity of Atherosclerosis and Serum Lipoprotein Levels in a Welsh Population. *Arterioscl. Thromb* 1994; 14:1090-1097.

[201]Thorn JA, Chamberlain JC, Alcolado JC, Oka K, Chan L,Stocks J, Galton DJ. Lipoprotein and hepatic lipase gene variants in coronary atherosclerosis. *Atherosclerosis* 1990; 85:55-60.

[202]Wang XL, McCredie RM, Wilcken DEL. Common DNA Polymorphisms at Lipoprotein Lipase Gene. Association With Severity of Coronary Artery Disease and Diabetes. *Circulation* 1996; 93:1339-1345.

[203]Wittrup HH, Nordestgaard BG, Sillesen H, Schnohr P, Tybjærg-Hansen A. A Common Mutation in lipoprotein lipase confers a 2-Fold increase in risk of ischemic cerebrovascular disease in women but not in men. *Circulation* 2000; 101:2393-2397.

[204]Shimo-Nakanishi Y, Urabe T, Hattori N, Watanabe Y, Nagao T, Yokochi M, Hamamoto M, Mizuno Y. Polymorphism of the lipoprotein lipase gene and risk of atherothrombotic cerebral infarction in the Japanese. *Stroke* 2001; 32:1481-1486.

[205]Zhao SP, Tong QG, Xiao ZJ, Cheng YC, Zhou HN, Nie S. The lipoprotein lipase Ser447Ter mutation and risk of stroke in the Chinese. *Clinica Chimica Acta* 2003; 330: 161-164.

[206]Fidani L, Hattzitolios AI, Goulas A, Savopoulos C, Basayannis C, Kotsis A. Cholesteryl ester transfer protein Taq I B and lipoprotein lipasi Ser 447Ter gene polymorphisms are not associated with ischaemic stroke in Greek patients. *Neuroscience Letters* 2005; 384: 102-105.

[207]Morrison AC, Ballantyne CM, Bray M, Chambless LE, Sharrett AR, Boerwinkle E. LPL polymorphism predicts stroke risk in men. *Genetic Epidemiology* 2002; 22: 223-242.

[208]Schmidt H, Schmidt R, Niederkorn K, Gradert A, Schumacher M, Watzinger N, Hartung HP, Kostner GM.Paraoxonase PON1 polymorphism leu-Met54 is associated

with carotid atherosclerosis: results of the Austrian Stroke Prevention Study. *Stroke* 1998;29:2043-2048.

[209]Baum L, Ng HK, Woo KS, Tomlinson B, Rainer TH, Chen X, Cheung WS, Chan DK, Thomas GN, Tong CS, Wong KS. Paraoxonase 1 gene Q192R polymorphism affects stroke and myocardial infarction risk. *Clin. Biochem*. 2006; 39:191-195.

[210]Imai Y, Morita H, Kurihara H, Sugiyama T, Kato N, Ebihara A, Hamada C, Kurihara Y, Shindo T, Oh-hashi Y, Yazaki Y. Evidence for association between paraoxonase gene polymorphisms and atherosclerotic diseasee. *Atherosclerosis* 2000; 149: 435-442.

[211]Ueno T, Shimazaki E, Matsumoto T, Watanabe H, Tsunemi A, Takahashi Y, Mori M, Hamano R, Fujioka T, Soma M, Matsumoto K, Kanmatsuse K. Paraoxonase 1 polymorphism Leu-Met55 is associated with cerebral infarction in Japanese population. *Med. Sci. Monit.* 2003; 9: 260-264.

[212]Pasdar A, Grant FA, Whalley LJ, Hakonarson H, Thorsteindottir U, Kong A, Gulcher J, Stefansson K, MacLeod MJ. Asspciation between the Gene Encoding 5-Lipoxygenase-Activating Protein and Stroke Replicated ina Scottish Population. *Am. J. Hum. Genet.* 2005; 76: 505-509.

[213]Huang Q, Liu YH, Yang QD, Xiao B, Ge L, Zhang N, Xia J, Zhang L, Liu ZJ. Human serum paraoxonase gene polymorphisms, Q192R and L55M, are not associated with the risk of cerebral infarction in Chinese Han population. *Neurol. Res.* 2006; 28:549-554.

[214]Schiavon R, Turazzini M, De Fanti E, Battaglia P, Targa L, Del Colle R, Fasolin A, Silvestri M, Biasioli S, Guidi G.PON1 activity and genotype in patients with arterial ischemic stroke and in healthy individuals. *Acta Neurol. Scand.* 2007; 116:26-30.

[215]Shin BS, Oh SY, Kim YS, Kim KW. The paraoxonase gene polymorphism in stroke patients and lipid profile. *Acta Neurol. Scand*. 2008;117:237-243.

[216]Can Demirdöğen B, Türkanoğlu A, Bek S, Sanisoğlu Y, Demirkaya S, Vural O, Arinç E, Adali O. Paraoxonase/arylesterase ratio, PON1 192Q/R polymorphism and PON1 status are associated with increased risk of ischemic stroke. *Clin. Biochem*. 2008;41:1-9.

[217]Voetsch B, Benke KS, Damasceno BP, Siqueira LH. Paraoxonase 92 Gln->Arg polymorphism: an independent risk factor for nonfatal arterial ischemic stroke among young adults. *Stroke* 2002; 33:1459-1464.

[218]Voetsch B, Benke KS, Panhuysen CI, Damasceno B, Loscalzo J. The combined effect of paraoxonase promoter and coding region polymorphisms on the risk of arterial ischemic stroke among young adults. *Arch Neurol.* 2004; 61:351-356.

[219]Bevan S, Porteous L, Sitzer M, Markus HS. Phosphodiesterase 4D Gene, Ischemic Stroke, and Asymptomatic Carotid Atherosclerosis. *Stroke* 2005; 36: 949-953.

[220]Gretarsdottir S, Sveinbjornsdottir S, Jonsson HH, Jakobsson F, Einarsdottir E, Agnarsson U, Shkolny D, Einarsson G, Gudjonsdottir HM, Valdimarsson EM, Einarsson OB, Thorgeirsson G, Hadzic R, Jonsdottir S, Reynisdottir ST, Bjarnadottir SM, Gudmundsdottir T, Gudlaugsdottir GJ, Gill R, Lindpaintner K, Sainz J, Hannesson HH, Sigurdsson GT, Frigge ML, Kong A, Gudnason V, Stefansson K, Gulcher JR. Localization of a susceptibility gene for common forms of stroke to 5q12 *Am. J. Hum. Genet*. 2002; 70:593-603.

[221]Gretarsdottir S, Thorleifsson G, Reynisdottir ST, Manolescu A, Jonsdottir S, Jonsdottir T, Gudmundsdottir T, Bjarnadottir SM, Einarsson OB, Gudjonsdottir HM, Hawkins M, Gudmundsson G, Gudmundsdottir H, Andrason H, Gudmundsdottir AS, Sigurdardottir M, Chou TT, Nahmias J, Goss S, Sveinbjornsdottir S, Valdimarsson EM, Jakobsson F, Agnarsson U, Gudnason V, Thorgeirsson G, Fingerle J, Gurney M, Gudbjartsson D, Frigge ML, Kong A, Stefansson K, Gulcher JR. The gene encoding phosphodiesterase 4D confers risk of ischemic stroke. *Nat. Genet.* 2003; 35:131-138.

[222]Meschia JF, Brott TG, Brown RD, Crook R, Worrall BB, Kissela B, Brown M, Rich S, Case LD, Evans EW, Hague S, Singleton A, Hardy Jon behalf of the SWISS, ISGS and MSGD Investigators. Phosphodiesterase 4D and 5-Lypoxygenase Activating Protein in Ischemnic Stroke. *Ann. Neurol.* 2005; 58:351-361.

[223]Alberts MJ. Stroke Genetics Update. *Stroke* 2003; 34: 342-344.

[224]Nilsson-Ardnor S, Wiklund P-G, Lindgren P, Nilsson AK, Janunger T, Escher SA, Hallbeck B, Stegmayr B, Asplund K, Holmberg D. Linkage of ischemic Stroke to the PDE4D Region on 5q in a Swedish population. *Stroke* 2005; 36:1666-1671.

[225]Van Rijin MJE, Slooter AJC, Scht AFC, Isaacs A, Aulchenko YS, Snijders PJLM, Kappelle LJ, van Swieten JC, Oostra BA, van Duijn CM. Familial aggregation, the PDE4D gene, and ischemic stroke ina genetically isolated population. *Neurology* 2005; 65: 1203-1209.

[226]Lõhmussaar E, Gschwendtner A, Mueller JC, Org T, Wichmann E, Hamann G, Meitinger T, Dichgans M. AloX5Ap Gene and the PDE4D Gene in a Central European Population of Stroke Patients *Stroke* 2005; 36: 731-736

[227]Saleheen D, Bukhari S, Haider SR, Nazir A, Khanum S, Shafqat S, Anis MK, Frossard P. Association of phosphodiesterase 4D gene with ischemic stroke in a Pakistani population. *Stroke* 2005 ;36: 2275-2277.

[228]Brophy VH, Ro SK, Rhees BK, Lui LY, Lee JM, Umblas N, Bentley LG, Li J, Cheng S, Browner WS, Erlich HA. Association of phosphodiesterase 4D polymorphisms with ischemic stroke in a US population stratified by hypertension status. *Stroke* 2006; 37:1385-1390.

[229]Zee RY, Brophy VH, Cheng S, Hegener HH, Erlich HA, Ridker PM. Polymorphisms of the phosphodiesterase 4D, cAMP-specific (PDE4D) gene and risk of ischemic stroke: a prospective, nested case-control evaluation. *Stroke* 2006;37:2012-2017.

[230]Staton JM, Sayer MS, Hankey GJ, Thakkinstian A, Yi Q, Cole VJ,Baker R, Eikelboom JW. Association between phosphodiesterase 4D gene and ischaemic stroke. *J. Neurol. Neurosurg. Psychiatr.* 2006;77:1067-1069.

[231]Kuhlenbäumer G, Berger K, Huge A, Lange E, Kessler C, John U, Funke H, Nabavi DG, Stögbauer F, Ringelstein EB, Stoll M.Evaluation of single nucleotide polymorphisms in the phosphodiesterase 4D gene (PDE4D) and their association with ischaemic stroke in a large German cohort. *J. Neurol. Neurosurg. Psychiatry* 2006;77:521-524.

[232]Nakayama T, Asai S, Sato N, Soma M. Genotype and haplotype association study of the STRK1 region on 5q12 among Japanese: a case-control study. *Stroke* 2006;37:69-76.

[233]Rosand J, Altshuler D. Human genome sequence variation and the search for genes influencing stroke. *Stroke* 2003; 34:2512-2517.

[234]Song Q, Cole JW, O'Connell JR, Stine OC, Gallagher M, Giles WH, Mitchell BD, Wozniak MA, Stern BJ, Sorkin JD, McArdle PF, Naj AC, Xu Q, Gibbons GH, Kittner SJ. Phosphodiesterase 4D polymorphisms and the risk of cerebral infarction in a biracial population: the Stroke Prevention in Young Women Study. *Hum. Mol. Genet.* 2006;15: 2468-2478

[235]Bevan S, Dichgans M, Gschwendtner A, Kuhlenbäumer G, Ringelstein EB, Markus HS. Variation in the PDE4D Gene and Ischemic Stroke Risk. A Systematic Review and Meta-analysis on 5200 Cases and 6600 Controls. *Stroke* 2008 Apr 17

[236]Helgadottir A, Manolescu A, Thorleifsson G, Gretarsdottir S, Jonsdottir H, Thorsteinsdottir U, Samani NJ, Gudmundsson G, Grant SF, Thorgeirsson G, Sveinbjornsdottir S, Valdimarsson EM, Matthiasson SE, Johannsson H, Gudmundsdottir O, Gurney ME, Sainz J, Thorhallsdottir M, Andresdottir M, Frigge ML, Topol EJ, Kong A, Gudnason V, Hakonarson H, Gulcher JR, Stefansson K. The gene encoding 5-lipoxygenase activating protein confers risk of myocardial infarction and stroke. *Nat. Genet.* 2004; 36:233-239.

[237]Dixon RA, Diehl RE, Opas E, Rands E, Vickers PJ, Evans JF, Gillard JW, Miller DK Requirement of a 5-lipoxygenase-activating protein for leukotriene synthesis. *Nature* 1990; 343: 282-284.

[238]Meharabian M, Allayee H, Wong J, Shih W, wang XP, Shaposhnik Z, Funk CD, Lusis AJ. Identification of 5-Lipoxygenaseas a Major Gene Contributing to Atherosclerosis Susceptibility in Mice. *Circ. Res.* 2002; 91:120-126.

[239]Spanbroek R, Gräbner R, Lötzer K, Hildner M, Urbach A, Rühling K, Moos MP, Kaiser B, Cohnert TU, Wahlers T, Zieske A, Plemz G, Robenek H, Salbach P, Kühn H, Samulesson B, Habenicht AJR. Expanding expression of the 5-lipoxygenase pathway within the arterial wall during human atherogenesis. *PNAS* 2003; 100: 1238-1243.

[240]Helgadottir A, Gretarsdottir S, St Clair D, Manolescu A, Cheung J, Thorleifsson G, Pasdar A, Grant SF, Whalley LJ, Hakonarson H, Thorsteinsdottir U, Kong A, Gulcher J, Stefansson K, MacLeod MJ.Association between the gene encoding 5-lipoxygenase-activating protein and stroke replicated in a Scottish population. *Am. J. Hum. Genet.* 2005;76:505-509.

[241]Kaushal R, Pal P, Alwell K, Haverbusch M, Flaherty M, Moomaw C, Sekar P, Kissela B, Kleindorfer D, Chakraborty R, Broderick J, Deka R, Woo D. Association of ALOX5AP with ischemic stroke: a population-based case-control study. *Hum. Genet.* 2007 121:601-607.

[242]Goldstein LB, Adams R, Alberts MJ, Appel LJ, Brass LM, Bushnell CD, Culebras A, Degraba TJ, Gorelick PB, Guyton JR, Hart RG, Howard G, Kelly-Hayes M, Nixon JV, Sacco RL; American Heart Association/American Stroke Association Stroke Council; Atherosclerotic Peripheral Vascular Disease Interdisciplinary Working Group; Cardiovascular Nursing Council; Clinical Cardiology Council; Nutrition, Physical Activity, and Metabolism Council; Quality of Care and Outcomes Research Interdisciplinary Working Group; American Academy of Neurology. Primary prevention of ischemic stroke: a guideline from the American Heart

Association/American Stroke Association Stroke Council: cosponsored by the Atherosclerotic Peripheral Vascular Disease Interdisciplinary Working Group; Cardiovascular Nursing Council; Clinical Cardiology Council; Nutrition, Physical Activity, and Metabolism Council; and the Quality of Care and Outcomes Research Interdisciplinary Working Group: the American Academy of Neurology affirms the value of this guideline. *Stroke* 2006; 37:1583-1633.

[243] Altmuller J, Palmer LJ, Fischer G, Scherb H, Wjst M. Genomewide scans of complex human diseases: true linkage is hard to find. *Am. J. Hum. Genet.* 2001 Nov; 69:936-950.

[244] Wang WY, Barratt BJ, Clayton DG, Todd JA. Genome-wide association studies: theoretical and practical concerns. *Nat. Rev. Genet.* 2005;6:109-118

[245] The Wellcome Trust Case Control Consortium. Genome-wide association study of 14,000 cases of seven common diseases and 3,000 shared controls. *Nature* 2007; 447: 661-678.

In: Cerebral Ischemia in Young Adults
Editors: A. Pezzini and A. Padovani

ISBN 978-1-60741-627-2

Chapter 23

Mitochondrial Diseases

***Massimiliano Filosto*[1*] *and Michelangelo Mancuso*[2]**

1. Dipartimento di Scienze Mediche e Chirurgiche, Clinica Neurologica, Università degli Studi di Brescia, Brescia, Italia
2. Dipartimento di Neuroscienze, Università di Pisa, Pisa, Italia

Abstract

Mitochondrial diseases (MD) are disorders caused by an impairment of the mitochondrial respiratory chain function. They are usually progressive, isolated or multi-system diseases and have variable times of onset between birth and senescence.

Mitochondria have their own DNA called mitochondrial DNA (*mtDNA*). Therefore MD have the unique characteristic that they can be caused by mutations in both *mtDNA* and nuclear DNA (*nDNA*). The complexity of mitochondrial genetics is in part responsible for the intra- and inter-familiar clinical heterogeneity of this class of diseases.

MD are currently classified according to the location of the genetic defect either on *mtDNA* (sporadic or of maternal inheritance) or on *nDNA* (autosomic inheritance).

Among the variety of symptoms and signs caused by respiratory chain deficiency, stroke may be secondary to classical vascular and non-vascular mechanisms.

Vascular mechanisms include atherothrombotic and cardioembolic processes linked to classical vascular risk factors which are present in many MD patients. Non-vascular mechanisms are typical of MELAS, which is characterized by stroke-like lesions located in the cortical posterior regions of the brain with a distribution that does not respect vascular territories. Stroke-like episodes are most likely related to the increased hyperexcitability and susceptibility of cortical neurons to excitotoxic injury.

* Correspondence: Massimiliano Filosto, Pz.le Spedali Civili 1, 25123 Brescia, Italia. Phone 0039 030 3995632, Fax 0039 030 3384086. E-mail filosto@med.unibs.it.

Mitochondrial Medicine

Mitochondrial diseases (MD) are caused by mutations in either mitochondrial (*mtDNA*) or nuclear (*nDNA*) DNA resulting in impaired respiratory chain activity.

They are usually progressive, isolated or multi-system diseases that can manifest anytime between birth and senescence [1]. Tissues with high-energy demand, for instance skeletal muscle, central and peripheral nervous systems (CNS and PNS), endocrine glands, heart, ears, eyes, gastrointestinal tract, liver, kidneys, bone marrow and dermis, are frequently involved [1, 2]. Of these, skeletal muscle and CNS are the most commonly affected systems, for which the term encephalomyopathy is used [1, 2].

The first studies on mitochondrial diseases date back to 1988 when Holt et al. and Wallace et al. reported large-scale single deletions in patients with "mitochondrial myopathy" [3] and a point mutation in the gene encoding subunit 4 of complex I in a family with Leber's hereditary optic neuropathy [4].

In 1989, Zeviani et al described a progressive external ophtalmoplegia inherited as an autosomal dominant trait and associated with multiple *mtDNA* deletions in muscle [5]. This was the first example of a mitochondrial disorder caused by a primary nuclear mutation that impaired *mtDNA* integrity.

Over the next few years, a growing number of pathogenic point mutations and rearrangements on *mtDNA* have been reported [6].

In the last years, the renewed interest for the *nDNA* role in regulating mitochondrial function stimulated research on *nDNA* defects that are directly or indirectly responsible for respiratory chain dysfunction.

Epidemiology of Mitochondrial Diseases

Many epidemiological studies have shown that mitochondrial diseases are very common genetic disorders.

The minimum point-prevalence of the Mitochondrial Encephalomyopathy with Lactic Acidosis and Stroke-like episodes (MELAS) A3243G mutation in the general population was estimated to be 16.3:100,000 in Finland [7]. A minimum point-prevalence of 6.57:100,000 on adults with suspected mitochondrial disease was found in England [8].

In Leber Hereditary Optic Neuropathy (LHON) a prevalence of 11.82 every 100,000 individuals was reported, therefore establishing LHON as a very frequent cause of visual loss in young adults [9].

A swedish study gave a minimum point prevalence for MD of 4.7 in 100,000 children [10] while australian data showed a minimum birth prevalence of childhood respiratory chain diseases as 5.0 per 100,000 infants [11].

By combining the results of these data on childhood and adult mitochondrial diseases, the minimum prevalence is about 1 in 5000.

Mitochondrial Biology and Genetics

Mitochondria contain two membranes, an outer membrane (OMM) and an inner membrane (IMM) that invaginates to form cristae. Albeit traditionally considered individual organelles, mitochondria form complex branching networks owing to their ability to move, fuse and split. The abundance of mitochondria varies from tissues to tissues depending on their dependence on oxidative phosphorylation. Neurones as well as cardiac and skeletal muscle have a high density of mitochondria, which explains why they are particularly vulnerable to energy-dependent defects resulting from mitochondrial abnormalities.

Besides their role in producing ATP, mitochondria are involved in the response mechanisms to oxidative stress, are a source of toxic free radicals and play a role in apoptosis [12-14]. Apoptosis appears to be a feature of mitochondrial disease and to correlate with clinical severity and percentage of mutant *mtDNA* [14-16].

Human *mtDNA* is a 16,569-kb circular, double-stranded molecule that contains 37 genes: 2 *rRNA* genes, 22 *tRNA* genes and 13 structural genes which are encoding subunits of the mitochondrial respiratory chain (Figure 1) [1].

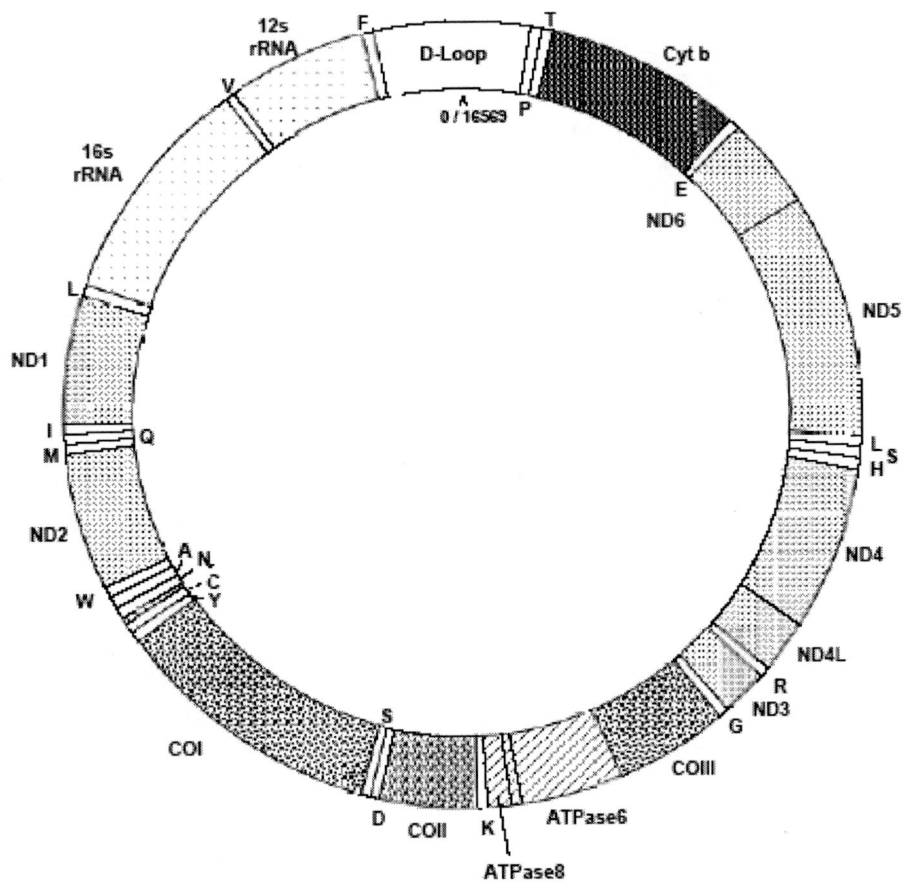

Modified from MITOMAP: http://www.mitomap.org

Figure 1. Mitochondrial DNA.

Reducing equivalents produced in the ß-oxidation spirals and Krebs cycle are passed along a series of protein complexes (the electron transport chain) embedded in the IMM and consisted of four multimeric complexes (I to IV), plus two small electron carriers, coenzyme Q (or ubiquinone) and cytochrome c. Energy generated by the electron transport chain is used to pump protons from the mitochondrial matrix into the space between the IMM and OMM. This creates an electrochemical proton gradient which is utilized by complex V (ATP synthase) to generate ATP as protons flow back into the matrix through its membrane-embedded F0 portion, the rotor of the turbine [2].

Mitochondria are the only organules in the eukaryotic cells that have their own DNA distinct from nuclear DNA. This accounts for MD's unique characteristic to be caused by mutations in both *mtDNA* and *nDNA.*

The main characteristics of the genetics of mitochondrial diseases are briefly reported below:

1) *mtDNA* mutations can be sporadic or inherited; in the latter case, since mitochondria derive exclusively from the oocyte, mutations of *mtDNA* are typically inherited from the mother [1, 2, 17]. Schwartz and Vissing described a paternal-inheritance of *mtDNA* in a patient suffering from a myopathy due to a microdeletion in the ND2 gene [18]. However, further studies have not found any evidence of paternal inheritance in other subjects; therefore such an inheritance modality should be considered a rare exception [19, 20].
2) Cells have variable amounts of mitochondria, each of which contains many (*polyplasmy*) identical (*homoplasmy*) copies of *mtDNA* [2]. Mutations located in all the mitochondrial genomes are defined as being *homoplasmic*; they may be rarely responsible for heterogeneous disorders [21], but are usually silent polymorphisms. On the contrary, *heteroplasmic mutations*, which are harboured only in part of *mtDNA* genomes, are often responsible for disease phenotypes.
3) Molecules of mutated and wild-type *mtDNA* can coexist in the same cell and mutated genomes are randomly distributed among daughter cells so that their amount will vary in the different mitotic cycles (*different mitotic segregation).*
4) Symptoms appear when mutated molecules, following successive mitoses, are numerous enough to cause energy deficiency (*threshold effect)* [2].

The most significant consequence of the complexity and peculiar characteristics of mitochondrial genetics is the heterogeneity of the clinical pictures associated with *mtDNA* defects. The same genetic defect may result in different phenotypes in different individuals or families (intra- and inter-familial clinical heterogeneity); vice versa, homogeneous phenotypes could be expression of different mutations. Clinical expression of mutations and age of onset can depend on the degree of heteroplasmy, tissue distribution and vulnerability of different tissues to a specific mutation [22]. Those tissues particularly dependent on oxidative metabolism or having a low mitotic rate, i.e. skeletal and cardiac muscle, central nervous system, retina and kidneys, are especially vulnerable to alterations of the mitochondrial function; in these tissues a relatively small amount of mutated genome may be sufficient to cause disease. Mitotic segregation could explain the time-related changes of clinical characteristics sometimes observed in MD.

mtDNA mutations can be divided into two main groups: major rearrangements (deletions and single duplications) and point mutations. Deletions may be single or multiple and may cover various parts of *mtDNA*.

Single Deletions

The dimensions of single deletions can vary from less than 2000 bp to more than 10 kb [23, 24]. The most frequent single deletion, called "common deletion", is 4977 bps long and is located among position 8470 (subunit 8 of the *ATPase* gene) and position 13447 (*ND5* gene) [24].

Analysis of the deletions and their location has allowed to determine as a very elevated number of single deletions, around 70%, have the common characteristic of being flanked by a homologous sequence of repeated bases, in numbers that vary among deletions (it is 13 bp for the common deletion). This feature differentiates the single deletions in two groups [25]:

1) Class I - those flanked by repetitive sequences;
2) Class II - deletions that do not present repetitive sequences or that present them in incomplete form

Multiple Deletions

Multiple *mtDNA* deletions have been reported in patients with autosomal dominant and recessive disorders.

Single Duplications

Duplications of *mtDNA* are generally associated with the presence of deletions [26]. The pathological significance of these alterations remains uncertain, and maternal inheritance has been shown in cases where duplications and deletions coexist [27].

Point Mutations

tRNA and rRNA Gene Point Mutations

While rRNA gene mutations are rare, *tRNA* gene mutations are quite numerous and are the cause of most phenotypically defined syndromes. The greatest part of *tRNA* gene mutations determines multi-systemic clinical pictures, although cases where only one tissue is involved (usually skeletal muscle) have been reported. Many of these mutations have a maternal transmission but sporadic transitions have been also reported [28].

Point Mutation in Genes of Structural Protein of the Respiratory Chain Complexes

There are many descriptions of mutations in *mtDNA* genes that codify for structural proteins of the respiratory chain. The consequences are often isolated biochemical defects of the involved complexes. The most frequent are mutations in *ATPase*, *Cytochrome b* and *complex I* genes.

Clinical-genetic Classification of Mitochondrial Diseases

Certain well-defined nosological syndromes are often associated with specific mutations. However, in many cases, phenotypes are heterogeneous and polymorphous and may range from pure myopathy to multisystemic disorders, which makes it difficult to establish a precise genotype/phenotype correlation. New developments in this field have led to frequent revisions of the nosology of this class of diseases.

Table 1. Genetic classification of *mtDNA*-related diseases

SYNDROMES DUE TO REARRANGEMENTS
Sporadic
Kearns-Sayre syndrome (KSS)
Pearson syndrome
Sporadic chronic progressive external ophtalmoplegia (cPEO)
Diabetes and deafness
Maternal-inherited
cPEO
Multisystemic syndromes
SYNDROMES DUE TO POINT MUTATIONS
Sporadic
cPEO
Mitochondrial encephalomyopathy with lactic acidosis and stroke-like episodes
(MELAS)
Exercise intolerance
Isolated myopathy
Maternal-inherited
Point Mutation in polypeptide-encoding genes
- Leber hereditary optic neuropathy (LHON)
- Neuropathy, ataxia, retinitis pigmentosa syndrome (NARP)
- Leigh syndrome
Point Mutation in genes encoding tRNAs
- MELAS
- Myoclonic epilepsy with ragged red fibers (MERRF)
- Cardiomyopathy and myopathy (MIMyCa)
- cPEO
- Isolated myopathy
- Diabetes and deafness
- Sensorineural deafness
- Hypertrophic cardiomyopathy
- Tubulopathy
Point Mutations in genes encoding rRNAs
- Aminoglycosides-induced non syndromic deafness
- Hypertrophic cardiomyopathy

Modified from Filosto and Mancuso, 2007.

Table 2. Genetic classification of mitochondrial diseases caused by disorders of nuclear genome

DEFECTS OF GENES ENCODING FOR STRUCTURAL PROTEINS OF THE COMPLEXES
Leigh Syndrome
Cardiomyopathy
Paraganglioma
Multisystemic Syndromes
DEFECTS OF "ASSEMBLY GENES"
Leigh Syndrome
Multisystemic Syndromes
DEFECTS OF INTERGENOMIC COMMUNICATION
Autosomal cPEO
Early-onset parkinsonism
Multisystemic syndromes
Mitochondrial neurogastrointestinal encephalomyopathy (MNGIE)
mtDNA depletion syndromes
COENZYME Q10 DEFICIENCY
DEFECTS OF THE LIPID MILIEU
Barth syndrome
DEFECTS OF MITOCHONDRIAL RIBONUCLEIC ACID MODIFICATIONS
Mitochondrial myopathy and sideroblastic anemia (MLASA)
DEFECTS OF MITOCHONDRIAL TRANSLATION
MRPS16 mutation syndrome
DEFECTS OF MITOCHONDRIAL FISSION OR FUSION
Autosomal dominant optic atrophy (ADOA)

Modified from Filosto and Mancuso, 2007.

To date, a classification based on the location of the genetic defect, either on *mtDNA* (sporadic or of maternal inheritance) or *nDNA* (autosomal inheritance), respectively, seems to be the most helpful [1, 2]. An updated classification of *mtDNA*- and *nDNA*-related diseases based on genetic defects is summarized in Tables 1 and 2.

Herein we report a description of the main phenotypes; a more detailed description is beyond the purpose of this chapter. A comprehensive review of the main clinical pictures can be found in Filosto and Mancuso, 2007.

SYNDROMES LINKED TO DEFECTS OF THE MITOCHONDRIAL GENOME

These can be sporadic or maternally-inherited (Table 1).

Sporadic Rearrangements (Single Large Scale Deletions)

Chronic Progressive External Ophthalmoplegia (CPEO)

CPEO is usually characterized by palpebral ptosis, a progressive limitation of eye movements and generalized weakness. Time of onset varies, sometimes before the age of 20 years. Signs of multisystem involvement (intolerance to exercise, cardiomyopathy, cataracts, cerebellar dysfunction, retinopathy, sensorineural deafness) may be present (CPEO plus) [24].

Deletions causing CPEO may differ in both size and location; the "common deletion" is found in more than one-third of patients [29].

Kearns-Sayre Syndrome (KSS)

KSS is clinically characterized by progressive external ophthalmoplegia and pigmentary retinopathy. At least one of the following conditions must be concomitant: cardiac conduction defects, cerebellar ataxia or hyperproteinorrachia. Onset often occurs before 20 years of age. Additional features may include retarded growth, endocrinopathies, deafness, muscle weakness, renal dysfunction, heart block and hyperlactacidemia [30].

Maternally-Inherited Point Mutations

Point Mutations in Genes Encoding Structural Proteins

Leber Hereditary Optic Neuropathy (LHON)

LHON is a retrobulbar neuritis associated with pseudopapilledema, retinal blood vessel alteration, and, in some cases, cerebellar ataxia, peripheral neuropathy and defects in cardiac conduction [31]. Typically, onset is between 18 and 30 years of age with monocular loss of vision that is followed within weeks or months by the same problems affecting the contralateral eye. At least five pathogenic point mutations in genes encoding subunits of complex I are associated with the disease (primary mutations). Certain mutations cannot cause LHON alone, but, if associated with primary mutations, can modulate its phenotype (secondary mutations).

Maternally-Inherited Leigh Syndrome (MILS)

MILS generally manifests during the first year of life [32]. The infants may present with motor retardation, hypotonia, ataxia, epileptic seizures, myoclonus, neuropathy, optic atrophy, pigmentary retinopathy, lactic acidosis or psychomotor regression (or a combination of any of these). MILS is usually associated with point mutations in the *APTase6* gene (complex V of the respiratory chain), especially at nucleotide 8993 [23]. If the percentage of mutant *mtDNA* is less than 90% (between 70 – 90%), the clinical outlook is more benign, there will be a later onset and the disease is characterized by neuropathy, ataxia and pigmentary retinopathy (NARP syndrome) [32].

Point Mutations in Genes Encoding tRNAs

Mitochondrial Encephalomyopathy with Lactic Acidosis and Stroke-like Episodes (MELAS)

MELAS consists of a progressive encephalomyopathy characterized by repeated stroke-like events, recurring headaches, intolerance to exercise, seizures and lactic acidosis [33] (see below). Mutations most frequently associated with this condition are located in *tRNALeu(UUR)* [23]. This gene is therefore considered a "hot-spot" for MELAS [1].

Myoclonic Epilepsy with Ragged Red Fibers (MERRF)

MERRF has a variable age of onset and is most frequently characterized by generalized seizures, myoclonus and lactic acidosis [22]. It is associated with various point mutations, the most frequent of which are A8344G and T8356C in *tRNALys* [23]. The A8344G mutation can determine other clinical pictures such as Leigh Syndrome, pure myopathy, cPEO and multiple symmetrical lypomatosis [1, 22].

A point mutation in the *tRNAPhe* has been reported in a patient with a typical MERRF clinical picture [34].

Point Mutations in Genes Encoding rRNAs

Mitochondrial Non-Syndromic Sensorineural Deafness (mtNSSND)

mtNSSND linked to ototoxicity of aminoglycosidic medication has been associated with mutations in the 12S ribosomal RNA gene [23].

SYNDROMES LINKED TO NUCLEAR GENOME DEFECTS

Being secondary to a nuclear mutation, these defects are transmitted in an dominant or recessive autosomal manner. There are different *nDNA* defects involved in MD [1, 2, 35, 36]:

- defects in genes encoding structural subunits of the respiratory chain
- defects in genes encoding factors responsible for the maintenance and the replication of *mtDNA (i*ntergenomic communication).
- defects in genes encoding proteins assembling respiratory chain complexes
- defects in genes that import mitochondrial proteins
- defects of the lipid milieu
- defects of mitochondrial ribonucleic acid modifications
- defects of mitochondrial translation, fission or fusion
- defects in genes encoding proteins indirectly related to OXPHOS
- defects of Coenzyme Q10

Here we briefly discuss main groups of defects.

Defects of Nuclear Genes Encoding Structural Subunits of the Respiratory Chain

Mutations of genes encoding subunits of respiratory chain complexes cause heterogeneous clinical pictures. Complex I subunit mutations cause Leigh Syndrome, cardiomyopathy, encephalomyopathy and myoclonic epilepsy [37-40]. Mutations in the gene encoding the flavoprotein subunit of Complex II (*SDHA*) cause optic atrophy, ataxia and proximal myopathy [41] as well as Leigh Syndrome [42]. Mutations in *SDHC and SDHD* (gene encoding *"cybS protein" cytochrome b small subunit*) have been reported in cases of hereditary paragangliomas [43, 44].

Defects of Assembly Genes

Assembly genes encode proteins that assemble subunits of the complexes of the respiratory chain [45]. Pathogenic mutations have been reported more frequently in the "assembly genes" of complex IV (cytochrome oxidase, COX), *SURF-1* (the most frequent cause of Leigh Syndrome-COX [LS-COX]), *SCO2* (in cases of cardioencephalomyopathy) , *SCO1* (in cases of neonatal liver dysfunction and encephalopathy), *COX 10* (in cases of leucoencephalopathy, myopathy, ataxia, seizures and proximal tubulopathy) and *COX15* (in one patient with severe neonatal cardiomyopathy and in two with rapidly fatal and slowly progressive Leigh syndrome) [46, 47].

Defects of Intergenomic Communication

Mutations of nuclear genes encoding factors involved in maintaining the integrity and stability of *mtDNA* and in *mtDNA* replication i.e. polymerases, elicases, ligases, factors of regulation for transcription and pool of nucleotides, usually lead to multiple deletions or depletion of *mtDNA* [1, 35, 36].

At least ten genes are involved:

- *POLG1* encodes the Polymerase γ–alpha subunit and *POLG2* encodes the Polymerase γ-beta subunit (p55 accessory subunit); both of them are involved in multiple deletion and depletion syndromes.
  Polymerase γ is a hetererodimeric multienzymatic complex located in the inner mitochondrial membrane and is necessary for *mtDNA* replication [48]. *POLG1* transitions are the most frequently observed causes of both dominant and recessive autosomal PEO [48, 49]. Mutations can alter the activity of Polymerase γ, therefore causing a slowing down or blockage of replication and predisposing *mtDNA* to the formation of deletions [35].
- *ANT-1* encodes Adenine Nucleotide Translocator 1 which forms a homodimeric channel in the inner mitochondrial membrane and play a fundamental role in regulating adenine nucleotide concentrations in cytoplasm and mitochondria [50]. *ANT-1* mutations are likely to cause blockage of replication and synthesis of intermediates pairing in inappropriate ways by unbalancing the pool of mitochondrial nucleotides. Since ANT-1 protein is a component of mitochondrial

permeability transition pores (MPTP), which are implicated in the mitochondria-mediated apoptosis, gene mutations could also alter the MPTP opening mechanism.

- *C10orf2* encodes the mitochondrial helicase Twinkle, which is a mitochondrial protein homologous to "phage T7 primase/helicase" [51]. Mutations in *C10orf2* likely alter the replication processes of *mtDNA* and therefore cause *mtDNA* multiple deletions.
- *TP*, the thymidine phosphorylase gene, is involved in Mitochondrial Neurogastrointestinal Encephalomyopathy (MNGIE). Thymidine phosphorylase is an enzyme that catabolizes thymidine to thymine and deoxyribose-1-phosphate. Mutations reduce enzymatic activity and increase the plasma levels of thymidine [52]. The accumulation of thymidine, probably through an alteration of the nucleotide pool, causes an impairment of *mtDNA* replication and of the repair mechanism and, consequently, *mtDNA* depletion and multiple deletions.
- the genes of deoxyguanosine kinase (*dGK*), beta subunit of the ADP-forming succinyl-CoA synthetase ligase (*SUCLA2*), MPV17 inner mitochondrial membrane protein (*MPV17*), thymidine kinase 2 (*TK2*) and cytosolic p53-inducible ribonucleotide reductase small subunit (*RRM2B*) are involved in the *mtDNA* depletion syndromes.

Since dGK and TK2 phosphorylate deoxynucleotides, mutations in their genes are likely to cause a mitochondrial dNTP pool imbalance [53, 54].

MPV17 is a mitochondrial inner membrane protein and its dysfunction has been shown to cause oxidative phosphorylation failure and *mtDNA* depletion in *MPV17*(-/-) mice [55].

Dysfunctions of Succinyl-CoA synthetase ligase, encoded by *SUCLA2*, cause a marked decrease in succinyl-CoA synthetase (SCAS) activity [56]. Since SCAS links to the mitochondrial nucleotide diphosphate kinase, mutations in *SUCLA2* may cause defects in mitochondrial dNTP metabolism and, consequently, *mtDNA* depletion.

Ribonucleotide reductase, whose cytosolic p53-inducible small subunit is encoded by the *RRM2B* gene, is a heterotetrameric enzyme responsible for conversion of ribonucleoside 5'-diphosphates into deoxyribonucleoside 5'-diphosphates, essential for DNA synthesis [57].

Main clinical pictures are briefly discussed below.

- Autosomal Chronic Progressive External Ophthalmoplegia (aPEO) with multiple deletions of *mtDNA* can be inherited both in a dominant (adPEO) or recessive fashion (arPEO) [48]. It is caused by mutations in *ANT-1*, *C10ORF2* and *POLG* genes.

  ANT-1 phenotypes are substantially homogeneous and mainly characterized by adPEO and muscle weakness beginning anytime between 17 and 30 years of age. A bipolar affective disorder in addition to adPEO has been described in a family harbouring the *Leu98Pro* substitution [58]. The first recessive mutation in *ANT-1* has been reported in a patient with multiple deletions of *mtDNA*, hypertrophic cardiomyopathy, exercise intolerance and lactic acidosis, but no ophthalmoplegia [59].

C10ORF2 clinical features are relatively homogeneous: adPEO and muscle weakness may, in some cases, be associated with myalgia and exercise intolerance, motoneuron disease-like conditions, psychiatric symptoms or peripheral neuropathy [60]. Age of onset varies from late adolescence to 30 years, although in some patients the first symptoms appeared at an earlier age (12 years).

Phenotypes of patients with *POLG1* mutations are more heterogeneous and often more serious than those of carriers of *ANT-1* and *C10orf2* defects [49, 61, 62]. Besides aPEO and weakness, the clinical picture may include psychiatric disorders, dysphagia, dysphonia, facial dyplegia, neuropathy, ataxia, diabetes mellitus, bladder and erection dysfunctions, hypogonadism, gastrointestinal dysmotility and extrapyramidal symptoms [49, 63, 61, 62].

SANDO, a recessive syndrome characterized by sensory ataxia, neuropathy, dysarthria and ophthalmoplegia, has recently been linked to *POLG1* mutations [64].

In 2006, Longley et al described the first heterozygous dominant mutation in *POLG2* that causes multiple *mtDNA* deletions and aPEO [65]. In vitro studies on the Polymerase γ–β subunit have shown defective stimulation of the catalytic subunit due to compromised interactions and altered DNA-binding strength of the alpha-beta complex.

- *MNGIE* is caused by mutations in *TP*. It usually begins anytime between 15 months and 43 years of age; it is transmitted as an autosomal recessive trait and is characterized by ophthalmoplegia, serious gastrointestinal dysmotility, neuropathy and leucoencephalopathy [52].
- mtDNA depletion syndromes begin weeks or months after birth (early onset) or during the first twenty years of age (late onset) and are transmitted as an autosomal recessive trait [53, 55-57, 66, 67]. The clinical picture is characterized by the involvement of skeletal muscles (hypotonia, weakness, palpebral ptosis, ophthalmoplegia), motoneurons (rare SMA-like clinical picture), brain (seizures, cortical atrophy, white matter alterations, partial agenesis of the corpus callosum), nerves (axonal neuropathy), liver (steatosis, cirrhosis), heart (cardiomyopathy) and kidneys (tubulopathies). Three main syndromes have been described: the hepatocerebral form is associated with mutations in *dGK* and *MPV17*, the myopathic form with mutations in *TK2* and *RRM2B* and the encephalomyopathic form with *SUCLA2*.

  Early identification of a genetic defect is essential in those forms that involve a single organ. Transplants represent a possible therapeutic solution, although the possible appearance of *mtDNA* depletion in other organs in later years still has to be studied [68].
- Alpers Syndrome, a rare poliodystrophic encephalopathy associated with hepatopathy, manifests in infancy or adolescence and is characterized by refractory epileptic seizures, progressive neurological deterioration and liver dysfunction [69]. It was recently linked to mutations in the *POLG1* gene and depletion of *mtDNA* [70].

Coenzyme Q10 Deficiency

It is inherited as a recessive autosomal trait. A mutation in the Para-Hydroxybenzoate-Polyprenyl transferase gene (*COQ2*) has been identified in children affected with a severe primary deficiency of CoQ10 [71]. Three main clinical phenotypes have been described: myopathy which involves the central nervous system, infantile encephalomyopathy with renal dysfunction and ataxia with cerebellar atrophy [72]. Patients may respond promptly to the administration of CoQ10 and show rapid improvement of symptoms.

General Diagnostic Principles

The diagnosis of mitochondrial diseases is based, first of all, on the clinical evaluation. Codified clinical-pathological criteria may be useful but their use is very difficult in practice due to the wide clinical and genetic heterogeneity of this group of diseases [73]. Some tests may support the diagnostic hypothesis; however, none of these can be taken as unequivocal proof of mitochondrial disease, and the lack of confirmation cannot exclude clinical suspicion.

The following tests can be helpful:

- Determination of plasma lactate. High levels should be considered suspect.
- Lactate/pyruvate ratio. A ratio higher than 25:1 is common in respiratory chain diseases.
- Creatine kinase levels. They can be normal or only moderately high. Important exceptions are patients with myopathies linked to *mtDNA* depletion, where CK is often higher than 1000 UI.
- MR spectroscopy. It can be used to assess encephalic lactate and phosphocreatine/ inorganic phosphate ratios in muscle at rest, during exercise or during the recovery phase [74].

Histopathological Aspects

A muscle biopsy is usually an early procedure in establishing the diagnosis of a possible mitochondrial disease. It can provide diagnostic clues even when skeletal muscle is not primarily affected.

Histological and histochemical studies on frozen muscle sections usually include modified Gomori's trichrome, succinate dehydrogenase (SDH), nicotinamide adenine dinucleotide-tetrazolium reductase (NADH-TR) and double cytochrome-c-oxidase (COX)-SDH stains.

Modified Gomori trichrome stain easily shows ragged-red fibers (RRFs), which are myofibers appearing with a reddish stain in their subsarcolemmal region and containing a high percentage of mutated genomes and structurally altered mitochondria [75]. RRFs are more often present when there is an alteration of functional proteins (for instance, tRNAs), but rarely when structural genes are involved (such as in LHON and NARP/MILS) [22, 76].

SDH and NADH-TR staining specifically show ragged-red fibers, which then become "ragged-blue fibers" (Figure 2b). COX staining may show a variable number of COX-negative fibers. Scattered COX-negative fibers represent the most frequent pattern observed in a muscle biopsy; they are not specific for a definite complex defect and may occur in all the respiratory chain disorders (Figure 2a).

The use of anti-COX subunit antibodies makes possible a comparison between nuclear protein synthesis (COX IV) and mitochondrial protein synthesis (COX I, II and III) in single fibers and enables to find the site of the dysfunction (nuclear or mitochondrial).

Histopathological studies can be supported by ultrastructural studies that show an accumulation of structurally abnormal mitochondria in myofibers.

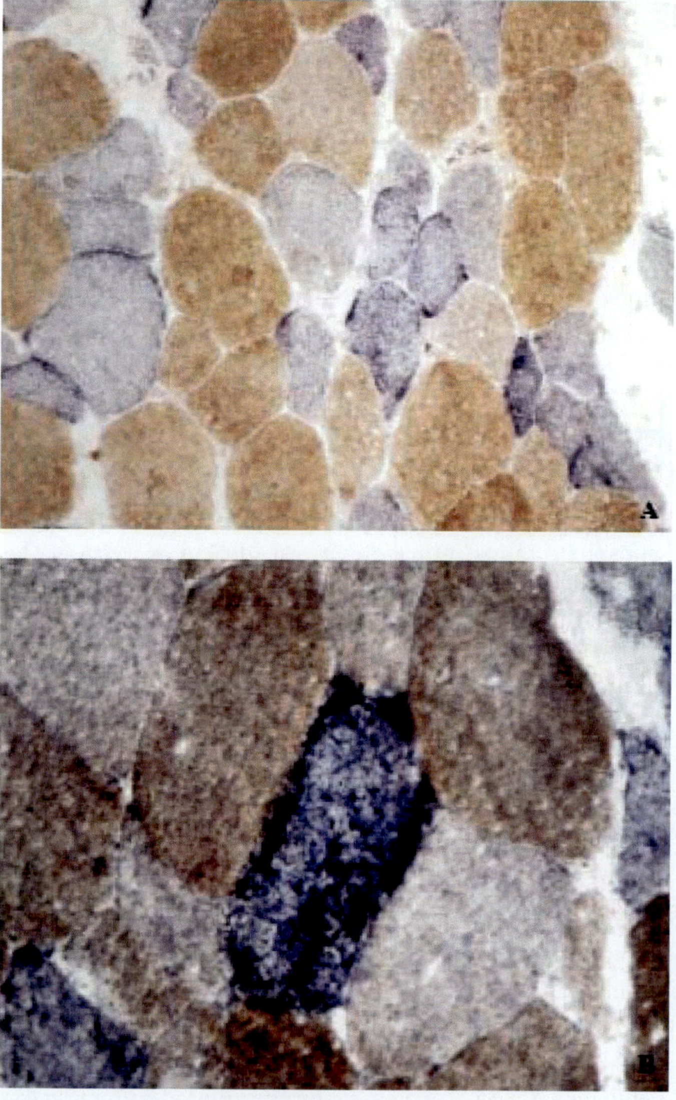

Figure 2. Muscle biopsy from a patient with MELAS: A - COX negative fibers (COX-SDH double staining). B - ragged blue fiber (COX-SDH staining).

Biochemical Aspects

Respiratory chain enzyme assay can detect complex defects. The deficiency can be limited to a single complex if the mutations are located on a subunit-encoding gene but it can involve multiple complexes if the mutations in tRNAs, deletions or depletion impair mitochondrial protein synthesis [75].

Genetic Aspects

A clinical assessment along with histological and biochemical data determine the successive genetic analysis. Southern Blot analysis to look for rearrangements will be performed in case of sporadic or autosomally-transmitted CPEO. A *mtDNA* single deletion in a sporadic case indicates a diagnosis of "classical" CPEO. *mtDNA* multiple deletions or depletion require the study of related genes based on clinical presentation..

In case of maternally-inherited CPEO or other defined syndromes (MELAS, MERRF, etc), the known mutations will be searched by *Polymerase Chain Reaction-Restriction Fragment Length Polymorphism analysis (PCR-RFLP)*. Biochemical data may help in finding new *mtDNA* mutations through direct genetic sequencing or denaturing high performance liquid chromatography (DHPLC).

Mithocondrial Diseases and Stroke

Respiratory chain impairment may cause stroke by classical vascular and non-vascular mechanisms due to energy failure within the brain [77].

Classical vascular mechanisms are usually secondary to damage in organs different from the brain. Many patients with mitochondrial defects present with various alterations including diabetes mellitus, dyslipidemia, carotid atheromasia and hypertension, all of which are well-known risk factors of atherothrombotic stroke [78]. In some mitochondriopathies, respiratory chain damage causes liver damage, which may be responsible for coagulopathies, and renal tubular dysfunctions that induce proteinuria and imbalance of coagulation factors, therefore favouring the formation of thrombi or haemorrhaging [78]. Cardioembolic stroke is often the consequence of cardiac involvement (dilated cardiomyopathy or dysrhythmia, decreased cardiac output, left ventricular hypokinesis, ventricular hypertrophy and valvular prolapse) which causes an increased risk of the formation of atrial thrombi [79].

Potentially, almost all the mitochondrial diseases can cause stroke via these mechanisms, particularly those syndromes that have significant multisystem involvement, such as MELAS, MERRF and KSS [80].

Among the mitochondrial diseases, MELAS is frequently associated with clinical or pathologic findings suggestive of “true” cerebral infarction. Cardiomyopathy is frequently seen in MELAS and some infarctions can have a cardioembolic origin [81].

Cases of cardioembolic stroke have also been reported in patients with KSS, whether or not they have previously documented cardiomyopathy and/or dysrhythmia [82-84].

Non-vascular mechanisms are typical of MELAS and they are not yet completely understood. Stroke-like lesions are often located in the cortical posterior regions of the brain and their distribution does not respect vascular territories [80, 85].

Vascular changes could be important in the pathogenesis of stroke-like episodes and contribute to the pathogenic bases of brain lesions [85-88]. The so-called "primary vascular hypothesis" is based on evidence that, in MELAS patients, muscle and brain arterioles and epithelial cells of the choroids plexus strongly react to SDH staining, thereby indicating abnormal mitochondrial accumulation, aggregation and respiratory chain impairment [88, 89]. Moreover, high levels of A3243G mutation in COX deficient vessels has been reported [88, 89]. This angiopathy causes a narrowing of capillary lumens and aberrant vascular tone which could be directly responsible for impaired cerebral blood flow and local cortical ischemia following increases in metabolic demand [87, 88, 90].

An extension of this hypothesis, based on the evidence of COX deficiency and structural abnormalities in the choroids plexus, suggests a role for the blood brain barrier damage in the development of pathological changes [88, 89, 91]. However, the primary vascular hypothesis alone cannot explain the selective location and distribution of lesions because respiratory chain-deficient vessels have been found in all regions of the examined MELAS brains, even when they seemed not involved in the pathological process.

Selectivity of lesion distribution could be explained by the simultaneous respiratory chain failure within some populations of neurones (the so-called "metabolic hypothesis"). Gilchrist et al. provided electron microscopic evidence of abnormal mitochondria within neurones other than smooth muscle and endothelial cells [86]. Magnetic resonance spectroscopy (MRS) showed increased lactate and impaired oxidative metabolism within the cortical lesions during acute episodes with a return to normal after clinical resolution [92, 93]. According to the metabolic hypothesis, the distribution of the infarct-like lesions in the posterior temporal and occipital cortices could be related to a greater metabolic demand on cortical cells in these areas as compared to other regions of the brain. It is unclear whether there is a greater metabolic demand on neurones in the gyral crests (peculiarly susceptible to MELAS pathology) than in the sulci [85]. Some authors have suggested that mitochondrial defects in brain cells different from neurones could play a role in contributing to neuron loss and development of infarct-like lesions [85].

An alternative hypothesis explains stroke-like episodes by an increased hyperexcitability and susceptibility of cortical neurons to excitotoxic injury [94]. Migraine, which may be triggered by neuronal hyperexcitability within the trigeminovascular system and is a frequent early symptom of stroke-like episodes, has been considered as illustrative of MELAS physiopathology [85].

Impaired oxidative phosphorylation within the grey matter could be the cause of destabilization of neuronal membranes that, in turn, causes hyperexcitability [95]. Several mechanisms used by the endothelial cells of cerebral vessels and the epithelial cells of the choroid plexus to create blood–brain and blood–CSF barriers are energy dependent, including the maintenance of ion homeostasis. Impaired oxidative metabolism and ATP production, which leads to increased potassium and calcium concentrations in the extracellular and cerebrospinal fluid, has been mentioned as an explanation for the initial destabilization of neuronal membranes [89].

Once neuronal hyperexcitability has developed in a localized brain region as a result of mitochondrial dysfunction in the capillary endothelial cells, neurons or astrocytes, destabilization of neuronal membranes potentially may depolarize the adjacent neurons resulting in the spread to the cortex surrounding the focus area [94, 96]. This spreading process is assumed to be closely related to epileptic seizure activity [94, 96]. On cerebral magnetic resonance imaging, stroke-like episodes start from a temporal focal lesion and usually move to the surrounding parietal or occipital areas over a few weeks [96].

Increased capillary permeability caused by epileptic activities in the presence of mitochondrial capillary angiopathy may cause edematous brain lesions mainly involving the cortex [94]. The process may result in neuronal loss with a laminar distribution in susceptible cortex areas [94, 96]. Cortical laminar necrosis is present in all the patients who have experienced prolonged seizures [96]. These data suggest that seizures play an important role in the progression of a stroke-like episode and support the notion that membrane instability may serve as a trigger. Seizure activity, especially when it is prolonged or repetitive, also can increase the risk of glutamate and calcium related excitotoxic free radical injury [95].

MELAS

Clinical Findings

MELAS is probably the most common maternally-inherited MD. It is a progressive encephalomyopathy characterized by repeated stroke-like events typically involving the occipital and parietal lobes regardless of the distribution of vascular territories. Onset may range from childhood to adulthood [80, 97, 98].

Stroke-like episodes usually recur and manifest clinically as focal weakness, speech disturbance, homonymous hemianopsia, hemispatial neglect, cortical blindness, impaired visual acuity, hemihypoesthesia or seizures [85, 99]. They are often preceded by migraine phenomena [96, 99]. Myopathy, recurrent migraine-like headaches and vomiting, exercise intolerance, short stature and lactic acidosis are frequently described [80]. Other clinical features such as myoclonus, neuropathy, personality change, dementia, cerebellar ataxia, optic atrophy, pigmentary retinopathy, deafness, diabetes, hypoparathyroidism, hypopituitarism, dilative or hypertrophic cardiomyopathy, CPEO, multiple lipoma, paralytic ileus or renal failure may also be present (Table 3) [80, 99]. A recently described cardiac abnormality of A3243G mutants is a left ventricular hypertrabeculation [100]. Skin manifestations of MELAS are scaly, pruritic diffuse erythema, reticular pigmentation, moderate hypertrichosis, seborrheic eczema or vitiligo [101]. Rarely, MELAS may present with ketoacidosis [102].

A clinical diagnosis should be suspected when at least the following features are present: (1) stroke-like episodes that typically begin before age 40; (2) seizures and cognitive impairment; and (3) mitochondrial dysfunction as shown by the presence of lactic acidosis, ragged-red fibers or both [33].

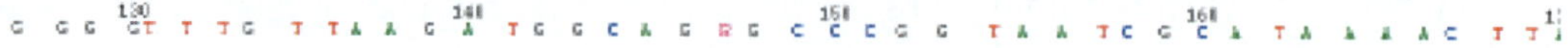

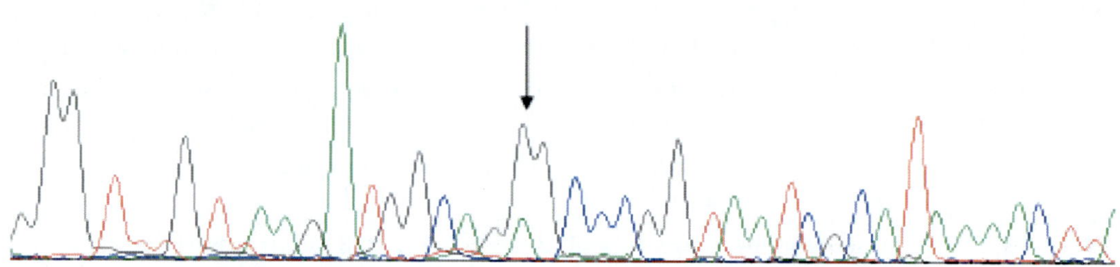

Figure 3. Electropherogram of the mtDNA region encompassing the A3243G mutation (arrow) in the tRNA Leu(UUR) gene. Mutation is in heteroplasmy. In green: wild-type A; in black: mutated G.

MELAS Mutations and Phenotypic Variability

A number of point mutations have been described in association with MELAS phenotype. They arise most frequently in *tRNA* genes. The most frequently reported mutations are the A3243G and T3271C in *tRNA Leu (UUR)* [2]. Approximately 80% of MELAS patients carry the A3243G mutation (Figure 3) [98].

In the other patients, MELAS is caused by *mtDNA* point mutations in the *tRNAPhe, tRNAVal, tRNALys, COXIII, ND1, ND5* or *rRNA* genes or by small-scale *mtDNA* deletions in the *cytb* gene [23].

The phenotypic expression of the A3243G mutation is highly variable ranging from absent expression to mild or severe phenotypes (Table 3) [103]. Severe phenotypes can be either well-defined clinical syndromes, such as MELAS syndrome [104], MERRF syndrome [105], MELAS/MERRF overlap syndrome [106], chronic external ophthalmoplegia (CPEO) [103], Kearns-Sayre syndrome (KSS) [104], maternally-inherited diabetes and deafness (MIDD) [107] and Leigh syndrome (LS) [108], or non-syndromic mitochondrial disorders (floppy infant, enteromyopathy, hypertrophic cardiomyopathy, cluster headache, pancreatitis and liver failure) [80].

Whether the A3243G mutation is associated with an increased risk of malignancy is not known, but single cases suggest involvement in carcinogenesis [109]. The A3243G mutation has been found in a colon cancer cell line as well as in kidney cell carcinoma tissue [109, 110].

Clinical manifestations of the A3243G mutation had different frequence in a study on 111 carriers: myopathy in 53%, seizures in 50%, stroke-like episodes in 48%, deafness in 44%, CPEO in 28%, dementia in 27%, ataxia in 24%, diabetes in 15%, short stature in 15%, pigmentary retinopathy in 15%, myoclonus in 8%, polyneuropathy in 5%, gastrointestinal abnormalities in 3%, cardiomyopathy in 3%, extrapyramidal abnormalities in 3%, optic atrophy in 1%, and lipomatosis in 1% of these patients [111].

Table 3. Main clinical manifestations of MELAS A3243G mutation

Central nervous system
Stroke-like-episodes
Headache, migraine
Cluster headache
Seizures
Neuropsychological deficits
Chorea-ballism
Lethargy, apathy
Cerebellar ataxia
Autism
Parkinson syndrome
Peripheral nervous system
Polyneuropathy
Myopathy, facial and limb weakness
Exercise intolerance, easy fatigability
Muscle cramps
Ophthalmoparesis, ptosis
Hypotonia, floppy infant
Respiratory muscle weakness
Endocrine glands
Multihormonal hypopituitarism, short stature
Hashimoto thyroiditis
Hypoparathyroidism
Diabetes mellitus
Addison's disease
Ovarian failure, abortion, miscarriage
Heart
Hypertrophic cardiomyopathy
Left ventricular hypertrabeculation
Arterial hypertension
Aortic rupture
Ear
Sensorineural hearing loss
Eye
Pigmentary retinopathy
Macula dystrophy
Optic atrophy
Visual field defects
Gastrointestinal manifestations
Constipation, diarrhea
Nausea, cyclic or episodic vomiting
Intestinal pseudoobstruction (ileus)

Table 3. Main clinical manifestations of MELAS A3243G mutation (Continued)

Abdominal pain, epigastralgia
Dysphagia
Gastric dysmotility
Kidney
Focal glomerulosclerosis
Renal cysts
Tubular dysfunction
Nephrotic syndrome
Dermal
Lipoma
Atopic dermatitis, local melanoderma

Modified from Finsterer, 2007.

The mutation load increases with age in most tissues. However, in blood lymphocytes the mutation load decreases with age [112]. This is explained by the preferred selection of cells containing high levels of wild-type *mtDNA* [113].

A high mutation load in the muscle is associated with stroke-like episodes, but some patients carrying over 80% A3243G remain stroke-free, which suggests that additional environmental or genetic factors, such as the background *mtDNA* sequence variation, influence phenotype expression [111, 114].

The risk of stroke-like episodes in A3243G patients seems to increase in the presence of the homoplasmic A12308G polymorphic variant in *mtDNA* [115]. Together with the A11467G and G12372A polymorphisms, the A12308G polymorphism defines the super-haplogroup U/K [115]. However, the absence of a relationship between the U super-haplogroup and the frequency of stroke-like episodes in 107 patient carriers of the A3243G mutation do not support an influence of the *mtDNA* background on phenotypic expression [116]. The A3243G mutation has all the evolutionary features expected from a deleterious *mtDNA* mutation and the role of *mtDNA* background in modulating the phenotype is still unclear [117].

There is increasing evidence that the A3243G mutation is also influenced by the nuclear background [118]. Microarray method revealed several differentially expressed genes on eight patients with the A3243G mutation [118].

Molecular Pathogenesis

After transcription, tRNAs undergo important post-transcriptional modifications, such as folding into a cloverleaf, methylation, and aminoacylation [80, 119]. The primary sequence of tRNALeu (UUR) allows a secondary folding with stems and loops and contains conserved and semi-conserved nucleotides involved in the tertiary folding [119].

The A3243G mutation affects structure stabilization, amino-acylation, methylation and codon recognition [120, 121] and results in incorrect processing and polypeptide maturation such as deficient pre-tRNA processing [120], impaired post-transcriptional base modification [122] and impaired translation [123, 124].

Mutation primarily disrupts the tertiary interaction between the highly conserved np A14 (>90% for adenine) and U8, a binding that stabilizes the L-shaped tertiary fold [125]. Consequently, tRNA transcripts are only partially folded into the L-shaped structure with a floppy anticodon branch [126]. It also seems to induce a profound change in the tRNA quaternary structure by promoting the formation of a dimeric complex by introduction of a palindromic hexa-nucleotide sequence within the D-stem/loop [127].

Mutation impedes normal taurine modification of 5-taurino-methyl-2- thio-uridine at the first (wobble) position of the anticodon (tRNA) that the third letter of the codon (mRNA) pairs with; therefore, it impairs the pairing of the mutant mitochondrial tRNALeu (UUR) anticodon with the mRNA codon [128, 129]. Uridine modifications at the wobble position are necessary for accurate and efficient codon recognition, because taurine modification lack results in a deficient translation, especially deficient UUG decoding, termination of polypeptide elongation, generation of premature proteins, decreased rates of protein synthesis, decreased enzyme activity and severe respiratory defects [128-130].

Overall, the A3243G mutation results in a high glycolytic rate, increased lactate production, reduced glucose oxidation, impaired NADH response, reduced mitochondrial membrane potential, markedly reduced ATP production, deranged cell calcium handling with an increased cytosolic calcium load, increased amount of reactive oxygen species in cybrid cells, reduced insulin secretion, premature aging and deregulation of genes involved in the metabolism of amino groups and urea genesis [80].

Neuroimaging and Neurophysiological Studies

Imaging studies have shown lesions of the occipital and parietal lobes mimicking ischemia but with a distribution pattern that does not correspond to any vascular territory [131]. Lesions are often limited to the cortex with relative sparing of deep white matter. The involvement of white matter has been occasionally reported in the form of non-specific periventricular white matter abnormalities or corpus callosum involvement [131]. Widespread cerebral or cerebellar atrophy, basal ganglia calcification, altered signals in the brainstem or cerebellum may also be present [132]. Watershed hyperintensities have rarely been described [133].

Magnetic resonance spectroscopy can be helpful in diagnosing mitochondrial diseases [131]; in particular, ^{1}H-MRS is able to detect increased lactate levels in cerebrospinal fluid and cortical matter. ^{31}P-MRS of skeletal muscle is the optimal use of MRS [134] because it permits to study oxidative and glycolytic muscle metabolism during rest, exercise and recovery. It can detect reduced ATP, phosphocreatine (PCr) and inorganic phosphate (Pi) production [131]. Increase in Pi and decrease in PCr with a reduced PCr/Pi ratio at rest and delayed post-exercise recovery are considered the most probable indicators of a mitochondrial disorder [134].

Use of the Pcr/Pi ratio at rest alone gives ambiguous results because of its presence also in other neuromuscular diseases, among which are muscular dystrophies [131].

^{31}P-MRS of the myocardium in A3243G mutants with thickened myocardium can reveal reduced cardiac ATP production [135].

EEG can show diffuse or focal slowing, or generalized or focal paroxysmal activity [75]. Latencies of visually evoked potentials may be prolonged in patients with or without clinical or morphological central nervous system manifestations [2, 75].

Nerve conduction tests may be normal or may reveal axonal or demyelinating polyneuropathy in the absence of established causes of polyneuropathy [136]. In a study on 30 patients carrying the A3243G mutation, nerve conduction analysis was abnormal in 77% [137]. Neuropathy was predominantly axonal, sensory and mainly present in the legs; it occurred mainly in old age and in males.

Neuropathology

CNS pathology features in MD are neuronal damage, vasculo-necrotic changes and spongy degeneration [89, 138-141]. Gliosis and demyelination are also frequently reported [89, 139-141].

Neuronal involvement may range from diffuse atrophy to neuronal loss. Vasculo-necrotic lesions are mainly characterized by focal softening of tissue, astrocytosis or cavitation. Spongy degeneration is characterized by splitting of the myelin sheath which results in vacuolation and sieve-like appearance, while oligodendrocytes are often preserved.

These lesions are not specific of MD; they can display a vast spectrum of severity regardless of the phenotype and are widely expressed throughout the CNS [138]. However, they usually present with a distinctive distribution and different degrees of severity which are often typical of a specific disorder. Therefore, the *per se* non-specific CNS lesions constitute pathological patterns that are sufficiently characteristic to suggest a specific diagnosis. On the basis of the predominant involvement of either the grey or white matter, two main groups of diseases can be distinguished (Table 4).

Table 4. Main phenotypes associated with both grey or white matter involvement

Grey matter involvement
MELAS
MERRF
Leigh Syndromes (LS)
Alpers Syndrome
White matter involvement
Kearns-Sayre Syndrome (KSS)
mtDNA Depletion Syndrome linked to *dGK* mutations
Some cases of LS

Modified from Filosto et al, 2007

Grey matter pattern mainly is characterized by vasculo-necrotic multifocal lesions and neuronal loss (often prominent in specific neuronal populations), while white matter pattern is characterized by demyelination and spongy degeneration. Gliosis can be found in both grey and white matter with various degrees of severity. Table 2 shows the main phenotypes associated with either grey or white matter lesions.

MELAS belongs to the group with prominent grey matter involvement. The most common neuropathological pattern in MELAS is given by multifocal infarct-like lesions in the occipital, parietal and temporal cortices associated with neuronal loss and gliosis that do not respect vascular territories [138]. Neuronal loss can also be observed in the basal ganglia, thalamus, cerebellum and brain stem [89, 139-141]. There have been reports of mineral deposits in blood vessels of the basal ganglia and capillary proliferation [85, 142]. The most severe COX deficiency associated with the highest proportion of mutated *mtDNA* was found in the walls of the leptomeningeal and cortical blood vessels in every brain region [90]. There is neuronal loss of either sub-cortical grey structures or brainstem and spinal cord nuclei. It is not yet known whether these changes are secondary to primary cortical events or whether this condition should be considered a multi-system degeneration.

Muscle biopsy typically shows moderate variability of fiber size, ragged-red fibers, and speckled, patchy negative cytochrome c-oxidase staining [1, 2, 138]. Type I muscle fibers may be those predominantly affected. There can also be COX-positive ragged-red muscle fibers. Smooth muscle cells of intramuscular small arteries may show succinate dehydrogenase (SDH) hyper-reactivity. Biochemical tests on the various tissues can reveal reduced activity of any respiratory chain complex and often of multiple complexes [1]. Complexes I and IV are most frequently affected by the A3243G mutation.

Treatment and Management

There is no causative therapy for MELAS.

Individual patients carrying an A3243G mutation may benefit from physiotherapy, vitamin supplements, coenzymes or hormones, symptomatic therapy for any of the abnormalities described above or from surgery. Because of the complex clinical manifestations, it is important to adopt an integrated, multi-disciplinary approach that includes specialist nurses, speech, occupational, or physical therapists, as well as medical professionals in neurology, ophthalmology, oto-rhino-laryngology, internal medicine, dermatology, psychiatry and anesthesiology. In addition, it is important to avoid certain drugs that impair respiratory chain activity such as valproic acid, barbiturates, biguanides, tetracyclines, chloramphenicol, zidovudin, certain local anesthetics and phenothiazines.

Exercise training has been suggested as a way to improve physical capacity and the quality of life in patients with *mtDNA* mutations [143]. Physical training and exercise are well tolerated by patients and can improve exercise endurance; consequently, they induce physiological adaptations able to reverse the effects of deconditioning and improve the underlying mitochondrial defect [143].

Concerning the anaesthetic management of A3243G mutants, care should be taken when administering non-depolarizing muscle relaxants. Frequently, there is a deterioration of clinical signs following general anaesthesia, possibly induced by stress, inflammatory responses to an infection or surgery, or the anaesthetics themselves. Methoxyflurane should be avoided as it causes nephrotoxicity due to the formation of methoxydifluoro-acetic acid and DCA [144].

Symptomatic treatment of MELAS includes anticonvulsants for seizures, dietary or pharmacological therapy for diabetes mellitus, cochlear implants for neurosensory hearing loss, psychotropic drugs for patients with psychiatric symptoms [145].

Some strategies for treating MELAS are as follows:

- drugs to remove noxious metabolities:
  Dichloroacetic acid (DCA), a potent lactate lowering agent, acts by inhibiting pyruvate dehydrogenase (PDH) kinase thus favouring pyruvate metabolism and lactate oxidation. It has been shown to relieve the symptoms in A3243G mutants. In a group of four A3243G patients, DCA resolved headache, weakened abdominal pain and stroke-like episodes but it has been shown to cause toxic neuropathy that overshadows any potential beneficial effects [146].
- drugs to manage electron acceptors:
  Quinone derivatives are among the rare compounds successfully used in the treatment of mitochondrial disorders. Their effect appears to depend on their side chain, which presumably governs their interaction with the respiratory chain. Beneficial effects have been reported with coenzyme Q10 and its short-chain variant idebenone in coenzyme-Q10 deficiency [72].
- oxygen radical scavengers, metabolities and cofactors:
  An improved aerobic oxidative function of mitochondria following creatine administration has been reported [147]. Recent studies have shown that l-arginine, a nitric oxide precursor, improves endothelial functions and may be beneficial for stroke-like episodes in MELAS patients [148]. Some authors have reported that humanin, an endogenous peptide that suppresses apoptosis, appears a possible therapeutic agent for A3243G mutants. Humanin induce an increase in ATP not related to mitochondrial proliferation, because it rather suppresses *mtDNA* replication. This suppression may be useful in the treatment of affected cells in MELAS, since the mutant *mtDNAs* that increase during compensatory *mtDNA* replication for ATP deficiency cause excessive formation of reactive oxygen species, leading to further energy crisis [149].
- gene therapy approach:
  A possible future strategy is to force a shift in heteroplasmy to reduce the ratio of mutant to wild-type genomes (gene shifting) by inhibiting replication of mutant genomes with peptide nucleic acids or by importing RNAs or polypeptides into mitochondria [145].

Acknowledgment

We kindly thank Dr. Giuliano Tomelleri and Dr. Paola Tonin from University of Verona and Prof. G. Siciliano from University of Pisa for their fundamental role in our professional growth.

References

[1] Filosto M, Mancuso M. Mitochondrial diseases: a nosological update. *Acta Neurol. Scand.* 2007; 115: 211-221

[2] DiMauro S, Schon EA Mitochondrial respiratory-chain diseases. *N. Engl. J. Med.* 2003; 348: 2656-2668

[3] Holt IJ, Harding AE and Morgan Hughes JA. Deletions of muscle mitochondrial DNA in patients with mitochondrial myopathies. *Nature* 1988; 331: 717-719

[4] Wallace DC, Singh G, Lott MT, Hodge JA, Schurr TG, Lezza AM, Elsas LJ 2nd, Nikoskelainen EK. Mitochondrial DNA mutation associated with Leber's hereditary optic neuropathy. *Science* 1988; 242: 1427-1430

[5] Zeviani M, Servidei S, Gellera C, Bertini E, DiMauro S, DiDonato S. An autosomal dominant disorder with multiple deletions of mitochondrial DNA starting at the D-loop region. *Nature* 1989; 339: 309-311

[6] Schon EA. 2003 Rearrangements of mitochondrial DNA. In: I. Holt, Editors, *Genetics of Mitochondrial Diseases*, Oxford University Press, Oxford, 111

[7] Majamaa K, Moilanen JS, Uimonen S, Remes AM, Salmela PI, Kärppä M, Majamaa-Voltti KA, Rusanen H, Sorri M, Peuhkurinen KJ, Hassinen IE. Epidemiology of A3243G, the mutation for mitochondrial encephalomyopathy, lactic acidosis, and strokelike episodes: prevalence of the mutation in an adult population. *Am. J. Hum. Genet.* 1998; 63: 447-454

[8] Chinnery PF, Johnson MA, Wardell TM, Singh-Kler R, Hayes C, Brown DT, Taylor RW, Bindoff LA, Turnbull DM. Epidemiology of pathogenic mitochondrial DNA mutations. *Ann. Neurol.* 2000; 48; 188-193

[9] Man PY, Griffiths PG, Brown DT, Howell N, Turnbull DM, Chinnery PF. The epidemiology of leber hereditary optic neuropathy in the north East of England. *Am. J. Hum. Genet.* 2003, 72: 333-339

[10] Darin N, Oldfors A, Moslemi AR, Holme E, Tulinius M. The incidence of mitochondrial encephalomyopathies in childhood: clinical features and morphological, biochemical, and DNA abnormalities. *Ann. Neurol.* 2001; 49: 377-383

[11] Skladal D, Halliday J, Thorburn DR. Minimum birth prevalence of mitochondrial respiratory chain disorders in children. *Brain* 2003; 126: 1905-1912

[12] Filosto M, Tonin P, Vattemi G, Spagnolo M, Rizzuto N, Tomelleri G. Antioxidant agents have a different expression pattern in muscle fibers of patients with mitochondrial diseases. *Acta Neuropathol.* 2002; 103: 215-220

[13] Kroemer G. Mitochondrial implication in apoptosis. Towards an endosymbiont hypothesis of apoptosis evolution. *Cell Death Differ.* 1997; 4: 443-456

[14] Mirabella M, Di Giovanni S, Silvestri G, Tonali P, Servidei S. Apoptosis in mitochondrial encephalomyopathies with mitochondrial DNA mutations: a potential pathogenic mechanism. *Brain* 2000; 123: 93-104

[15] Asoh S, Mori T, Hayashi J, Ohta S. Expression of the apoptosis-mediator Fas is enhanced by dysfunctional mitochondria. *J. Biochem.* 1996; 120: 600-607

[16] Wolvetang EJ, Johnson KL, Krauer K, Ralph SJ, Linnane AW. Mitochondrial respiratory chain inhibitors induce apoptosis. *FEBS Lett.* 1994; 339: 40-44
[17] Mancuso M, Filosto M, Choub A, Tentorio M, Broglio L, Padovani A, Siciliano G. Mitochondrial DNA-related disorders. *Biosci. Rep.* 2007; 27: 31-37
[18] Schwartz M, Vissing J. Paternal inheritance of mitochondrial DNA. *N. Engl. J. Med.* 2002; 347: 576-580
[19] Filosto M, Mancuso M, Vives-Bauza C, Vilà MR, Shanske S, Hirano M, Andreu AL, DiMauro S. Lack of paternal inheritance of muscle mitochondrial DNA in sporadic mitochondrial myopathies. *Ann. Neurol.* 2003; 54: 524-526
[20] Taylor RW, McDonnell MT, Blakely EL, Chinnery PF, Taylor GA, Howell N, Zeviani M, Briem E, Carrara F, Turnbull DM. Genotypes from patients indicate no paternal mitochondrial DNA contribution. *Ann. Neurol.* 2003; 54: 521-524
[21] Limongelli A, Schaefer J, Jackson S, Invernizzi F, Kirino Y, Suzuki T, Reichmann H, Zeviani M. Variable penetrance of a familial progressive necrotising encephalopathy due to a novel tRNA(Ile) homoplasmic mutation in the mitochondrial genome. *J. Med. Genet.* 2004; 41: 342-349
[22] DiMauro S, Hirano M, Kaufmann P, Tanji K, Sano M, Shungu DC, Bonilla E, DeVivo DC. Clinical features and genetics of myoclonic epilepsy with ragged red fibers. *Adv. Neurol.* 2002; 89: 217-229
[23] Mitomap 2007. A Human Mitochondrial Genome Database. http://www.mitomap.org.
[24] Moraes CT, DiMauro S, Zeviani M, Lombes A, Shanske S, Miranda AF, Nakase H, Bonilla E, Werneck LC, Servidei S, et al. Mitochondrial DNA deletions in progressive external ophthalmoplegia and Kearns-Sayre syndrome. *N. Engl. J. Med.* 1989; 320: 1293-1299
[25] Mita S, Rizzuto R, Moraes CT, Shanske S, Arnaudo E, Fabrizi GM, Koga Y, DiMauro S, Schon EA. Recombination via flanking direct repeats is a major cause of large-scale deletions of human mitochondrial DNA. *Nucleic Acids Res.* 1990; 11: 561-567
[26] Rotig A, Bessis JL, Romero N, Cormier V, Saudubray JM, Narcy P, Lenoir G, Rustin P, Munnich A. Maternally inherited duplication of the mitochondrial genome in a syndrome of proximal tubulopathy, diabetes mellitus, and cerebellar ataxia. *Am. J. Hum. Genet.* 1992; 50: 364-370
[27] Manfredi G, Vu T, Bonilla E, Schon EA, DiMauro S, Arnaudo E, Zhang L, Rowland LP, Hirano M. Association of myopathy with large-scale mitochondrial DNA duplications and deletions: which is pathogenic? *Ann. Neurol.* 1997; 42: 180-188
[28] Filosto M, Tonin P, Scarpelli M, Savio C, Greco F, Mancuso M, Vattemi G, Govoni V, Rizzuto N, Tupler R, Tomelleri G. Novel mitochondrial tRNA(Leu(CUN)) transition and D4Z4 partial deletion in a patient with a facioscapulohumeral phenotype. *Neuromuscul. Disord.* 2008; 18: 204-209
[29] Schon EA, Rizzuto R, Moraes CT, Nakase H, Zeviani M, DiMauro S. A direct repeat is a hotspot for large-scale deletions of human mitochondrial DNA. *Science* 1989; 244: 346-349
[30] Hirano M, DiMauro S. 1996 Clinical features of mitochondrial myopathies and encephalomyopathies. In: Lane RJ, editor. Handbook of muscle disease. New York: Marcel Dekker, 479.

[31] Carelli V, Ross-Cisneros FN, Sadun AA. Mitochondrial dysfunction as a cause of optic neuropathies. *Prog. Retin. Eye Res.* 2004; 23: 53-89

[32] Schon EA, DiMauro S. 2001 Primary disorders of mitochondrial DNA and the pathophysiology of mtDNA-related disorders. In: Lemasters JJ, Nieminen A., eds, Mitochondria in pathogenesis. New York: Kluwer Academic/Plenum Publishers, 53

[33] Hirano M, Ricci E, Koenigsberger MR, Defendini R, Pavlakis SG, DeVivo DC, DiMauro S, Rowland LP. MELAS: an original case and clinical criteria for diagnosis. *Neuromusc. Disord.* 1992; 2: 125-135

[34] Mancuso M, Filosto M, Mootha VK, Rocchi A, Pistolesi S, Murri L, DiMauro S, Siciliano G. A novel mitochondrial tRNAPhe mutation causes MERRF syndrome. *Neurology* 2004; 62: 2119-2121

[35] Hirano M, Marti R, Ferreiro-Barros C, Vilà MR, Tadesse S, Nishigaki Y, Nishino I, Vu TH. Defects of intergenomic communication: autosomal disorders that cause multiple deletions and depletion of mitochondrial DNA. *Semin. Cell Dev. Biol.* 2001; 12: 417-427

[36] Spinazzola A, Zeviani M. Disorders of nuclear-mitochondrial intergenomic communication. *Biosci. Rep.* 2007; 27: 39-51

[37] Benit P, Chretien D, Kadhom N, de Lonlay-Debeney P, Cormier-Daire V, Cabral A, Peudenier S, Rustin P, Munnich A, Rötig A. Large-scale deletion and point mutations of the nuclear NDUFV1 and NDUFS1 genes in mitochondrial complex I deficiency. *Am. J. Hum. Genet.* 2001; 68:1344-1352

[38] Budde SM, Van Den Heuvel LP, Janssen AJ, Smeets RJ, Buskens CA, DeMeirleir L, Van Coster R, Baethmann M, Voit T, Trijbels JM, Smeitink JA. Combined enzymatic complex I and III deficiency associated with mutations in the nuclear encoded NDUFS4 gene. *Biochem. Biophys. Res. Commun.* 2000; 275: 63-68

[39] Loeffen J, Elpeleg O, Smeitinik J, Smeets R, Stöckler-Ipsiroglu S, Mandel H, Sengers R, Trijbels F, van den Heuvel L. Mutations in the complex I NDUFS2 gene of patients with cardiomyopathy and encephalomyopathy. *Ann. Neurol.* 2001; 49: 195-201

[40] Schuelke M, Smeitink J, Mariman E, Loeffen J, Plecko B, Trijbels F, Stöckler-Ipsiroglu S, van den Heuvel L. Mutant NDUFV1 subunit of mitochondrial complex I causes leukodystrophy and myoclonic epilepsy. *Nat. Genet.* 1999; 2: 260-261

[41] Birch-Machin MA, Taylor RW, Cochran B. Late-onset optic atrophy, ataxia, and myopathy associated with a mutation of a complex II gene. *Ann. Neurol.* 2000; 48: 330-335

[42] Bourgeron T, Rustin P, Chretien D, Birch-Machin M, Bourgeois M, Viegas-Péquignot E, Munnich A, Rötig A. Mutation of a nuclear succinate dehydrogenase gene results in mitochondrial respiratory chain deficiency. *Nat. Genet.* 1995; 11:144-149

[43] Baysal BE, Ferrell RE, Willett-Brozick JE, Lawrence EC, Myssiorek D, Bosch A, van der Mey A, Taschner PE, Rubinstein WS, Myers EN, Richard CW 3rd, Cornelisse CJ, Devilee P, Devlin B. Mutations in SDHD, a mitochondrial complex II gene, in hereditary paraganglioma. *Science* 2000; 287: 848-851

[44] Niemann S, Muller U. Mutations in SDHC cause autosomal dominant paraganglioma, type 3. *Nat. Genet.* 2000; 26: 268-270

[45] Petruzzella V, Tiranti V, Fernandez P, Ianna P, Carrozzo R, Zeviani M. Identification and characterization of human cDNAs specific to BCS1, PET112, SCO1, COX15, and COX11, five genes involved in the formation and function of the mitochondrial respiratory chain. *Genomics* 1998; 54: 494-504

[46] Valnot I, Osmond S, Gigarel N, Mehaye B, Amiel J, Cormier-Daire V, Munnich A, Bonnefont JP, Rustin P, Rötig A. Mutations of the SCO1 gene in mitochondrial cytochrome c oxidase deficiency with neonatal-onset hepatic failure and encephalopathy. *Am. J. Hum. Genet.* 2000; 67:1104-1119

[47] Zhu Z, Yao J, Johns T, Fu K, De Bie I, Macmillan C, Cuthbert AP, Newbold RF, Wang J, Chevrette M, Brown GK, Brown RM, Shoubridge EA. SURF1, encoding a factor involved in the biogenesis of cytochrome c oxidase, is mutated in Leigh syndrome. *Nat. Genet.* 1998; 20: 337-343

[48] Van Goethem G, Dermaut B, Lofgren A, Martin JJ, Van Broeckhoven C. Mutations of POLG is associated with progressive external ophthalmoplegia characterized by mtDNA deletions. *Nat. Genet.* 2001; 28: 211-212

[49] Filosto M, Mancuso M, Nishigaki Y, Pancrudo J, Harati Y, Gooch C, Mankodi A, Bayne L, Bonilla E, Shanske S, Hirano M, DiMauro S. Clinical and genetic heterogeneity in progressive external ophthalmoplegia due to mutations in polymerase gamma. *Arch Neurol.* 2003b; 60: 1279-1284

[50] Kaukonen J, Juselius JK, Tiranti V, Kyttälä A, Zeviani M, Comi GP, Keränen S, Peltonen L, Suomalainen A. Role of adenine nucleotide translocator 1 in mtDNA maintenance. *Science* 2000; 289: 782-785

[51] Spelbrink JN, Li FY, Tiranti V, Nikali K, Yuan QP, Tariq M, Wanrooij S, Garrido N, Comi G, Morandi L, Santoro L, Toscano A, Fabrizi GM, Somer H, Croxen R, Beeson D, Poulton J, Suomalainen A, Jacobs HT, Zeviani M, Larsson C. Human mitochondrial DNA deletions associated with mutations in the gene encoding Twinkle, a phage T7 gene 4-like protein localized in mitochondria. *Nat. Genet.* 2001; 28: 223-231

[52] Nishino I, Spinazzola A, Hirano M. Thymidine phosphorylase gene mutations in MNGIE, a human mitochondrial disorder. *Science* 1999 ; 283: 689-692

[53] Mandel H, Szargel R, Labay V, Elpeleg O, Saada A, Shalata A, Anbinder Y, Berkowitz D, Hartman C, Barak M, Eriksson S, Cohen N. The deoxyguanosine kinase gene is mutated in individuals with depleted hepatocerebral mitochondrial DNA. *Nat. Genet.* 2001; 29: 337-341

[54] Saada A, Ben-Shalom E, Zyslin R, Miller C, Mandel H, Elpeleg O. Mitochondrial deoxyribonucleoside triphosphate pools in thymidine kinase 2 deficiency. *Biochem. Biophys. Res. Commun.* 2003; 310: 963-966

[55] Spinazzola A, Viscomi C, Fernandez-Vizarra E, Carrara F, D'Adamo P, Calvo S, Marsano RM, Donnini C, Weiher H, Strisciuglio P, Parini R, Sarzi E, Chan A, DiMauro S, Rötig A, Gasparini P, Ferrero I, Mootha VK, Tiranti V, Zeviani M. MPV17 encodes an inner mitochondrial membrane protein and is mutated in infantile hepatic mitochondrial DNA depletion. *Nat. Genet.* 2006; 38: 570-575

[56] Elpeleg O, Miller C, Hershkovitz E, Bitner-Glindzicz M, Bondi-Rubinstein G, Rahman S, Pagnamenta A, Eshhar S, Saada A. Deficiency of the ADP-forming succinyl-CoA synthase activity is associated with encephalomyopathy and mitochondrial DNA depletion. *Am. J. Hum. Genet.* 2005; 76: 1081-1086

[57] Bourdon A, Minai L, Serre V, Jais JP, Sarzi E, Aubert S, Chrétien D, de Lonlay P, Paquis-Flucklinger V, Arakawa H, Nakamura Y, Munnich A, Rötig A. Mutation of RRM2B, encoding p53-controlled ribonucleotide reductase (p53R2), causes severe mitochondrial DANN depletion. *Nat. Genet.* 2007; 39: 776-780

[58] Siciliano G, Tessa A, Petrini S, Mancuso M, Bruno C, Grieco GS, Malandrini A, DeFlorio L, Martini B, Federico A, Nappi G, Santorelli FM, Murri L. Autosomal dominant external ophthalmoplegia and bipolar affective disorder associated with a mutation in the ANT-1 gene. *Neuromuscul. Disord.* 2003; 13:162-165

[59] Palmieri L, Alberio S, Pisano I, Lodi T, Meznaric-Petrusa M, Zidar J, Santoro A, Scarcia P, Fontanesi F, Lamantea E, Ferrero I, Zeviani M. Complete loss-of-function of the heart/muscle-specific adenine nucleotide translocator is associated with mitochondrial myopathy and cardiomyopathy. *Hum. Mol. Genet.* 2005; 14:3079-3088

[60] Deschauer M, Kiefer R, Blakely EL, He L, Zierz S, Turnbull DM, Taylor RW. A novel Twinkle gene mutation in autosomal dominant progressive external ophthalmoplegia. *Neuromuscul. Disord.* 2003; 13: 568-572

[61] Mancuso M, Filosto M, Bellan M, Liguori R, Montagna P, Baruzzi A, DiMauro S, Carelli V. POLG mutations causing ophthalmoplegia, sensorimotor polyneuropathy, ataxia, and deafness. *Neurology* 2004b; 62: 316-318

[62] Mancuso M, Filosto M, Oh SJ, DiMauro S. A novel polymerase gamma mutation in a family with ophthalmoplegia, neuropathy, and Parkinsonism. *Arch Neurol.* 2004c; 61:1777-1779

[63] Luoma P, Melberg A, Rinne JO, Kaukonen JA, Nupponen NN, Chalmers RM, Oldfors A, Rautakorpi I, Peltonen L, Majamaa K, Somer H, Suomalainen A. Parkinsonism, premature menopause, and mitochondrial DNA polymerase gamma mutations: clinical and molecular genetic study. *Lancet* 2004; 364: 875-882

[64] Spinazzola A, Zeviani M. Disorders of nuclear-mitochondrial intergenomic signaling. *Gene* 2005; 354: 162-168

[65] Longley MJ, Clark S, Yu Wai Man C, Hudson G, Durham SE, Taylor RW, Nightingale S, Turnbull DM, Copeland WC, Chinnery PF. Mutant POLG2 disrupts DNA polymerase gamma subunits and causes progressive external ophthalmoplegia. *Am. J. Hum. Genet.* 2006; 78: 1026-1034

[66] Saada A, Shaag A, Mandel H, Nevo Y, Eriksson S, Elpeleg O. Mutant mitochondrial thymidine kinase in mitochondrial DNA depletion myopathy. *Nat. Genet.* 2001; 29: 342-344

[67] Filosto M, Mancuso M, Tomelleri G, Rizzuto N, Dalla Bernardina B, DiMauro S, Simonati A. Hepato-cerebral sindrome: genetic and pathological studies in an infant with a dGK mutation. *Acta Neuropathol.* 2004; 108: 168-171

[68] Salviati L, Sacconi S, Mancuso M, Otaegui D, Camaño P, Marina A, Rabinowitz S, Shiffman R, Thompson K, Wilson CM, Feigenbaum A, Naini AB, Hirano M, Bonilla E, DiMauro S, Vu TH. Mitochondrial DNA depletion and dGK gene mutations. *Ann. Neurol.* 2002; 52: 311-317

[69] Simonati A, Filosto M, Tomelleri G, Savio C, Tonin P, Polo A, Rizzuto N. Central-peripheral sensory axonopathy in a juvenile case of Alpers-Huttenlocker disease. *J. Neurol.* 2003; 250: 702-706

[70] Ferrari G, Lamantea E, Donati A, Filosto M, Briem E, Carrara F, Parini R, Simonati A, Santer R, Zeviani M. Infantile hepatocerebral syndromes associated with mutations in the mitochondrial DNA polymerase-gamma A. *Brain* 2005; 128: 723-731

[71] Quinzii C, Naini A, Salviati L, Trevisson E, Navas P, Dimauro S, Hirano M. A mutation in Para-hydroxybenzoate-polyprenyl transferase (COQ2) causes primari coenzyme Q10 deficiency. *Am. J. Hum. Genet.* 2006; 78: 345-349

[72] Musumeci O, Naini A, Slonim AE, Skavin N, Hadjigeorgiou GL, Krawiecki N, Weissman BM, Tsao CY, Mendell JR, Shanske S, De Vivo DC, Hirano M, DiMauro S. Familial cerebellar ataxia with muscle coenzyme Q10 deficiency. *Neurology* 2001; 56: 849-855

[73] Bernier FP, Boneh A, Dennett X, Chow CW, Cleary MA, Thorburn DR. Diagnostic criteria for respiratory chain disorders in adult and children. *Neurology* 2002; 59: 1406-1411

[74] Gillis L, Kaye E. Diagnosis and management of mitochondrial diseases. *Ped. Clin. North America* 2002: 49: 203-219

[75] DiMauro S, Bonilla E, De Vivo DC. Does the patient have a mitochondrial encephalomyopathy? *J. Child Neurol.* 1999; 14: S23-S35

[76] DiMauro S, Schon EA. Mitochondrial DNA mutations in human disease. *Am. J. Med. Genet.* 2001;106: 19-26

[77] Michelson DJ, Ashwal S. The pathophysiology of stroke in mitochondrial disorders. *Mitochondrion* 2004; 4: 665-674

[78] Gerbitz KD, van den Ouweland JM, Maassen JA, Jaksch M. Mitochondrial diabetes mellitus: a review. *Biochim. Biophys. Acta* 1995; 1271: 253-260

[79] Anan R, Nakagawa M, Miyata M, Higuchi I, Nakao S, Suehara M, Osame M, Tanaka H. Cardiac involvement in mitochondrial diseases. A study on 17 patients with documented mitochondrial DNA defects. *Circulation* 1995; 91: 955-961

[80] Finsterer J. Genetic, pathogenetic, and phenotypic implications of the mitochondrial A3243G tRNALeu(UUR) mutation. *Acta Neurol. Scand.* 2007; 116:1-14

[81] Sparaco M, Simonati A, Cavallaro T, Bartolomei L, Grauso M, Piscioli F, Morelli L, Rizzuto N. MELAS: clinical phenotype and morphological brain abnormalities. *Acta Neuropathol.* 2003; 106: 202-212

[82] Chabrol B, Paquis V. Cerebral infarction associated with Kearns-Sayre syndrome. *Neurology* 1997; 49: 308

[83] Kosinski C, Mull M, Lethen H, Töpper R. Evidence for cardioembolic stroke in a case of Kearns-Sayre syndrome. *Stroke* 1995; 26: 1950-1952

[84] Provenzale JM, VanLandingham K. Cerebral infarction associated with Kearns-Sayre syndrome-related cardiomyopathy. *Neurology* 1996; 46: 826-828

[85] Betts J, Jaros E, Perry RH, Schaefer AM, Taylor RW, Abdel-All Z, Lightowlers RN, Turnbull DM. Molecular neuropathology of MELAS: level of heteroplasmy in individual neurones and evidence of extensive vascular involvement. *Neuropathol. Appl. Neurobiol.* 2006; 32: 359-373

[86] Gilchrist JM, Sikirica M, Stopa E, Shanske S. Adult-onset MELAS. Evidence for involvement of neurons as well as cerebral vasculature in stroke-like episodes. *Stroke* 1996; 27: 1420-1423

[87] Goto Y. Clinical features of MELAS and mitochondrial DNA mutations. *Muscle Nerve* 1995; 3: S107-112

[88] Ohama E, Ohara S, Ikuta F, Tanaka K, Nishizawa M, Miyatake T. Mitochondrial angiopathy in cerebral blood vessels of mitochondrial encephalomyopathy. *Acta Neuropathol.* 1987; 74: 226-233

[89] Tanji K, Kunimatsu T, Vu TH, Bonilla E. Neuropathological features of mitochondrial disorders *Semin. Cell Dev. Biol.* 2001; 12: 429-439

[90] Clark JM, Marks MP, Adalsteinsson E, Spielman DM, Shuster D, Horoupian D, Albers GW. MELAS: Clinical and pathologic correlations with MRI, xenon/CT, and MR spectroscopy. *Neurology* 1996; 46: 223-227

[91] Ohama E, Ikuta F. Involvement of choroid plexus in mitochondrial encephalomyopathy (MELAS). *Acta Neuropathol.* 1987b; 75: 1-7

[92] Kamada K, Takeuchi F, Houkin K, Kitagawa M, Kuriki S, Ogata A, Tashiro K, Koyanagi I, Mitsumori K, Iwasaki Y. Reversible brain dysfunction in MELAS: MEG, and (1)H MRS analysis. *J. Neurol. Neurosurg. Psychiatry* 2001; 70: 675-678

[93] Mathews PM, Andermann F, Silver K, Karpati G, Arnold DL. Proton MR spectroscopic characterization of differences in regional brain metabolic abnormalities in mitochondrial encephalomyopathies. *Neurology* 1993; 43: 2484-2490

[94] Iizuka T, Sakai F. Pathogenesis of stroke-like episodes in MELAS: analysis of neurovascular cellular mechanisms. *Curr. Neurovasc. Res.* 2005; 2: 29-45

[95] Cock H, Schapira AH. Mitochondrial DNA mutations and mitochondrial dysfunction in epilepsy. *Epilepsia* 1999; 40 Suppl 3: 33-40

[96] Iizuka T, Sakai F, Kan S, Suzuki N. Slowly progressive spread of the stroke-like lesions in MELAS. *Neurology* 2003; 61: 1238-1244

[97] Kanaumi T, Hirose S, Goto Y, Naitou E, Mitsudome A. An infant with a mitochondrial A3243G mutation demonstrating the MELAS phenotype. *Pediatr Neurol.* 2006; 34: 235-238

[98] Shanske S, Pancrudo J, Kaufmann P, Engelstad K, Jhung S, Lu J, Naini A, DiMauro S, De Vivo DC.Varying loads of the mitochondrial DNA A3243G mutation in different tissues: implications for diagnosis. *Am. J. Med. Genet.* 2004; 130: 134-137

[99] Finsterer J. Central nervous system manifestations of mitochondrial disorders. *Acta Neurol. Scand.* 2006; 114: 217-238.

[100]Finsterer J, Stöllberger C, Schubert B. Acquired left ventricular hypertrabeculation/ noncompaction in mitochondriopathy. *Cardiology* 2004;102: 228-230

[101]Carmi E, Defossez C, Morin G, Fraitag S, Lok C, Westeel PF, Canaple S, Denoeux JP. MELAS syndrome (mitochondrial encephalopathy with lactic acidosis and stroke-like episodes). *Ann. Dermatol. Venereol.* 2001; 128: 1031-1035

[102]Strachan J, McLellan A, Kirkpatrick M, Hume R, Mechan D. Ketoacidosis: an unusual presentation of MELAS. *J. Inherit. Metab. Dis.* 2001; 24: 409-410

[103]Koga Y, Akita Y, Takane N, Sato Y, Kato H. Heterogeneous presentation in A3243G mutation in the mitochondrial tRNA(Leu(UUR)) gene. *Arch Dis. Child.* 2000; 82: 407-411

[104]Chae JH, Hwang H, Lim BC, Cheong HI, Hwang YS, Kim KJ. Clinical features of A3243G mitochondrial tRNA mutation. *Brain Dev.* 2004; 26: 459-462

[105]Fabrizi GM, Cardaioli E, Grieco GS, Cavallaro T, Malandrini A, Manneschi L, Dotti MT, Federico A, Guazzi G. The A to G transition at nt 3243 of the mitochondrial tRNALeu(UUR) may cause an MERRF syndrome. *J. Neurol. Neurosurg. Psychiatry* 1996; 61: 47-51

[106]Campos Y, Martin MA, Lorenzo G, Aparicio M, Cabello A, Arenas J. Sporadic MERRF/MELAS overlap syndrome associated with the 3243 tRNA(Leu(UUR)) mutation of mitochondrial DNA. *Muscle Nerve* 1996; 19: 187-190

[107]van den Ouweland JM, Lemkes HH, Ruitenbeek W, Sandkuijl LA, de Vijlder MF, Struyvenberg PA, van de Kamp JJ, Maassen JA. Mutation in mitochondrial tRNA(Leu)(UUR) gene in a large pedigree with maternally transmitted type II diabetes mellitus and deafness. *Nat. Genet.* 1992; 1: 368-371

[108]Yang YL, Sun F, Zhang Y, Qian N, Yuan Y, Wang ZX, Qi Y, Xiao JX, Wang XY, Qi ZY, Zhang YH, Jiang YW, Bao XH, Qin J, Wu XR. Clinical and laboratory survey of 65 chinese patients woth Leigh Syndrome. *Chin. Med. J.* 2006; 119: 373-377

[109]Lorenc A, Bryk J, Golik P, Kupryjańczyk J, Ostrowski J, Pronicki M, Semczuk A, Szołkowska M, Bartnik E. Homoplasmic MELAS A3243G mtDNA mutation in a colon cancer sample. *Mitochondrion* 2003; 3: 119-124

[110]Sangkhathat S, Kusafuka T, Yoneda A, Kuroda S, Tanaka Y, Sakai N, Fukuzawa M. Renal cell carcinoma in a pediatric patient with an inherited mitochondrial mutation. *Pediatr Surg. Int.* 2005; 21: 745-748

[111]Chinnery PF, Howell N, Lightowlers RN, Turnbull DM. Molecular pathology of MELAS and MERRF. The relationship between mutation load and clinical phenotypes. *Brain* 1997; 120:1713-1721

[112]Sue CM, Quigley A, Katsabanis S, Kapsa R, Crimmins DS, Byrne E, Morris JG. Detection of MELAS A3243G point mutation in muscle, blood and hair follicles. *J. Neurol. Sci.* 1998; 161: 36-39

[113]Rahman S, Poulton J, Marchington D, Suomalainen A. Decrease of 3243 A-->G mtDNA mutation from blood in MELAS syndrome: a longitudinal study. *Am. J. Hum. Genet.* 2001; 68: 238-240

[114]Chinnery PF, Howell N, Lightowlers RN, Turnbull DM. MELAS and MERRF. The relationship between maternal mutation load and the frequency of clinically affected offspring. *Brain* 1998;121: 1889-1894

[115]Pulkes T, Sweeney MG, Hanna MG. Increased risk of stroke in patients with the A12308G polymorphism in mitochondria. *Lancet* 2000; 356: 2068-2069

[116]Deschauer M, Chinnery PF, Schaefer AM, Turnbull DM, Taylor RW, Zierz S, Shanske S, DiMauro S, Majamaa K, Wilichowski E, Thorburn DR. No association of the mitochondrial DNA A12308G polymorphism with increased risk of stroke in patients with the A3243G mutation. *J. Neurol. Neurosurg. Psychiatry* 2004; 75: 1204-1205

[117]Torroni A, Campos Y, Rengo C, Sellitto D, Achilli A, Magri C, Semino O, García A, Jara P, Arenas J, Scozzari R. Mitochondrial DNA haplogroups do not play a role in the variable phenotypic presentation of the A3243G mutation. *Am. J. Hum. Genet.* 2003; 72: 1005-1012

[118]Crimi M, Bordoni A, Menozzi G, Riva L, Fortunato F, Galbiati S, Del Bo R, Pozzoli U, Bresolin N, Comi GP. Skeletal muscle gene expression profiling in mitochondrial disorders. *FASEB J.* 2005; 19: 866-888

[119]Helm M, Florentz C, Chomyn A, Attardi G. Search for differences in post-transcriptional modification patterns of mitochondrial DNA-encoded wild-type and mutant human tRNALys and tRNALeu(UUR). *Nucleic Acids Res.* 1999; 27: 756-763

[120]Levinger L, Oestreich I, Florentz C, Mörl M. A pathogenesis-associated mutation in human mitochondrial tRNALeu(UUR) leads to reduced 3'-end processing and CCA addition. *J. Mol. Biol.* 2004; 337: 535-544

[121]Jacobs HT, Holt IJ. The np 3243 MELAS mutation: damned if you aminoacylate, damned if you don't. *Hum. Mol. Genet.* 2000; 9: 463-465

[122]Yasukawa T, Suzuki T, Ueda T, Ohta S, Watanabe K. Modification defect at anticodon wobble nucleotide of mitochondrial tRNAs(Leu)(UUR) with pathogenic mutations of mitochondrial myopathy, encephalopathy, lactic acidosis, and stroke-like episodes. *J. Biol. Chem.* 2000; 275: 4251-4257

[123]Chomyn A, Martinuzzi A, Yoneda M, Daga A, Hurko O, Johns D, Lai ST, Nonaka I, Angelini C, Attardi G. MELAS mutation in mtDNA binding site for transcription termination factor causes defects in protein synthesis and in respiration but no change in levels of upstream and downstream mature transcripts. *Proc. Natl. Acad. Sci. USA* 1992; 89: 4221-4225

[124]Schon EA, Koga Y, Davidson M, Moraes CT, King MP. The mitochondrial tRNA(Leu)(UUR)) mutation in MELAS: a model for pathogenesis. *Biochim. Biophys. Acta* 1992; 1101: 206-209

[125]Roy MD, Wittenhagen LM, Kelley SO. Structural probing of a pathogenic tRNA dimer. *RNA* 2005; 11: 254-260

[126]Sohm B, Frugier M, Brulé H, Olszak K, Przykorska A, Florentz C Towards understanding human mitochondrial leucine aminoacylation identity. *J. Mol. Biol.* 2003; 328: 995-1010

[127]Wittenhagen LM, Kelley SO. Dimerization of a pathogenic human mitochondrial tRNA. *Nat. Struct. Biol.* 2002; 9: 586-590

[128]Suzuki Y, Nishimaki K, Taniyama M, Muramatsu T, Atsumi Y, Matsuoka K, Ohta S. Lipoma and opthalmoplegia in mitochondrial diabetes associated with small heteroplasmy level of 3243 tRNA(Leu(UUR)) mutation. *Diabetes Res. Clin. Pract.* 2004; 63: 225-229

[129]Kirino Y, Yasukawa T, Ohta S, Akira S, Ishihara K, Watanabe K, Suzuki T. Codon-specific translational defect caused by a wobble modification deficiency in mutant tRNA from a human mitochondrial disease. *Proc. Natl. Acad. Sci. USA* 2004; 101: 15070-15075

[130]Yasukawa T, Kirino Y, Ishii N, Holt IJ, Jacobs HT, Makifuchi T, Fukuhara N, Ohta S, Suzuki T, Watanabe K. Wobble modification deficiency in mutant tRNAs in patients with mitochondrial diseases. *FEBS Lett.* 2005; 579: 2948-2952

[131]Bianchi MC, Sgandurra G, Tosetti M, Battini R, Cioni G. Brain magnetic resonance in the diagnostic evaluation of mitochondrial encephalopathies. *Biosci. Rep.* 2007; 27: 69-85

[132]Huang CC, Kuo HC, Chu CC, Liou CW, Ma YS, Wei YH. Clinical phenotype, prognosis and mitochondrial DNA mutation load in mitochondrial encephalomyopathies. *J. Biomed. Sci.* 2002; 9: 527-533

[133]Apostolova LG, White M, Moore SA, Davis PH. Deep white matter pathologic features in watershed regions: a novel pattern of central nervous system involvement in MELAS. *Arch Neurol.* 2005; 62: 1154-1156

[134]Kuhl CK, Layer G, Träber F, Zierz S, Block W, Reiser M. Mitochondrial encephalomyopathy: correlation of P-31 exercise MR spectroscopy with clinical findings. *Radiology* 1994;192: 223-230

[135]Lodi R, Rajagopalan B, Blamire AM, Crilley JG, Styles P, Chinnery PF. Abnormal cardiac energetics in patients carrying the A3243G mtDNA mutation measured in vivo using phosphorus MR spectroscopy. *Biochim. Biophys. Acta* 2004; 1657: 146-150

[136]Finsterer J. Mitochondrial neuropathy. *Clin. Neurol. Neurosurg.* 2005; 107: 181-186

[137]Kaufmann P, Pascual JM, Anziska Y, Gooch CL, Engelstad K, Jhung S, DiMauro S, De Vivo DC. Nerve conduction abnormalities in patients with MELAS and the A3243G mutation. *Arch Neurol.* 2006; 63: 746-748

[138]Filosto M, Tomelleri G, Tonin P, Scarpelli M, Vattemi G, Rizzuto N, Padovani A, Simonati A. Neuropathology of mitochondrial diseases. *Biosci. Rep.* 2007; 27: 23-30

[139]Sparaco M, Bonilla E, DiMauro S, Powers JM. Neuropathology of mitochondrial encephalomyopathies due to mitochondrial DNA defects. *J. Neuropathol. Exp. Neurol.* 1993; 52: 1-10

[140]Brown GK, Squier MV. Neuropathology and pathogenesis of mitochondrial diseases. *J. Inherit. Metab. Dis.* 1996; 19: 553-572

[141]Betts J, Lightowlers RN, Turnbull DM. Neuropathological aspects of mitochondrial DNA disease. *Neurochem. Res.* 2004; 29: 505-511

[142]Shapira Y, Cederbaum SD, Cancilla PA, Nielsen D, Lippe BM. Familial poliodystrophy, mitochondrial myopathy, and lactate acidemia. *Neurology* 1975; 25: 614-621

[143]Gardner JL, Craven L, Turnbull DM, Taylor RW. Experimental strategies towards treating mitochondrial DNA disorders. *Biosci. Rep.* 2007; 27: 139-150

[144]Kharasch ED, Schroeder JL, Liggitt HD, Ensign D, Whittington D. New insights into the mechanism of methoxyflurane nephrotoxicity and implications for anesthetic development (part 2): Identification of nephrotoxic metabolites. *Anesthesiology* 2006; 105: 737-745

[145]DiMauro S, Mancuso M. Mitochondrial diseases: therapeutic approaches. *Biosci. Rep.* 2007; 27: 125-137

[146]Kaufmann P, Engelstad K, Wei Y, Jhung S, Sano MC, Shungu DC, Millar WS, Hong X, Gooch CL, Mao X, Pascual JM, Hirano M, Stacpoole PW, DiMauro S, De Vivo DC. Dichloroacetate causes toxic neuropathy in MELAS: a randomized, controlled clinical trial. *Neurology* 2006; 66: 324-330

[147]Komura K, Hobbiebrunken E, Wilichowski EK, Hanefeld FA. Effectiveness of creatine monohydrate in mitochondrial encephalomyopathies. *Pediatr Neurol.* 2003; 28: 53-58

[148]Koga Y, Akita Y, Nishioka J, Yatsuga S, Povalko N, Katayama K, Matsuishi T. MELAS and L-arginine therapy. *Mitochondrion* 2007; 7: 133-139

[149]Kariya S, Hirano M, Furiya Y, Ueno S. Effect of humanin on decreased ATP levels of human lymphocytes harboring A3243G mutant mitochondrial DNA. *Neuropeptides* 2005; 39: 97-101

In: Cerebral Ischemia in Young Adults
Editors: A. Pezzini and A. Padovani
ISBN 978-1-60741-627-2

Chapter 24

Prognosis after Cerebral Infarction among Young Adults

Halvor Naess*
Department of Neurology, Haukeland University Hospital,
University of Bergen, Bergen, Norway

Abstract

In recent years several studies have been published shedding light on both short-term and long-term prognosis among young adults suffering from cerebral infarction. In general, prognosis is better among young than among older patients with cerebral infarction both regarding mortality, recurrence of cerebral infarction, functional outcome, and post-stroke depression. However, long-term mortality is 10 times higher among young adults with cerebral infarction than among age and sex matched controls. Furthermore, both long-term mortality and recurrence of cerebral infarction are highly associated with traditional risk factors such as hypertension, smoking, diabetes mellitus, and cardiac disease. In contrast, long-term mortality and recurrence of cerebral infarction are low among patients with no traditional risk factors, among patients with cerebral infarction due to dissection of the neck vessels, and among patients with cerebral infarction due to classical migraine. Aggressive secondary preventive treatment is especially important among patients at high risk.

Introduction

Studies on prognosis after cerebral infarction among young adults are usually short-term. Most studies report data on the case fatality rate (usually within 30 days). Few studies have reported short-term complications such as the frequency of recurrent stroke, other vascular

* Correspondence: Halvor Naess, N-5021 Bergen, Norway. Tel.: +47-55975045, fax: +47-55975164, e-mail: halvor.naess@haukeland.no.

events, or seizures. Although most studies on short-term prognosis are hospital-based, there are a few population-based studies.

Information on long-term prognosis after suffering cerebral infarction is especially important among young patients in order to make informed decisions about education, work, family etc. Shedding light on factors contributing to non-employment after cerebral infarction is required. Aetiology, risk factors, neurological deficits, cognitive deficits, post-stroke depression, epilepsy, and fatigue are stroke-related factors possibly contributing to long-term functional outcome, and employment. Factors unrelated to cerebral infarction such as pre-stroke depression, level of education, and social status also need to be evaluated regarding long-term outcome. Identifying patients at high risk of long-term complications such as mortality, recurrent stroke, and other vascular events is important in order to target appropriate secondary preventive treatment.

Most studies of long-term prognosis after cerebral infarction among young adults are hospital-based and few studies have followed the patients more than 6 years. The only population-based study with a mean follow-up longer than 11 years was performed in Hordaland County, Norway.

Short-term Prognosis

Mortality

Among patients irrespective of age, a population-based study in Norway showed that case-fatality rate within 30 days for patients with cerebral infarction was 10.9% [1]. A population-based study in Greece including patients irrespective of age with cerebral infarction showed that case-fatality rate within 28 days was 20.4% [2].

A hospital-based study in Lund, Sweden including 60 patients aged 16-40 years with cerebral infarction showed that the case fatality rate within 30 days was 3.3% [3]. The cause of death was increased intracranial pressure with herniation. A hospital-based study in Minnesota, USA including 61 patients aged 16-49 years with cerebral infarction reported acute death among 6.9% [4]. A hospital-based study in Santander, Spain included 38 patients aged ≤50 years with cerebral infarction [5]. The case fatality rate within 30 days of stroke onset was 7.9%. The main cause of death was herniation. A hospital-based study in Bari, Italy included 56 patients aged 17-45 years with cerebral infarction or TIA [6]. The case fatality rate within 30 days was 7%. A hospital-based study in L'Aquila, Italy including 192 patients aged 15-44 years with cerebral infarction showed that the case-fatality rate within 30 days was 3.6% [7]. A hospital-based study in Atlanta, USA included 112 black patients aged 15-44 years with cerebral infarction [8]. In hospital-mortality was 12%. A hospital-based study in Iowa, USA including 296 patients aged 15-45 years with cerebral infarction showed that 7% died as a direct cause of the initial stroke [9]. A hospital-based study in Madrid, Spain including 272 patients aged 15-45 years with cerebral infarction showed that 3% died as a result of their initial stroke [10]. A hospital-based study in Karachi, Pakistan including 118 patients aged 15-45 years with ischemic stroke reported that the in-hospital mortality was 11% [11].

A population-based study in Florence, Italy included 18 patients aged 15-44 years with cerebral infarction [12]. The case-fatality rate within 30 days was 6%. A population-based study in Israel including 204 patients aged 17-49 years with cerebral infarction showed that the case fatality rate within 30 days was 4.9% [13]. The Northern Manhattan Stroke Study, a population-based study including 33 patients aged 20-44 years with cerebral infarction, showed that the case fatality rate within 30 days was 6% [14]. A population-based study in Northern Sweden included 88 patients aged 18-44 years with cerebral infarction [15]. Case-fatality rate within 28 days was 5.7% (n = 5). Three patients died from herniation, one patient died from severe brainstem infarction, and one patient died because of myocardial infarction. A population-based study in Hordaland County, Norway included 232 patients aged 15-49 years with cerebral infarction [16]. The case-fatality rate within 30 days was 3.4% (n = 8). Six patients died because of herniation due to malignant middle cerebral infarction, one patient died because of secondary hemorrhagic transformation after thrombolytic treatment, and one patient died because of acute myocardial infarction.

Comments

Early mortality is considerably lower among young adults with cerebral infarction than among older patients. Thus, the case-fatality rate within 30 days varies from 3-7% in most hospital-based and population-based studies among young adults. However, a study comprising black patients in USA showed an in-hospital mortality of 12%. Most deaths within 30 days of stroke onset seem to be a direct effect of the initial stroke by herniation. The underlying aetiologies of cerebral infarction causing early death most likely include large-vessel vasculopathy such as dissection or atherosclerosis, and cardiac embolism. Due to increasing use of decompressive craniectomy in malignant middle cerebral artery infarction among young adults, early mortality nowadays is probably considerably lower than in most published studies, perhaps as low as 1%.

Functional Outcome

Functional outcome is often considered the most important variable as to outcome after stroke. The most commonly used functional outcome scale is the modified Rankin Scale (mRS) (0-6 points). Zero points represent complete recovery while 6 points represent death. Patients scoring 0-2 points are functionally independent while patients scoring 3-5 points are functionally dependent.

A hospital-based study in Karachi, Pakistan including 118 patients aged 15-45 years with ischemic stroke reported that short-term outcome was excellent in 27%, good in 50% and poor in 23% [11]. A hospital-based study in Atlanta, USA included 112 black patients aged 15-44 years with cerebral infarction [8]. It was found that 82% were independent, and 6% were dependent on discharge while 12% had died.

A population-based study in Israel included 204 patients aged 17-49 years with cerebral infarction [13]. Seven patients (3.4%) recovered completely, 15 (7.4%) had a minimal impairment that did not interfere with their return to all pre-stroke activities, and 172 (84.3%)

had an impairment that resulted in disability (minor in 96 (47.1%), moderate in 38 (18.6%), and severe in 38 (18.6%)). Fifty-three patients (26%) were referred to inpatient rehabilitation.

A population-based study in Hordaland County, Norway included 232 patients aged 15-49 years with cerebral infarction [16]. Among survivors 25 (11%) patients had mRS = 0, 61 (27%) had mRS = 1, 100 (45%) had mRS = 2, 29 (13%) had mRS = 3, 9 (4%) had mRS = 4, and none had mRS = 5. Functional outcome on discharge was significantly better among patients with infarction in the posterior circulation than in the anterior circulation system. Only 1 (1.3%) of the patients with posterior circulation infarction had mRS = 4. None needed nursing home [16]. Favourable outcome (mRS ≤2) was found among 71% of the patients with cardiac embolism, 67% of the patients with atherosclerosis, 100% of the patients with small vessel disease, 79% of the patients with dissection, 94% of the patients with prothrombotic states, and 77% of the patients with unknown aetiology [17].

Comments

Few studies have reported short-term functional outcome after cerebral infarction among young adults. Only one study used a validated scale and showed that 83% had favourable functional outcome (mRS ≤ 2) on discharge. Functional outcome seems to be better among patients with posterior circulation than anterior circulation infarctions. As to aetiologies, small vessel disease seems to have the best short-term prognosis.

Complications other than Mortality

Little is reported on short-term complications other than mortality. A population-based study in Hordaland County, Norway included 232 patients aged 15-49 years with cerebral infarction [16]. During the hospital stay for the qualifying stroke 5 patients (2.2%) had recurrence of cerebral infarction, 1 patient (0.4%) had acute myocardial infarction, 10 patients (4.3%) suffered from pneumonia, 5 patients (2.2%) developed venous thromboembolism, and 7 patients (3.0%) had epileptic seizures.

Long-term Prognosis

Mortality

Mortality Rate

Population-based studies including patients with cerebral infarction irrespective of age have shown that long-term mortality among young patients is relatively much higher than the mortality of old patients compared to age and sex matched controls. Thus, a population-based study in Perth comprising 251 patients with stroke disclosed that 13 patients <45 years with stroke (including TIA, cerebral infarction, intracerebral hemorrhage and subarachnoidal hemorrhage) had a 78-fold higher mortality than individuals of the same sex and age in the general population during a 10-year follow-up period [18]. However, the confidence interval was large due to a low number of young adults included in the study. In comparison, the mortality of stroke patients aged 65-74 years was 4-fold higher than individuals of the same sex and age in the general population during a 10 year period [18].

A few follow-up studies including young patients only have been reported. Most of these studies have been hospital-based and the mortality rate has differed considerably. A French study including 287 patients aged 15-45 years with cerebral infarction showed that 7.7% with cerebral infarction had died after a mean follow-up of 3 years [19]. A hospital-based study in USA including 296 patients aged 14-45 years with cerebral infarction disclosed that 21% had died after a mean follow-up period of 6 years [9]. However, that study was referral based possibly including many serious cases. A hospital-based study from Switzerland including 203 patients aged 16-45 years with cerebral infarction showed that 10 patients (4.9%) had died after a mean follow-up period of 26 months [20]. A hospital-based study in Taiwan included 231 patients aged 25-49 years with cerebral infarction [21]. The study included only patients with cerebral infarction due to atherosclerosis, small artery occlusion, or undetermined cause. On follow-up at a mean time of 29 months after the index stroke only 9 patients (3.6%) had died.

A few studies have included patients with either TIA or cerebral infarction. Thus, a study from Italy including 155 patients aged 16-45 years showed that 9 patients (5.8%) had died after a mean follow-up period of 6 years [22]. Another study from Italy including 330 patients aged 15-44 years with TIA or cerebral infarction showed that 9.1 % had died after a mean follow-up period of 8 years [23]. The mortality rate was about 10 times higher than among the general population of the same age. A study from Portugal including 215 patients ≤45 years with TIA or cerebral infarction showed that 6 patients (2.8%) had died after a mean follow-up period of 33 months [24].

Three studies had follow-up periods longer than 10 years. A small study from Sweden including 74 patients aged 16-40 years with cerebral infarction showed that 12 patients (16%) had died after a mean follow-up period of 16 years [25]. A large study from Spain including 272 patients aged 15-45 years with cerebral infarction showed that 16% had died after mean follow-up period of 11.7 years [10].

The only population-based long-term follow-up study after cerebral infarction was performed in Hordaland County, Norway. That study included 232 patients aged 15-49 year and showed that 19.4 % had died after a mean follow-up period of 11 years [26]. In an age and sex matched control group only 2.0% had died ($P<.001$). Thus, the mortality rate was 10 times higher among the patients than among the controls during the follow-up period.

The mortality rate is highest during the first year after the cerebral infarction. In hospital-based studies the first-year mortality has been reported to be 4.5% [19], 6.3% [23], and 4.9% [10]. One study including 140 TIA patients showed that 0.7% died during the first year [23]. In a population-based study in Hordaland County, Norway the first-year mortality after cerebral infarction was 5.2% [26].

Following the first year, the annual average mortality rate after first-ever cerebral infarction in hospital-based studies has been reported to be 1.6% [19], 0.8% [23] and 0.8% [10]. One study including 140 TIA patients showed that the annual average mortality rate after the first year was 0.4% over a 5 year period [23]. In a population-based study in Hordaland County, Norway the average annual mortality rate following the first year of first-ever cerebral infarction was 1.8% over a 10 year period. In comparison, the annual average mortality rate among age and sex matched controls was 0.15% during the same period.

Predictors for Mortality

A hospital-based study from Iowa, USA showed that long-term mortality was significantly higher among patients with cerebral infarction because of large-vessel atherosclerosis [9]. On univariate analyses a hospital-based study from Italy including patients with either TIA or cerebral infarction showed that long-term mortality was significantly associated with male gender (HR 2.6), age >35 years (HR 3.7), cerebral infarction (HR 4.2), cardiac diseases (HR 4.5), and hypertension (HR 2.3). On multivariate analysis long-term mortality was associated with cerebral infarction (HR 3.3) and cardiac diseases (HR 3.7) [23]. A hospital-based study from Spain including patients with cerebral infarction showed that long-term mortality was significantly associated with male gender (RR 1.9), age >35 years (RR 2.0), and severe handicap at discharge (RR 5.1). No patient with cerebral infarction due to dissection of extra-cranial vessels died during follow-up (P<.01) [10].

In a population-based study including patients with first-ever cerebral infarction in Hordaland County, Norway a first follow-up was performed on average 6 years after stroke onset. Though 9.9% had died, neither hypertension, diabetes mellitus, smoking, age nor sex were significantly associated with time to death [17]. A second follow-up was performed on average 11 years after stroke onset. Between the first and second follow-up another 9.5% had died. Multivariate analysis showed that mortality between the first and second follow-up was independently associated with malignant tumor, alcoholism, coronary atherosclerosis, living alone, and seizures. Between the first and second follow-up 22% of patients living alone, 24% of heavy smokers, 60% of alcoholics, 27% of patients with coronary atherosclerosis, 28% of patients with epilepsy, 54% of patients with malignant tumors, and 47% of patients with peripheral artery disease had died (all P≤.001, log-rank test) [26].

Comments

First year mortality after first ever cerebral infarction is about 5% while annual average mortality after the first year ranges from 0.8 to 1.8%. The long-term mortality rate is about 10 times higher than among age and sex matched controls. As to aetiology, long-term mortality is linked to cardiac diseases and large vessel atherosclerosis while long-term mortality seems to be low among patients with dissection of neck vessels. Modifiable risk factors such as hypertension, smoking and alcoholism have been shown to be significantly associated with long-term mortality. This indicates the need for appropriate long-term preventive treatment among patients at risk.

Recurrence of Cerebral Infarction and other Vascular Events

Recurrency Rate of Cerebral Infarction

More than 30% of patients with first-ever cerebral infarction irrespective of age suffered from recurrence of cerebral infarction during a five-year follow-up period in Perth, Australia [27]. The recurrency rate among old patients with cerebral infarction is about 10% the first year and subsequently 5% per year [28, 29].

A small hospital-based study in France including 71 patients <45 years with cerebral infarction showed that 6.2% had recurrent cerebral infarction during an average 32 months follow-up period [30]. None were fatal. Another hospital-based study in France including 287 patients aged 15-45 years with cerebral infarction showed that 3.5% had recurrent cerebral infarction during a 3 year follow-up period [19]. None were fatal. A hospital-based study in Lisbon, Portugal including 172 patients ≤45 years with cerebral infarction or TIA showed that 6 patients (3.5%) had recurrent cerebral infarction during a mean follow-up period of 3.3 years [24]. A hospital-based study in Iowa, USA including 296 patients aged 15-45 years with cerebral infarction showed that 9% had recurrent cerebral infarction during a mean follow-up period of 6 years [9]. Nine recurrent strokes (39%) were fatal. A study from Bergamo, Italy included 135 patients aged 16-45 years with cerebral infarction [31]. Fifteen (11.1%) suffered from recurrent ischaemic stroke during a mean follow-up period of 27 months. None were fatal. A hospital-based study from Switzerland including 203 patients aged 16-45 years with cerebral infarction showed that 15 patients (7.4%) developed recurrent stroke during a mean follow-up period of 26 months [20]. Two strokes were fatal. TIA was suffered by 6 patients (3%) during the follow-up period. A hospital-based study in Taiwan included 231 patients aged 25-49 years with cerebral infarction [21]. The study included only patients with cerebral infarction due to atherosclerosis, small artery occlusion, or undetermined cause. On follow-up at a mean time of 29 months after the index stroke 28 patients (12.1%) had suffered from recurrent stroke.

A few studies have included both patients with cerebral infarction and TIA. Thus, a hospital-based study in Italy including 330 patients aged 15-44 years with cerebral infarction or TIA showed that 3.2% had recurrent cerebral infarction during a follow-up period of 96 months [23]. Another study in Italy including 155 patients aged 16-45 years with cerebral infarction or TIA showed that 3% had recurrent cerebral infarction during a mean follow-up period of 5.8 years [22]. Half of the recurrent strokes were fatal.

Three studies had follow-periods more than 10 years. A small hospital-based study in Sweden including 74 patients aged 16-40 years with cerebral infarction showed that 8% had recurrent cerebral infarction during a mean follow-up period of 16 years [25]. Half of the recurrent strokes were fatal. A hospital-based study in Madrid, Spain including 272 patients aged 15-45 years with cerebral infarction showed that 25% had recurrent cerebral infarction during a mean follow-up of 12 years [10]. Ten patients (3.7%) died because of recurrent stroke.

A long-term population-based study including 232 patients aged 15-49 years with cerebral infarction was performed in Hordaland County, Norway [17]. A first follow-up was performed at a mean time of 6 years after stroke onset. Recurrent cerebral infarction was disclosed among 23 patients (9.9%). Two patients had more than one recurrent cerebral infarction, and one patient had fatal recurrent cerebral infarction. A second follow-up was performed at a mean time of 12 years after stroke onset [32]. Among surviving patients on follow-up 26% had suffered from recurrent cerebral infarction.

In hospital-based studies the recurrency rate of cerebral infarction during the first year after the index stroke was 1.4% [19], and 2.75% [23]. In a hospital-based study including 140 TIA patients none suffered from cerebral infarction during the first year [23]. In a population-based study in Hordaland County, Norway the recurrency rate during the first year after the index stroke was 2% [32].

A study from Bergamo, Italy reported the annual incidence rate of recurrent ischaemic stroke including the first year to be 2.3% during a mean follow-up period of 27 months [31]. A study from Switzerland reported the annual incidence rate of recurrent stroke including the first year to be 3.0% during a mean follow-up period of 26 months [20]. The combined annual rate for recurrent stroke and TIA was 5.9%.

Following the first year after the index stroke, the average annual recurrency rate of cerebral infarction in hospital-based studies have been reported to be 1.0% [19] and 0.43% [23]. Following the first year after TIA the average annual frequency of cerebral infarction was reported to be 0.18% in a hospital-based study [23].

The only population-based study including patients with first-ever cerebral infarction showed that the average annual frequency of cerebral infarction during a mean follow-up period of 12 years was 2.2% for surviving patient [32]. The average annual frequency of stroke among sex and age matched controls was 0.42% per year.

Patent Foramen Ovale

Patent foramen ovale (PFO) has been associated with cerebral infarction of undefined aetiology [33- 35]. A multi-center study (Patent Foramen Ovale in Cryptogenic Stroke Study) assessed the frequency of recurrent ischemic stroke among patients with and without PFO [36]. Mean age was 59 years. There was no significant difference in the time to primary endpoint (recurrent ischemic stroke or death) between those with and those without PFO (14.8% versus 15.4% 2-year event rate). There was no difference between patients with isolated PFO and patients with PFO in association with atrial septum aneurysm [36]. Another multi-center study included 581 patients aged 18-55 years with cerebral infarction of unknown origin [37]. After 4 years, 2.3% of the patients with isolated PFO, 15.2% of the patients with both PFO and atrial septum aneurysm, and 4.2% of the patients with no cardiac abnormalities had suffered from recurrent cerebral infarction.

Predictors for recurrent cerebral infarction or composite vascular outcome events

Most studies have either included too few patients or had too short follow-up periods to disclose any predictors for recurrent cerebral infarction. However, a hospital-based study in

Bergamo, Italy reported that recurrence of ischaemic stroke was significantly associated with Partial Anterior Circulation Syndrome (PACS) and haematological abnormalities including antiphospholipid antibodies, protein S, and protein C deficiency [31]. In a hospital-based study in Madrid, Spain the frequency of recurrent cerebral infarction was significantly higher among patients with cardiovascular risk factors (RR 1.6), diabetes mellitus (RR 2.3), stroke in the carotid territory (RR 1.7), and atherosclerosis (RR 1.9) while dissection of neck vessels (RR 0.4) and stroke associated with classical migraine (RR 0.4) were significantly associated with lower recurrence rate of cerebral infarction [10]. A hospital-based study in Italy showed that a composite outcome event comprising stroke, myocardial infarction and death was significantly associated with male gender, age >35 years, cardiac diseases, carotid abnormalities and hypertension [23]. A hospital-based study from Switzerland reported recurrence of stroke to be significantly associated with TIA prior to the index stroke [20].

The only population-based long-term study was performed in Hordaland County, Norway and had a first follow-up at a mean time of 6 years after the index stroke. Diabetes mellitus was the only variable significantly associated with recurrence of cerebral infarction [17]. A composite outcome event comprising recurrent cerebral infarction or post-stroke myocardial infarction was defined. The composite outcome event was significantly associated with the following variables present before the index stroke: diabetes mellitus, myocardial infarction, angina pectoris, intermittent claudication, and smoking [38]. Furthermore, the composite outcome event was significantly associated with small vessel disease. The proportion of patients with 0-5 traditional risk factors present before stroke onset (hypertension, smoking, hypercholesterolemia, diabetes mellitus, myocardial infarction, angina pectoris, and peripheral artery disease) and composite outcome event was 2.1%, 6%, 19%, 26%, 30%, and 67% ($p<.001$) [38]. The average annual frequency of the composite outcome event among patients with no traditional risk factor was only 0.35% per year. A second follow-up was performed at a mean time of 12 years after the index stroke [32]. A comparison was made between surviving patients who had suffered from arterial events comprising recurrent cerebral infarction, symptomatic coronary heart disease, or symptomatic peripheral artery disease, and patients who had not suffered from any arterial event after the index stroke. Multivariate analysis showed that arterial events were independently associated with age (OR 1.1), family history of coronary heart disease (OR 3.7), current smoking on follow-up (OR 7.5), ex-smoking (OR 4.8), and diabetes mellitus (OR 5.5). Another comparison was made between patients without arterial events during follow-up and age and sex matched controls. There were no significant differences as to smoking, hypertension, diabetes mellitus, body mass index, or family history of coronary heart disease [32].

Other Vascular Events

A hospital-based study in Italy including 190 patients with cerebral infarction showed that none had myocardial infarction during the first year after the index stroke. From the second year after the index stroke the average annual frequency of myocardial infarction was 0.72% per year [23]. A hospital-based study in Madrid, Spain including 272 patients with cerebral infarction showed that 10% had non-cerebral cardiovascular events (angina pectoris, myocardial infarction, cardiac failure, and arrhythmia) during a mean follow-up time of 12 years [10]. Non-cerebral cardiovascular events were significantly associated with male gender, age > 35 years, diabetes mellitus and atherosclerosis. Dissection, migraine and non-atherosclerotic vasculopathy were significantly associated with low frequency of non-cerebral vascular events [10]. A hospital-based study in Bologna, Italy including 135 patients with TIA or cerebral infarction showed that 1.5% suffered from myocardial infarction during a mean follow-up of 5.8 years [22]. A hospital-based study in Lille, France including 287 patients with cerebral infarction showed that 0.7% had myocardial infarction during a mean follow-up period of 3 years [19]. A hospital-based study in Taiwan included 231 patients aged 25-49 years with cerebral infarction [21]. The study included only patients with cerebral infarction due to atherosclerosis, small artery occlusion, or undetermined cause. On follow-up at a mean time of 29 months after the index stroke 2 patients (0.9%) had suffered from myocardial infarction.

A population-based study in Hordaland County, Norway including 232 patients had a first follow-up at a mean time of 6 years after the index stroke [17]. In total, 4.3% had suffered from myocardial infarction after the index stroke. At a second follow-up performed on average 12 years after the index stroke among 144 surviving patients 13.2% reported symptomatic coronary heart disease and 11.8% peripheral artery disease [32].

Comments

The recurrence rate of cerebral infarction among young adults is lower than among older patients, but significantly higher than the incidence of first-ever stroke in the general population of the same age. Thus, the frequency of recurrent cerebral infarction the first year after the index stroke ranges from 1.4 to 2.75% in different studies. The average annual frequency of recurrent cerebral infarction after the first year ranges from 0.43 to 2.2% per year. In one study, the rate of recurrent cerebral infarction was 5 times higher than the rate of first ever infarction among age and sex matched controls [32]. Several studies have shown that recurrence of cerebral infarction is highly associated with modifiable risk factors such as hypertension, diabetes mellitus, symptomatic atherosclerosis, and smoking. The risk of recurrent vascular events (including cerebral infarction and myocardial infarction) is strongly linked to the number of traditional risk factors. Thus, an aggressive approach to secondary preventive treatment should comprise antihypertensive medication, statins, appropriate antithrombotic treatment (antiplatelets or warfarin depending on the aetiology), smoking cessation, and careful regulation of blood glucose. One study has shown recurrence of ischaemic stroke to be associated with haematological abnormalities. TIA prior to the index stroke is also associated with higher recurrence rate of stroke. The rate of recurrent cerebral infarction among patients with isolated PFO and no other defined aetiology is probably in the low range.

Several studies indicate that there is a large subgroup with excellent prognosis. This subgroup includes patients with no traditional risk factors. Furthermore, patients with cerebral infarction associated with dissection of neck vessels or migraine have low rate of recurrent cerebral infarction. Among these patients, long-term secondary preventive medication is possibly not indicated.

Post-stroke Seizures

Patients suffering cerebral infarction affecting the cerebral cortex are at risk of developing focal epilepsy [39, 40]. In a study comprising mainly older patients the frequency of post-stroke epilepsy was 11.5% within 5 years after the stroke [39]. It is common to differentiate between early and late seizures after the stroke because of differences in prognosis. Seven days after stroke onset has been proposed as the cut-off point [41]. Prognosis as to recurrence of seizures is thought to be better among patients with early onset seizures.

A study in Auckland, New Zealand including 66 patients aged 11-39 years with cerebral infarction reported that 5 (7.6 %) developed epilepsy during a mean follow-up interval of 3 years [42]. The seizures were difficult to control in one patient. In a study from Lille, France 19 (6.6%) of 287 patients aged 15-45 years with cerebral infarction developed epileptic seizures during a 3 years follow-up period. First seizure was within one year of stroke onset among 15 (79%) of these patients [19]. Another study from France including 65 surviving patients aged 15-45 years with cerebral infarction showed that post-stroke seizures occurred in 7 (11%) patients during a mean follow-up period of 31.7 months [30]. All had the index stroke in the anterior circulation territory. A small study including 62 surviving patients aged 16-40 years with cerebral infarction showed that 8 (13%) had developed post-stroke epilepsy during a mean follow-up time of 17.7 years [25]. The frequency of post-stroke epilepsy among the patients who died during follow-up was higher (25%) (P=.04) [25]. A study in Madrid, Spain including 272 patients aged 15-45 years with cerebral infarction showed that 10% had developed seizures during a follow-up period of 12 years [10].

A population-based study in Hordaland County, Norway including 232 patients aged 15-49 years disclosed that 24 (10.5%) patients had developed post-stroke seizures within a first follow-up performed on average 6 years after the index stroke [17]. Four (1.8%) patients experienced early onset seizures while 20 (8.8%) patients had late onset seizures. In total 22 (92%) patients were seizure-free on follow-up. About 80% developed post-stroke seizures within two years of the index stroke. In all but one patient the index stroke was located in the cerebrum. One third of the patients with severe neurological deficits on admission for the index stroke developed post-stroke seizures [17]. A second follow-up was performed on average 11 years after the index stroke [26]. In total, 28% of the patients with epilepsy still alive on the first follow-up had died within the second follow-up (P=.001). On multivariate analysis the hazards ratio for dying between the first and second follow-up was 3.5 for patients with epilepsy compared with patients without epilepsy (P=.04) [26].

A study from France including 581 patients aged 18-55 years with cryptogenic cerebral infarction showed that 2.4% developed early seizures and 5.5% developed late seizures during a follow-up period of 3 years [41]. Most were seizure free at the end of the follow-up period. Early seizures, cortical signs and large infarction were independent risk factors for late seizures.

Comments

The frequency of post-stroke epilepsy on long-term follow-up seems to be similar among young and old patients with cerebral infarction (10-13%). Patients with large infarctions in the cerebrum have the highest risk of developing post-stroke epilepsy. Most patients develop post-stroke epilepsy within two years of the index stroke and most patients become seizure-free. However, two studies have shown that long-term mortality is significantly higher among patients with post-stroke epilepsy than among patients without post-stroke epilepsy. Whether chronic antiepileptic treatment should be introduced after early seizures to prevent late seizures is not settled [41].

Functional Outcome

Functional outcome is often considered the most important variable as to outcome after stroke. The most commonly used functional outcome scale is the modified Rankin Scale (mRS) (0-6 points). Zero points represent complete recovery while 6 points represent death. Patients scoring 0-2 points are functionally independent while patients scoring 3-5 points are functionally dependent. However, some studies used other outcome scales such as the Glasgow Outcome Scale (GOS) that makes comparison between different studies difficult.

A population-based study from Greece including patients with cerebral infarction irrespective of age showed that 26% of males and 37% of females were functionally dependent on one-year follow-up [43].

A study in Iowa, USA including 296 patients aged 15-45 years with cerebral infarction showed that 76% had minimal or no problems, 17% had moderate handicaps and 7% had major handicaps after a mean follow-up of 6 years based on GOS [9]. A study in Lisbon, Portugal including 172 patients ≤45 years with cerebral infarction showed that 12% were severely disabled (mRS 4-5) after a mean follow-up of 43 months [24]. Disability on follow-up was significantly associated with major index stroke ($P<.0001$). A study in Lille, France including 287 patients aged 15-45 years with cerebral infarction showed that 151 (53%) patients had completely recovered (mRS=0), while 72 (25%) patients scored mRS=1, and 26 (9%) scored mRS=2 after a mean follow-up of 3 years [19]. Among the functionally dependent, 10 (3.5%) scored mRS = 3, 2 (0.7%) scored mRS = 4 and 4 (1.4%) scored mRS = 5 [19]. Dependence on follow-up (mRS 3-5) was significantly associated with higher age, alcoholism, diabetes mellitus, and hypercholesterolemia. Another study in France including 71 patients aged 15-45 years with cerebral infarction showed that 65% had good functional outcome (mRS 0-1), 21% had moderate functional outcome (mRS 2-3), and 14% had poor functional outcome (mRS 4-5) after a mean follow-up of 32 months [30]. Poor functional outcome was associated with anterior circulation territory infarction. A study in Madrid, Spain including 272 patients aged 15-45 years with cerebral infarction showed that 27% had recovered completely (mRS = 0), 85% were functionally independent (mRS ≤ 2), and 15% were functionally dependent (mRS 3-5) after a mean follow-up of 12 years [10]. Age ≥35 years and severe handicaps at discharge for the index stroke were significantly associated with functional dependence on follow-up. A hospital-based study from Switzerland including

203 patients aged 16-45 years with cerebral infarction showed that outcome was favourable in 67% (mRS 0-1), and unfavourable in 33% (mRS 2-5) after a mean follow-up period of 26 months [20]. Based on the OCSP classification of the index stroke it was found that 28% with TACS, 74% with PACS, 88% with LACS and 69% with POCS had favourable outcome (mRS $\leq$1) [20]. Logistic regression showed that diabetes mellitus, a high NIHSS score on admission for the index stroke, and TACS were independently associated with unfavourable outcome (mRS $\geq$2). Age, sex, risk factors other than diabetes mellitus, and stroke aetiology had no predictive value for the clinical outcome.

A population-based study in Hordaland County, Norway included 232 patients aged 15-49 years with cerebral infarction [17]. On follow-up 6 years mean time after the index stroke independent functional outcome (mRS $\leq$ 2) was found among 77.9% of all 232 patients. On univariate analyses significant predictors for unfavourable outcome (mRS $\geq$ 3) were anterior circulation territory infarction, diabetes mellitus, severe neurological deficits on admission for the index stroke, and post-stroke seizures. On multivariate analysis only diabetes mellitus (odds ratio 7, $p = .001$) and severe neurological deficits on admission for the index stroke (odds ratio 13, $p < .001$) remained independently associated with unfavourable outcome on follow-up. Time to follow-up for survivors did not influence on functional outcome [17].

Comments

Compared to studies including old patients the long-term functional outcome is better among young patients. Among survivors about 85% are functionally independent on long-term follow-up (mRS $\leq$ 2). Variables associated with unfavourable functional outcome (mRS 3-5) include higher age, severe index stroke, diabetes mellitus, alcoholism, and anterior circulation territory infarction. The most important predictor for unfavourable functional outcome seems to be the severity of the index stroke.

Post-stroke Depression

Post-stroke depression is an important factor contributing to morbidity in patients after suffering from cerebral infarction [44]. In studies including older patients the prognosis is worsened both regarding mortality and functional outcome [45] while antidepressive treatment seems to improve outcome [46,47]. Some investigators have found early post-stroke depression to be associated with cerebral infarction in the left hemisphere among older patients [48-50]. However, this association is controversial [45]. The frequency of long-term post-stroke depression has been reported to be about 40% among older patients [51-53]. Several studies have shown the frequency of major post-stroke depression to be 15-20% among older patients [51,52,54,55]. Higher prevalence of post-stroke depression with increasing time after the index stroke has been reported among older patients [49].

A hospital-based study in Sweden including 62 surviving patients aged 16-40 years with cerebral infarction showed that 7 (11%) were depressed on follow-up on average 18 years after the index stroke [25]. Three of the patients had had depression prior to the index stroke. A hospital-based study in Iowa, USA including 296 patients aged 15-45 years with cerebral infarction showed that 28% reported depression on follow-up 6 years mean time after the index stroke [9]. However, based on the SF-36 Health Status questionnaire 46% were classified as depressed. Approximately 55% reported that they had had periods of depression after their index stroke [9]. A hospital-based study in France included 71 patients aged 15-45 years with cerebral infarction [30]. On follow-up at a mean time of 32 months after the index stroke 48% of the patients were classified as depressed according to the DSM-IIIR criteria of depression. Depression was significantly associated with infarction in the anterior circulation territory. A study in Madrid, Spain including 272 patients aged 15-45 years with cerebral infarction showed that 22% had depression as assessed by a psychiatrist on follow-up at a mean time of 12 years after the index stroke [10].

A population-based study in Hordaland County, Norway included 232 patients aged 15-49 years with cerebral infarction [56]. Based on the Montgomery Asberg Depression Rate Scale 29% reported depression on follow-up at a mean time of 6 years after the index stroke. Mild depression was found among 25%, moderate depression among 4% while none had major depression. Univariate analyses showed that depression on follow-up was significantly associated with depressive symptoms any time before the index stroke, alcoholism before the index stroke, being unmarried on follow-up, loss of employment after the index stroke, and lower education. Time to follow-up was not associated with depression. There was no association between the hemispheric side of the index stroke and depression. Multivariate analysis showed that depression on follow-up was independently associated with depressive symptoms before the index stroke, alcoholism before the index stroke, and severe neurological deficits on admission for the index stroke.

In the population-based study in Hordaland County, Norway the patients were compared with age and sex matched controls as to the frequency of depressive symptoms [56]. The presence of depressive symptoms was based on the emotional reaction subscore of the Nottingham Health Profile. Depressive symptoms were reported by 39% of the patients and 24% of the controls (p = .002).

Comments

It is difficult to compare studies of post-stroke depression among young adults with cerebral infarction because of different study designs. Four hospital-based studies reported that 11-48% of the patients were depressed on long-term follow-up. In a population-based study only 29% were depressed on follow-up and most had mild depression. Predictors for depression on long-term follow-up include depressive symptoms any time before the index stroke, alcoholism, severe stroke, and infarction in the anterior circulation territory.

Health Related Quality of Life

Health related quality of life (HRQoL) should assess at least physical, functional, mental, and social health [57]. HRQoL is often used to evaluate the effectiveness of healthcare and medical treatment [58]. There have been few studies including HRQoL analyses among young adults with cerebral infarction.

A hospital-based study in Iowa, USA including 296 patients aged 15-45 years with cerebral infarction assessed HRQoL by means of parts of the SF-36 Health Status questionnaire (SF-36) on follow-up at a mean time of 6 years after the index stroke [9]. It was found that 28% reported poor outcome as to physical functioning, 27% reported poor outcome as to social functioning, and 19% reported poor outcome as to emotional problems. A hospital-based study in France including 60 patients aged 15-45 years with cerebral infarction assessed HRQoL by means of parts of the Sickness Impact Profile (SIP) on follow-up at a mean time of 32 months after the index stroke [30]. It was found that 23% reported poor outcome as to sleep and rest, 17% reported poor outcome as to emotional behaviour, 44% reported poor outcome as to alertness behaviour, 13% reported poor outcome as to communication, 40% reported poor outcome as to recreation and pastimes, and 25% reported poor outcome as to social interaction. On multivariate analyses poor quality of life was associated with major stroke, depression, and employment [30].

A population-based study in Hordaland County, Norway included 232 patients aged 15-49 years with cerebral infarction [59]. On follow-up at a mean time of 6 years after the index stroke HRQoL was assessed by means of the SF-36 among 190 patients, and among 215 controls. The patients scored significantly lower than the controls on several subscales including physical functioning, role limitations due to physical problems, general health perceptions, vitality, and social functioning. However, the mean difference was less than one standard deviation in all subscale scores indicating that cerebral infarction had only moderate effect on self-reported HRQoL. The largest difference between patients and controls was related to physical functioning. Subgroup analyses among the patients showed clinically significant reduction of HRQoL among patients who were depressed, unemployed, unmarried, functionally dependent (mRS 3-5), and suffered from fatigue. There was no difference between men and women. Multivariate analyses showed that fatigue, but not depression was independently associated with physical functioning [59].

Comments

It is difficult to compare different studies among young adults with cerebral infarction as to HRQoL because of different study design. A population-based study showed that the difference in HRQoL between patients and controls at the group level was not large. However, several studies show that HRQoL is poor among important subgroups of the patients. Predictors for poor HRQoL at long-term follow-up are depression, fatigue, functional dependence (mRS 3-5), unemployment, and being unmarried.

Post-stroke Fatigue

The subjective sensation of fatigue is defined as an overwhelming sense of tiredness, lack of energy, or feeling of exhaustion [60,61]. Fatigue is a frequent symptom in chronic neurological diseases such as multiple sclerosis, Parkinson's disease, and poliomyelitis [60,61]. Fatigue is also a common symptom of depression, but many patients experience fatigue without other symptoms that are characteristic of depression [62,63]. A study including older patients with cerebral infarction showed an association between fatigue and higher mortality [63]. Another study including older patients suggested that there is an association between fatigue and brainstem and thalamic lesions [60]. A study including older patients with stroke reported that fatigue was present in 70% as assessed by the Fatigue Severity Scale (FSS) one year after the index stroke [64]. The mean FSS score was 4.7.

The only study of fatigue among young patients with cerebral infarction was a population-based study in Hordaland County, Norway including 232 patients age 15-49 years with cerebral infarction [65]. Fatigue was assessed by means of the FSS score on follow-up at a mean time of 6 years after the index stroke among 192 patients and 212 controls. The frequency of fatigue was 37% among the patients and 23% among the controls ($p = .01$). The mean FSS score was 4.1 among the patients and 3.4 among the controls ($p < .001$). Multivariate analysis including patients only showed that fatigue was independently associated with depression and unfavourable functional outcome (mRS 3-5). In addition, large infarction in the brainstem and cerebellum seemed to have higher impact on fatigue than large infarction in the cerebrum [65]. Assessment by means of the SF-36 among the patients showed that the presence of fatigue had a clinically important deleterious impact on the quality of life on follow-up [59]. This pertained especially to the subscales including physical functioning, bodily pain and general health.

Comments

Several studies support the existence of primary posts-stroke fatigue without coexisting depression both among young patients and older patients with cerebral infarction. Fatigue is less severe among young adults with cerebral infarction than among patients with multiple sclerosis and Parkinson's disease [65]. Fatigue also seems to be less severe among younger patients with stroke than older patients. However, the presence of fatigue has important deleterious impact on quality of life among young patients with cerebral infarction on long-term follow-up. Independent predictors for post-stroke fatigue include unfavourable functional outcome, depression, and possibly infarction in the posterior circulation territory.

Post-stroke Pain

There have been few studies systematically evaluating the development of post-stroke pain among young adults with cerebral infarction. Studies including older patients with stroke suggest that post-stroke pain often develops more than 3 months after stroke onset [66].

A study compared quality of life by means of the Nottingham Health Profile scale (comprising six subscales) between 191 young adults aged 15-49 years with cerebral infarction and 337 multiple sclerosis patients with secondary progressive course [67]. The patients with cerebral infarction were assessed at a mean time of 6 years after the index stroke and the patients with multiple sclerosis were assessed at a mean time of 5 years after the onset of secondary progressive course. At the time of assessment, the mean age of the patients with cerebral infarction was 48 years and the mean age of the patients with multiple sclerosis was 45 years. Comparing the patients with cerebral infarction and the patients with multiple sclerosis adjusting for physical mobility showed that both pain and sleep disturbances were significantly more pronounced among the patients with cerebral infarction. Pain was associated with sleep disturbances and energy level, but not depressive symptoms [67].

Comments

Pain may be a serious long-term affliction among young adults with cerebral infarction. This pertains especially to patients with significant reduction in physical abilities. Possible consequences of post-stroke pain include sleep disturbances, and fatigue. Because post-stroke pain often develops more than 3 months after stroke onset long-term follow-up is needed. Appropriate treatment of post-stroke pain in addition to pain relief may have beneficial effect on sleep and vitality.

Cognitive Dysfunction

Although about 85% of young patients with cerebral infarction are functionally independent (mRS ≤2) on long-term follow-up many suffer from mild to moderate cognitive dysfunction. The high fraction of patients on disability pension after cerebral infarction may partially be explained by cognitive dysfunction [17]. However, there has been little systematic investigation of cognitive function on long-term follow-up after cerebral infarction among young adults. A population-based study including patients irrespective of age showed that 38% had Mini-Mental State Examination (MMSE) ≤ 23 on long-term follow-up [68].

A hospital-based study including 296 patients aged 15-45 years with cerebral infarction was performed in Iowa, USA [9]. On follow-up at a mean time of 6 years after the index stroke, MMSE was performed among 71 patients. It was found that 71% had MMSE = 28-30, 20% had MMSE = 24-27, and 9% had MMSE = 0-23. A population-based study in Hordaland County, Norway included 232 patients aged 15-49 years with cerebral infarction [56]. On follow-up at a mean time of 6 years after the index stroke, MMSE was assessed among 193 patients. The mean score was 28.0 (range 15-30). It was found that 31% had MMSE = 30, 73% had MMSE = 28-30, 19% had MMSE = 25-27, and 8% had MMSE ≤ 24.

Comments

Compared to older patients with cerebral infarction, cognitive dysfunction as measured by MMSE seems to be milder among young patients. Two studies show that about 70% of young patients with cerebral infarction have MMSE = 28-30 on long-term follow-up while less than 10% have MMSE ≤24. However, the MMSE has limited specificity. For example, it does not evaluate executive function, which is critical to informed decision-making. Future studies of long-term outcome among young adults with cerebral infarction should include an appropriate neuropsychological battery.

Employment

Young patients have often the primary responsibility for generating income for the family. Suffering from stroke at a young age may therefore have serious consequences for the whole family if the stroke leads to inability of resuming employment. Information on factors contributing to loss of employment is therefore important.

A hospital-based study in Bari, Italy included 56 patients aged 17-45 years with cerebral infarction or TIA [6]. On follow-up at a mean time of 4 years after the index stroke 41% continued in the same job, 29% were employed in a different type of work, and 30% were out of work. A hospital-based study in Malmoe, Sweden including 74 patients aged 16-40 years showed that 63% had full working capacity while 11% were working part-time on follow-up at a mean time of 18 years after the index stroke [25]. A hospital-based study in Bologna, Italy including patients aged 16-45 years with cerebral infarction (n=85) or TIA (n=70) showed that 91% had resumed work after a mean follow-up of 6 years [22]. A hospital-based study in Lisbon, Portugal included 172 patients aged ≤45 years with cerebral infarction [24]. On follow-up at a mean time of 3.3 years after the index stroke, 59% were full- or part-time workers. The employment rate was 64% among the patients with minor stroke and 40% among the patients with major stroke. Predictors for employment were drinking <60g pr day of alcohol, and minor stroke. A hospital-based study in Iowa, USA included 296 patients aged 15-45 years with cerebral infarction [9]. On long-term follow-up at mean time of 6 years after the index stroke only 42% were employed, and in 23% of them adjustments in their occupation were necessary. A hospital-based study in Italy included 330 patients aged 15-44 years with cerebral infarction or TIA. On follow-up at a mean time of 8 years after the index stroke 56% had returned to work [23]. A hospital-based study in Lille, France included 287 patients aged 15-45 years with cerebral infarction [19]. On follow-up at a mean time of 3 years after the index stroke 50% had returned to the same work (7% of them with adjustment in their occupation) while 11% had found a new job. Another hospital-based study from France included 71 patients aged 15-45 years with cerebral infarction [30]. On follow-up at a mean time of 32 months after the index stroke 73% had returned to work, and in 26% of them adjustments were necessary (other work or part-time employment). The mean time of returning to work was 7.8 months (range 0-40 months). Univariate analyses showed that not returning to work was significantly associated with high NIHSS score, aphasia, epilepsy, and depression. Only 5% with a NIHSS score <10 did not return to work while 71% with NIHSS score ≥10 did not return to work [30]. A hospital-based study in Messina, Italy included 55 patients aged 17-45 years with cerebral infarction or TIA [69]. On follow-up at mean time of 6 years after the index stroke, 69% had returned to work, although adjustments (other job or part-time employment) were necessary for 27% of them. A hospital-based study in Spain included 272 patients aged 15-45 years with cerebral infarction [10]. On follow-up at mean time of 12 years after the index stroke 53% had returned to work. Of these, 23% needed to make occupational adjustments (another job or part-time employment). In total 35% were considered to be unable to work for medical reasons. Not being able to return to work was significantly associated with severe handicap at discharge, and cardioembolic stroke [10].

A population-based study in Hordaland County, Norway included 232 patients aged 15-49 years with cerebral infarction [17]. On follow-up at a mean time of 6 years after the index stroke, 58% were employed. Before the index stroke 85% were employed. More patients were part-time employed on follow-up than before stroke onset (18% vs 11%, $p = .03$). Disability pension was awarded to 33%. Multivariate analysis showed that loss of employment was associated with increasing age, unfavourable functional outcome (mRS 3-5) on discharge, being unmarried on follow-up, and low education [17]. Among patients employed before the index stroke 80% with MMSE ≤ 24, 45% with MMSE = 25-27, and 24% with MMSE ≥ 28 had not returned to work on follow-up [56].

Comments

The range of young patients with cerebral infarction returning to work on long-term follow-up goes from 42% to 91% in different studies. However, the percentage in most studies seems to be about 60%. About 25% of the patients resuming work need job adjustment such as finding a new job or working part-time. Predictors for unemployment on long-term follow-up include major stroke, aphasia, epilepsy, low score on MMSE, depression, increasing age, and low education.

Pregnancy

Cerebral infarction is associated with pregnancy [70]. A retrospective study in Toronto, Canada identified 13 cerebral infarctions of approximately 50 700 admissions for delivery [70]. All survived. A study in Houston, USA included 79 301 deliveries [71]. Five deliveries were associated with cerebral infarction. All survived. A study in France included 373 women aged 15-40 years with cerebral infarction [72]. The risk of recurrent stroke was 1% within one year and 2.3% within 5 years. There were 187 pregnancies after the index stroke. Recurrent stroke were associated with two pregnancies (1.1%). The authors concluded that young women with a history of cerebral infarction have a low risk of recurrent cerebral infarction in subsequent pregnancies [72].

Comments

The mortality of cerebral infarction associated with pregnancy seems to be low. A history of cerebral infarction among young women is no contraindication for subsequent pregnancies.

Conclusion

Both short-term and long-term prognoses are better among young adults with cerebral infarction than among older patients with cerebral infarction. Case-fatality rate within 30 days of stroke onset is 3-7% and about four fifths of the survivors are functionally independent on discharge. Early death is most often caused by stroke related herniation. Long-term mortality rate is about 10 times higher than the mortality rate in the age matched general population. Long-term mortality is associated with risk factors such as atherosclerosis, hypertension, smoking, and alcoholism. Dissection of the neck vessel is associated with low mortality. Recurrence rate of cerebral infarction is about 2% per year. Recurrence of cerebral infarction is highly associated with modifiable risk factors such as atherosclerosis, hypertension, smoking, and diabetes mellitus. A large subgroup seems to have good long-term prognosis both as to death and recurrent cerebral infarction. This group comprises patient with no traditional risk factors, patients with migraine, or patients with dissection of the neck vessels. About 10% develop post-stroke epilepsy, and in most cases within 2 years of the index stroke. Most become seizure-free. Post-stroke depression is frequent although mostly mild. Post-stroke depression is associated with severe stroke, stroke in the anterior circulation territory, alcoholism, and depression any time before the index stroke. Predictors for poor health related quality of life at long-term follow-up are depression, fatigue, functional dependence, unemployment, and being unmarried. Pain, fatigue, and sleep disturbances are other frequent long-term afflictions after cerebral infarction. About 60% resume employment after the index stroke. However, about 25% of the patients resuming work need job adjustments. Predictors for unemployment after cerebral infarction include major stroke, aphasia, epilepsy, cognitive dysfunction, depression, increasing age, and low education.

The most important findings as to long-term prognosis after cerebral infarction among young adults are that both long-term mortality and recurrence of cerebral infarction are highly associated with traditional risk factors such as hypertension, diabetes mellitus, cardiac diseases, and smoking. Thus, aggressive long-term secondary preventive treatment has a potentially huge beneficial effect among patients with traditional risk factors.

References

[1] Ellekjaer H, Holmen J, Indredavik B, Terent A. Epidemiology of stroke in Innherred, Norway, 1994 to 1996. Incidence and 30-day case-fatality rate. *Stroke* 1997;28:2180-4.

[2] Vemmos K, Bots ML, Tsibouris PK, Zis VP, Grobbee DE, Stranjalis GS, Stamatelopoulos S. Stroke incidence and case fatality in southern Greece: the Arcadia stroke registry. *Stroke* 1999;30:363-70.

[3] Hindfelt B, Nilsson O. The prognosis of ischemic stroke in young adults. *Acta Neurol. Scand.* 1977;55:123-30.

[4] Snyder BD, Ramirez-Lassepas M. Cerebral infarction in young adults. *Stroke* 1980; 11:149-153.

[5] Leno C, Berciano J, Combarros O, Polo JM, Pascual J, Quintana F, Merino J, Sedano C, Martín-Durán R, Alvarez C, et al. A prospective study of stroke in young adults in Cantabria, Spain. *Stroke* 1993;24:792-5.

[6] Federico F, Calvario T, Di Turi N, Paradiso F. Ischaemic cerebral infarction in young adults. *Acta Neurol. (Napoli).* 1990;12:101-8.

[7] Carolei A, Marini C, Ferranti E, Frontoni M, Prencipe M, Fieschi C. A prospective study of cerebral ischemia in the young. Analysis of pathogenic determinants. The National Research Council Study Group. *Stroke* 1993; 24:362-7.

[8] Qureshi AI, Safdar K, Patel M, Janssen RS, Frankel MR. Stroke in young black patients. Risk factors, subtypes, and prognosis. *Stroke* 1995;26:1995-8.

[9] Kappelle LJ, Adams HP Jr, Heffner ML, Torner JC, Gomez F, Biller J. Prognosis of young adults with ischemic stroke. A long-term follow-up study assessing recurrent vascular events and functional outcome in the Iowa Registry of Stroke in Young Adults. *Stroke* 1994;25:1360-5.

[10] Varona JF, Bermejo F, Guerra JM, Molina JA. Long-term prognosis of ischemic stroke in young adults. Study of 272 cases. *J. Neurol.* 2004; 251:1507-14.

[11] Razzaq AA, Khan BA, Baig SM. Ischemic stroke in young adults of South Asia. *J. Pak. Med.. Assoc.* 2002;52:417-22.

[12] Nencini P, Inzitari D, Baruffi MC, Fratiglioni L, Gagliardi R, Benvenuti L, Buccheri AM, Cecchi L, Passigli A, Rosselli A, et al. Incidence of stroke in young adults in Florence, Italy. *Stroke* 1988;19:977-81.

[13] Rozenthul-Sorokin N, Ronen R, Tamir A, Geva H, Eldar R. Stroke in the young in Israel. Incidence and outcomes. *Stroke* 1996;27:838-41.

[14] Jacobs BS, Boden-Albala B, Lin IF, Sacco RL. Stroke in the young in the northern Manhattan stroke study. *Stroke* 2002;33:2789-93.

[15] Kristensen B, Malm J, Carlberg B, Stegmayr B, Backman C, Fagerlund M, Olsson T. Epidemiology and etiology of ischemic stroke in young adults aged 18 to 44 years in northern Sweden. *Stroke* 1997;28:1702-9.

[16] Naess H, Nyland HI, Thomassen L, Aarseth J, Nyland G, Myhr KM. Incidence and short-term outcome of cerebral infarction in young adults in Norway. *Stroke* 2002; 33:2105-8.

[17] Naess H, Nyland HI, Thomassen L, Aarseth J, Myhr KM. Long-term outcome of cerebral infarction in young adults. *Acta Neurol. Scand.* 2004;110:107-12.

[18] Hardie K, Hankey GJ, Jamrozik K, Broadhurst RJ, Anderson C. Ten-year survival after first-ever stroke in the perth community stroke study. *Stroke* 2003;34:1842-6.

[19] Leys D, Bandu L, Hénon H, Lucas C, Mounier-Vehier F, Rondepierre P, Godefroy O. Clinical outcome in 287 consecutive young adults (15 to 45 years) with ischemic stroke. *Neurology* 2002;59:26-33.

[20] Nedeltchev K, der Maur TA, Georgiadis D, Arnold M, Caso V, Mattle HP, Schroth G, Remonda L, Sturzenegger M, Fischer U, Baumgartner RW. Ischaemic stroke in young adults: predictors of outcome and recurrence. *J. Neurol. Neurosurg. Psychiatry* 2005; 76(2):191-5.

[21] Yeh PS, Lin HJ, Li YH, Lin KC, Cheng TJ, Chang CY, Ke DS. Prognosis of young ischemic stroke in Taiwan: impact of prothrombotic genetic polymorphisms. *Thromb Haemost*. 2004;92:583-9.

[22] Lanzino G, Andreoli A, Di Pasquale G, Urbinati S, Limoni P, Serracchioli A, Lusa A, Pinelli G, Testa C, Tognetti F. Etiopathogenesis and prognosis of cerebral ischemia in young adults. A survey of 155 treated patients. *Acta Neurol. Scand*. 1991;84:321-5.

[23] Marini C, Totaro R, Carolei A. Long-term prognosis of cerebral ischemia in young adults. National Research Council Study Group on Stroke in the Young. *Stroke* 1999; 30:2320-5.

[24] Ferro J, Crespo M. Prognosis after transient ischemic attack and ischemic stroke in young adults. *Stroke* 1994;25:1611-6.

[25] Hindfelt B, Nilsson O. Long-term prognosis of ischemic stroke in young adults. *Acta Neurol. Scand*. 1992;86:440-5.

[26] Waje-Andreassen U, Naess H, Thomassen L, Eide GE, Vedeler CA. Long-term mortality among young ischemic stroke patients in Norway. *Acta Neurol. Scand*. 2007 116:150-6.

[27] Hardie K, Jamrozik K, Hankey GJ, Broadhurst RJ, Anderson C. Trends in five-year survival and risk of recurrent stroke after first-ever stroke in the Perth Community Stroke Study. *Cerebrovasc. Dis*. 2005;19:179-85.

[28] Burn J, Dennis M, Bamford J, Sandercock P, Wade D, Warlow C. Long-term risk of recurrent stroke after a first-ever stroke. The Oxfordshire Community Stroke Project. *Stroke* 1994;25:333-7.

[29] Eriksson SE, Olsson JE. Survival and recurrent strokes in patients with different subtypes of stroke: a fourteen-year follow-up study. *Cerebrovasc. Dis*.2001;12:171-80.

[30] Neau J, Ingrand P, Mouille-Brachet C, Rosier MP, Couderq C, Alvarez A, Gil R. Functional recovery and social outcome after cerebral infarction in young adults. *Cerebrovasc. Dis*. 1998;8:296-302.

[31] Camerlingo M, Casto L, Censori B, Ferraro B, Caverni L, Manara O, Finazzi G, Radice E, Drago G, De Tommasi SM, Gotti E, Barbui T, Mamoli A. Recurrence after first cerebral infarction in young adults. *Acta Neurol. Scand*. 2000;102:87-93.

[32] Waje-Andreassen U, Naess H, Thomassen L, Eide GE, Vedeler CA. Arterial events after ischemic stroke at a young age: a cross-sectional long-term follow-up of patients and controls in Norway. *Cerebrovasc. Dis*. 2007; 24:277-82.

[33] Lechat P, Mas JL, Lascault G, Loron P, Theard M, Klimczac M, Drobinski G, Thomas D, Grosgogeat Y. Prevalence of patent foramen ovale in patients with stroke. *N. Engl. J. Med*. 1988;318:1148-52.

[34] Webster MW, Chancellor AM, Smith HJ, Swift DL, Sharpe DN, Bass NM, Glasgow GL. Patent foramen ovale in young stroke patients. *Lancet* 1988;2:11-2.

[35] Di Tullio M, Sacco RL, Gopal A, Mohr JP, Homma S. Patent foramen ovale as a risk factor for cryptogenic stroke. *Ann. Intern. Med*. 1992;117:461-5.

[36] Homma S, Sacco RL, Di Tullio MR, Sciacca RR, Mohr JP. Effect of medical treatment in stroke patients with patent foramen ovale: patent foramen ovale in Cryptogenic Stroke Study. *Circulation* 2002;105:2625-31.

[37] Mas JL, Arquizan C, Lamy C, Zuber M, Cabanes L, Derumeaux G, Coste J; Patent Foramen Ovale and Atrial Septal Aneurysm Study Group. Recurrent cerebrovascular events associated with patent foramen ovale, atrial septal aneurysm, or both. *N. Engl. J. Med.* 2001;345:1740-6.

[38] Naess, H, Waje-Andreassen U, Thomassen L, Nyland H, Myhr KM. Do all young ischemic stroke patients need long-term secondary preventive medication? *Neurology* 2005; 65:609-11.

[39] Burn J, Dennis M, Bamford J, Sandercock P, Wade D, Warlow C. Epileptic seizures after a first stroke: the Oxfordshire Community Stroke Project. *Bmj* 1997;315:1582-7.

[40] Lossius MI, Rønning OM, Mowinckel P, Gjerstad L. Incidence and predictors for post-stroke epilepsy. A prospective controlled trial. The Akershus stroke study. *Eur. J. Neurol.* 2002;9:365-8.

[41] Lamy C, Domigo V, Semah F, Arquizan C, Trystram D, Coste J, Mas JL; Patent Foramen Ovale and Atrial Septal Aneurysm Study Group. Early and late seizures after cryptogenic ischemic stroke in young adults. *Neurology* 2003;60:400-4.

[42] Chancellor AM, Glasgow GL, Ockelford PA, Johns A, Smith J. Etiology, prognosis, and hemostatic function after cerebral infarction in young adults. *Stroke* 1989;20:477-82.

[43] Vemmos KN, Bots ML, Tsibouris PK, Zis VP, Takis CE, Grobbee DE, Stamatelopoulos S. Prognosis of stroke in the south of Greece: 1 year mortality, functional outcome and its determinants: the Arcadia Stroke Registry. *J. Neurol. Neurosurg. Psychiatry* 2000;69:595-600.

[44] Parikh RM, Robinson RG, Lipsey JR, Starkstein SE, Fedoroff JP, Price TR. The impact of poststroke depression on recovery in activities of daily living over a 2-year follow-up. *Arch Neurol.* 1990;47:785-9.

[45] Pohjasvaara T, Vataja R, Leppävuori A, Kaste M, Erkinjuntti T. Cognitive functions and depression as predictors of poor outcome 15 months after stroke. *Cerebrovasc. Dis.* 2002;14:228-33.

[46] Lipsey JR, Robinson RG, Pearlson GD, Rao K, Price TR. Nortriptyline treatment of post-stroke depression: a double-blind study. *Lancet* 1984;1:297-300.

[47] Andersen G, Vestergaard K, Lauritzen L. Effective treatment of poststroke depression with the selective serotonin reuptake inhibitor citalopram. *Stroke* 1994;25:1099-104.

[48] Robinson RG, Price TR. Post-stroke depressive disorders: a follow-up study of 103 patients. *Stroke* 1982;13:635-41.

[49] Astrom M, Adolfsson R, Asplund K. Major depression in stroke patients. A 3-year longitudinal study. *Stroke* 1993;24:976-82.

[50] Spalletta G, Guida G, De Angelis D, Caltagirone C. Predictors of cognitive level and depression severity are different in patients with left and right hemispheric stroke within the first year of illness. *J. Neurol.*2002;249:1541-51.

[51] Kotila M, Numminen H, Waltimo O, Kaste M. Depression after stroke: results of the FINNSTROKE Study. *Stroke* 1998;29:368-72.

[52] Pohjasvaara T, Leppävuori A, Siira I, Vataja R, Kaste M, Erkinjuntti T. Frequency and clinical determinants of poststroke depression. *Stroke* 1998;29:2311-7.

[53] Kauhanen ML, Korpelainen JT, Hiltunen P, Nieminen P, Sotaniemi KA, Myllylä VV. Domains and determinants of quality of life after stroke caused by brain infarction. Arch *Phys. Med. Rehabil.* 2000;81:1541-6.

[54] Morris PL, Raphael B. Depressive disorder associated with physical illness. The impact of stroke. *Gen. Hosp. Psychiatry* 1987;9:324-30.

[55] Tateno A, Murata Y, Robinson RG. Comparison of cognitive impairment associated with major depression following stroke versus traumatic brain injury. *Psychosomatics* 2002;43:295-301.

[56] Naess H, Nyland HI, Thomassen L, Aarseth J, Myhr KM. Mild depression in young adults with cerebral infarction at long-term follow-up: a population-based study. *Eur. J. Neurol.* 2005;12:194-8.

[57] de Haan R, Aaronson N, Limburg M, Hewer RL, van Crevel H. Measuring quality of life in stroke. *Stroke* 1993;24:320-7.

[58] Anderson C, Laubscher S, Burns R. Validation of the Short Form 36 (SF-36) health survey questionnaire among stroke patients. *Stroke* 1996;27:1812-6.

[59] Naess H, Waje-Andreassen U, Thomassen L, Nyland H, Myhr KM. Health-related quality of life among young adults with ischemic stroke on long-term follow-up. *Stroke* 2006; 37:1232-6.

[60] Staub F, Bogousslavsky J. Fatigue after stroke: a major but neglected issue. *Cerebrovasc. Dis*. 2001;12:75-81.

[61] Herlofson K, Larsen JP. Measuring fatigue in patients with Parkinson's disease - the Fatigue Severity Scale. *Eur. J. Neurol.*2002; 9:595-600.

[62] van der Werf SP, van den Broek HL, Anten HW, Bleijenberg G. Experience of severe fatigue long after stroke and its relation to depressive symptoms and disease characteristics. *Eur. Neurol.* 2001;45:28-33.

[63] Glader EL, Stegmayr B, Asplund K. Poststroke fatigue: a 2-year follow-up study of stroke patients in Sweden. *Stroke* 2002;33(5):1327-33.

[64] Schepers VP, Visser-Meily AM, Ketelaar M, Lindeman E. Prediction of social activity 1 year poststroke. *Arch Phys. Med. Rehabil.* 2005;86:1472-6.

[65] Naess H, Nyland HI, Thomassen L, Aarseth J, Myhr KM. Fatigue at long-term follow-up in young adults with cerebral infarction. *Cerebrovasc. Dis*. 2005;20:245-50.

[66] Widar M, Samuelsson L, Karlsson-Tivenius S, Ahlström G. Long-term pain conditions after a stroke. *J. Rehabil. Med.* 2002;34:165-70.

[67] Naess H, Beiske AG, Myhr KM. Quality of life among young patients with ischaemic stroke compared with patients with multiple sclerosis. *Acta Neurol. Scand.* 2008; 117: 181-5.

[68] Patel MD, Coshall C, Rudd AG, Wolfe CD. Cognitive impairment after stroke: clinical determinants and its associations with long-term stroke outcomes. *J. Am. Geriatr.* Soc. 2002;50:700-6.

[69] Musolino R, La Spina P, Granata A, Gallitto G, Leggiadro N, Carerj S, Manganaro A, Tripodi F, Epifanio A, Gangemi S, Di Perri R. Ischaemic stroke in young people: a prospective and long-term follow-up study. *Cerebrovasc. Dis*. 2003;15:121-8.

[70] Jaigobin C, Silver F.L. Stroke and pregnancy. *Stroke* 2000;31:2948-51.

[71] Witlin AG, Friedman SA, Egerman RS, Frangieh AY. Cerebrovascular disorders complicating pregnancy--beyond eclampsia. *Am. J. Obstet. Gynecol.* 1997;176:1139-45; discussion 1145-8.

[72] Lamy C, Hamon JB, Coste J, Mas JL. Ischemic stroke in young women: risk of recurrence during subsequent pregnancies. French Study Group on Stroke in Pregnancy. *Neurology* 2000;55(2):269-74.

In: Cerebral Ischemia in Young Adults
Editors: A. Pezzini and A. Padovani

ISBN 978-1-60741-627-2

Chapter 25

Stroke Rehabilitation in Young Ischemic Stroke Survivors

Stefano Paolucci**, *Francesca Romana Fusco, Luca Pratesi, Maura Bragoni, Paola Coiro, Domenico De Angelis, and Vincenzo Venturiero
Fondazione I.R.C.C.S. Santa Lucia,
Via Ardeatina,Rome, Italy.

Abstract

Rehabilitation plays a relevant role in the treatment of sequelae of cerebrovascular events even in the younger age groups. However, literature data have essentially been focused on the role of aging in influencing rehabilitative results. Thus, data on the course of rehabilitation program in younger patients are less exhaustive. In the rehabilitation of younger patients several aspects other than independence in activities of daily living must be taken into account, such as returning to work, sexuality and driving. In the few papers that stratified patients according to classes of age, younger patients had significantly better functional outcome and rehabilitation results than the older groups.

Introduction

It is commonly believed that young patients have a favourable recovery form stroke. However, even if a complete functional recovery is achieved by most of younger cases [1-3], there are many cases who need specific rehabilitation treatment.

In stroke survivors, rehabilitation treatment may reduce disability and improve quality of life. Stroke rehabilitation is an active process that begins during hospitalisation in the acute

* Correspondence: Stefano Paolucci, Via Ardeatina, 306, 00179 Rome, Italy. tel. 06.51501001 - 06.515011, fax 06.51501004 - 06.5032097. e-mail: s.paolucci@hsantalucia.it.

phase, progresses through a systematic program of rehabilitation services and continues after the individual returns to the community. Cerebral reorganisation is considered to be the principle process responsible for recovery after stroke, and different interventions like physiotherapy, occupational therapy, speech therapy, electrical stimulation, etc. may facilitate such changes [4].

In this paper, we describe several factors that need to be taken into account when approaching the complex problem of neurological rehabilitation of young stroke patients.

Impact of Aging on Functional Outcome

To evaluate the role of any prognostic factor upon a specific dependent variable, it is first necessary to clearly define the correct measure of outcome. In rehabilitation medicine, this is still an unresolved problem. In fact, even if several measures are available, none of them can be considered the perfect one to identify changes due to the rehabilitation therapy. In fact, some of these end-points, as mortality or return home or to work, are associated with overall functional status, but poorly explain the rehabilitation process. The improvement in functional score in one of the most commonly used rating scale is a classic measure. However, the real impact of rehabilitation is influenced not only by ordinal characteristic of scales, but also by their floor and ceiling effects. In rehabilitation, the most widely used scale are disability scales [5], such as the Barthel Index or the FIM (Functional Instrument Measure), that evaluate the independence in ADL (Activities of Daily Living) [6-8]. Other measures, such as rehabilitation effectiveness and rehabilitation efficiency, have been proposed [9,10]. Rehabilitation effectiveness and rehabilitation efficiency provide a basis for measuring the success of rehabilitation, both in terms of individual patient performance and of rehabilitation center adequacy. Rehabilitation efficiency relates to the amount of improvement averaged over the duration of rehabilitation and can be regarded as the average increase in functional ability per day, but it is influenced by the length of rehabilitation. Therefore, rehabilitation efficiency is not truly an outcome measure and cannot be compared with other outcome measures.

Rehabilitation effectiveness is a measure of improvement that adjusts for functional score at admission, and reflects the proportion of potential improvement actually obtained during rehabilitation. Rehabilitation effectiveness is calculated as actual improvement divided by maximum potential improvement times 100% [9,10]. Thus, rehabilitation effectiveness = (discharge score – admission score)/(maximum score-admission score) x 100%. The main problem with rehabilitation effectiveness as an outcome measure is that it is overly sensitive at the upper end. So, to have a wider knowledge of rehabilitation results it is preferable to use a battery of measures.

Rehabilitation treatment is quite long and expensive. Thus, several studies have been performed, in the recent years that aimed at identifying reliable prognostic factors on functional outcome and rehabilitation results.

Most of these studies evaluated age factor, but they mainly were focused on the role of aging. Thus, literature data on the role of aging on functional recovery is enough exhaustive, with general consensus on aging as an unfavourable risk factor for functional outcome [10-20]. Few papers described opposite results [21,22].

A Finnish study compared stroke features and poststroke disability between younger (55 to 70 years) and older (71 to 85 years) ischemic stroke patients (486 cases) and found that this latter group was more dependent 3 months after stroke than the younger ones [23].

The data of Copenhagen Stroke Study, a prospective, community-based study, showed that a 10-year increase in age was associated with a 7% decrease in gain on the Barthel Index [14]. In other report of the same study, patients with most severe strokes who achieved a good functional outcome were generally characterized by younger age [24].

Similarly, Sanchez-Blanco and co-workers observed that patients <70 years of age had twice the probability of achieving independent ambulation [19].

In 2002, Bogousslavsky and Pierre, evaluating 202 younger patients (≤45 yrs) out of 1638 (12.3%) ischemic stroke patients from Lausanne stroke registry, found a better prognosis in patients <30 years as comparison with the other [25].

In 2003, Kugler et al., evaluating a cohort study of 2.219 patients, found that patients younger than 55 years, in comparison with older ones, had not only a better recovery (67% of the maximum possible improvement vs. 50%), but also a faster one [26].

Recently, Black-Schaffer and Winston, evaluating the effect of advancing age on rehabilitation results in 979 stroke rehabilitation patients at a long-term acute care rehabilitation hospital, found a strong relationship of increasing age to poorer outcome in all patient with basal severe disability (admission FIM score <40), but no relationship of age to the outcome measures in patients with basal mild disability (admission FIM score >80) [27].

Moreover, Patel et al. observed that patients aged 75 and older had a higher risk (OR, 2.5; 95% CI, 1.5 to 4.2) of cognitive impairment 3 months after stroke as compared with younger ones [28].

Lastly, age ≥65 years was associated with a higher risk (OR, 3.93; 95% CI, 1.73 to 8.95) of functional worsening at 1 year follow-up [29].

Current opinion is that younger patients reach a better functional improvement as compared with older ones because of higher neuroplasticity and compensatory abilities. The poorer functional outcome typical of elderly stroke patients might be due to age-associated factors, such as greater stroke severity, co-morbidity, frailty, and social factors [30].

Rehabilitation Studies in Young Stroke Patients

As previously reported, findings focused on rehabilitation results in young ischemic stroke survivors are quite scarce. Recovery and rehabilitation from stroke represent important challenges for the younger survivors (one day fit and well, the next greatly disabled). The stroke survivor must come to terms with physical and emotional changes as well as significant lifestyle adjustments - mobility, work, income, dependence, relationships - everything changes. Thus, young stroke survivors in rehabilitation often present with complex social problems including marital break-up, unemployment, childcare difficulties, loss of independence and dependence on relatives. In the stroke rehabilitation program a crucial role is related to involvement of relatives. In the early phases of care, the rehabilitation team develops a treatment plan with the patient and his/her family. Staff members then teach the family how to assist with specific therapeutic activities. In this process, family members develop skills to help during hospital treatment and after discharge. A relevant point is that of transition from rehabilitative hospital stay to outpatient rehabilitative treatment. Because stroke management is aimed at facilitating community reintegration, it would be logical that the sooner the patient can be discharged, the sooner such reintegration can begin. While this point is true for all patients, it is crucial for younger patients. However, many patients and families perceive the end of rehabilitation hospital stay as the end of the recovery process. Ongoing education and support are even more critical during the transition phase as patients and families are actively dealing with these issues. A policy of early hospital discharge and home-based rehabilitation for patients with stroke can reduce the use of hospital rehabilitation beds without compromising clinical patient outcomes. Thus, a recent Cochrane review underscored the effectiveness of outpatient rehabilitation treatment in improving independence in personal ADL [31]. However, policy of early hospital discharge and home-based rehabilitation, even if does not compromise clinical patient outcomes, may be accompanied by a potential risk of poorer mental health on the part of caregivers [32]. So, education regarding the challenges of transition to home and the stroke recovery process should begin in the acute rehabilitation phase. Moreover, younger patients often find it difficult, for instance, to have access to the right rehabilitation facilities, which are often designed for elderly people. They may also need family support—in relation to what has happened to their children or with parenting.

The importance of rehabilitation in these patients is also related to objective of reducing indirect cost due to stroke, prevalent and enormous in young survivors. In fact, some years ago, Taylor and co-workers found that in USA in 1990 an ischemic male patient of 25 years of age had a mean lifetime cost of 406.000 $, a male patient of 45 yrs of 296.000 $, in comparison with 46.000 $ of male patient of 65 yrs and 7.000 for a male of 85 yrs of age [33]. For female patients, the costs are lower, but with similar distribution [33]. An adequate rehabilitation treatment could reduce functional disability and therefore indirect costs.

The question regarding the return to work will be described in the following chapter of this book, while in this chapter we give details on rehabilitative results in young survivors and on driving. Driving is often a major concern after a stroke. It's not unusual for stroke survivors to be willing to drive. Being able to get around after a stroke is very important. But while safety is always an issue when a person gets behind the wheel, it's even more important after a stroke.

In 1992 Adunsky et al published data regarding rehabilitation results of thirty young stroke patients (range of age 23-40 years), after hospitalization and during prolonged follow-up (31 ± 8 months). During hospitalization, patients showed significant improvements in activities of daily living, including transfer, standing, sitting and walking abilities, while during the follow-up period a further improvement was observed for standing and walking abilities. The mean length was quite long (87 ± 17 days), because patients were discharged only when multidisciplinary team judged that patient had had the maximum results obtainable not only on functional but also on psychological status. However, the main data showed a generally good prognosis for this series of patients: in fact, while no deaths was observed during the study period, on one hand, more than 80 % (81%) resumed their previous or other jobs six months after discharge, on the other [34].

In 1994 Falconer at al compared rehabilitation results of older stroke adults (≥ 75 years) with that of young adults (< 65 years) and young-old adults (65-74 years). Even if in this series there was no distinction in patients under 65 between young (<45 years) and young adults (45-64 years), however, the younger classes of patients had significantly longer rehabilitation stays (36.1 days *vs* 35.2 and 30.2, respectively) and were more frequently discharged to community (78% *vs* 75% and 58%, respectively) [30].

In the same year, Alexander et al., evaluating 520 patients in rehabilitation, found a highly significant effect of age both on rehabilitation results and discharge destination: in particular, not only none of the 44 patients under 55 years of age (12%) were discharged to nursing home (in comparison with 20.7% of 65-74 yrs class of age, 27.7% of 75-84 yrs and 32.7 for ≥85 years), but they also had a high probability of excellent improvement (FIM change >40) [35].

A favourable functional outcome was observed by Kong et al. in 57 young stroke patients (aged 45 years and below) admitted to a rehabilitation centre in Singapore [36].

In 1997, it has published a Japanese paper, on 487 consecutive patients (mean age 64.4 ± 13.1 years) with unilateral supratentorial infarction, on prediction of locomotion function at one month after stroke [37]. The study showed the prognosis depended on age, level of consciousness, size of brain lesion and severity of paresis. In particular, as shown in Table 1, a very small percentage of <50 years patients did not reach any sort of walking (5.8% remained in wheelchair and 1.5% in bed), as compared with higher percentages of other classes of age.

Teasell et al., on a whole case series of 563 patients admitted to the rehabilitation unit over the 10 year period, studied the social issues in the rehabilitation of 83 (15%) younger stroke patients (<50 years of age). Of the 55 patients with spouses, 8 (14.5%) separated within 3 months of hospital discharge. Fifteen of the 83 patients (18.1%) were not able to return to their premorbid place of residence; 4 (4.8%) required institutionalization [38].

In the same year, Jackson and co-workers published a report on 152 stroke patients (median age 54), unable to walk three months after onset, admitted consecutively in a rehabilitation unit. With intensive specialist input, seventy-five patients (49%) regained the ability to walk independently between 3 and 11 months, though late walkers may follow a slower recovery course [39].

Table 1. Locomotion function at one month after stroke [37]

	<50 yrs	50-65	65- 80	>80
Normal	18.8	12.8	12.7	2.2
Walking alone	53.1	44.2	37.5	15.2
Walking with aids	18.8	17.9	14.5	10.9
Wheelchair	5.8	19.2	21.7	26.1
Bedridden	1.5	5.8	13.6	45.6

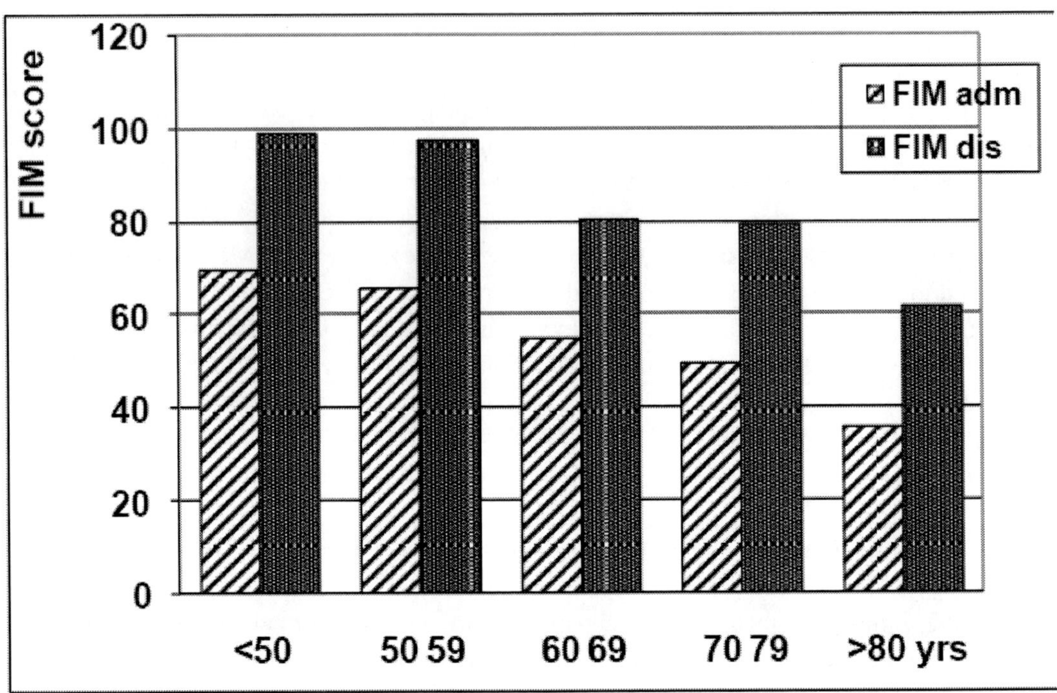

Inouye, 2001.

Figure 1. Admission and discharge FIM score in a Japanese rehabilitation series.

In another Japanese series, Inouye et al., stratifying 464 stroke patients into five groups of age (≤ 49, 50-59, 60-69, 70-79, and ≥ 80 yrs), observed, as shown in Figure 1, that younger classes (≤49, 50-59 yrs) had higher FIM score, both at admission and at discharge from rehabilitation hospital in comparison with other classes of age [40]. However, they also found, using stepwise multiple regression analyses, that the model for patients aged 60-69 yrs had the best predictive capacity and explained 76% of variation for discharge FIM. The model for stroke patients aged ≤49 yrs accounted for 72% of the variance in outcome [40]. Therefore, although equations can predict with a sufficient degree of accuracy functional recovery for each class of age, there is always uncertainty in determining the actual outcome of each individual.

Recently, we conducted a case-comparison study to assess the specific influence of age on basal functional status and rehabilitation results. We enrolled 150 stroke inpatients, matched for severity of stroke (measured by Canadian Neurological Scale - CNS) and onset admission interval (within 3 days) and divided into five subgroups according to age: ≤50; 51-64; 65-74; 75-84; and ≥85 years.

Even if basal severity of stroke was the same (CNS score 5.93±2.34), younger age was associated either with admission minor disability in both ADL, evaluated by means of BI, and mobility, and with better rehabilitation results [41]. In particular, as shown in Table 2, despite the same functional pre-stroke historical finding and the same neurological severity, at admission younger patients had a significant higher BI score. The same differences were found at discharge from rehabilitation hospital, with discharge BI score of oldest patients nearly less than half that of the ≤50 year old subgroup.

Table 2. ADL status before and after rehabilitative hospital stay [41]

Class of age	Before stroke	rehabilitation admission	Rehabilitation discharge	effectiveness
≤50	100 ± 0.00	46.17 ± 24.87	87.41± 9.88	73.72 ± 25.68
51-64	100 ± 0.00	42.00 ± 29.23	77.5 ± 23.41	68.39 ± 27.92
65-74	99.8 ± 0.91	33.83 ± 22.23	62.93 ± 28.23	47.57 ±33.99**
75-84	99.5 ± 1.53	25.67 ± 26.64	55.58 ± 34.68	46.79 ± 33.41**
≥85	99.3 ± 0.1.73	19.67 ± 26.64	38.08 ± 32.34	27.96 ± 27.64****††

Tukey HSD Test vs. ≤50 years subgroup: ** p<0.01; and ****p<0.001; vs. 51-64 years subgroup †† p<0.001.

Table 3. Mobility status before and after rehabilitative hospital stay [41]

Class of age	Before stroke	rehabilitation admission	Rehabilitation discharge	effectiveness
≤50	15.00 ±0.00	4.17±4.36	11.62±2.13	64.85±23.45
51-64	15.00± 0.00	3.90±3.99	9.53±4.51	56.06±31.14
65-74	14.93±0.25	2.87±3.23	7.45±4.82	40.76±31.31**
75-84	14.90±0.03	1.97±3.41	5.96±4.71	32.26±27.50****
≥85	14.03±0.41	1.93±3.02	4.19±3.94	18.64±24.02****††‡

Tukey HSD Test vs. ≤50 years subgroup: ** p<0.01; and ****p<0.001; vs. 51-64 years subgroup † p <0.05, †† p<0.001 vs. 51-64 years subgroup ‡ p <0.05.

Moreover, patients ≤50 years of age had significantly higher effectiveness on BI than all other groups (except 51-64 year old group) [41].

Similar data were observed for mobility. As shown in Table 3, patients ≤50 yrs of age were discharged with a mean Rivermead Mobility Index [42] score of 11.62 (±2.13) out of 15, score that implies the possibility of picking up something from the floor and walk back, in comparison with 7.45 (±4.82) for patients aged between 65 and 74, with 5.96 (±4.71) for patients aged 75-84 and 4.19 (±3.94) for ones ≥85 yrs. Moreover, patients ≤50 yrs had a significant higher effectiveness on mobility than older classes of patients, with the exclusion of patients aged 51-64 years. In particular, younger patients had an effectiveness on mobility nearly twice greater than that of patients aged 75-84 yrs (64.85% vs 32.26%, respectively) and nearly three times and half than that of patients aged ≥85 years.

Furthermore, in younger patients the percentage of *"low responders"* patients was smaller. As previously reported, we considered as *"low responders"* those patients whose treatment effectiveness on ADL and mobility was lower than the mean minus/plus 1 SD [17].

Increasing age, as shown in Figure 2, was associated with increasing percentage of low response to treatment. In particular, in younger patient less than 7% showed a low therapeutic response, in comparison with nearly thirty percent of patients aged 75-84 and with nearly fifty percent of oldest patients.

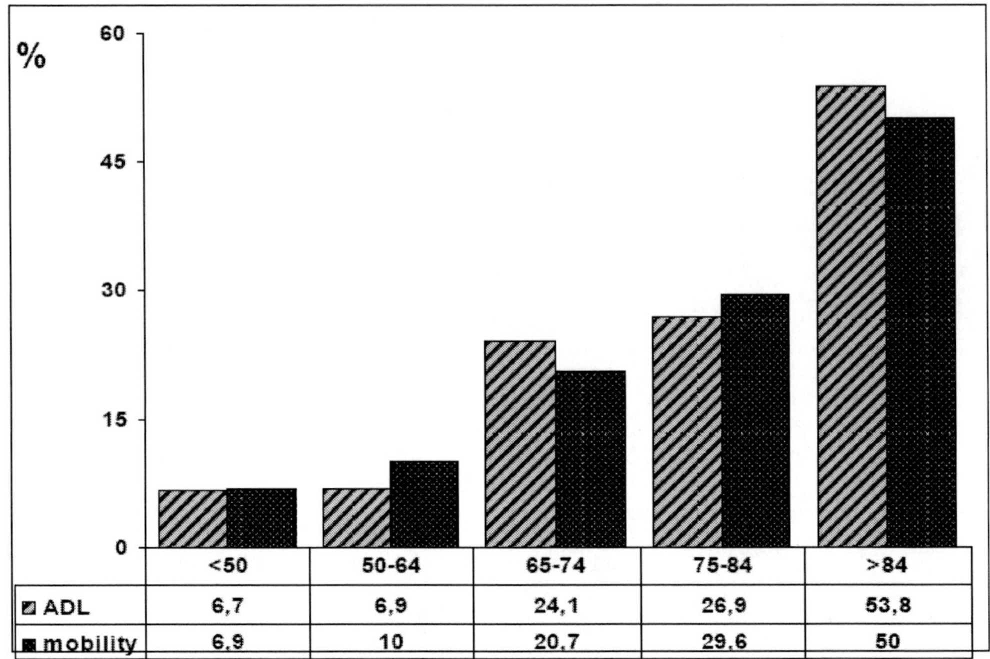

Figure 2. Percentage of low responders patients after rehabilitative hospital treatment [41].

Another relevant difference was observed in the frequency of urinary incontinence (UI): in our series, younger patients had a significantly lower percentage of UI at admission in comparison with older classes of age (75-84 and $\geq$85), and none of them had UI at discharge (*vs* 15.4 in patients 75-84 and 38.5% in patients $\geq$85 years, respectively; $p<0.001$) [17]. The association between UI and age had also been observed by Patel and co-workers, who found in multivariate analyses a very high risk of UI in patients aged >75 years (OR, 15.9; 95% CI, 2.2 to 116.2) [43].

In our sample, we did not find any difference among subgroups for percentage of home discharge. This data is in disagreement with previously cited studies [30,35], but is consistent with another study conducted in Italy [44].

More recently, O'Connor et al., evaluating an Irish younger stroke sample (range 47-59), admitted to a late multidisciplinary rehabilitation (mean interval, 112 days), found a relevant functional improvement, with reduction of cases fully wheelchair dependent, from 65.2% of admission to 32.6% [45].

During hospital rehabilitative phase, younger patients (<65 year) are less likely to die or be transferred than the older ones: a significant difference (30.9% vs 43.8%, $p<0.01$) was observed in the case series of Wright and coworkers [46], a favourable trend for younger patients in Italian series [41] and no death in Israelian one [34].

Another relevant point is the risk hip fracture, because it has reported that the risk of fracture is two to seven times greater in stroke patients than in nonstroke patients [47,48]. Hip fracture occurs most commonly on the paretic side and is usually trochanteric, most likely due to a higher risk of falling on the affected side. Moreover, the risk is greater in women [48]. Even if the relative risk still substantially increased at all ages, it has been reported, for any fracture requiring hospitalization, that the risk ratio (RR) was greatest in the younger age groups (RR, 2.38 to 4.69) and declined with age. The highest risks were seen in young women [47]. The increase in risk was most marked immediately after the stroke, intermediate at 6 months, and lowest at 4 years. Similar data was observed for hip fracture, but with much higher risk: in particular, the risk of any fracture requiring hospitalization immediately after stroke was 3.72 in women aged 50 to 54 years, while the risk for hip fracture was 11.75 [47].

Returning to Work

Returning persons to work is considered one of the main goals of rehabilitation process. However, many stroke patients fail to resume vocational activities: the reported rates of return to work range from 3% to 84% [18]. This large variation is due to the different definitions of "return to work" as well as the many factors influencing it. A young stroke patient may not be able to return to heavy labour but could be trained for a more sedentary job.

As stated earlier, this topic will be fully discussed in the following chapter of this book.

Sexuality

Stroke survivors often report a decrease in sexual desire and activity [49]. Some people stop having sex after experiencing stroke as they feel undesirable and embarrassed or because they are apprehensive about the health risks. In particular, the younger persons who have had a stroke may feel that their disabilities or the emotional acceptance of their stroke has considerable effect on their sex life. The issue of sexuality may be overlooked in rehabilitation programs, or the person who has had a stroke and their partner may be embarrassed in asking questions about sex. In fact, in the initial stages of recovery from a stroke, sex is less important than issues of mobility or speech.

However, as recovery progresses, and survivors and their spouses begin to have sexual feelings again, an informed and positive approach to the effects of stroke on sexuality can enhance recovery and strengthen self-esteem.

Several men have decreased ability to achieve an erection on a regular basis. For some of them this is due to the emotional effects of stroke. This is often related to the fear not only of not being able to achieve an erection, but also of having another stroke during intercourse. For others, a decreased ability to achieve an erection may be due to the action of antihypertensive drugs, while a delay in ejaculation may be due to serotonergic antidepressants.

Generally, females report a strong decrease in vaginal lubrication and the ability to have an orgasm. Lastly, sexual life may be further complicated by muscle spasms or stiffness, bowel or bladder incontinence, fatigue, vision problems, and lack of balance.

Korpelainen et al., prospectively evaluating sexual life in 50 young/adult stroke patients (38 men, 12 women, aged 32 to 65 years) and in their spouses during 6-month follow-up, found that 14% patients at 6 months had stopped their sexual intercourse and underscored the multifactorial aetiology for sexual dysfunction, with including both organic and psychosocial factors [50]. The same author found that the most important explanatory factors were the general attitude toward sexuality, fear of impotence, inability to discuss sexuality, reluctance to participate in sexual activity, and the degree of functional disability [51].

Physicians should provide exhaustive informations about sexual issues, and/or arranging for sex counselling if necessary, or by prescribing an antidepressant if depression is a factor. Stroke sequelae may require adjustments in seeking a comfortable position for sex or the use of other types of sexual expression, such as tenderness or touching.

Driving

Recovery of driving capacity may be essential for improvement of freedom and independence in all stroke survivors, but mainly for younger patients. However, the question of returning to driving must be carefully evaluated, because it can affect the safety and lives of the driver and many others.

Driving is a complex task that requires an intact set of skills and experiences in the areas of motor, language, visual, perceptual, cognitive or executive functions. Any impairment in these areas may affect this specific ability.

About 30 to 42 percent of stroke survivors are able to resume safe driving [52]. Even if cognitive abilities are today judged as the most important predictive test, a suggested by Marshall et al. in a recent review [53], younger age plays also a relevant role. In fact, Fisk et al., evaluating 290 stroke survivors 3 months up to 6 years poststroke, found that 30% percent of stroke survivors who drove before the stroke resumed driving after the stroke.

Younger stroke survivors are more likely to resume driving after stroke (OR, 0.96; 95% CI, 0.94 to 0.99), with stroke survivors being 4% less likely to drive with each increasing year of age [52]. The importance of age in predicting the decision of driving ability in stroke patients has been observed also in a Belgian series, and explained by impairment of vision and reactions due to aging [54].

Conclusions

Literature data confirm on one hand the unfavorable influence of age on functional outcome and on the other that inpatient rehabilitation is more effective in younger patients than in older ones.

However, in the rehabilitation of younger patients several aspects other than independence in activities of daily living must be taken into account, such as returning to work, sexuality and driving.

References

[1] Leys D, Bandu L, Henon H, Lucas C, Mounier-Vehier F, Rondepierre P, Godefroy O. Clinical outcome in 287 consecutive young adults (15 to 45 years) with ischemic stroke. *Neurology* 2002;*59*:26-33.

[2] Neau JP, Ingrand P, Mouille-Brachet C, Rosier MP, Couderq C, Alvarez A, Gil R. Functional recovery and social outcome after cerebral infarction in young adults. *Cerebrovasc. Dis*. 1998;*8*:296-302.

[3] Nedeltchev K, der Maur TA, Georgiadis D, Arnold M, Caso V, Mattle HP, Schroth G, Remonda L, Sturzenegger M, Fischer U, Baumgartner RW. Ischaemic stroke in young adults: predictors of outcome and recurrence. *J. Neurol. Neurosurg. Psychiatry* 2005; *76*: 191-195.

[4] Aichner F, Adelwohrer C, Haring HP. Rehabilitation approaches to stroke. *J. Neural. Transm. Suppl.* 2002;59-73.

[5] Haigh R, Tennant A, Biering-Sorensen F, Grimby G, Marincek C, Phillips S, Ring H, Tesio L, and Thonnard JL. The use of outcome measures in physical medicine and rehabilitation within Europe. *J. Rehabil. Med.*2001;*33*:273-278.

[6] Mahoney F, Barthel DW. Functional evaluation: the Barthel Index. *Md. State Med. J.* 1965;*14*:61-65.

[7] Granger CV, Cotter AC, Hamilton BB, Fiedler RC. Functional assessment scales: a study of persons after stroke. *Arch Phys. Med. Rehabil.* 1993;*74*:133-138.

[8] Ottenbacher KJ, Hsu Y, Granger CV, Fiedler RC. The reliability of the functional independence measure: a quantitative review. *Arch Phys. Med. Rehabil.* 1996;*77*:1226-1232.

[9] Shah S, Vanclay F, Cooper B. Efficiency, effectiveness and duration of stroke rehabilitation. *Stroke* 1990;*21*:241-246.

[10] Vanclay F. Functional outcome in stroke rehabilitation. *Stroke* 1991;*22*:105-108.

[11] Granger CV, Hamilton BB, Fiedler RC. Discharge outcome after stroke rehabilitation. *Stroke* 1992;*23*:978-982.

[12] Johnston KC, Connors AF Jr, Wagner DP, Knaus WA, Wang X, Haley EC Jr. A predictive risk model for outcomes of ischemic stroke. *Stroke* 2000;*31*:448-455.

[13] Chamie M. What does morbidity have to do with disability? *Disabil. Rehabil.*1995;*17*: 323-337.

[14] Nakayama H, Jorgensen HS, Raaschou HO, Olsen TS. The influence of age on stroke outcome. The Copenhagen Stroke Study. *Stroke* 1994;*25*:808-813.

[15] Kalra L, Crome P. Inpatient rehabilitation in elderly stroke patients. *J. Am. Geriatr. Soc.* 1994;*42*:1027.

[16] Ween JE, Alexander MP, D'Esposito M, Roberts M. Factors predictive of stroke outcome in a rehabilitation setting. *Neurology* 1996;*47*:388-392.

[17] Paolucci S, Antonucci G, Pratesi L, Traballesi M, Lubich S, Grasso MG. Functional outcome in stroke inpatient rehabilitation: predicting no, low and high response patients. *Cerebrovasc. Dis*. 1998;*8*:228-234.

[18] Flick CL. Stroke rehabilitation. 4. Stroke outcome and psychosocial consequences. *Arch Phys. Med. Rehabil*. 1999;*80*:S21-S26.

[19] Sanchez-Blanco I, Ochoa-Sangrador C, Lopez-Munain L, Izquierdo-Sanchez M, Fermoso-Garcia J. Predictive model of functional independence in stroke patients admitted to a rehabilitation programme. *Clin. Rehabil.* 1999;*13*:464-475.

[20] Bagg S, Pombo AP, Hopman W. Effect of age on functional outcomes after stroke rehabilitation. *Stroke* 2002;*33*:179-185.

[21] Feigenson JS, McDowell FH, Meese P, McCarthy ML, Greenberg SD. Factors influencing outcome and length of stay in a stroke rehabilitation unit. Part 1. Analysis of 248 unscreened patients-- medical and functional prognostic indicators. *Stroke* 1977, *8*:651-656.

[22] Luk JK, Cheung RT, Ho SL, Li L. Does age predict outcome in stroke rehabilitation? A study of 878 Chinese subjects. *Cerebrovasc. Dis*. 2006;*21*.229-234.

[23] Pohjasvaara T, Erkinjuntti T, Vataja R, Kaste M. Comparison of stroke features and disability in daily life in patients with ischemic stroke aged 55 to 70 and 71 to 85 years. *Stroke* 1997;*28*:729-735.

[24] Jorgensen HS, Reith J, Nakayama H, Kammersgaard LP, Raaschou HO, Olsen TS. What determines good recovery in patients with the most severe strokes? The Copenhagen Stroke Study. *Stroke* 1999;*30*:2008-2012.

[25] Bogousslavsky J, Pierre P. Ischemic stroke in patients under age 45. *Neurol. Clin.* 1992; *10*:113-124.

[26] Kugler C, Altenhoner T, Lochner P, Ferbert A. Does age influence early recovery from ischemic stroke? A study from the Hessian Stroke Data Bank. *J. Neurol*. 2003;*250*:676-681.

[27] Black-Schaffer RM, Winston C. Age and functional outcome after stroke. *Top Stroke Rehabil.* 2004;*11*:23-32.

[28] Patel MD, Coshall C, Rudd AG, Wolfe CD. Cognitive impairment after stroke: clinical determinants and its associations with long-term stroke outcomes. *J. Am. Geriatr. Soc.* 2002; *50*, 700-706.

[29] Paolucci S, Grasso MG, Antonucci G, Troisi E, Morelli D, CoiroP, Bragoni M. One-year follow-up in stroke patients discharged from rehabilitation hospital. *Cerebrovasc. Dis*. 2000;*10*:25-32.

[30] Falconer JA, Naughton BJ, Strasser DC, Sinacore JM. Stroke inpatient rehabilitation: a comparison across age groups. *J. Am. Geriatr. Soc.* 1994;*42*:39-44.

[31] Outpatient Service Trialists. Therapy-based rehabilitation services for stroke patients at home. *Cochrane Database Syst. Rev*. 2003, CD002925.

[32] Anderson C, Rubenach S, Mhurchu CN, Clark M, Spencer C, Winsor,A. Home or hospital for stroke rehabilitation? results of a randomized controlled trial : I: health outcomes at 6 months. *Stroke* 2000;*31*:1024-1031.

[33] Taylor TN, Davis PH, Torner JC, Holmes J, Meyer JW, Jacobson MF. Lifetime cost of stroke in the United States. *Stroke* 1996;*27*:1459-1466.

[34] Adunsky A, Hershkowitz M, Rabbi R, Asher-Sivron L, Ohry A. Functional recovery in young stroke patients. *Arch Phys. Med. Rehabil.* 1992;*73*:859-862.

[35] Alexander MP. Stroke rehabilitation outcome. A potential use of predictive variables to establish levels of care. *Stroke* 1994;*25*:128-134.

[36] Kong KH, Chan KF, Tan ES. Functional outcome in young strokes. *Ann. Acad. Med. Singapore* 1995;*24*:172-176.

[37] Matsunaga A, Kurokawa Y, Kanda T, Sakai F. Prediction of Locomotion Function at One Month after Stroke. *J. Phys. Ther. Sci.* 1997;*9*:93-97.

[38] Teasell RW, McRae MP, Finestone HM. Social issues in the rehabilitation of younger stroke patients. *Arch Phys. Med. Rehabil.* 2000;*81*:205-209.

[39] Jackson D, Thornton H, Turner-Stokes L. Can young severely disabled stroke patients regain the ability to walk independently more than three months post stroke? *Clin. Rehabil.* 2000;*14*:538-547.

[40] Inouye M. Predicting models of outcome stratified by age after first stroke rehabilitation in Japan. *Am. J. Phys. Med. Rehabil.* 2001;*80*:586-591.

[41] Paolucci S, Antonucci G, Troisi E, Bragoni M, Coiro P, De Angelis D, Pratesi L, Venturiero V, Grasso MG. Aging and stroke rehabilitation. A case-comparison study. *Cerebrovasc. Dis.* 2003;*15*:98-105.

[42] Collen FM, Wade DT, Robb GF, Bradshaw CM. The Rivermead Mobility Index: a further development of the Rivermead Motor Assessment. *Int. Disabil. Stud.* 1991; *13*: 50-54.

[43] Patel M, Coshall C, Rudd AG, Wolfe CD. Natural history and effects on 2-year outcomes of urinary incontinence after stroke. *Stroke* 2001;*32*:122-127.

[44] Tesio L, Franchignoni FP, Perucca L, Porta GL. The influence of age on length of stay, functional independence and discharge destination of rehabilitation inpatients in Italy. *Disabil. Rehabil.* 1996;*18*:502-508.

[45] O'Connor RJ, Cassidy EM, Delargy MA. Late multidisciplinary rehabilitation in young people after stroke. *Disabil. Rehabil.* 2005;*27*:111-116.

[46] Wright RE, Rao N, Smith RM, Harvey RF. Risk factors for death and emergency transfer in acute and subacute inpatient rehabilitation. *Arch Phys. Med. Rehabil.* 1996; *77*: 1049-1055.

[47] Kanis J, Oden A, Johnell O. Acute and long-term increase in fracture risk after hospitalization for stroke. *Stroke* 2001;*32*:702-706.

[48] Whitson HE, Pieper CF, Sanders L, Horner RD, Duncan PW, Lyles KW. Adding injury to insult: fracture risk after stroke in veterans. *J. Am. Geriatr. Soc.* 2006;*54*:1082-1088.

[49] Giaquinto S, Buzzelli S, Di Francesco L, Nolfe G. Evaluation of sexual changes after stroke. *J. Clin. Psychiatry* 2003;*64*:302-307.

[50] Korpelainen JT, Kauhanen ML, Kemola H, Malinen U, Myllyla VV. Sexual dysfunction in stroke patients. *Acta Neurol. Scand.* 1998;*98*:400-405.

[51] Korpelainen JT, Nieminen P, Myllyla VV. Sexual functioning among stroke patients and their spouses. *Stroke* 1999;*30*:715-719.

[52] Fisk GD, Owsley C, Pulley LV. Driving after stroke: driving exposure, advice, and evaluations. *Arch Phys. Med. Rehabil.* 1997;*78*:1338-1345.

[53] Marshall SC, Molnar F, Man-Son-Hing M, Blair R, Brosseau L, Finestone HM, Lamothe C, Korner-Bitensky N, Wilson KG. Predictors of driving ability following stroke: a systematic review. *Top Stroke Rehabil.* 2007;*14*:98-114.

[54] Akinwuntan AE, Feys H, DeWeerdt W, Pauwels J, Baten G, Strypstein E. Determinants of driving after stroke. *Arch Phys. Med. Rehabil.* 2002;*83*:334-341.

Index

4

A

B

C

D

E

F

G

H

I

J

K

L

M

N

O

P

Q

R

S

T

U

V

W

X

Y